Evidence Based Gastroenterology and Hepatology

MEDICAL LIBRARY
HEMEL HEMPSTEAD HOSPITAL
HILLFIELD ROAD
HEMEL HEMPSTEAD
HERTS HP2 4AD

EVIDENCE BASED GASTROENTEROLOGY AND HEPATOLOGY

Edited by

John WD McDonald
Professor of Medicine, Gastroenterology Service, London Health Sciences Centre, London, Ontario, Canada

Andrew K Burroughs
Consultant Physician/Hepatologist, Royal Free Hospital, London, UK

Brian G Feagan
Professor of Medicine, Gastroenterology Service, London Health Sciences Centre, London, Ontario, Canada

BMJ
Books

BMJ Books in an imprint of the BMJ Publishing Group

First published in 1999
by BMJ Books, BMA House, Tavistock Square,
London WCIH 9JR

www.bmjbooks.com

British Library Cataloguing in Publication Data

A catalogue record for this book is available from the British Library

ISBN 0-7279-1182-1

Typeset by Latimer Trend & Company Ltd, Plymouth
Printed and bound in Great Britain by MPG Books Ltd, Bodmin, Cornwall

Contents

Contributors

Paul C Adams
Department of Medicine, University of Western Ontario, London, Ontario, Canada

Piero Almasio
Istituto di Clinica Medica, University of Palermo, Italy

Vicente Arroyo
Liver Unit, Institut de Malalties Digestives, Hospital Clinic, Barcelona, Spain

Therese Bevers
The University of Texas, MD Anderson Cancer Center, Houston, Texas, USA

Calogero Cammà
ISMEDA-CNR, Palermo, Italy

Roger WG Chapman
Department of Gastroenterology, John Radcliffe Hospital, Oxford, UK

Naoki Chiba
Surrey GI Clinic, Guelph, Ontario, Canada

Nicholas Church
Gastrointestinal Unit, Western General Hospital, Edinburgh, UK

Massimo Colombo
Divisione e Cattedra Medicina Interna, IRCCS Ospedale Maggiore, Universitá degli Studi di Milano, Italy

Ann Cranney
Division of Rheumatology, Ottawa Civic Hospital, Ottawa, Canada

Antonio Craxì
Cattedra di Medicina Interna, Istituto di Clinica Medica, University of Palermo, Italy

Lucy Dagher
Department of Liver Transplantation and Hepatobiliary Medicine, Royal Free Hospital, London, UK

Douglas A Drossman
Division of Digestive Diseases and Nutrition, Department of Medicine, University of North Carolina, Chapel Hill, USA

Catherine Dube
Division of Gastroenterology, Department of Medicine, Ottawa Hospital – Civic Campus, Ottawa, Canada

Peter Ferenci
Department of Internal Medicine IV, Gastroenterology and Hepatology, University of Vienna, Vienna, Austria

Pere Ginès
Liver Unit, Institut de Malaties Digestives, Hospital Clinic, Barcelona, Spain

Marco Giunta
Cattedra di Medicina Interna, Istituto di Clinica Medica, University of Palermo, Italy

John Goulis
Department of Liver Transplantation and Hepatobiliary Medicine, Royal Free Hospital, London, UK

James Gregor
Gastroenterology Services, London Health Sciences Centre, London, Ontario, Canada

Jenny Heathcote
Department of Medicine, University Health Network, Toronto Western Hospital, University of Toronto, Toronto, Ontario, Canada

Richard H Hunt
Division of Gastroenterology, McMaster University, Hamilton, Ontario, Canada

Gary Jeffrey
Department of Medicine, University of Western Australia, Perth, Australia

Derek P Jewell
Gastroenterology Unit, Radcliffe Infirmary, Oxford, UK

Jarol B Knowles
Division of Digestive Diseases and Nutrition, Department of Medicine, University of North Carolina, Chapel Hill, USA

Bret A Lashner
Center for Inflammatory Bowel Disease, Cleveland Clinic Foundation, Cleveland, Ohio, USA

Calvin HL Law
General Surgery, St Joseph's Hospital, McMaster University, Hamilton, Ontario, Canada

Bernard Levin
University of Texas, The MD Anderson Cancer Center, Houston, Texas, USA

Andreas Maetzel
Division of Gastroenterology, Department of Medicine, University of Ottawa, Ottawa, Canada

Michael Peter Manns
Department of Gastroenterology and Hepatology, Medizinische Hochschule, Hannover, Germany

Patrick Marcellin
Service d'Hépatologie, Centre de Recherche Claude Bernard sur les Hépatites Virales, Hôpital Beaujon, Clichy, France

Philippe Mathurin
University of Southern California, School of Medicine, Los Angeles, California, USA

Stephen A Mitchell
Department of Gastroenterology, Wycombe Hospital, High Wycombe, UK

Christian Müller
Department of Internal Medicine IV, Gastroenterology and Hepatology, University of Vienna, Vienna, Austria

Nick Murphy
Intensive Care Unit, Guy's Hospital, London, UK

Kelvin Palmer
Gastrointestinal Unit, Western General Hospital, Edinburgh, UK

Thierry Poynard
Groupe Hospitalier Pitie-Salpetriere, France

Juan Rodés
Liver Unit, Institut de Malaties Digestives, Hospital Clinic, Barcelona, Spain

Nancy Rolando
Department of Liver Transplantation and Hepatobiliary Medicine, The Royal Free Hospital, London, UK

Alaa Rostom
Division of Gastroenterology, Department of Medicine, University of Ottawa, Ottawa, Canada

Andreas Schüler
Department of Gastroenterology and Hepatology, Medizinische Hochschule, Hannover, Germany

William J Sandborn
Inflammatory Bowel Disease Clinic, Division of Gastroenterology, Mayo Clinic and Mayo Foundation, Rochester, Minnesota, USA

Jonathon Springer
Division of Gastroenterology, Mount Sinai Hospital, Department of Medicine, University of Toronto, Toronto, Ontario, Canada

Hillary Steinhart
Division of Gastroenterology, Mount Sinai Hospital, Department of Medicine, University of Toronto, Toronto, Ontario, Canada

Lloyd R Sutherland
University of Calgary, Calgary, Alberta, Canada

Véd R Tandan
Surgical Outcomes Research Centre, St Joseph's Hospital and Department of Surgery, Department of Clinical Epidemiology and Biostatistics, McMaster University, Hamilton, Ontario, Canada

Peter Tugwell
Department of Medicine, Ottawa Hospital, Ottawa, Canada

Sander JO Veldhuyzen Van Zanten
Division of Gastroenterology, Department of Medicine, Dalhousie University, Halifax, Canada

Jim J Wade
Dulwich Public Health Laboratory, and Department of Medical Microbiology, King's College School of Medicine & Dentistry, London, UK

Alastair JM Watson
Department of Medicine, Section of Gastroenterology, Hope Hospital, Salford, UK

George Wells
Department of Medicine and Clinical Epidemiology Unit, University of Ottawa, Ottawa, Canada

Julia Wendon
Institute of Liver Studies, King's College Hospital, London, UK

Preface

This important new book emphasizes the approaches of evidence based medicine to gastroenterology and hepatology. Traditional textbooks emphasize the basic sciences of pathology, biochemistry, and physiology. Following the publication of the highly successful *Evidence Based Cardiology*, this book utilizes clinical epidemiology, 'the basic science of clinical medicine' to present the strongest and most current evidence for interventions for the major diseases of the gastrointestinal tract and liver. Leading gastroenterologists have summarized the evidence for important interventions in a manner that allows the reader to make better informed decisions about which treatments to offer to their patients.

The strength of evidence which supports various treatment recommendations is made clear. The emphasis is on the analysis of randomized trials, and systematic reviews of these trials. However, lower levels of evidence, such as case-control and cohort studies, sometimes provide the only available evidence or provide important supporting evidence for efficacy of particular interventions. The authors of several chapters have also included these kinds of evidence where appropriate. A notation in the margin or the text indicates the strength of the evidence. Where it is recommended that an intervention be adopted into practice, this is also highlighted.

R
Grade A

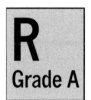

The speed with which new information becomes available results in rapid obsolescence for traditional textbooks. Readers of *Evidence Based Gastroenterology* will be able to access updates on the BMJ website as new evidence comes to the attention of the authors and editors.

Grading of recommendations and levels of evidence used in *Evidence Based Gastroenterology and Hepatology*

GRADE A

- Evidence from large randomized clinical trials (RCTs) or systematic reviews (including meta-analyses) of multiple randomized trials which collectively have at least as much data as one single well-defined trial
- Evidence from at least one "All or None" high quality cohort study; in which ALL patients died/failed with conventional therapy and some survived/succeeded with the new therapy (eg chemotherapy for tuberculosis, meningitis, or defibrillation for ventricular fibrillation): or in which many died/failed with conventional therapy and NONE died/failed with the new therapy (eg penicillin for pneumococcal infections)
- Evidence from at least one moderate sized RCT or a meta-analysis of small trials which collectively only has a moderate number of patients
- Evidence from at least one RCT

GRADE B

- Evidence from at least one high quality study of non-randomized cohorts who did and did not receive the new therapy
- Evidence from at least one high quality case control study
- Evidence from at least one high quality case series

GRADE C

- Opinions from experts without reference or access to any of the foregoing (eg argument from physiology, bench research or first principles)

R
Grade A

A comprehensive approach would incorporate many different types of evidence (eg RCTs, non-RCTs, epidemiologic studies, and experimental data), and examine the architecture of the information for consistency, coherence, and clarity. Occasionally the evidence does not completely fit into neat compartments. For example, there may not be an RCT that demonstrates a reduction in mortality in individuals with stable angina with the use of beta-blockers, but there is overwhelming evidence that mortality is reduced following MI. In such cases, some may recommend use of beta-blockers in angina patients with the expectation that some extrapolation from post-MI trials is warranted. This could be expressed as Grade A/C. In other instances (e.g. smoking cessation or a pacemaker for complete heart block), the non-randomized data are so overwhelmingly clear and biologically plausible that it would be reasonable to consider these interventions as Grade A.

Recommendation grades appear either in a shaded margin box with an "R" logo as shown, or within the text, for example [Grade A].

Glossary

AAA	aromatic amino acids
AC	acyclovir
AFP	α-fetoprotein
AGA	antigliadin antibodies
AIH	autoimmune hepatitis
ALD	alcoholic liver disease
ALF	acute liver failure
ALT	alanine aminotransferase
AMA	antimitochondrial antibodies
ANA	antinuclear antibodies
ApoA-I	apolipoprotein A-I
ARA	antireticulin antibodies
ARDS	acute respiratory distress syndrome
ARR	absolute risk reduction
ASA	aminosalicylic acid (aspirin)
AZA	azathioprine
BCAA	branched chain amino acids
bid	twice daily
BMC	bone mineral content
BMD	bone mineral density
CAH	chronic active hepatitis
CBD	common bile duct
CBDS	common bile duct stones
CD	Crohn's disease
CDAI	Crohn's Disease Activity Index
CI	confidence interval
CLD	chronic liver disease
CMV	cytomegalovirus
CSOP	corticosteroid-induced osteoporosis
DSRS	distal splenorenal shunt
DU	duodenal ulcer
DXA	dual energy X-ray absorptiometry
ERCP	endoscopic retrograde cholangiopancreatography
ES	endoscopic sphincterotomy
EMA	(smooth) muscle endomysium antibodies (antiendomysial antibody)
ENRD	endoscopy negative reflux disease

FAP	familial adenomatous polyposis
FHF	fulminant hepatic failure
GCV	gancyclovir
GERD	gastroesophageal reflux disease
GI	gastrointestinal
GSRS	Gastrointestinal Symptom Rating Scale
GU	gastric ulcer
HAI	Hepatic Activity Index
HB[C,D]V	hepatitis B[C,D] virus
HCC	hepatocellular carcinoma
HE	hepatic encephalopathy
HIV	human immunodeficiency virus
HLA	human leukocyte antigen
HNPCC	hereditary non-polyposis colorectal cancer
HO	hepatic osteodystrophy
H_2RA	H_2-receptor antagonist
HRS	hepatorenal syndrome
HVPG	hepatic venous pressure gradient
IBD	inflammatory bowel disease
IBS	irritable bowel syndrome
IFN	interferon
IOC	intraoperative cholangiogram
IPPA	ileal pouch–anal anastomosis
ITT	intention to treat
LC	laparoscopic cholecystectomy
LCBDE	laparoscopic common bile duct exploration
LES	lower esophageal sphincter
MALT	mucosa-associated lymphoid tissue
MHC	major histocompatibility complex
MRC	magnetic resonance cholangiography
MTX	methotrexate
NAC	N-acetylcysteine
NCCP	non-cardiac chest pain
NCT	number connection test
NNT	number needed to treat
nocte	at bedtime
NSAIDs	non-steroidal anti-inflammatory drugs
OC	open cholecystectomy
OCBDE	open common bile duct exploration
od	once daily
OLT	orthotopic liver transplantation
OM	osteomalacia
OR	odds ratio
OTC	over-the-counter
pANCA	perinuclear anti-neutrophil cytoplasmic antibodies
PAF	platelet activating factor
PBC	primary biliary cirrhosis
PCR	polymerase chain reaction
PCP	*Pneumocystis carinii* pneumonia
PCS	portacaval shunt

PCHGS	portacaval H graft shunt
PDAI	Pouchitis Disease Activity Index
PEEP	positive end expiratory pressure
PEI	percutaneous ethanol injection
PGWB	psychological general well being
PIIIP	procollagen III propeptide
POR	pooled odds ratio
PPI	proton pump inhibitors
PSC	primary sclerosing cholangitis
PTH	parathyroid hormone
qid	four times daily
ROC	receiver operating characteristic
RRR	relative risk reduction
QCT	quantitative computed tomography
QOL	quality of life
SASP	salazopyrine
SBD	selective bowel decontamination
SBP	spontaneous bacterial peritonitis
SCFA	short chain fatty acids
SDD	selective decontamination of the digestive tract
SIP	sickness impact profile
SIRS	systemic inflammatory response syndrome
SMA	smooth muscle antibodies
SPS	sulphasalazine
SSRI	selective serotonin reuptake inhibitors
TACE	transcatheter arterial chemo-embolization
TEN	total enteral nutrition
TGF	transforming growth factor
tid	three times daily
TIPS	transjugular intrahepatic portosystemic shunt
TNF	tumor necrosis factor
TPN	total parenteral nutrition
UBT	urea breath test
UC	ulcerative colitis
UCA	human umbilical cord
UDCA	ursodeoxycholic acid
UGI	upper gastrointestinal
US	ultrasound
VILI	ventilator induced lung injury

Evidence based gastroenterology and hepatology: an introduction

1

JOHN WD MCDONALD, BRIAN G FEAGAN, ANDREW K BURROUGHS

Over the past three decades the emergence of evidence based medicine (EBM) has had a substantial impact on clinical practice. In the first half of the twentieth century, diagnostic tests or treatments, usually based on a strong scientific rationale and experimental work in animals, were routinely introduced into clinical care without good scientific proof of efficacy in people. Some of these interventions, such as gastric freezing for the treatment of ulcers and penicillamine therapy for primary biliary cirrhosis, were ultimately shown to be ineffective[1,2] and harmful. There is little doubt that the widespread acceptance by physicians of unproven treatments has been detrimental to the wellbeing of many patients.

Fortunately, the need for a more critical approach to medical practice was recognized. In 1948 the first randomized controlled trial (RCT) in humans was performed under the direction of the British Medical Research Council.[3] Epidemiologists and statisticians, notably Sir Richard Doll and Sir Bradford Hill, provided scientific leadership to the medical community, which responded with improvements in the quality of clinical research. The use of randomized allocation to control for confounding variables and to minimize bias was recognized as invaluable for the performance of valid studies of treatments. The initiation of these landmark experiments defined a new era in clinical research; the RCT soon became the benchmark for the evaluation of medical and surgical interventions. Gastroenterologists played an important part in these early days. In 1955 Professor Sidney Truelove performed the first randomized trial in the discipline of gastroenterology.[4] He and his colleagues proved that cortisone was more effective than a placebo for the treatment of ulcerative colitis. As noted in Chapter 9, this treatment has stood the test of time. The ascendancy of the RCT was accompanied by a call for greater scientific rigor in the usual practice of clinical medicine. Strong advocates of the application of epidemiological principles to patient care emerged and found a growing body of support among clinicians.

As the number of randomized trials grew to the point of becoming unmanageable, the need became recognized to provide summaries of the evidence provided by these trials for the use of practitioners, who frequently lack both time and expertise to consult the primary research. Busy clinicians may consult local experts, with the tacit assumption that they will make recommendations based on evidence. Liberati and colleagues[5] provided evidence that this approach led to inappropriate care for many women with breast cancer. Subsequently, convincing evidence became available through the work of Antman and Chalmers[6] and of Mulrow[7] that the conventional review article and the traditional textbook chapter are seldom comprehensive, and are frequently biased. Recently Jefferson[8] reinforced this conclusion, on the basis of a survey concerning recommendations for vaccination for cholera which appeared in editorials and review articles. He pointed out that authors of editorials and reviews frequently resort to the "desk drawer" technique, pulling out evidence with which they are very familiar, but failing to assemble and review all of the evidence in a systematic way.

In the United Kingdom Archie Cochrane, as early as 1979, made a compelling case that there was a need to prepare and maintain summaries of all randomized trials.[9] Cochrane's challenge to the medical community to use scientific methods to identify, evaluate, and systematically summarize the world's medical literature pertaining to all health care interventions is now being met. From its inception in 1993, the electronic database prepared by the volunteer members of the Cochrane Collaboration and published as the Cochrane Library[10] has grown exponentially. Cochrane reviews are now widely utilized by clinicians in the daily practice of medicine, by researchers and by the public. Accordingly, data from systematic reviews published in the Cochrane Library are featured prominently in several chapters in *Evidence Based Gastoenterology and Hepatology*. Unfortunately, coverage in the Cochrane Library of topics in gastroenterology and hepatology is still far from complete.

Several other clinical epidemiologists played important roles in the evolution of evidence based medicine. Beginning in the 1970s, David Sackett encouraged practicing physicians to become familiar with the basic principles of critical appraisal. Criteria developed by Sackett and others for the evaluation of clinical studies assessing therapy, causation, prognosis, and other clinical topics were widely published.[11,12] His text *Clinical Epidemiology: a basic science for clinical medicine*, co-authored by colleagues Gordon Guyatt, Brian Haynes, and Peter Tugwell, introduced many physicians to the concepts of EBM.[13] In the United States Alvin Feinstein called attention to the need for increased rigor in the design and interpretation of observational studies and explored the scientific principles of diagnostic testing.[14,15] Among gastroenterologists, Thomas Chalmers, an early strong advocate for the RCT,[16] was responsible for introducing gastroenterologists and others to the importance of randomized trials in gastroenterology and hepatology[17] and to the concept of systematic reviews and meta-analysis as a means of summarizing data from these studies.[18]

Despite the opposition of some,[19] the popularity of EBM continues to grow. Although the explanations for this phenomenon are complex, one factor is that many practitioners recognize that ethical patient care should be based on the best possible evidence. For this and other reasons the fundamental concept behind EBM – the use of the scientific method in the practice of clinical medicine – has been widely endorsed by medical opinion leaders, patients, and governments.

WHAT IS EVIDENCE BASED GASTROENTEROLOGY AND HEPATOLOGY?

Evidence based gastroenterology and hepatology is the application of the most valid scientific information to the care of patients with gastrointestinal and hepatic diseases. Physicians who treat patients with digestive diseases must provide their patients with the most appropriate diagnostic tests, the most accurate prognosis, and the most effective and safe therapy. To meet this high standard individual clinicians must have access to and be able to evaluate scientific evidence. Although many practitioners argue that this has always been the standard of care in clinical medicine, a great deal of evidence exists to the contrary. Wide variances in practice patterns among physicians have been documented for many treatments, despite the presence of good data from widely publicized RCTs and the promotion of practice guidelines by content experts. For example, Scholefield *et al.* performed a survey of British surgeons, who were questioned regarding the performance of screening colonoscopy for colon cancer.[20] Although this study was performed in 1998 (after publication of the results of the RCTs described in Chapter 13 which demonstrated a benefit of this practice), many of these physicians failed to make appropriate recommendations for screening patients at risk. What is the explanation for this finding? One possibility is that many clinicians rely for information on their colleagues, on local experts, or on review articles or textbook chapters that are not written based on the principles of EBM.

Two important points about EBM should be emphasized. First, use of the principles of EBM in the management of patients is complementary to traditional clinical skills and will never supersede the recognized virtues of careful observation, sound judgment, and compassion for the patient. It is noteworthy that many good doctors have intuitively utilized the basic principles of EBM. Hence, the promotion of such well known clinical aphorisms as "go where the money is" and "do the last test first". Knowledge of EBM enables physicians to understand why these basic rules of clinical medicine are valid through the use of a quantitative approach to decision making. This paradigm can in no way be considered detrimental to the doctor–patient relationship.

Second, although RCTs are the most valuable source of data for evaluating health care interventions, other kinds of evidence must frequently be utilized. In some instances, most obviously in studies of causation, it is neither possible nor ethical to perform RCTs. Here, data from methodologically rigorous observational studies are extremely valuable. A dramatic example was the demonstration by several authors (quoted in Chapter 18) that the relative risk of hepatocellular carcinoma in chronic carriers of the hepatitis B virus is dramatically higher than in persons who are not infected. Although these data are observational, the strength of the association is such that it is exceedingly unlikely that a cause other than hepatitis B virus is responsible for the development of cancer in these people. Case–control studies are especially useful for studying rare diseases and for the initial development of scientific hypotheses regarding causation. The etiological role of non-steroidal anti-inflammatory drugs in the development of gastric ulcers[21] was recognized using this methodology. Finally, case series can provide compelling evidence for the adoption of a new therapy in the absence of data from RCTs, if the natural history of disease is both well characterized and severe. An example is the identification of orthotopic liver transplantation as a dramatically effective intervention for patients with advanced liver disease.

Table 1.1 shows a generally agreed approach to ranking the strength of evidence that arises from various types of studies of health care interventions, and this system is used throughout the book. This ranking of evidence has appeared in a number of publications; we have chosen to reproduce it from *Evidence Based Cardiology*,[22] along with the system used by its editors, Yusuf *et al.*, for making recommendations on the basis of these levels of evidence. Throughout this book marginal notations based on this table indicate the level of evidence that supports the statements in the text about the effectiveness of interventions. Recommendations for adoption of a specific intervention are frequently highlighted with the marginal notation "**R**" as well as the level of evidence on which this recommendation is made.

Table 1. 1 Grading of recommendations and levels of evidence used in *Evidence Based Gastroenterology and Hepatology*

GRADE A

- Evidence from large randomized clinical trials (RCTs) or systematic reviews (including meta-analyses) of multiple randomized trials which collectively have at least as much data as one single well-defined trial
- Evidence from at least one "All or None" high quality cohort study; in which ALL patients died/failed with conventional therapy and some survived/succeeded with the new therapy (eg chemotherapy for tuberculosis, meningitis, or defibrillation for ventricular fibrillation): or in which many died/failed with conventional therapy and NONE died/failed with the new therapy (eg penicillin for pneumococcal infections)
- Evidence from at least one moderate sized RCT or a meta-analysis of small trials which collectively only has a moderate number of patients
- Evidence from at least one RCT

GRADE B

- Evidence from at least one high quality study of non-randomized cohorts who did and did not receive the new therapy
- Evidence from at least one high quality case control study
- Evidence from at least one high quality case series

GRADE C

- Opinions from experts without reference or access to any of the foregoing (eg argument from physiology, bench research or first principles)

R
Grade A

A comprehensive approach would incorporate many different types of evidence (eg RCTs, non-RCTs, epidemiologic studies, and experimental data), and examine the architecture of the information for consistency, coherence, and clarity. Occasionally the evidence does not completely fit into neat compartments. For example, there may not be an RCT that demonstrates a reduction in mortality in individuals with stable angina with the use of beta-blockers, but there is overwhelming evidence that mortality is reduced following MI. In such cases, some may recommend use of beta-blockers in angina patients with the expectation that some extrapolation from post-MI trials is warranted. This could be expressed as Grade A/C. In other instances (e.g. smoking cessation or a pacemaker for complete heart block), the non-randomized data are so overwhelmingly clear and biologically plausible that it would be reasonable to consider these interventions as Grade A.

Recommendation grades appear either in a shaded margin box with an "R" logo as shown, or within the text, for example [Grade A].

CLINICAL DECISION MAKING IN GASTROENTEROLOGY AND HEPATOLOGY

Clinical decision making by gastroenterologists usually falls into one of the following categories:

- Deciding whether to apply a specific diagnostic test in arriving at an explanation of a patient's problem, or determining the status of the patient's disease.

- Offering a prognosis to a patient.
- Deciding among a number of interventions available for managing a patient's problem. In this category, the first question is "Does a given intervention do more good than harm?" The second is "Does it do more good than other effective interventions?" The third is "Is it more or less cost-effective than other interventions?"

Application of a diagnostic test

Example: *A 4-year-old child is experiencing diarrhea and has a positive family history of celiac disease. Should a serological test for antiendomysial antibody be performed?*

Chapter 7 includes an extensive treatment of this topic with a summary (Table 7.1) of studies that included various groups of patients with a greater or lesser probability of having celiac disease (ranging from patients with GI symptoms to patients in whom celiac disease was suspected on clinical grounds). At least one of the studies in Table 7.1, that of Cataldo *et al.*,[23] is relevant to this patient. When evaluating this test the reader may wish to adopt the approach of Kitching, Sackett, and Yusuf[24] for deciding on the clinical usefulness of a diagnostic test (Figure 1.1).

The criteria listed in Figure 1.1 for validity of a diagnostic test were clearly met in Cataldo's study. In Chapter 7 James Gregor explores the utility of the test and points out that tests with high positive likelihood ratios (LR >10) and low negative likelihood ratios (LR <0.1) are generally considered to be clinically useful. The EMA test clearly falls into this category. Gregor draws attention to the fact that the probability that a specific patient actually has celiac disease (based on a positive test), or does not have it (based on a negative test), also depends on the *pretest odds* of the patient having the disease (see Table 1.2).

If the child in question, whose pretest likelihood of celiac disease is estimated to be 8%, has a negative test it may be concluded that the child almost certainly does not have celiac disease; on the other hand, if the child has a positive test, the likelihood of him/her having celiac disease is still only 65%.

As Gregor points out, the implications of misdiagnosis must be considered carefully. In the circumstance of a positive test in the child with non-specific symptoms the physician and the child's parents should consider whether it is now reasonable to proceed to intestinal biopsy to confirm the diagnosis, rather than recommending a gluten-free diet, presumably for life. If a search for other clinical or laboratory clues reveals that celiac disease is very likely to be the correct diagnosis, the pretest likelihood may be as high as 50%. This would raise the post-test likelihood to 97%. The physician and parents may be comfortable accepting the diagnosis and proceed to a trial of a gluten-free diet, rather than subjecting a young child to intestinal biopsy. This is an excellent example of how a skilled clinician must integrate the principles of evidence based medicine with traditional clinical skills and judgment.

Offering a prognosis

Example: *A 50-year-old woman with recently diagnosed celiac disease has learned at a meeting of the local Celiac Society that patients with celiac disease have a substantial increase in the risk of developing a number of cancers and that this cancer risk is reduced by strict adherence to a gluten-free diet.*

Chapter 7 describes the types of studies which are relevant to determination of prognosis and discusses the strengths and weaknesses of case–control and cohort studies. The

- **Are the study results valid?**

1 Was there an independent blind comparison (or unbiased comparison) with a reference ("gold") standard of diagnosis?
2 Was the diagnostic test evaluated in an appropriate spectrum of patients (like those seen in the reader's practice)?
3 Was the reference standard applied regardless of the diagnostic test result?

- **What are the results?**

Cataldo F, Ventura A, Lazzari R *et al.* Antiendomysium antibodies and celiac disease: solved and unsolved questions. An Italian multicentre study. *Acta Paediatr* 1995; **84**(10): 1125–31.

A study of IgA endomysium antibodies (EMA) in 1485 children with gastrointestinal disease (688 with celiac disease confirmed by intestinal biopsy)

Results for antiendomysial antibody (EMA) test

	Number of patients with biopsy proven celiac disease		
	Present	Absent	Totals
EMA positive	645	20	665
	a	b	a+b
EMA negative	c	d	c+d
	43	777	810
	a+c	b+d	a+b+c+d
Totals	688	797	1485

Sensitivity = a/(a+c) = 645/688 = 0.94
Specificity = d/(b+d) = 777/797 = 0.97
Likelihood ratio (positive result) = sensitivity/(1–specificity) = 0.94/(1–0.97) =31
Likelihood ratio (negative result) = (1–sensitivity)/specificity = (1–0.94)/0.97 = 0.06
Positive predictive value = a/(a+b) = 645/665 = 0.97
Negative predictive value = d/c+d = 777/810 = 0.96

Figure 1.1 Approaches to evaluating evidence about diagnosis

Table 1.2 The antiendomysial antibody test for celiac disease. Dependence of post-test likelihood of celiac disease on pretest likelihood, assuming positive LR = 31, negative LR = 0.06

Pretest likelihood of celiac disease	Post-test likelihood with a positive EMA test	Post-test likelihood with a negative EMA test
8% (non-specific symptoms, positive family history)	65%	0.5%
50% (more specific symptoms)	97%	6%
0.25% (population screen)	8%	0.02%

Data from Chapter 7

author points out that certain case–control studies which reported very high mortality rates and malignancy rates may have been subject to selection bias (inclusion of particularly ill or refractory patients) and measurement bias (patients with abdominal symptoms being more likely to undergo investigations such as small bowel biopsy which may lead to a diagnosis of celiac disease). He refers to a British study in which a cohort of patients with celiac disease was assembled and followed for 10 years. This design attempts to minimize the biases that are inherent in the case–control studies. Table 1.3 shows that the risk of certain cancers is increased compared to the risk in the general population. Table 1.4 shows that strict adherence to a gluten-free diet significantly reduced this risk and may have eliminated the excess risk for several of the identified cancers.

On the basis of this evidence it is reasonable to advise the patient that her disease does carry with it an increased risk of certain relatively uncommon cancers and that adherence to a strict gluten-free diet appears to minimize this increased risk.

Table 1.3 Cancer mortality in 210 patients with celiac disease at the end of 1985

Site of cancer	ICD8	O	E	O/E	*P*
All sites	140–208	31	15.48	2.0	**
Mouth and pharynx	141–147	3	0.31	9.7	*
Oesophagus	150	3	0.24	12.3	*
Non-Hodgkin's lymphoma	200, 202	9	0.21	42.7	**
GI tract	151–154	3	3.07	1.0	NS
Remainder		13	11.65	1.1	NS

O, observed numbers; E, expected numbers.
**P*<0.01; ***P*<0.001.
Source: Holmes GKT, Prior R, Lane MR *et al*. Malignancy in celiac disease: effect of a gluten-free diet. *Gut* 1989; **30**: 333–8.

Table 1.4 Cancer morbidity by diet group

Site of cancer	Diet group	N	O	E	O/E	*P*
All sites	1	108	14	9.06	1.5	
	2	102	17	6.42	2.6	**
Mouth, pharynx, esophagus	1	108	1	0.33	3.0	
	2	102	5	0.22	22.7	**
Non-Hodgkin's lymphoma	1	108	2	0.12	16.7	*
	2	102	7	0.09	77.8	**
Remainder	1	108	11	8.61	1.3	
	2	102	5	6.11	0.8	

Diet group 1, strict adherence to gluten-free diet; group 2, reduced gluten diet or normal diet.
**P*<0.01; ***P*<0.001.
Source: Holmes GKT, Prior R, Lane MR *et al*. Malignancy in celiac disease: effect of a gluten-free diet. *Gut* 1989; **30**: 333–8.

Recommendations concerning therapy

We have provided examples of how evidence concerning the use of diagnostic tests and prognosis can be analyzed and incorporated into clinical practice. Most chapters in this book deal more extensively with evidence concerning therapy and rely heavily on data from randomized trials and meta-analyses.

Example: *Should a 28-year-old woman who has had an uncomplicated resection of the terminal ileum for Crohn's disease receive maintenance therapy with a 5-ASA product? Prior to the surgery she had had steroid dependent disease and had failed treatment with both azathioprine and methotrexate.* A search of the literature for placebo controlled randomized trials of 5-ASA for maintenance of remission in patients with a surgically induced remission of disease would reveal several trials. The largest published trial is that of McLeod and colleagues,[25] who randomized 163 adult patients to receive either 3 g/day of 5-ASA or a placebo following surgery. The primary outcome of interest was the recurrence of active Crohn's disease as defined by the recurrence of symptoms and the documentation of active disease either radiologically or endoscopically. At the end of the follow-up period (maximum duration 72 months, median duration 34 months), 31% of patients who received active treatment remained in remission compared with 41% of those who received a placebo ($P = 0.031$). 5-ASA was well tolerated. A low proportion of patients developed adverse reactions in the control and active treatment groups. One patient treated with 5-ASA developed pancreatitis that was attributed to the study drug. The results of this study can be evaluated using the guidelines described in Figure 1.2, which is modelled after the approach of Kitching *et al.*[24]

ARE THE RESULTS OF THIS STUDY VALID?

A review of the methods section of the article confirms that an appropriate method of randomization was employed (computer generated in permutated blocks), which insured concealment of the randomization code. Furthermore, inspection of the baseline characteristics of the treatment and control groups shows that they are well balanced with respect to such confounding variables as the time from surgery to randomization. This information further supports the legitimacy of the randomization process. Assessment of the method of randomization is important, because non-randomized designs are especially vulnerable to the effects of bias. Studies which employ "quasi-randomization" schemes such as allocation to treatment according to the day of the week or alphabetically by the patient's surname have been shown to consistently overestimate the treatment effect identified by RCTs that employ a valid randomization scheme.[26,27] However, it may be noted that 87 patients were randomized to 5-ASA, compared to only 76 patients in the control group. This observation raises the concern that the analysis might not have been performed according to the "intent to treat" principal which specifies that patients are analyzed in the group to which they were originally assigned, irrespective of the treatment that was ultimately received. The use of this strategy reduces the possibility of bias, which might occur if investigators selectively withdrew from the analysis patients who had done poorly or experienced toxicity. For this reason, the intent to treat principal yields a conservative estimate of the true benefit of the treatment. However, detailed review shows that in this study the discrepancy in patient numbers occurred because five patients who were randomized to the active treatment group withdrew consent prior to receiving the study medication and were not included. Thus it appears that the analysis was based on the intent to treat principle.

- **Are the results valid?**

1 Was the assignment of patients to treatment really randomized (and the randomization code concealed)?
2 Were all patients who entered the study accounted for at its conclusion?
3 Were the clinical outcomes measured blindly?

- **Is the therapeutic effect important?**

1 Were both statistical and clinical significance considered?
2 Were all clinically important outcomes reported?

- **What are the results?**

McLeod RS, Wolff BG, Steinhart AH *et al.* Prophylactic mesalamine treatment decreases postoperative recurrence of Crohn's disease. *Gastroenterology* 1995; **109**: 404–13.

Randomized controlled trial in which 163 patients with Crohn's disease who had all visible disease resected were randomized to receive mesalamine (Pentasa) 3 g daily or a placebo for a median period of 34 months. Primary outcome was recurrent Crohn's disease defined by recurrence of symptoms and radiographic or endoscopic documentation of recurrence.

	Recurrent Crohn's disease		Risk	ARR	RRR
	Yes	No			
5-ASA	27	60	31%	10%	24%
Placebo	31	45	41%	–	–

ARR, absolute risk reduction; RRR, relative risk reduction.

- **Are the results relevant to my patient?**

1 Were the study patients recognizably similar to my own?
2 Is the therapeutic maneuver feasible in my practice?

Figure 1.2 Elements of a valid and useful randomized trial

Approximately 10% of patients in both treatment groups had incomplete follow-up. Methodologically rigorous studies have a very low proportion of patients for whom data are missing. This issue is important, since patients who are lost to follow-up usually have a different prognosis than those for whom complete information is available. If a substantial proportion of patients have incomplete follow-up data, the results are uninterpretable.[28]

Turning to an assessment of the outcomes in this study, both the patients and investigators were unaware of the treatment allocation. Blinding is used to reduce bias in the interpretation of outcomes. This is especially important when a subjective outcome is evaluated.[29] In this study objective demonstration of recurrent disease (endoscopy and/or radiology) was required in addition to the more subjective measure of the introduction of treatment for recurrent symptoms. Thus the reader can be satisfied that the primary outcome measure was both clinically meaningful and objectively assessed.

Finally, the data analysis and results should be examined. A great deal of useful information can be obtained by reviewing the assumptions that were used in the sample size calculation. In this study, which analyzes a difference in proportions, the investigators had to define four variables: the alpha (type 1) error rate, the beta (type 2) error rate, the expected proportion of patients who would be expected to relapse in the placebo group, and the minimum difference in the rate of relapse which the investigator wished to detect. In this publication these parameters are easily identified. The rate of symptomatic recurrence was estimated to be 12.5% per year and it was anticipated that treatment with 5-ASA would reduce this rate by 50% to an absolute value of 6.25% per year. In contrast to the expected 50% relative risk reduction which was anticipated, the 3-year *actuarial* risk of recurrence was 26% in the treatment group compared with 45% in the group that received 5-ASA ($P = 0.039$). Therefore, the relative risk reduction ([45%–26%]/45% = 42%) is slightly lower than the figure which the investigators considered to be clinically meaningful. Furthermore, the probability of a type 1 error is described as a one-tailed value of $P = 0.05$. This implies that one-tailed statistical testing was used to derive the P value of 0.039. The use of one-sided statistical testing raises legitimate concerns regarding the statistical inferences made in the study.[30] It is inappropriate to hypothesize that 5-ASA therapy could *only* be beneficial, given that the drug can cause diarrhea and colitis.[31] For these reasons, uncertainty exists regarding both the clinical and statistical interpretation of these data.

ARE THE RESULTS OF THIS VALID STUDY IMPORTANT?

To assess the importance of this result it is necessary to quantify the magnitude of the treatment effect. How the evidence is presented may influence both physicians and patients in making choices. The most basic means of expressing the magnitude of a treatment of fact is the absolute risk reduction (ARR), which is defined as the proportion of patients in the experimental group with a treatment success minus the proportion of patients with this outcome in the control group. In this instance the annual rate of relapse in the placebo treated patients was 15% (success rate of 85%) compared with 8.7% (success rate of 91.3%) in those who received the active treatment. This yields an ARR of 6.3%. The number needed to treat (NNT), the number of patients with Crohn's disease who would have to be treated with 3 g/day of 5-ASA to maintain a remission over a year, can be calculated as the reciprocal of this number, and is 16. Alternative ways of describing effectiveness include calculating the observed relative risk reduction (RRR = 6.3/15) of 42%, or even stating that about 90% of patients respond to maintenance therapy, ignoring the substantial placebo effect which is evident. The evidence presented as the ARR or NNT, rather than the numbers which show the treatment in a more favorable light, may still lead the physician to recommend this form of treatment and cause the patient to choose to accept this strategy over no intervention. However, the expectations of the physician and patients are likely to be more realistic[32] than they may be if the physician accepts and promotes in an uncritical way the information that 90% of patients who receive 5-ASA maintenance therapy will remain in remission over 1 year.

ARE THESE RESULTS APPLICABLE TO MY PATIENT?

Following an assessment of the validity of the evidence using the criteria described in the preceding paragraphs it is necessary to decide whether the conclusions of the study are relevant and important to the individual patient. An initial step is to evaluate the demographic characteristics of the patients in the RCT and compare them to those of the patient in question. If the patient for whom maintenance therapy is being considered is similar to the patients who were evaluated in the trial, it is reasonable to assume that she will experience the same benefit of therapy and is at no greater risk for the development of adverse drug reactions. Alternatively, this patient may have characteristics that make it unlikely that a benefit from 5-ASA will be realized. For example, if the patient had residual active Crohn's disease it would be difficult to generalize the results of the study of McLeod *et al.*,[25] since the patients in this trial had resection of all visible disease prior to study entry.

At this point, if we accept that the results are generalizable to our patient example, the relative risks and benefits of the therapy must be weighed and the patient's preferences should be considered. Evaluation of the data reveals that the trial was methodologically rigorous and evaluated an important outcome. However, it is doubtful whether conventional statistical significance was demonstrated. This raises the question of whether the observed differences between the treatment groups might have occurred by chance. Furthermore, the magnitude of the treatment effect is relatively small. In presenting to the patient the benefit of an annual reduction in the risk of recurrence of 6.3% it is also necessary to consider the cost and inconvenience of taking medication for an asymptomatic condition. One observation in favor of recommending the treatment is that the risk of serious toxicity with 5-ASA appears to be low.

Because there is a degree of uncertainty concerning the true benefit of 5-ASA maintenance therapy based on analysis of this single RCT, it would be prudent to review additional published data. A recent meta-analysis of 5-ASA therapy has been published.[33] Meta-analysis, the process of combining the results of multiple RCTs using quantitative methods, is an important tool for the practitioner of EBM. Pooling the results of multiple RCTs increases statistical power and thus may resolve the contradictory results of individual studies. Combining data from RCTs statistically also increases the precision of the estimate of a treatment effect. Moreover, the greater statistical power afforded by meta-analysis may allow insight into the benefits of treatment for specific subgroups of patients. These properties are particularly relevant to the case under consideration, given the previously identified concerns.

The meta-analysis summarized data from 15 RCTs which evaluated the efficacy of 5-ASA maintenance therapy in 1371 patients with quiescent Crohn's disease. Patients were randomly assigned to receive either 5-ASA or placebo for treatment periods of 4–48 months. Although 5-ASA was superior to placebo in 13 of the 15 studies, the results of only two trials were statistically significant. Separate analyses were performed using data from the four trials that included patients with a surgically induced remission (Figure 1.3) in distinction to those that evaluated patients after a medically induced remission. Sensitivity analyses assessed the response to therapy in specific subgroups of patients. The overall analysis concluded that 5-ASA has a statistically significant benefit; the risk of symptomatic relapse in patients who received 5-ASA was reduced by 6.3% (95% confidence interval –10.4% to –2.1%, $2P = 0.0028$), which corresponds to an NNT of 16. Importantly, the greatest benefit was observed in the four trials that evaluated patients following a surgical resection. In these studies there was a 13.1% reduction in the risk of a relapse (95% CI –21.8% to –4.5%, $2P = 0.0028$), which corresponds to an NNT of 8. No statistically significant effect was demonstrable in the analysis, which was restricted to the patients with medically induced remission.

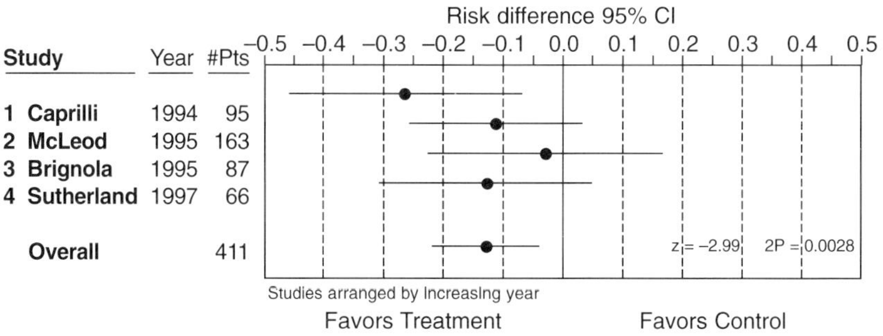

Figure 1.3 Meta-analysis of the four RCTs of mesalamine for prevention of clinical relapse in quiescent Crohn's disease after surgically induced remission. Cumulative risk diffference and the respective 95% CIs are plotted on the graph. (Reproduced with permission from Camma C, Giunta M, Rosselli M *et al.* Mesalamine in the maintenance treatment of Crohn's disease: a meta-analysis adjusted for confounding variables. *Gastroenterology* 1997; **113**: 1469)

- ***Are the results of this overview valid and reliable?***

1 Is it an overview of randomized trials of treatments?
2 Does it include a methods section that describes:
   (a) finding and including all the relevant trials?
   (b) assessing their individual validity?
   (c) using valid statistical methods that compared "like with like" stratified by study?
3 Were the results consistent from study to study?
4 Are the conclusions based on sufficiently large amounts of data to exclude a spurious difference (type 1 error) or missing a real difference (type II error).

- ***Are these applicable to your patient?***

Differences between subgroups should only be believed if you can say "yes" to all of the following:
1 Was it hypothesized before the study began (rather than the product of dredging the data), and has it been confirmed in other, independent studies?
2 Was it one of just a few subgroups analyses carries out in this study?
3 Is the difference both clinically (beneficial for some but useless or harmful for others) and statistically significant?
4 Does it really make biologic and clinical sense?

Figure 1.4 Approaches to evaluating evidence concerning overviews. (Reproduced from Yusuf S, Cairns JA, Camm AJ *et al.* (eds). *Evidence Based Cardiology.* London: BMJ Books, 1998, p 20)

ARE THE RESULTS OF THIS META-ANALYSIS VALID AND RELIABLE?

Figure 1.4 provides some useful guidelines for the interpretation of overview analyses. It is important that a comprehensive search strategy be performed since publication bias, the selective publication of studies with positive results, is an important threat to the validity of meta-analysis.[34] This criterion was met. Camma and colleagues' review of the literature was extensive and not limited to English language publications. The investigators also searched review articles, primary studies, and abstracts by hand. Quality scores were used to evaluate the validity of the individual studies and a sensitivity analysis was performed which assessed the effect of trial quality on the result. No important change in the overall result was noted when studies of lower quality were excluded from consideration. However this type of analysis was not performed in the analysis of the subgroups of four trials (411 patients) which evaluated 5-ASA after a surgically induced remission.

One of the included studies, that of Caprilli *et al.*,[35] which involved 95 patients, showed a greater benefit for 5-ASA than any other trial, medical or surgical, which has been performed. An important methodological deficiency of this RCT was the failure to conceal the treatment allocation from the investigators. Since these physicians were aware of the treatment assignment, and the definition of relapse used required clinical interpretation, it is possible that the 27% reduction in the risk of relapse identified is an overestimation of the true treatment effect. Accordingly, the inclusion of the results of this study in the subgroup analysis of the surgical studies may overestimate the true benefit of 5-ASA. Furthermore, Camma *et al.* did not include an additional trial by Lochs[36] which was only available as a preliminary report at the time the meta-analysis was performed. This study, which is the largest RCT to evaluate 5-ASA following surgery, assigned 318 patients to receive either 4 g of active drug or a placebo for 18 months. Although Camma and colleagues described this study as "confirming" a benefit of 5-ASA after surgery, the results are not impressive. Only a 6.9% reduction in the rate of relapse was observed in patients who received the active treatment (24.5% 5-ASA compared with 31.4% placebo). This difference was not statistically significant.

This example underscores the importance of updating systematic reviews as new information becomes available, which is the approach of the Cochrane Collaboration, but not of reviews in conventional publications. If the data provided by Lochs *et al.* were aggregated with those of the other trials, the overall estimate of benefit for 5-ASA would be less. Based on these data it can be concluded that 5-ASA may be an effective maintenance therapy following surgery, but the magnitude of the treatment effect is modest at best.

ARE THESE RESULTS APPLICABLE TO OUR PATIENT EXAMPLE?

The meta-analysis of surgical trials performed by Camma provides important information to the clinician who must decide whether or not to offer patients 5-ASA for maintenance therapy. The concern regarding statistical significance raised by the critique of the McLeod study has been reduced. It seems likely that the beneficial effect of 5-ASA following surgery is real. However, although the majority of the criteria outlined in Figure 1.4 have been met, the issue of clinical relevance remains. The most optimistic estimate of the size of the treatment effect, derived from the meta-analysis, is an NNT of 8. However, given the possibility of bias in the study of Caprilli, a more conservative estimate could be based on the data of Lochs and colleagues from the single large randomized trial which yielded an NNT of 15.

In presenting this information to the patient the following points should be emphasized:

1 The existing data suggest that 5-ASA is effective but the benefit of treatment is small (with NNT estimates ranging from 8 to 15).
2 The annual risk of relapse following surgery is relatively low without treatment.
3 5-ASA therapy is safe.
4 The cost of 5-ASA therapy is approximately $70 (US) per month.
5 To derive a benefit from the treatment the medication must be taken on a regular basis. This requires the patient to take six pills each day.

Patients undoubtedly will react in different ways to this information. Our patient chose not to accept this therapy.

RATIONALE FOR A BOOK ON EVIDENCE BASED GASTROENTEROLOGY AND HEPATOLOGY

Gastroenterologists, hepatologists, and general surgeons are fortunate to have many excellent textbooks that provide a wealth of information regarding digestive diseases. Such traditional textbooks concentrate on the pathophysiology of disease and are comprehensive in their scope. *Evidence Based Gastroenterology and Hepatology* is not intended to replace these texts, since its focus is on clinical evidence.

Excellent electronic databases are available, and many traditional publications contain relevant research evidence and important summaries and reviews to support evidence based practice. However, Cumbers and Donald[37] have found that physicians in clinical practice find the acquisition of data from these sources time consuming. Their study revealed that even locating relevant articles required on average 3 days for practitioners with an onsite library and a week for those without such a facility. This book has been written for the purpose of saving valuable time for busy practitioners of gastroenterology, hepatology, and general surgery.

The book cannot claim to be comprehensive; for example, the reader will not find chapters on the management of achalasia or Ogilvie's syndrome. While we would have preferred to provide our readers with a more complete coverage of topics, we had to establish a list of priority areas where we felt that there was important evidence to be reviewed and summarized on one hand and available authors with the required expertise on the other. We hope that future editions will expand the number of topics that are included.

A limitation of any textbook is the timeliness of the information that it is possible to provide in print form. New evidence accumulates rapidly in clinical medicine and it is impossible to include the most up-to-date information in a textbook because of the time required for production. For example, it is pointed out in Chapter 21 that a meta-analysis of the effects of ursodeoxycholic acid in primary biliary cirrhosis was not available for critical appraisal by the author during the writing of this chapter. To meet the needs of our readers for the most timely information it is planned to produce electronic updates of chapters at regular intervals. These updates, like those for the companion book *Evidence Based Cardiology*, will appear on the BMJ webpage (http: //www.bmj.com).

REFERENCES

1 Ruffin JM, Grizzle JE, Hightower NC *et al.* A co–operative double–blind evaluation of gastric "freezing" in the treatment of duodenal ulcer. *N Engl J Med* 1969; **281**(1): 16–19.

2 Dickson ER, Fleming TR, Wiesner RH *et al.* Trial of penicillamine in advanced primary biliary cirrhosis. *N Engl J Med* 1985; **312**(16): 1011–15.

3 A Medical Research Council Investigation. Streptomycin treatment of pulmonary tuberculosis. *Br Med J* **1948**: 770–82.

4 Truelove SC, Witts LJ. Cortisone in ulcerative colitis. Final report on a therapeutic trial. *Br Med J* **1955**: 1041–8.

5 Liberati A, Apolone G, Nicolucci A *et al.* The role of attitudes, beliefs, and personal characteristics of Italian physicians in the surgical treatment of early breast cancer. *Am J Publ Hlth* 1991; **81**: 38–41.

6 Antman EM, Lau J, Kupelnick B *et al.* A comparison of results of meta-analyses of randomized control trials and recommendations of clinical experts. *JAMA* 1992; **268**: 240–8.

7 Mulrow CD. The Medical Review Article: state of the science. *Ann Intern Med* 1987; **106**: 485–8.

8 Jefferson T. What are the benefits of editorials and non-systematic reviews? *Br Med J* 1999; **318**: 135.

9 Cochrane AL. Archie Cochrane in his own words. Selections arranged from his 1972 introduction to "Effectiveness and Efficiency: Random Reflections on the Health Services". *Controlled Clinical Trials* 1989; **10**(4): 428–33.

10 The Cochrane Library (database on disk and CD-ROM). Oxford: The Cochrane Collaboration. Update Software, 1999.
11 Sackett DL. Clinical epidemiology. *Am J Epidemiol* 1969; **89**(2): 125–8.
12 Sackett DL. Interpretation of diagnostic data: 1. How to do it with pictures. *Can Med Assoc J* 1983; **129**(5): 429–32.
13 Sackett DL, Haynes RB, Guyatt GH *et al. Clinical epidemiology. A basic science for clinical medicine*, 2nd edn. Boston, MA: Little Brown and Co., 1991.
14 Reid MC, Lachs MS, Feinstein AR. Use of methodological standards in diagnostic test research. *JAMA* 1995; **274**(8): 645–51.
15 Ransohoff DF, Feinstein AR. Problems of spectrum and bias in evaluating the efficacy of diagnostic tests. *N Engl J Med* 1978; **299**(17): 926–30.
16 Chalmers TC. Randomization of the first patient. *Med Clin North Am* 1975; **59**(4): 1035–8.
17 Resnick RH, Iber FL, Ishihara AM *et al.* A controlled study of the therapeutic portacaval shunt. *Gastroenterology* 1974; **67**(5): 843–57.
18 Sacks HS, Berrier J, Reitman D *et al.* Meta-analyses of randomized controlled trials. *N Engl J Med* 1987; **316**(8): 450–5.
19 Kernick DP Lies, damned lies, and evidence-based medicine. Jabs and Jibes. *Lancet* 1998; **351**: 1824.
20 Scholefield JH, Johnson AG, Shorthouse AJ. Current surgical practice in screening for colorectal cancer based on family history criteria. *Br J Surg* 1998; **85**: 1543
21 Gabriel SE, Jaakkimainen L, Bombardier C. Risk for serious gastrointestinal complications related to use of nonsteroidal anti-inflammatory drugs. A meta-analysis. *Ann Intern Med* 1991; **115**: 787–96.
22 Yusuf S, Cairns JA, Camm AJ *et al.* (eds). *Evidence based cardiology*. London: BMJ Books, 1998.
23 Cataldo F, Ventura A, Lazzari R *et al.* Antiendomysium antibodies and celiac disease: solved and unsolved questions. An Italian multicentre study. *Acta Paediatr* 1995; **84**: 1125–31.
24 Kitching A, Sackett D, Yusuf S. Approaches to evaluating evidence. In: *Evidence based cardiology*. London: BMJ Books,1998.
25 McLeod RS, Wolff BG, Steinhart AH *et al.* Prophylactic mesalamine treatment decreases postoperative recurrence of Crohn's disease. *Gastroenterology* 1995; **109**: 404–13.
26 Chalmers TC, Celano P, Sacks HS *et al.* Bias in treatment assignment in controlled clinical trials. *N Engl J Med* 1983; **309**: 1358–61.
27 Schulz KF, Chalmers I, Hayes RJ *et al.* Empirical evidence of bias. Dimensions of methodological quality associated with estimates of treatment effects in controlled trials. *JAMA* 1995; **273**: 408–12.
28 ICH Harmonised Tripartite Guideline. *Statistical principles for clinical trials: section 5.3 – missing values and outliers*. ICH Steering Committee, 5 February 1998.
29 Feagan BG, McDonald JWD, Koval JJ. Therapeutics and inflammatory bowel disease: a guide to the interpretation of randomized controlled trials. *Gastroenterology* 1996; **110**: 275–83.
30 Koch GG. One-sided and two-sided tests and *P* values. *J Biopharm Stat* 1991; **1**: 161–70.
31 Kapur KC, Williams GT, Allison MC. Mesalazine induced exacerbation of ulcerative colitis. *Gut* 1995; **37**: 838–9.
32 Naylor CD, Chen E, Strauss B. Measured enthusiasm: does the method of reporting trial results alter perceptions of therapeutic effectiveness? *Ann Intern Med* 1992; **117**: 916–21.
33 Camma C, Giunta M, Rosselli M *et al.* Mesalamine in the maintenance treatment of Crohn's disease: a meta-analysis adjusted for confounding variables. *Gastroenterology* 1997; **113**: 1465–73.
34 Oxman AD, Cook DJ, Guyatt GH. User's guides to the medical literature. VI: How to use an overview. Evidence-Based Medicine Working Group. *JAMA* 1994; **272**: 1367–71.
35 Caprilli R, Andreoli A, Capurso L *et al.* Oral mesalazine (5-aminosalicylic acid; Asacol) for the prevention of post-operative recurrence of Crohn's disease. *Aliment Pharmacol Ther* 1994; **8**: 35–43.
36 Lochs H, Mayer M, Fleig WE *et al.* Prophylaxis of postoperative relapse in Crohn's disease with Pentasa. Results of the European Cooperative Crohn's Disease Study I. *Gastroenterology* (in press).
37 Cumbers B, Donald A. Evidence-based practice. Data day. *Health Service J* 1999; **109**: 30–1.

2 Gastroesophageal reflux disease

Naoki Chiba, Richard H Hunt

INTRODUCTION

Gastroesophageal reflux occurs physiologically in all persons, when gastric contents reflux into the esophagus. However, due to acid neutralization by saliva and prompt esophageal clearance of refluxate, symptoms occur in a minority of people. The typical symptoms of GERD are heartburn, acid regurgitation and dysphagia. It is difficult to determine at what point reflux results in disease. Many patients may regard some degree of heartburn as normal and only a small proportion of patients seek medical care, conceptually outlined in Castell's "iceberg".[1] Reflux also may result in extra-esophageal manifestations such as asthma, non-cardiac chest pain (NCCP), posterior laryngitis and hoarseness which are beyond the scope of this chapter, where discussions focus on the esophageal symptoms of reflux.

Early literature often used the terms hiatus hernia and gastroesophageal reflux synonymously, a nomenclature that is incorrect. Hiatus hernia is a structural abnormality and reflux is a functional or mechanical event. Subsequently, reflux disease was considered to be present when abnormally prolonged acid refluxate resulted in esophageal damage, either macroscopic (endoscopic esophagitis) or microscopic (histological esophagitis). However, more recently, it has been recognized that symptomatic gastroesophageal reflux without obvious damage, "endoscopy negative reflux disease" (ENRD), is an important part of the spectrum of reflux disease. Moreover, patients will often present not only with reflux symptoms but also with epigastric pain and/or discomfort, symptoms associated with "dyspepsia" rather than GERD.

EPIDEMIOLOGY

With inconsistency of definitions and methods of diagnosis, it is difficult to determine the current prevalence of GERD in the general population. Heartburn is experienced by 4–7% of the population on a daily basis and by 34–44% of the population at least once a month (Table 2.1).[2–6] The overall prevalence of reflux esophagitis in Western countries has been estimated to be about 2%.[7] Twenty-seven per cent of adults self treat with antacids more than twice a month, and 84% of this group have objective evidence of reflux esophagitis if investigated.[8]

The incidence of GERD is estimated to be 4.5 per 100 000, with a dramatic increase in persons over the age of 40.[9] A Canadian study found that heartburn occurred at least

Table 2.1 Population based questionnaire studies of heartburn prevalence

Study	Daily (%)	At least once weekly (%)	At least once a month (%)	Total at least once a month (%)
Nebel, 1976[2]	7	14	15	36
Thompson, 1982[3]	4	10	21	35
Gallup, 1988[4]	—	—	—	44
Isolauri, 1995[5]	5	15	21	41
Locke, 1997[6]	—	18	—	42

once a week in 19% of persons aged over 60 years, compared to 4.8% of persons less than age 27.[3]

Nebel *et al* in 1976[2] studied the point prevalence and precipitating factors associated with symptomatic gastroesophageal reflux using a questionnaire in 446 hospitalized patients and 558 outpatients (Table 2.1). Age, gender, or hospitalization did not significantly affect prevalence. Fried or "spicy" foods and alcohol were the most common precipitating factors. In a more recent Finnish study of 1700 adults, of symptomatic patients, only 16% reported taking medications and only 5% had sought medical care.[5]

ESOPHAGEAL COMPLICATIONS OF GERD

Complications of GERD include bleeding (<2%), ulceration (around 5%), and strictures (from 1.2% to 20%).[10–12] Patients with strictures are older and more frequently have a hiatus hernia.[10] Barrett's esophagus has been identified in 10–20% of GERD patients.[13] Six of 50 patients (12%) developed Barrett's esophagus during approximately 20 years of follow-up, a crude incidence of 0.6% per year.[14]

Heading estimated that GERD patients would require 10 operations per 100 000 persons/year and that 5–10% of patients seen by gastroenterologists would require fundoplication.[12] However, this observation was made before the introduction of proton pump inhibitors (PPI), which have dramatically changed the approach to medical therapy for GERD.

For patients with mild esophagitis, the course of the disease may be benign, with only 23% progressing to more severe esophagitis, while 31% improve and 46% spontaneously heal with no further episodes.[15] Patients with endoscopic esophagitis diagnosed more than 10 years earlier were contacted by postal questionnaire and phone interview.[11] Of the respondents, over 70% continued to have significant symptoms of reflux, 40–50% were still taking acid suppressive medications regularly and had reduced quality of life (lower SF-36, physical and social function domain scores). Thus, GERD is a chronic disease with significant morbidity and impacts negatively on the quality of life. A Finnish cohort study reported data from 17- to 22-year follow-up in 60 GERD patients who were not receiving chronic acid suppressive treatment.[14] The severity of reflux symptoms declined in the long term, but objective testing with endoscopy and 24h pH studies documented that pathological reflux persisted in two-thirds of patients.

Despite frequent symptoms, even severe reflux disease has little effect on life expectancy, with almost no deaths directly due to GERD reported in long term follow-up.[9,11,14] However, a recent population based study identified GERD as a strong risk factor for esophageal adenocarcinoma but not squamous cell carcinoma.[16]

Table 2.2 Summary of diagnostic tests in GERD

Test	What does it measure?	Comments
Esophageal manometry	Measures lower esophageal sphincter (LES) pressure only	Too much overlap with normals to diagnose GERD Does not detect transient LES relaxation May be useful in pre/postoperative evaluation
	Low (<10 mmHg) LES pressure: 58% sensitivity and 84% specificity for abnormal acid exposure[25] Does not measure risk for reflux Does not assess esophagitis	
Radiology	Shows morphological findings (eg stricture) and may rule out other pathology (eg ulcers) Best test for dysphagia	Best test for this
	Detects gastroesophageal reflux. Some use abdominal compression	In patients with GERD detects reflux in 10–50%[26] Free reflux correlates best
	Can detect hiatus hernia	Unclear role in most patients with GERD Many with hiatus hernia have no symptoms
	Poor detection for mild esophagitis 0–53%[26]	For moderate esophagitis, sensitivity 79–93%[26](46) For severe esophagitis, sensitivity 95–100%[26]
	Does not assess symptoms	
Scintigraphy	Can show reflux	Sensitivity 14–86%[26] Limited utility as reflux is intermittent Requires radioactivity exposure
Endoscopy	Detects esophagitis Detects Barrett's esophagus Allows biopsy, but esophageal histology has limited utility	Lacks sensitivity
Bernstein (acid perfusion test)	Measures esophageal acid sensitivity, not a test for esophagitis Can be positive in patients with normal endoscopy and 24h pH studies Determines esophageal origin of pain May identify those with 'acid sensitive esophagus'	Sensitivity 42–100%, mean 77%[26] Specificity 50–100%, mean 86%[26] May be useful in patients with atypical symptoms and NCCP
24h esophageal pH monitoring	Quantifies gastroesophageal reflux Allows assessment of whether 'pathological reflux' occurs Does not detect mucosal damage	Normal in 14–29% of those with esophagitis Normal in 6–15% of patients with abnormal symptom index (SI)
Symptom index (SI) with 24h esophageal pH monitoring	Correlates symptoms with reflux events	Bimodal predictive value Can be positive when pH study is normal
Omeprazole test	Positive test detects acid reflux as probable cause of symptoms Tests reflux, acid damage, esophageal sensitivity	May be best overall test

PATHOPHYSIOLOGY

GERD is primarily a motility disorder of the esophagus which allows abnormal reflux of injurious gastric refluxate. This occurs as a failure of the antireflux barrier provided primarily by the lower esophageal sphincter (LES) and crural diaphragm. The two key abnormalities are abnormal transient lower esophageal sphincter relaxations (TLESRs),[17,18] precipitated by gastric distension in the postprandial period,[19] and poor basal LES tone.[17] The result is prolonged dwell time of gastric refluxate and increasing damage when the pH of the refluxate is below 3, which is optimal for pepsin activation.[20,21] A hiatus hernia may act as a reservoir for acid refluxate which can then reflux freely up the esophagus.[22,23]

DEFINING AND DIAGNOSING GERD

The diagnosis of GERD depends on the definition of "pathological" in diagnostic tests. Problems of definition have been recognized for more than two decades.[24] Methods of diagnosing GERD are outlined in Table 2.2. These tests evaluate different features of GERD, and none measures all aspects the disease. Tests such as barium studies, scintigraphy, and 24-hour (24h) esophageal pH studies show whether reflux occurs, endoscopy allows for the diagnosis of mucosal changes and assessments of complications, 24h pH studies can quantify the amount of acid exposure, and mucosal sensitivity can be assessed by the Bernstein test. The interpretation of tests is also important. For example, a patient with documented endoscopic esophagitis with a negative Bernstein test should not be regarded as having a "false negative" Bernstein test, but rather an acid insensitive esophagus. With variable patient populations, differences in definitions, techniques, and gold standards, it is impossible to compare sensitivity and specificity values.[27]

What are the symptoms of GERD?

The typical symptoms of GERD include heartburn (a rising retrosternal burning discomfort), acid regurgitation, and dysphagia. Many investigators consider that the diagnosis of GERD is based primarily on typical symptoms with the specificity of heartburn and acid regurgitation being 89% and 95% respectively.[28] An early study reported that when heartburn or regurgitation occurred daily, there was a positive predictive value of 59% and 66% respectively for the diagnosis of GERD.[29] When an abnormal pH-metry is the gold standard, symptoms have 72% sensitivity and 63% specificity.[30] Many patients have other symptoms, but according to recent concepts, these patients are probably more correctly classified as having dyspepsia rather than GERD.[31]

Symptoms as diagnostic predictors

An important study of patients with reflux-like dyspepsia was reported by Joelsson and Johnsson.[32] Erosive esophagitis (Savary–Miller grade 1 or worse) was identified in a third of patients with reflux symptoms. Whether the patient had erosive disease or not, the frequency of heartburn and acid regurgitation correlated with median esophageal acid

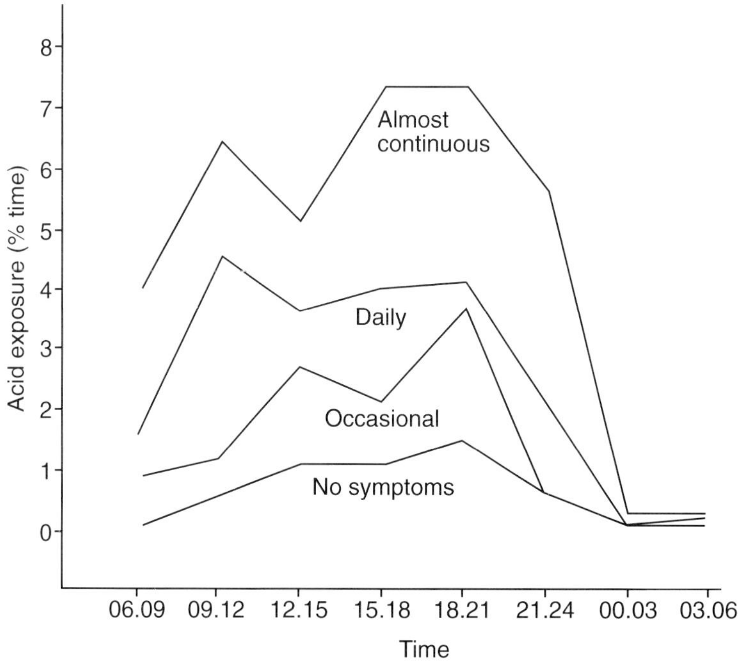

Figure 2.1 Acid exposure of the distal part of the esophagus during eight 3-hour periods expressed as median % time spent with pH <4 in 190 patients with different degrees of heartburn and acid regurgitation and 50 asymptomatic endoscopically normal subjects. Reproduced with permission.[32]

exposure time measured by 24h pH monitoring. Although patients with an endoscopically normal esophagus had lower overall median acid exposure, there was a trend towards more acid exposure in those with more severe symptoms. Figure 2.1 shows the relationship between severity of symptoms and acid exposure time. The authors concluded that reflux-like dyspepsia is accompanied by increased esophageal acid exposure, a concept that is supported by others.[33,34]

Unfortunately, severity of symptoms is a poor predictor of mucosal damage.[35–37] However, Johannessen[38] determined that heartburn showed the best discrimination for patients with esophagitis. Typical symptoms of GERD correlate with abnormal intraesophageal pH exposure in 56–73% of patients.[30,36]

In an effort to improve the diagnostic value of the history, investigators have applied structured questionnaires (Table 2.3). Using the questionnaire developed by Johnsson,[39] a positive response to all four questions is required to achieve a high positive predictive value, thus limiting usefulness. The description of symptoms, as opposed to using the term heartburn, may be a factor which improves the predictive value of this questionnaire.

DeMeester's study reported a retrospective review of 100 consecutive patients with symptoms of GERD.[40] The presence of grade 2 or 3 symptoms on their standardized questionnaire (Table 2.3) and endoscopic esophagitis, predicted increased acid exposure on 24h intraesophageal pH monitoring with a specificity of 97% and a positive predictive value of 98%.

The Carlsson–Dent questionnaire has been extensively validated for reflux esophagitis detected at endoscopy and abnormal 24h intraesophageal pH-metry.[41] The

Table 2.3 Validated GERD questionnaires

<table>
<tr><th>Study</th><th>Questionnaire</th></tr>
<tr><td>Johnsson, 1993[39]</td><td>Do you frequently experience a rising, spreading, uncomfortable feeling behind your breastbone?
Is this feeling often combined with a burning sensation in your chest?
Do antacids relieve your symptoms?
Have you had your symptoms during four or more days in the last week?
A positive response to all four questions above had a 85% probability that the patient would have erosive esophagitis and/or abnormal 24h pH study</td></tr>
<tr><td>Carlsson, 1998[41]</td><td>Weighted scores for each of the responses were added to obtain a final diagnostic score[a]
Which one of these four statements best describes the main discomfort you get in your stomach or chest (burning rising feeling, nausea, pain with swallowing, none of above)?
Having chosen one of the above, please now choose which one of the next three statements best describes the timing of your main discomfort (any time, within 2 hours of food, at a particular time not related to food)?
How do the following affect your main discomfort (larger than usual meals, fatty foods and strongly flavored/spicy food and whether these worsen, improve or have no effect)?
Which one of the following best describes the effect of indigestion medicines on your main discomfort (no benefit, relief <15 min, relief >15 min, not applicable)?
Which of the following best describes the effect of lying flat, stooping, or bending on your main discomfort (no effect, brings it on or makes worse, gives relief, don't know)?
Which of the following best describes the effect of lifting or straining (or any other activity that makes you breathe heavily) on your main activity (no effect, brings it on or makes worse, gives relief, don't know)?
If food or acid-tasting liquid returns to your throat or mouth what effect does it have on your main discomfort (no effect, brings it on or makes worse, gives relief, don't know)?
Symptom relief during treatment with omeprazole was predicted by the presence of heartburn "a burning feeling rising from the stomach or lower chest up towards the neck" and "relief from antacids"</td></tr>
<tr><td>Tefera, 1997[40]</td><td><table>
<tr><th>Symptom</th><th>Score</th><th>Severity</th></tr>
<tr><td>Heartburn</td><td>0</td><td>None</td></tr>
<tr><td></td><td>1</td><td>Minimal: occasional episodes</td></tr>
<tr><td></td><td>2</td><td>Moderate: primary reason for visit</td></tr>
<tr><td></td><td>3</td><td>Incapacitated: disabled for activities of daily life</td></tr>
<tr><td>Regurgitation</td><td>0</td><td>None</td></tr>
<tr><td></td><td>1</td><td>Mild: occasional, after straining or large meals</td></tr>
<tr><td></td><td>2</td><td>Moderate: predictable if lying down or straining</td></tr>
<tr><td></td><td>3</td><td>Incapacitated: associated with pulmonary aspiration</td></tr>
<tr><td>Dysphagia</td><td>0</td><td>None</td></tr>
<tr><td></td><td>1</td><td>Mild: occasional with coarse food, lasts seconds</td></tr>
<tr><td></td><td>2</td><td>Moderate: requires liquid to clear</td></tr>
<tr><td></td><td>3</td><td>Incapacitated: needs semisolid diet, meat impaction</td></tr>
</table>[This study used a composite score]</td></tr>
</table>

[a]Only the questions and abbreviated responses are given here, the exact responses to check off and scoring are not shown and readers are referred to the original paper.[41]

questionnaire has a maximum score of 18. In the endoscopic comparison, using a threshold of 4, the questionnaire had 70% sensitivity but only 46% specificity for diagnosis of esophagitis. When used in dyspeptic patients, the questionnaire had a sensitivity of 92% but a specificity of only 19% for diagnosis of GERD when compared to abnormal 24h intraesophageal pH monitoring. The mean score of 11 for GERD patients was higher than that observed in the dyspepsia cohort (mean 4.6). Symptom relief during treatment with omeprazole was predicted by the presence of heartburn, described as "a burning feeling rising from the stomach or lower chest up towards the neck" (OR 4) and "relief from antacids" (OR 2.2). In a non-ulcer dyspepsia study from which patients with predominant heartburn were excluded, 42% of the patients indicated that they had a "rising burning feeling", which defined heartburn in the Carlsson–Dent questionnaire. Even in this group of presumed non-GERD patients, those patients who answered positively to this key question had the best symptom relief with omeprazole.

Of dyspeptic patients identified as having heartburn (rising burning feeling) by this questionnaire, only 32% identified their primary complaint as heartburn when asked directly about heartburn. Thus, a descriptive definition of heartburn appears to be superior to the term heartburn itself for diagnosing reflux disease. This shows how difficult it can be to classify a patient into a specific symptom subgroup, and the overlap between GERD and reflux-like dyspepsia.

What role does a hiatus hernia play?

The mere presence of a hiatus hernia bears no relationship to the diagnosis of esophagitis and is frequently seen in those without esophagitis, and up to half the healthy population have a hiatus hernia.[24] Moreover, only half of the patients with symptoms of heartburn and regurgitation have a hiatus hernia.[42] Some studies have suggested that patients with a hiatus hernia have more severe reflux esophagitis than patients without.[43,44] A large hiatus hernia may act as a reservoir for acid that regurgitates readily when a swallow is initiated.[22,23]

A study in patients with pathological reflux (pH <4 for more than 5% of a 24h intraesophageal pH-metry study) identified hiatus hernia in 71% of patients with mild esophagitis compared to 39% in those without esophagitis.[45] Patients with a hiatus hernia also had higher 24h intraesophageal acid exposure compared to those without, particularly during the night. However, there were no differences in symptoms of heartburn or regurgitation whether or not patients had a hiatus hernia or esophagitis.

Manometry and lower esophageal pressure measurement

Lower esophageal sphincter pressures alone are not of diagnostic value as there is considerable overlap of LES pressures in those with and without esophagitis. In a review[25] of six studies, when the LES pressure was less than 10 mmHg, this correlated with an abnormal acid exposure with a sensitivity of only 58% and specificity of 84%. However, there may be some utility in low LES pressures as a predictor for identifying patients with the most severe reflux.[24] Manometry prior to surgery has been advocated to document a mechanically defective lower esophageal sphincter,[46] but there is no good evidence that this affects outcome.

Radiological diagnosis

A variety of outcome measures have been used in studies of radiology in GERD. Some have measured gastroesophageal reflux (with and without reflux provoking maneuvers) and correlated this with other measures of reflux such as esophageal pH studies. Others have examined the ability of radiological studies to identify esophagitis.

The radiological diagnosis of reflux esophagitis is generally considered to be unreliable. The diagnostic accuracy of barium radiography compared to endoscopy is 0–53% for mild, 79–93% for moderate and 95–100% for severe esophagitis.[26,47] Many of the early studies[48] compared radiological techniques to endoscopy as a gold standard. By 1980, it was recognized that about half the patients with symptomatic reflux did not have endoscopic esophagitis.[24,36] Thus, many patients would be expected to have normal barium studies. From a technical perspective, the gastroesophageal junction is not well visualized in up to a third of patients due to inadequate distention.[48,49]

Measuring reflux alone does not determine whether the patient suffers from GERD or correlates with the patient's symptoms. With provocative tests, reflux is seen in only 25–71% of symptomatic patients but is also seen in 20% of controls.[47] Low density contrast media are no better than regular barium.[50] Radiological studies are frequently falsely negative in patients in whom endoscopy or esophageal pH-metry studies are abnormal.

Measurement of the internal diameter of the cardiac esophagus was shown to predict 89% of patients with mild endoscopic esophagitis.[51] However, this was not confirmed in a study that found that the gastroesophageal junction could not be adequately visualized in 29% of patients.[48]

Free, severe reflux as seen on barium studies may by a highly specific predictor of reflux as confirmed by 24h esophageal pH monitoring.[25,48,52,53] However, esophagitis is rarely diagnosed radiographically in patients with abnormal intraesophageal pH studies.[54]

Scintigraphy

Reflux is assessed following ingestion of a liquid containing a radiolabeled pharmaceutical such as sulfur colloid or ^{99m}Tc in an acidified liquid suspension. This procedure is similar to the assessment of reflux during radiology, although scintigraphy may be superior.[42] Graded abdominal compression to detect reflux is unreliable with variable sensitivity of 14–90%.[26,42,47,48,55] The biggest problem appears to be the short duration of the imaging test, as reflux occurs intermittently. Overall, with the availability of endoscopy and 24h intraesophageal pH monitoring, there appears to be little value to this test in the diagnosis of GERD.

Upper gastrointestinal (UGI) endoscopy

Endoscopy provides the most accurate means of assessing mucosal detail of the esophagus, but is insensitive in diagnosing reflux. Definite endoscopic reflux esophagitis is unequivocal evidence that the patient suffers from GERD. Patients with an "acid sensitive" esophagus who experience symptoms in the absence of esophagitis cannot be diagnosed by endoscopy. The 24h intraesophageal pH study can be abnormal in 50% of patients with reflux symptoms and normal endoscopy.[36,56] Thus a negative endoscopy does not exclude

GERD. Histological diagnosis may be difficult due to either inadequate size of the biopsy,[57] patchy distribution of the histological findings[58] and minimal changes.[59]

Berstad and Hatlebakk[60] prospectively evaluated patients using their own unique endoscopic grading system. Those with true GERD have endoscopic findings according to their classification, but the presence of whitish exudate in the lesions and the width of the lesions were the only two endoscopic features that correlated with the severity of esophageal acid exposure as measured by 24h pH-metry.[61] Confirmatory data from other investigators using this classification are lacking.

The most widely applied esophagitis grading system has been the Savary–Miller classification in original and modified forms. A newer classification[62,63] which measures metaplasia, ulcer, stricture and erosions (MUSE classification) and records the degree of severity of each as absent, mild, moderate, and severe requires prospective evaluation.

Bernstein test (measures esophageal acid sensitivity)

This test was first described in 1958 to distinguish chest pain of esophageal from cardiac origin.[64] In an early (1978) prospective, comparative study of UGI endoscopy, UGI barium series, esophageal manometry, and the Bernstein test in patients with suspected reflux esophagitis, the Bernstein test had the greatest sensitivity (85%) for diagnosing esophagitis. However, there were many false positives as half the patients without esophagitis also had a positive Bernstein test. The lack of specificity for esophagitis is not so surprising, since most of these patients are now considered to have an acid sensitive esophagus, consistent with endoscopy negative reflux disease (ENRD). Another study found the sensitivity of the Bernstein test to be 70% in patients with typical reflux symptoms. However 97% of patients with a negative test had either endoscopic, histological or scintigraphic evidence of GERD.[65] In a review of seven studies,[66] the overall sensitivity of this test was 77% and specificity 86%. Although the Bernstein test does not establish that there is mucosal damage (esophagitis), and patient acceptance is limited, a positive test result implies that the esophagus is likely to be the origin of the pain.

24h ambulatory esophageal pH monitoring

Many experts consider that an abnormal 24h intraesophageal pH study is the gold standard for diagnosing GERD.[36] This test is useful in quantifying the amount and frequency of acid reflux that occurs. However, it is difficult to separate physiological from pathological reflux, and the threshold levels which separate "normal" from "abnormal" test results are not clear. Threshold levels suggested on the basis of separation from the mean by two standard deviations[36] or on the basis of receiver operating characteristic (ROC) analysis are listed in Table 2.4. ROC analysis correlates true and false positive rates for a series of cutoffs and is proposed as an alternative method of analysis to using means and standard deviations to define threshold abnormalities as GERD parameters are not normally distributed.

The test may be useful for investigating patients with atypical reflux symptoms or non-cardiac chest pain in whom GERD is suspected to be the cause of symptoms. The predictive value of specific threshold levels is age dependent.[67] The technique has many other limitations, including lack of availability, invasiveness, cost, lack of patient acceptability,

Table 2.4 Summary of 24h esophageal pH study criteria

Study	Parameter to define thresholds		Comments
DeMeester, 1980[36]		Normal value	They had relatively few controls to establish normal values
	No. of reflux episodes pH <4	<50	Abnormal score is placed 2 standard deviations above the mean. This may not be valid as values do not follow a normal distribution
	Total time pH <4	<4.2%	90% sensitivity and specificity
	Upright time pH <4	<6.3%	Others have not reported the same results with the same criteria[74]
	Supine time pH <4	<1.2%	
	No reflux episodes 5 min duration	3	
	Duration of longest reflux episode	9.2 min	
	Using these criteria they developed a composite scoring system		
Schindlbeck, 1987[68]	Upright time pH <4	<10.5%	They assessed all the same factors as DeMeester above
	Supine time pH <4	<6.0%	They performed ROC analysis
	One or both above threshold = abnormal		
Klauser, 1989[30]	Upright time pH <4	<8.2%	Same group as Schindlbeck but larger reference sample gave lower threshold values
	Supine time pH <4	<3.0%	
	One or both above threshold = abnormal		
Johnsson, 1987[69]	Total time pH <4	<3.4%	Complete separation between patients and controls with single determinant
			Sensitivity 87%, specificity 97%
Masclee, 1990[33]	Total time pH <4	<4.0%	Either equally predictive
	No. of reflux episodes	>30 in 24 h	
Jamieson, 1992[70]	Composite score as in DeMeester above		Used a combination of the composite score and ROC analysis
	Total time pH <4	<4.5%	
Mattox, 1990[71]	Upright time pH <4	<6.7%	These are 95th percentile figures for asymptomatic controls
	Supine time pH <4	<2.4%	
	Total time pH <4	<4.7%	
	Any of above threshold = abnormal		

ROC = receiver operating characteristic

debatable reproducibility, and technical problems such as improper placement of the pH probe, probe failures, and recording device failures.[67]

A cut-off pH of 4 to define pathological reflux has been validated.[27,69] Furthermore, this pH threshold makes physiological sense as proteolytic activity of pepsin is low at a pH above 4, while peptic activity is high below pH 3.[21] Unfortunately, even this cut-off may miss up to 50% of reflux episodes.[72]

DeMeester studied a large series of patients using the normal values in Table 2 4. Twenty-four-hour esophageal pH monitoring had a 90% sensitivity and specificity for acid reflux.[36] Other studies[27,73]using the same variables, reported sensitivity of 85–96% and specificity of 100%. However, another study using the same scoring system was able to distinguish only 41% of symptomatic patients from controls.[74] In these hospitalized patients, only 21% of those with a normal endoscopy had an abnormal intraesophageal pH, while in those with esophagitis, 71% had an abnormal study. A very important observation was that 93% of the endoscopy normal patients responded to antireflux therapy, and another explanation for the symptoms was found in only one patient. Thus, typical symptoms were important for predicting treatment response in spite of the endoscopic and esophageal pH findings.

A study of 45 outpatients with typical reflux symptoms and 42 asymptomatic controls[68] used ROC analysis to obtain maximum values for sensitivity of 93.3% and specificity of 92.9% using the following criteria: (a) only % of time with esophageal pH <4; (b) both the upright and supine reflux values are below threshold to define a normal test; and (c) thresholds levels of pH < 4 for 10.5% of the time in upright position and 6% in the supine position. A limitation of this retrospective study was the restriction to patients with typical symptoms.

When DeMeester's group refined their own analysis by using not only their composite score but but also the ROC analysis they reported values for sensitivity of 96% and specificity of 100%.[27]

Values for sensitivity of 79–95% and for specificity of 85–100% for extended esophageal pH monitoring were described in a comprehensive review[67] and supported by several individual studies.[33,36,69,73] While esophageal 24h pH-metry is often considered to be the gold standard for diagnosing GERD, the false negative rate can be as high as 14–29% in patients with endoscopic esophagitis.[34,36,74,75,76] These data raise doubt whether the pH-metry should be considered to be the gold standard test.

Symptom index

A quantitative method for correlating symptoms and esophageal acid reflux events was developed in1986 and called the "symptom index (SI)". This index was calculated as the number of times the symptom occurred when the pH was <4, divided by the total number of symptoms, multiplied by 100. Initial validation studies in 100 patients found the symptom index to be distributed in a bimodal fashion. Of patients with an SI above 75%, 97.5% had an abnormal esophageal pH study.[77] If the SI was less than 25%, the proportion of patients with a normal esophageal pH study was 81%, and 90% had a normal endoscopy.[78] Endoscopy was normal in nearly 30% of patients with a high SI. Thus, if endoscopy is found to be normal in the course of evaluating patients suspected of having GERD, an esophageal pH study measuring SI may be useful. There was very poor correlation between results of the Bernstein test and the SI. The negative predictive value of a low SI is useful.

Acid sensitive GERD

Further support for the concept that patients can have typical symptoms of reflux with a normal endoscopy comes from studies in which 6–15% of patients with symptomatic reflux had normal 24h esophageal pH-metry.[79–81] Pathological reflux has been identified in 21–61% of endoscopy negative patients.[33,36,74] In contrast, 71–91% of patients with endoscopic erosive esophagitis have pathological reflux.[33,36,74] The proportion of time below pH 4 increases over the spectrum from ENRD to worsening grades of esophagitis.[82]

Of 96 patients with normal 24h esophageal acid exposure, 12.5% were found to have a statistically significant association between symptoms and reflux episodes.[80] In these patients, the duration of reflux episodes was shorter and the pH of reflux episodes less acidic than in patients with typical GERD, suggesting that esophageal hypersensitivity is a cause for their symptoms.

An esophageal balloon distension study provided further experimental evidence of esophageal hypersensitivity in patients with normal acid exposure times with a value for SI of >50%.[79] These patients had significantly lower thresholds for initial perception and discomfort from esophageal balloon distention, compared both to normal controls and to patients with confirmed reflux.

Acid suppression as a diagnostic test

All of the diagnostic tests described above are cumbersome or invasive and detect different features of reflux. Proton pump inhibitors such as omeprazole are the most effective intervention for all grades of esophagitis and for treatment of symptoms such as heartburn. A therapeutic trial with a PPI may be useful in diagnosing GERD in a variety of patient populations, including patients with typical symptoms of GERD, patients with NCCP, and in those with positive and negative findings on endoscopy or pH monitoring. The variation of patients studied makes direct comparisons between studies impossible.

In a double-blind, placebo controlled study of patients with reflux symptoms (92% had heartburn) and only minor or no esophagitis at endsocopy, patients were randomized to receive omeprazole 40 mg od or a placebo for 14 days.[76] A 75% reduction in heartburn was considered to be a positive omeprazole test. There was a significant ($P = 0.04$) correlation between response to omeprazole and the results of the pH-metry. A response to omeprazole occurred in 68% of patients with abnormal reflux and in only 37% of patients with a normal pH study. Only 13% of patients responded to placebo.

A randomized trial of omeprazole 20 mg bid or placebo for 1 week tested the efficacy of omeprazole to determine reflux disease among dyspeptic patients.[83] A diagnosis of GERD was made on the basis of either grade II–III esophagitis or esophageal reflux with pH <4 for more than 4% of the esophageal pH monitoring time. Using this definition, 135 of 160 (84%) patients were found to have GERD. Of those with presumed ENRD, 63% had an abnormal pH study and 20% (18/92) of patients with esophagitis had normal pH studies. Using symptom improvement of at least one grade for the definition of a positive test, the "omeprazole test" had a sensitivity of 71–81% for diagnosing GERD compared to the sensitivity of placebo of 36–47%. With a more stringent definition for a positive test of total symptom relief, the sensitivity of omeprazole to diagnose reflux was lower at 48–59%, compared to 6–19% for placebo. Thus the difference became greater between omeprazole and placebo. However, the specificity of the test was low, and actually was higher with placebo than with omeprazole. Thus the test may be more useful for ruling out the diagnosis than ruling it in. Even in the patients who did not have GERD by definition, those treated with omeprazole had better symptom relief than with placebo. These may be patients with an acid sensitive esophagus who respond well to acid suppression despite their esophageal pH being within normal limits.

A recent UK study of 90 patients with dyspeptic symptoms suggestive of GERD evaluated the cost-effectiveness of an open course of treatment with omeprazole 40 mg daily for 14 days as a diagnostic test.[84] Only 74% of patients had heartburn at baseline, 51% had esophagitis at endoscopy, and 51% had an abnormal pH study. Ten patients (11%) could not tolerate pH monitoring. Patients were classified as responders if symptom severity improved at least two grades on a four-point scale or went from mild symptoms to none. Overall symptom improvement was seen in 82% of patients treated with omeprazole, and 59% had complete symptom relief by 3 days. Using symptom response to 2 weeks omeprazole the sensitivity of the omeprazole test was 69% and the specificity was 58%, using an abnormal esophageal pH test as the gold standard. When the omeprazole response was defined as those with heartburn improvement, sensitivity was improved to 89% but specificity fell to 35%. There was no significant correlation between endoscopic and pH monitoring findings. The cost per correct diagnosis was £47 for omeprazole (95% CI £40–59) compared to £480 for endoscopy (95% CI £396–608). The authors concluded that an empirical trial of omeprazole was cost-effective both for symptom relief and for diagnosing GERD in patients with typical symptoms.

In a small, 4-week, randomized placebo controlled crossover study[75] in patients with normal endoscopy and esophageal pH-metry but with an SI of >50, 10 of 12 (83 %) of patients with a positive SI showed improvement on omeprazole 20 mg bid for decreased symptom frequency, severity and consumption of antacids ($P<0.01$). The Medical Outcomes Study SF-36, quality of life (QOL) parameters for bodily pain and vitality also significantly improved. In the group with a negative SI only one patient clearly improved.

Thirty-three consecutive patients with symptoms of reflux, abnormal pH studies, but normal endoscopies[85] were sequentially allocated to receive ranitidine 150 mg bid, omeprazole 40 mg od, or omeprazole 40 mg bid for 7–10 days. During the last day of treatment an esophageal pH study was repeated and correlated with symptoms. Both doses of omeprazole were superior to ranitidine and correlated with reduction in mean acidity. Using a 75% reduction in symptoms as a positive test, and the pH test as the gold standard, the sensitivity of the omeprazole test using a dose of 40 mg bid was 83.3% while the sensitivity with omeprazole 40 mg od was only 27.2%. The authors concluded that the diagnosis of GERD could be practically ruled out if a patient failed to respond to a short course of high dose proton pump inhibitor.

In a small, 8-week, placebo controlled study of 36 patients with NCCP and abnormal esophageal 24h pH-metry, overall pain improvement was reported by 81 % of omeprazole and 6% of placebo treated patients.[86] Similar results were reported in another small study of 39 patients.[87] The omeprazole test correctly classified 78% of patients considered GERD patients by 24h esophageal monitoring and/or endoscopy and was positive in only 14% of GERD negative patients. Thus, an omeprazole trial may be useful in conditions other than typical GERD such as NCCP.

These lines of evidence indicate that a therapeutic trial of a proton pump inhibitor for 1–2 weeks may be reasonable to diagnose GERD. The advantages of this approach include simplicity, non-invasiveness, ease of prescription and consumption, tolerability, and savings in terms of direct costs and time lost by the patient. The therapeutic trial also predicts therapeutic response. These studies also support the notion that a symptom based diagnosis is reasonable for most patients with reflux disease.

TREATMENT OF GERD

Symptoms of gastroesophageal reflux are common, with significant adverse impact on QOL. The costs of disease include both drug acquisition costs, and indirect costs such as physician visits and time off work. Because of the difficulty in making a definitive diagnosis of GERD through investigations, the physician must make a presumptive diagnosis and initiate a management plan. The goals of therapy are to provide adequate symptom relief in all patients and prevent complications.

Recommended lifestyle modifications in GERD

- Raising the head of the bed has some efficacy.[89–92]
- Avoid food that transiently decreases LES pressure or may have direct irritative effects: fat,[93,94] chocolate,[95] peppermint,[96] spices,[97] raw onions,[98] caffeine,[1,99,100] alcohol,[1,101] orange juice, and tomato drink.[102]
- Avoid lying down within 3–4 hours of a meal.[90]
- Aggravating factors to be avoided: posture,[90] obesity,[1] cigarette smoking.[1,103]
- Avoid tight clothes.[1]
- Avoid certain drugs if possible: ß-blockers, anticholinergics including certain antidepressants, theophylline, calcium antagonists, nitrates.[1]

Antacids and lifestyle modifications

Although antacids and lifestyle modifications are frequently recommended, there is little evidence that these are of benefit. If a patient under the age of 50 has no serious "alarm symptoms", such as unexplained weight loss, dysphagia, or hematemesis, it is reasonable to start empirical therapy[85] as the most cost-effective approach.[88]

R Grade A

A small randomized placebo controlled trial of Maalox TC at a full dose of 15 ml seven times daily for 4 weeks in 32 patients showed no significant difference in symptom relief.[104] There appears to be marginal if any benefit of antacids and alginates over placebo, and antacids do not heal esophagitis.[105–107]

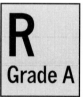

In an uncontrolled study of patients with grade I–III esophagitis healed with either an H_2-receptor antagonist (H_2RA) or omeprazole, patients were given alginate for symptomatic maintenance treatment.[108] At 6 months 76% were in remission. Those with more severe baseline esophagitis relapsed more frequently. In a randomized controlled trial, sodium alginate 10 ml qid was slightly more effective than cisapride 5 mg qid to reduce symptoms using a visual analogue scale (0–100) (alginate 29 ± 22, cisapride 35 ± 25, $P = 0.01$) and the number of reflux episodes in a 4-week period (alginate 2 ± 2, cisapride 3 ± 4, $P = 0.001$).[109] Conservative symptomatic therapy with alginate may be useful in some patients.

R Grade A

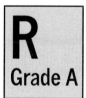

Acid suppression therapy for GERD

While transient relaxations of the LES and defective basal LES tone are thought to be primary determinants of reflux, damage to the esophagus and symptoms result from acidic reflux.[18] Thus, the focus of treatment has been on acid suppression.

Acid secretion can be controlled by various classes of drugs. Antimuscarinic agents are weak inhibitors of the parietal cell M3 cholinergic receptors and clinical use is limited by anticholinergic adverse effects. H_2RA inhibit parietal cell histamine receptors and thus acid inhibition can be partially overcome by stimulation of gastrin and cholinergic receptors as occurs when food is eaten.[110] Tolerance to H_2RAs develops and reduces their efficacy over time.[111] Proton pump inhibitors provide the most acid inhibition through covalent binding to the H^+,K^+-ATPase (acid or proton pump) located in the secretory canaliculus of the parietal cell. Inhibiting the proton pump, which is the final common pathway, blocks acid secretion to all known stimuli. The PPI have a long duration of action which depends on the rate of synthesis of new proton pumps by the parietal cell. These pharmacological differences predict that PPIs should be more effective than H_2RAs.

Studies of 24h intragastric acidity have been used extensively to assess the degree and duration of antisecretory drugs.[112,113] These studies have confirmed that PPIs are superior to H_2RAs in their ability to suppress food stimulated, daytime and total 24h acid secretion. Bell *et al*[112] have shown by meta-analysis, that the healing rate of erosive esophagitis correlated directly with the duration of acid suppression over the 24h period. The primary determinants of healing were the length of treatment, the degree of acid suppression, and the duration of acid suppression over the 24h period. There was also a highly significant correlation between the time that the pH in the esophagus was below 4 (ie below the threshold considered "normal") and the ability to heal erosive esophagitis. This work concluded that if intragastric acidity could be maintained above pH 4 for 20–22 hours of the day, 90% of patients with erosive esophagitis would be healed by 8 weeks. Thus, the superiority of the PPIs over H_2RAs was predicted based on their pharmacological ability to effectively suppress acid secretion.

Can symptom improvement predict esophagitis improvement?

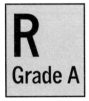

R Grade A

There is evidence that relief of symptoms by H_2RAs does not predict healing of mucosal damage. Patients with heartburn initially treated in a 4-week study with omeprazole or cimetidine,[114] were randomized to receive maintenance therapy with either omeprazole 10 mg od or cimetidine 800 mg qhs for 24 weeks.[115] Symptomatic remission, defined as no more than mild heartburn on 1 out of the 7 previous days was significantly more frequent with omeprazole (omeprazole 60%, cimetidine 24%, ARR 36%, NNT = 3). Erosive esophagitis was seen in only 10% of patients in symptomatic remission on omeprazole compared to 33% on cimetidine.

R Grade A

One-third of patients who relapsed by endoscopy during maintenance therapy with famotidine 40 mg bid were completely asymptomatic.[116]

A meta-analysis of relapse trials,[117] suggested that if heartburn resolved, only 4.5% of patients treated with omeprazole 20 mg od but 14.6% with ranitidine 150 g bid had asymptomatic relapse of endoscopic erosive esophagitis.

Symptomatic improvement on omeprazole may be a reliable indicator of healing of esophagitis, while damage may continue in spite of symptomatic improvement with H_2RAs as a consequence of lesser degree of acid suppression.

EROSIVE GERD: META-ANALYSIS OF HEALING AND SYMPTOM RELIEF WITH PPIS AND H_2RAs

Numerous high quality randomized trials have been performed and we have conducted a meta-analysis[118] of trials which included patients with more severe esophagitis (grade II in 61.8%, grade III in 31.7% and grade IV in 6.5%). A few studies have been published subsequently which support our original conclusions.[119–125]

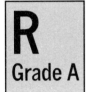

R Grade A

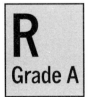

In this meta-analysis,[118] we demonstrated that the speed of healing, expressed as "% healed per week", was significantly superior with PPI therapy compared to H_2RA, particularly early in the course of treatment (weekly healing rate in first two weeks: PPI 32%, H_2RA 15%). The speed of healing slowed with increasing duration of treatment as fewer patients were still unhealed, but PPI remained superior to H_2RA. The overall healing proportions during 12 weeks, using pooled results irrespective of dose and duration were: PPI 84% (95% CI 79–88), H_2RA 52% (95% CI 47–57), sucralfate 39% (95% CI 4–75) and placebo 28% (95% CI 19–37). From these data we plotted rate of healing against time to create a "healing-time curve" (Figure 2.2). By the end of the second week, PPI had healed

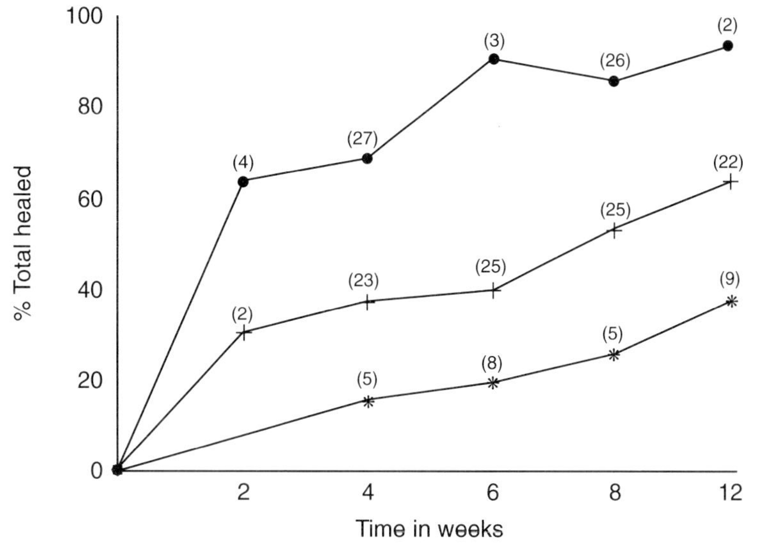

Figure 2.2 Healing-time curve expressed as the mean total healing for each drug class per evaluation time in weeks. By week 4, PPIs heal more patients than any other drug class, even after a much longer duration of treatment (12 weeks), implying a substantial therapeutic gain despite the fact that all drug classes achieve higher healing with longer durations of therapy. The number of studies is shown in parentheses. •, PPI; +, H_2RA, *, placebo. Reproduced with permission.[118]

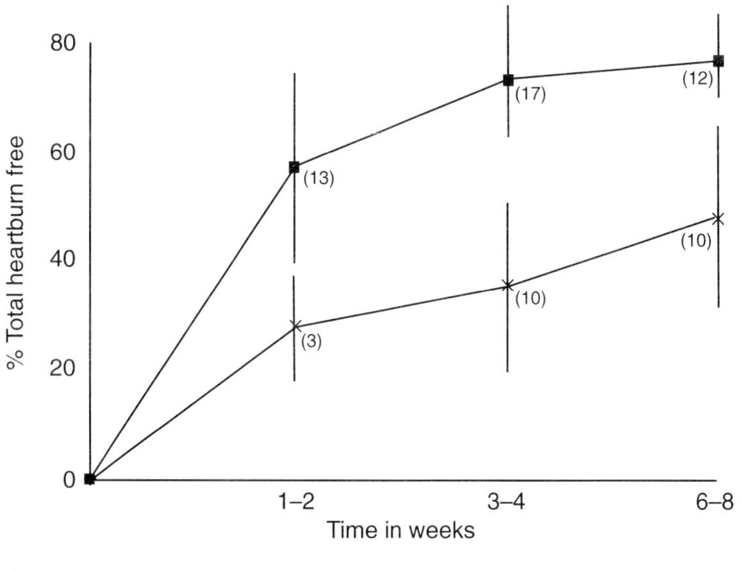

Figure 2.3 Symptom relief–time curve expressed as the mean total heartburn relief for each drug class corrected for patients free of heartburn at baseline at 1–2, 3–4, and 6–8 weeks. By week 2, more patients treated with PPIs are asymptomatic compared with H_2RA, even after a much longer duration of treatment (8 weeks), implying a substantial therapeutic gain despite the fact that both drug classes achieve greater symptom relief with longer durations of treatment. The number of studies is shown in parentheses. ■ ,PPI; ×, H_2RA. Reproduced with permission.[118]

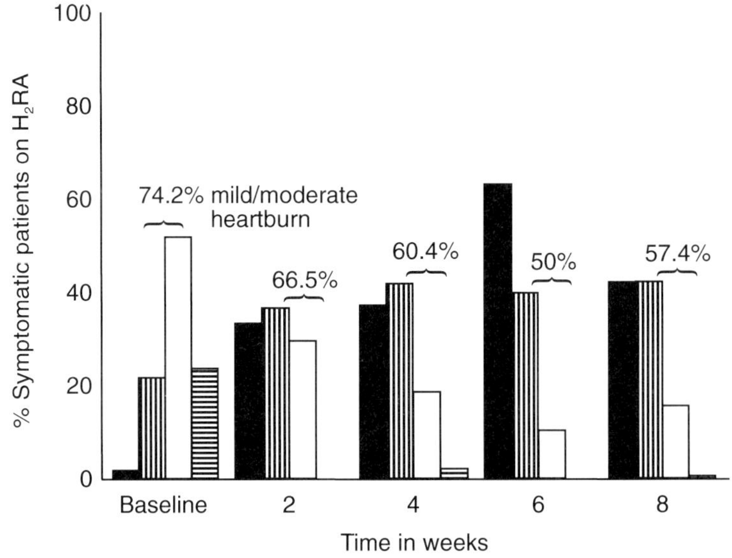

Figure 2.4 Shift in heartburn relief with H_2RAs. From studies using a symptom scale of none, mild, moderate, or severe, the shift in symptom severity with duration of treatment can be observed. With H_2RAs, although there is an increase in the number of patients completely heartburn free, at the end of the study, more than half of the patients still have mild to moderate symptoms. ■, None; ⊟, mild; □ ,moderate; ▥ ,severe. Reproduced with permission.[118]

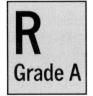

63.4 ± 6.6% of patients, while H_2RA required 12 weeks to achieve healing in a similar proportion (60.2 ± 5.9%). Linear regression analysis of individual study results showed that PPI heal with an overall rate of 11.7% per week (95% CI 10.7–12.6), twice as fast as H_2RA at 5.9% per week (95% CI 5.5–6.3) and four times faster compared to placebo (2.9, 95% CI 2.4–3.4).

R Grade A

Heartburn was present in all but 3.8% (95% CI 2.1–5.5) at baseline. Overall heartburn relief was seen in 77.4 ± 10.4% of patients treated with PPI and in 47.6 ± 15.5% treated with H_2RA. Data for heartburn relief were plotted against time to create a "symptom relief–time curve" (Figure 2.3). Linear regression analysis of the data showed an overall heartburn relief rate of 11.5% per week for PPI (95% CI 9.9–13.0) and 6.4% per week for H_2RA (95% CI 5.4–7.4).

Some studies measured heartburn in categories of none, mild, moderate, or severe, and reported the shift in heartburn relief with treatment (Figures 2.4 and 2.5). The proportion of patients with residual mild to moderate symptoms after 8 weeks of therapy was 11.1% for PPI and 57.4% for H_2RA.

This meta-analysis provides evidence that PPI are significantly better than H_2RA for both healing esophagitis and relieving symptoms in patients with moderately severe esophagitis. There is also RCT evidence for an effective role of PPI in healing persistent grade II–IV esophagitis after treatment failure with 12 weeks standard dose H_2RA.[126]

Randomized trials comparing two different PPIs (lansoprazole, omeprazole, pantoprazole, and rabeprazole) have failed to show a difference in healing rates with drugs used at their standard recommended doses.[121,123,127–132] There is some suggestion that lansoprazole provides better symptom relief than omeprazole early in treatment and this is consistent with their differences in pharmacology. However, symptom relief differences were no longer apparent at the end of the study.[121,128,129]

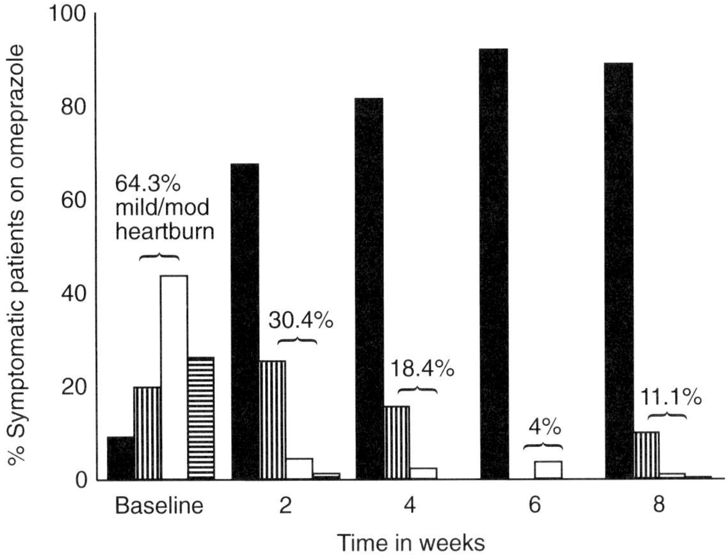

Figure 2.5 Shift in heartburn relief with PPIs. PPIs (omeprazole)-treated patients have a dramatic shift in the number of patients completely symptom free, particularly early in treatment, and at the end of the study, very few patients have any residual heartburn in contrast to patients treated with H_2RAs, ■, None; ⊟ mild; □, moderate; ◫, severe. Reproduced with permission.[118]

H_2-receptor antagonists (H_2RA)

INTERMITTENT/ON DEMAND THERAPY FOR MILD TO MODERATE SYMPTOMS

R Grade A

Acid suppressive therapy with H_2RA has been the mainstay of treatment for acid related disorders, and in many countries they are available for over-the-counter (OTC) use.[133] This permits intermittent, on demand use by the patient. A blinded crossover trial of famotidine 5, 10, and 20 mg versus placebo showed that all famotidine doses were more effective than placebo for the prevention of meal-induced heartburn and other dyspeptic symptoms.[134] This study established that heartburn severity peaked 1–2 hours after a meal. Thus, a small dose of H_2RA taken before eating may be useful to reduce symptoms induced by meals.

R Grade A

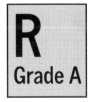

A unique formulation of a readily dissolving famotidine wafer (20 mg) was compared with a standard ranitidine 150 mg dose.[135] No difference in effect was demonstrated over 1–2 hours. A similar randomized trial in 377 patients, found a statistically significant, although clinically small, difference between ranitidine and famotidine for time to adequate symptom relief (ranitidine 15, famotidine 18.5 minutes, $P = 0.005$) and the proportion with symptom relief at 1 hour (ranitidine 92%, famotidine 84%, $P = 0.02$).[136] Thus for mild reflux symptoms, use of H_2RA on an as-needed basis is useful. However, in an open study reported in abstract form,[137] ranitidine effervescent tablets used on demand for one year in patients with grade I and II esophagitis revealed that the grade of esophagitis did not improve in spite of satisfaction with treatment by 84% of patients. Patients may be satisfied with their relief of symptoms, although damage to the esophagus continues.

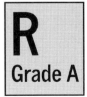

HIGH DOSE H_2RA

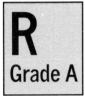

R Grade A

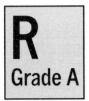

R Grade A

While standard doses of H_2RA heal more severe, grade II–IV esophagitis in about 52% of patients,[118] higher doses of H_2RA (150–300 mg qid) are more effective, healing 74–80% of patients in 12 weeks, under conditions in which the healing rate with placebo was 40–58%.[138,139] Silver *et al*[140] compared regimens of ranitidine 300 mg bid and 150 mg qid for treatment of erosive esophagitis. At 12 weeks, the healing proportion for the qid regimen was 77% and for the bid regimen, 66% (ARR 11%, NNT = 9). Ranitidine 150 mg qid was superior to standard dose ranitidine 150 mg bid or cimetidine 800 mg bid in patients with erosive esophagitis.[120] In another randomized trial in patients with erosive esophagitis,[141] healing with ranitidine 150 mg bid was 54% at 8 weeks compared to 75% with 300 mg qid (ARR 21%, NNT = 5). Famotidine is pharmacologically more potent than ranitidine and a large dose of 40 mg bid was superior to standard dose 20 mg bid or ranitidine150 mg bid in patients with erosive or worse esophagitis.[119]

PLACEBO HEALING RATES

Because healing of moderate to severe esophagitis with placebo therapy occurs in about 28% of patients,[118,142] the use of placebo controls has been important especially for the less effective drugs, such as H_2RA and prokinetics. For PPI, the therapeutic gain is so large that placebo controlled trials are less necessary.[118]

Prokinetic drugs

In a randomized, placebo controlled trial, metoclopramide and domperidone did not improve esophageal motility, duration of acid exposure or esophageal clearance, although both significantly increased lower esophageal sphincter (LES) pressure.[143] Cisapride is the only prokinetic drug that increases both esophageal clearance and enhances LES tone.[144–6] One study has reported that cisapride increased acid reflux in comparison to omeprazole and famotidine.[147]

R Grade A

R Grade A

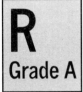

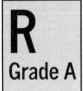

A randomized trial comparing cisapride 20 mg bid for 4 weeks with placebo in patients with reflux but no history of erosive esophagitis showed that cisapride significantly improved symptoms. The proportion of patients improved was not an end point, so the results cannot be compared with results of most conventional trials of PPI or H_2RA.[148] In patients with esophagitis, cisapride 10 mg qid for 12 weeks showed no significant benefit compared to placebo for global evaluation of symptoms, improvement in endoscopic esophagitis or for 24h acid exposure time.[146] Other studies confirmed that the cisapride 10 mg qid dosing was ineffective[149,150] and a larger dose of 20 mg qid for 12 weeks was required to obtain a small benefit over placebo for esophagitis healing (cisapride 51% placebo 36%, ARR 15%, NNT = 7, $P = 0.044$). Overall, placebo controlled trials show marginal benefit for cisapride in healing esophagitis.

For mild grades of esophagitis, cisapride is as effective as H_2RA for healing and symptom relief with comparable tolerability.[150–5] . Unfortunately, this drug requires prolonged use for up to 12 weeks before clinical benefit is seen.[149,150,152,154,156–8]

In one randomized trial in patients with milder GERD, omeprazole 10 or 20 mg daily was significantly more effective than cisapride 10 mg qid for relief of heartburn, regurgitation, and epigastric pain.[159] Quality of life improved in all treatment arms. This and other studies suggest that for symptomatic GERD, the degree of acid suppression is a more important determinant of symptom relief than prokinetic activity.

Combined prokinetic and acid suppression therapy

In healing grades I and II esophagitis, the addition of cisapride to omeprazole did not significantly increase efficacy over omeprazole alone.[160] In a randomized trial of moderate to severe esophagitis, ranitidine plus cisapride was more effective than ranitidine alone after 12 weeks' treatment (combination 82%, ranitidine 71%, ARR 11%, NNT = 9).[161] Thus, addition of cisapride to H_2RA, which does not suppress acid as effectively as PPI, produces only a modest enhancement of the response to H_2RA, while increasing costs substantially.

R Grade A

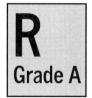

Cisapride as maintenance therapy

Randomized placebo controlled trials in milder forms of esophagitis showed that cisapride was effective as a maintenance therapy in preventing endoscopic and symptomatic recurrence.[158,160,162] However, in a study evaluating patients who had initially obtained relief with acid suppression, cisapride 20 mg at night or 20 mg bid was no more effective than placebo in delaying relapse.[163] Thus, stepping down to cisapride after healing with acid suppression has no proven value.

In Vigneri's study comparing five different maintenance therapies in patients with mild to moderate disease severity, cisapride and ranitidine were equally effective, but maintained remission in only about half the patients over 1 year.[164] Adding cisapride to ranitidine increased the proportion of patients maintained in remission (combined therapy 66%, ranitidine alone 49%, ARR 17%, NNT = 6). In contrast, omeprazole 20 mg daily was 80% effective (the number of patients needed to treat with omeprazole rather than ranitidine to maintain one additional patient in remission = 3). Adding cisapride to omeprazole did not significantly improve the remission rate. In patients with erosive esophagitis initially healed with antisecretory therapy, and in those with more severe baseline esophagitis, cisapride is not effective as maintenance treatment.[150,152,165,166]

R Grade A

R Grade A

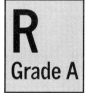

Cisapride has been associated with the development of serious cardiac arrhythmias including torsades de pointes, when used with other drugs that inhibit cytochrome P450 3A4. These include fluconazole, itraconazole, ketoconazole, erythromycin, clarithromycin, ritonavir, indinavir, nefazodone, tricyclic antidepressants, and certain tetracyclic antidepressants, certain antipsychotics, astemizole, terfenadine, and class 1A and III antiarrhythmics.[167] Although cisapride is as effective as H_2RA for milder forms of GERD, it is not recommended as first line therapy due to its greater potential for producing significant adverse events.

Sucralfate in GERD

For grade I–III GERD, there have been four small, randomized trials of sucralfate 1 g qid compared to standard dose H_2RA which did not show significant differences with respect to symptom resolution and healing.[168–71] However, none of these studies showed very large benefits with either medication. Heartburn relief ranged from 34 to 62% and healing from

31 to 64% of patients. Randomized trials of combined sucralfate and cimetidine have not shown statistically significant improvement compared to monotherapy with either drug, although only small numbers of patients were studied.[172,173]

Our meta-analysis of randomized trials of sucralfate for grade II–IV esophagitis yielded a pooled healing proportion of 39.2% compared to 28% for placebo.[118] Grade A However, the 95% CI was wide (3.6–74.8%).

In a 6 month study of grade I–II GERD, sucralfate was effective for preventing relapse compared to placebo (sucralfate 31%, placebo 65%, ARR 34, NNT = 3, P <0.001).[174] Grade A

It is interesting that sucralfate, which does not lower acid output, reduce esophageal acid exposure or improve esophageal transit time,[175] has any efficacy in this condition at all. The adverse effect of constipation, the need for four times daily dosing, and the modest treatment effect make sucralfate a less attractive choice than H_2RA or PPI.

TREATMENT OF GERD COMPLICATIONS

Esophageal peptic stricture, the most severe GERD complication, is difficult to manage. The H_2RA are marginally effective in reducing the need for repeat dilatations[176] compared to placebo.[177] There are two randomized trials comparing standard dose omeprazole 20 mg daily with H_2RA[178,179] and one with lansoprazole against high dose ranitidine.[180] Grade A

In one small study,[179] 34 patients with strictures were randomized to receive omeprazole 20 mg od, or ranitidine 150 mg or famotidine 20 mg bid. After 3 months, if esophagitis remained unhealed, the dose of medication was doubled and the patient was re-endoscoped at 6 months. At 3 months, there was no significant difference between PPI and H_2RA for esophagitis healing or relief of dysphagia, although there was a trend in favor of the PPI. By 6 months, omeprazole resulted in significantly better healing of esophagitis (omeprazole 100%, H_2RA 53%, ARR 47%, NNT = 2, P <0.01) and relief of dysphagia (omeprazole 94%, H_2RA 40%, ARR 54%, NNT = 2, P <0.01). Grade A Post hoc analysis also showed a trend to fewer dilatations required in omeprazole treated patients (omeprazole 41%, H_2RA 73%, P = 0.07). The number of dilatations required was significantly less for the omeprazole treated patients compared to the H_2RA arm (11 vs 31 dilatations, mean of 0.6 vs 2.1 sessions per patient, P <0.01). Cost-effectiveness analysis for healing and relief of dysphagia, which included costs of drugs, endoscopy, and dilatations, and of management of perforations, showed that omeprazole was 40–50% more cost-effective than H_2RA.

A further adequately powered study compared constant doses of omeprazole 20 mg od and ranitidine 150 mg bid for 1 year.[178] Endoscopy was done as required and at the end of the study. Repeat dilatation was required less frequently in omeprazole treated patients (omeprazole 30%, ranitidine 46%, ARR 16%, NNT = 6). Grade A Fewer dilatation sessions were required in omeprazole treated patients (omeprazole 0.48, ranitidine 1.08, P <0.01). Omeprazole was also superior with respect to the number of patients without stricture at end of study, esophagitis healing, and improved heartburn and dysphagia.

In a study of 158 patients over 6 months, lansoprazole 30 mg daily was more effective than ranitidine 300 mg bid for relieving dysphagia. Grade A There was a trend toward a reduction in the need for repeat dilatations (lansoprazole 30.8%, ranitidine 43.8%, P = 0.09) over 12 months.[180]

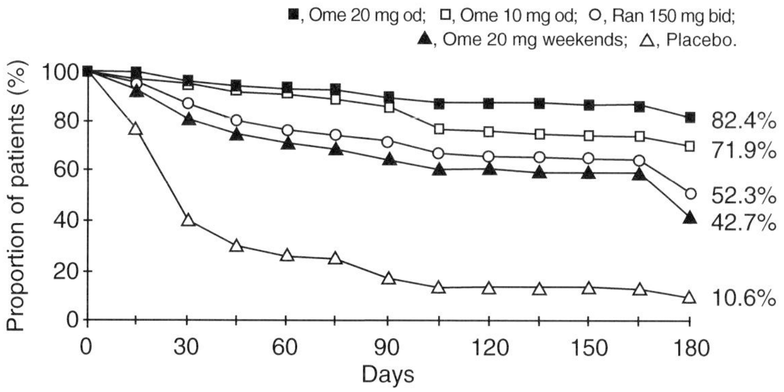

Figure 2.6 Actuarial life-table analysis. Estimated proportion of patients in endoscopic remission at the end of the 6 month follow-up period with maintenance treatment. Reproduced with permission.[98]

Thirty of 36 patients with reflux esophagitis and stricture treated openly with dilatation and omeprazole 20 mg bid for 6–8 weeks experienced healing of esophagitis and relief of dysphagia.[181] These patients were then randomized to receive omeprazole 20 mg bid, lansoprazole 30 mg bid or pantoprazole 40 mg bid (n = 10 each arm). After 4 weeks of treatment, significantly more omeprazole treated patients remained healed, but no difference was seen for the need to redilate strictures. Whether there is any true difference between the PPI is controversial because of the very limited sample size in this study.

MAINTENANCE THERAPY

For mild GERD, as seen at a community level, 46% of patients can spontaneously heal.[15] For moderately severe GERD, healing and symptom relief are readily obtained with PPI, but, within 6–12 months, irrespective of the initial healing agent, recurrences are reported in 36–82% of patients in the absence of maintenance therapy.[182–4]

After acute healing or stopping maintenance therapy, symptoms recur within a day, and erosive esophagitis can recur in most patients within 10 days[185] to 1 month.[186] Thus, maintenance therapy is required in most patients with GERD.

A meta-analysis of five omeprazole trials with 1154 patients (erosive GERD initially healed by omeprazole 20–40 mg) that have studied relapse of erosive esophagitis was reported by Carlsson *et al.*[117] Figure 2.6 shows the effects of various regimens. Omeprazole 20 mg daily which maintained 82.4% of patients in remission for 6 months was significantly better than omeprazole 10 mg daily (P = 0.04). Both of these regimens were significantly better than ranitidine 150 mg bid and omeprazole 20 mg on weekends. Thus, omeprazole should be given continuously and dosing intermittently for only 3 days per week is not adequate. Two trials assessed maintenance over 12 months. Omeprazole 20 mg daily was superior to ranitidine 150 mg bid (omeprazole 80.2%, ranitidine 39.4%, ARR 40.8%, NNT = 2). The proportions of patients with asymptomatic endoscopic esophagitis relapse were: omeprazole 20 mg 4.5%, omeprazole 10 mg 12.5%, and rantitidine 14.6%. Regression analysis identifed four risk factors for recurrence: pre-treatment severity of esophagitis, younger age, non-smoking status, and moderate to severe reflux pre-entry.

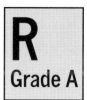

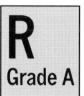

R Grade A

R Grade A

Table 2.5 RCTs of maintenance therapy in grade II–IV GERD

Study	Duration of treatment (months)	Treatment regimens	% relapse (no. relapsed/no. treated)
Simon, 1995[191]	6	F 40 mg bid	11 (8/72)
		F 20 mg bid	22 (15/69)
		Pla	61 (19/31)
Sontag, 1997[194]	6	O 20 mg od	30 (41/138)
		O 20 mg od, 3d/wk	66 (90/137)
		Pla	89 (116/131)
[a]Bardhan, 1998,[192]	6	O 10mg od	22 (28/130)
		Pla	57 (76/133)
Lundell, 1991[188]	12	O 20 mg od	32 (11/34)
		R 300 mg bid	88 (14/16)
Dent, 1994[195]	12	O 20 mg od	12 (5/43)
		O 20 mg od, 3d/wk	71 (34/48)
		R 150 mg bid	79 (38/48)
Hallerback, 1994[196]	12	O 20 mg od	28 (37/131)
		O 10 mg od	38 (51/133)
		R 150 mg bid	55 (70/128)
Bate, 1995[197]	12	O 20 mg od	32 (22/68)
		O 10 mg od	50 (30/60)
		Pla	90 (56/62)
Vigneri, 1995[164]	12	O 20 mg od	20 (7/35)
		R 150 mg tid	51 (18/35)
		C 10 mg tid	46 (16/35)
		R + C	34 (12/35)
		O + C	11 (4/35)
Gough, 1996[189]	12	L 30 mg od	20 (15/75)
		L 15 mg od	31 (27/86)
		R 300 mg bid	68 (50/74)
Robinson, 1996[193]	12	L 30 mg od	11 (6/56)
		L 15 mg od	22 (13/59)
		Pla	76 (42/55)
Sontag, 1996[186]	12	L 30 mg od	45 (22/49)
		L 15 mg od	34 (17/50)
		Pla	87 (41/47)
[b]Hatlebakk, 1997[198]	12	L 30 mg od	18 (4/22)
		L 15 mg od	44 (8/18)
[a]Bardhan, 1998[192]	12	O 10 mg od	38 (49/130)
		Pla	78 (104/133)
Carling, 1998[190]	12	O 20 mg od	9 (11/122)
		L 30 mg od	10 (12/126)

[a]Bardhan's study is the only one with 6 and 12 month relapse data.
[b]Data given for patients who had initial grade II esophagitis.
F, famotidine; Pla, placebo; O, omeprazole; R, ranitidine; C, cisapride; L, lansoprazole.

A previous systematic overview of continuous maintenance therapy in patients with initial grades II–IV esophagitis was updated for this chapter including only data from fully published papers.[187] The details of the studies are recorded in Table 2.5. For this review,

Table 2.6 Summary of pooled one-year GERD relapse

Drug regimen	No. trials	No. patients	1 yr relapse %	95% CI
Lansoprazole 30 mg od	5	328	18	14–22
Omeprazole 20 mg od	6	433	21	18–26
Lansoprazole 15 mg od	4	213	31	24–37
Omeprazole 10 mg od	3	323	40	35–46
H_2RA all doses	5	301	63	58–69
Placebo	3	295	72 (6 mth)	66–77
Placebo	4	297	82	77–86

patients in remission/relapse were derived from the numbers given or estimated from the all-evaluable patients life-table analysis. The pooled 1 year recurrence rates are shown in Table 2.6.

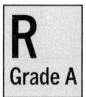

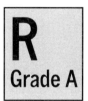

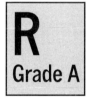

R Grade A

Most of the data were for relapse over 1 year. The therapy with the greatest degree of acid suppression consistently was most effective (Table 2.5). This held true even when high doses of H_2RA were used.[164,188,189] A small dose of lansoprazole (15 mg) daily was superior to a high dose of ranitidine (300 mg bid).[189] The best maintenance therapy was continuous omeprazole or lansoprazole at standard doses of 20 mg and 30 mg daily respectively, which maintained remission in approximately 80% of patients (Table 2.6). One trial directly compared lansoprazole 30 mg and omeprazole 20 mg od and found the same healing and symptom relief.[190] Smaller and intermittent doses of PPI were less effective (Table 2.6). The H_2RA are marginally superior to placebo when considering pooled data and data from the one trial in which a direct comparison of H_2RA (famotidine 20 mg or 40 mg bid) with placebo was made.[191]

R Grade A

Bardhan *et al*[192] treated patients with erosive esophagitis with omeprazole to produce healing and then randomized them to receive omeprazole 10 mg daily or a placebo. The small dose of omeprazole was effective for maintenance of remission for 18 months in 60% of patients. Symptomatic failures were well controlled on omeprazole 20 mg daily with relapse in only 9% of patients over 2 years. Scheduled endoscopy detected erosive changes in asymptomatic patients, accounting for a quarter of the relapses. A full dose of PPI is probably necessary to maintain better quality endoscopic and symptomatic remission.

R Grade A

The problem of healing the more severe grades of esophagitis is well known. The proportion of patients who experience acute healing for grade II esophagitis ranges from 76 to 100%, for grade III from 63 to 95%, and for grade IV from 56 to 75%.[187] Grade IV disease relapses more frequently than grade II and III disease.[186,193] In clinical practice, it is suggested that the dose of PPI can be titrated upwards to maintain healing in most patients.[194]

R Grade A/C

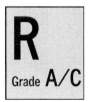

Cohort studies of long term therapy

The controlled trials show that most patients are maintained in remission for 1 year. However, 20% of patients still relapse. Klinkenberg-Knol *et al*[199] have followed a cohort of GERD patients for many years and reported that doubling the dose of omeprazole

R
Grade B

to 40 mg daily was effective to treat relapses. The long term omeprazole study has followed patients for up to 11 years on continuous therapy.[200] Of the 230 patients followed, one-third each had grade II, III, and IV disease. It was estimated that there was only one relapse for every 9 years of treatment, the median maintenance dose was 20 mg daily, and dose titration (range 20 mg q2d to 120 mg od) allowed most patients to remain in remission.

Cost-effectiveness of maintenance therapy

From the foregoing, it is clear that, overall, PPIs are the most effective treatments available to treat GERD, However, PPI are also more costly than H_2RA. Therefore cost-effectiveness analysis becomes important to assist in decision making. There are two well performed reviews of cost effectiveness in GERD.[201,202] Studies differ substantially with respect to methods, assumptions, interventions and outcomes being evaluated, the inclusiveness of cost items, and the jurisdiction to which the analyses are applied. No perfect cost-effectiveness study exists and new advances in therapy and changes in cost over time tend to render them out of date rather quickly.

However, despite these limitations, cost-effectiveness modeling studies are useful to put into perspective the role of existing interventions.

Many studies indicate that PPI are more cost-effective than H_2RA.[203–210] Cost-effectiveness data from Canada,[211] Sweden[212] and the US[213,214] arrived at similar conclusions. Maintenance PPI over a 1-year period is consistently the most effective but also the most costly intervention.[211–14] The Canadian study showed that intermittent omeprazole to treat symptomatic relapse was more cost-effective than continuous omeprazole therapy, although there was an increase in the number of symptomatic weeks per year. Maintenance ranitidine and cisapride therapy were least effective for controlling symptoms, but were of intermediate cost.

High dose H_2RA was more costly and less effective than PPI, with more frequent relapses that ultimately led to PPI maintenance therapy.[213] Harris *et al*[213] reported that treatment with continuous PPI becomes more cost-effective than H_2RA if patients with active symptoms of GERD experience a 9% decrement in QOL. When considering three different PPI maintenance strategies, starting continuous PPI after the second recurrence was least costly and least effective.[214] Continuous PPI started after the first recurrence added only a small increment of cost per recurrence prevented, compared to continuous PPI from the outset, which was10 times more costly.[214] However, for patients with a 22% decrement in QOL, continuous therapy became cost-effective when compared to maintenance after first relapse. All these strategies are modeled for only 1 year and may not be generalizable to life-long treatment.

A retrospective review of the UK MediPlus database (captures diagnostic procedures, prescribing patterns, specialist referrals, and other health care interventions) identified health care resources consumed by patients in their first six months of treatment.[215] A "step up" approach in which patients are initially treated with cisapride or an H_2RA represented a more cost-effective approach than the use of PPI for all patients. This analysis was retrospective, and hence the initial diagnosis of GERD and the determination whether the first episode was detected are uncertain. Reasons for use of a given medication can only be surmised. However, this project was an attempt to capture costs in the "real world" as opposed to the context of a clinical trial.

EFFECTS OF GERD ON QUALITY OF LIFE

Increased attention is being paid to quality of life (QOL) assessments as opposed to pathology of the esophagus. Several general health status and disease specific QOL instruments have been developed, validated, and used. They include: Medical Outcomes Study SF-36,[216] Psychological General Well Being (PGWB) index,[217] the Gastrointestinal Symptom Rating Scale (GSRS),[218–220] and the Quality of Life Reflux and Dyspepsia (QOLRAD) scale.[221]

Patients with gastrointestinal disorders have decreased functional status and well being.[222] Those with chronic gastrointestinal disorders and congestive heart failure have the poorest health perceptions, worse than for some other chronic conditions such as hypertension and arthritis.[218,222,223]

Studies have shown that successful treatment of GERD is associated with improvements in QOL.[224] Patients with severe reflux esophagitis have more impairment of QOL than those with endoscopy negative disease (ENRD), but QOL is significantly reduced in both groups of patients.[224] ENRD patients do not necessarily have objective markers such as endoscopic esophagitis or abnormal esophageal 24h pH-metry results that can be used to define treatment success. Symptom reduction to a level that does not cause significant impairment of health related QOL is essential. Both the PGWB and GSRS scores show good discriminative ability to reflect the severity of impairments in QOL in ENRD patients.[225] Improvements in health related QOL with treatment of ENRD and of erosive esophagitis have also been documented.[226,227]

TREATMENT OF ENDOSCOPY NEGATIVE REFLUX DISEASE

Endoscopy negative reflux disease (ENRD), as described in the diagnosis section, is present in patients without endoscopic findings who may have an abnormal 24h esophageal pH-metry result in 21–63%.[74,83] Others may have a positive Bernstein test, or a positive symptom index and improvement with acid suppressive therapy. These are patients with an acid sensitive esophagus.

A randomized trial compared omeprazole in doses of 20 or 10 mg daily and placebo in 509 patients with ENRD and heartburn as the predominant complaint.[219] Symptomatic remission of heartburn (no more than one day of mild symptoms in the week prior to the final visit) was significantly more frequent in 2–4 weeks with omeprazole in either dose, and the higher dose of omeprazole was more effective than the lower dose (Table 2.7). Symptom relief occurred in most patients by the end of the second week. With 4 weeks of treatment the proportion of patients indicating sufficient control of heartburn was 66% and 57% for the high and low doses of omeprazole respectively and only 31% for the placebo group. The more abnormal the initial pH study, the better the response to a greater degree of acid suppression. There was a significant correlation with acid reflux, age, and the presence of a hiatus hernia. No correlation was identified between body mass index and degree of acid exposure despite the widely held view that being overweight worsens reflux.

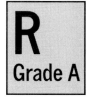

R
Grade A

Treatment of erosive esophagitis and ENRD

In a randomized trial in 221 patients[114] with heartburn as the predominant symptom (about half of whom had ENRD and half grade II or III esophagitis), omeprazole 20 mg

Table 2.7 RCTs of endoscopy negative reflux disease (ENRD) ± erosive esophagitis (non-primary care)

Study	Baseline characteristics	Treatments (no. patients)	Symptom relief	Comments/other findings
Lind, 1997,[219]	Heartburn predominant, ENRD only	OM 20 mg od (205) OM 10 mg od (199) Placebo (105) For 2–4 weeks	61% 49.3% 23.8% Symptomatic remission	63% had abnormal 24h pH study Omeprazole 20 mg more effective with worse rcflux 85% HB resolved if continued 20 mg daily for another 4 weeks Acid reflux correlated with presence of hiatus hernia
Bate ,1997[114]	Heartburn predominant, acute treatment, ENRD 46.6%, erosive GERD 53.4%	OM 20 mg od (112) CIM 400 mg qid (109) For 4 weeks	66% 31% Symptomatic remission	No correlation between HB severity and grade of esophagitis ENRD 51% Erosive GERD 59% Relief, P= NS
Bate, 1998[115]	Heartburn predominant, maintenance treatment of above study	OM 10 mg od (77) CIM 800 mg nocte (79) For 24 wk	60% 24% Maintained symptomatic remission	Complete relief of all symptoms 45% OM and 15% CIM, P= 0.0001 Median time to relapse 169 days for OM and 15 days for CIM, P= 0.0001 If in symptomatic remission: OM patients 10% EE, CIM 33% EE

Symptomatic remission = no more than 1 day of mild heartburn in the last 7 days.
HB, heartburn; OM, omeprazole; CIM, cimetidine; EE, erosive esophagitis.

daily produced significantly better heartburn relief than cimetidine 400 mg qid (Table 2.7). The entry grade of esophagitis did not correlate with heartburn severity and treatment benefit did not depend on presence or absence of esophagitis. Patients who were still symptomatic after the initial phase were treated with 4 weeks of omeprazole 20 mg daily and a further 67% (54/81) improved.

R
Grade A

Patients who improved in the acute study were randomized to receive maintenance therapy with omeprazole 10 mg daily or cimetidine 800 mg nocte for 6 months (Table 2.7).[115] Omeprazole maintained control of heartburn in more patients at both 3 months (omeprazole 69%, cimetidine 27%) and 6 months (omeprazole 60%, cimetidine 24%, ARR 36%, NNT = 3, P <0.0001). Seventy six percent of omeprazole treated patients compared to 46% of the cimetidine group were also free of regurgitation (P = 0.0002).

In another trial, 209 patients with mild grade I disease were randomized to receive a low dose of pantoprazole 20 mg daily or ranitidine 300 mg daily.[228] Pantoprazole was significantly more effective than ranitidine for symptom relief at 2 (pantoprazole 69%, ranitidine 48%, ARR 21%, NNT = 5, P <0.01) and 4 weeks (pantoprazole 80%, ranitidine 65%, ARR 15%, NNT = 7, P <0.05). Healing occurred significantly more frequently with pantoprazole than with ranitidine at 4 weeks (80% vs 64%, P <0.05) and 8 weeks (90% vs 73%, P <0.01). Thus, even a low dose of PPI is superior to H_2RA for symptom relief and healing of mild esophagitis.

R Grade A

STUDIES OF SYMPTOMATIC GERD IN FAMILY PRACTICE

Symptomatic GERD: empiric therapy

R Grade A

A randomized, 4 week trial involving 424 patients with a history of proven esophagitis enrolled from general practices in the UK[229] showed that omeprazole 20 mg od was more effective for relief of heartburn and regurgitation than ranitidine 150 mg bid (omeprazole 59%, ranitidine 27%, ARR 22%, NNT = 5) (Table 2.8). The prior history of esophagitis somewhat limits generalizability of this study to all patients in primary care practices, but the good relief of symptoms regardless of initial symptom severity is noteworthy.

R Grade A

In an American family practice study (Table 2.8), 590 patients with moderately severe symptomatic GERD were randomized without endoscopy to receive ranitidine 150 mg bid or a placebo.[230] Ranitidine rapidly and significantly improved heartburn severity scores, physician global assessment of the response to treatment, and the SF-36 score for physical functioning, bodily pain, and vitality dimensions. Using a heartburn specific questionnaire, a significant improvement in all dimensions – physical, heartburn pain, sleep, diet, social functioning, and mental health – was observed for ranitidine treated patients.

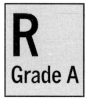

Symptomatic GERD: endoscopy positive and negative disease

The third large randomized trial in general practice was conducted by Venables *et al* in the UK in 994 patients with the predominant symptom of heartburn, which was at least moderate to severe in 70% of patients.[35] In contrast to the American study discussed above,[230] patients were all endoscoped and the grade of esophagitis established permitting symptom relief and mucosal healing assessments. Patients with ulcerative esophagitis were excluded. The majority of patients (68.2%) had ENRD. Patients were randomized to 4 weeks of omeprazole 10 or 20 mg od or ranitidine 150 mg bid. Overall relief of heartburn was defined as no more than 1 day of mild heartburn out of the preceding 7 days prior to the visit. Omeprazole 20 mg was the most effective therapy and the 10 mg omeprazole dose was also more effective than ranitidine (omeprazole 20 mg 61%, omeprazole 10 mg 49%, ranitidine 150 mg bid 40%, P <0.01). The NNT for the higher dose of omeprazole is approximately 9 when compared to the lower dose and 5 when compared to ranitidine. In the stratum of patients with erosive esophagitis, the comparable values for NNT are approximately 3 and 2. This study is generalizable to patients in primary care practices with either ENRD or esophagitis. It establishes omeprazole 20 mg daily as the most effective therapy for esophagitis healing and overall symptom relief.

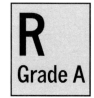

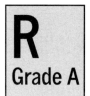

R Grade A

R Grade A

After the healing phase of this study, 495 patients with initial non-erosive GERD were randomized to receive omeprazole 10 mg or a placebo for 6 months.[231] Placebo treated patients were nearly twice as likely to discontinue treatment before the end of 6 months. Life-table estimates for cumulative remission at 6 months were 73% for omeprazole and 48% for placebo (ARR 25%, NNT = 4, P = 0.0001) (Table 2.8). QOL assessments showed a more significant deterioration in the GSRS reflux domain for placebo patients (P <0.05), but no significant differences were noted in PGWB. Thus, a continuous dose of omeprazole

Table 2.8 General practice (primary care) RCTs of GERD treatment

Study	Baseline characteristics	Treatments (no. patients)	Symptom relief	Comments/other findings
Continuous therapy				
Hungin, 1993[229]	Proven past history of reflux esophagitis, empiric tx	OM 20 mg od (215) RAN 150 mg bid (209) For 4 wk	OM 59% vs RAN 27% for heartburn OM 44% vs RAN 20% completely symptom free	If severe HB: OM 55% vs 11% RAN relief
Rush, 1995[230]	Symptomatic GERD, not scoped, empiric tx	RAN 150 mg bid (301) Placebo (289) For 6 wk	Overall symptom relief proportion not given	RAN significantly reduced HB pain scores and mean number of HB episodes within 48h RAN improved QOL scores
Venables, 1997[35]	Heartburn predominant, acute study, both ENRD (68.2%) and erosive esophagitis	OM 20 mg od (330) OM 10 mg od (338) RAN 150 mg bid (326) For 4 wk	61% 49% 40% Symptomatic remission	Severity of baseline heartburn correlated poorly with esophagitis grade Shift in HB severity from mod/severe to none/mild greatest with OM 20 mg
Venables, 1997[231]	Heartburn predominant, maintenance of above study with only ENRD	OM 10 mg od (242) Placebo (253) For 24 wk	73% 48% Maintained remission	6 mth maintenance with OM 10 mg od superior to placebo
Carlsson, 1998[232]	Carlsson–Dent questionnaire positive for GERD, 48.5% ENRD	ENRD patients OM 20 mg od (87) OM 10 mg od (86) Placebo (88) For 4 wk	Complete control/ sufficient control 29/60% 31/49% 19/35%	More endoscopy positive patients had HB at baseline and responded better to treatment than ENRD GSRS improved after treatment
		Erosive GERD OM 20 mg od (138) OM 10 mg od (139)	48/81% 37/70%	
Intermittent therapy				
Bardhan, 1997[233]	Heartburn predominant, both ENRD (31.3%) and esophagitis	RAN 150 mg bid (229) OM 10 mg od (227) OM 20 mg od (221) For 2 wk	26% 40% 55%	After initial relief, followed in maintenance phase with intermittent therapy (IT) for relapse IT unacceptable as strategy in only 9%

Symptomatic remission = no more than 1 day of mild heartburn in the last 7 days.
tx, treament; HB, heartburn; OM, omeprazole; RAN, ranitidine; EE, erosive esophagitis.

10 mg daily is effective maintenance therapy for the majority of patients with heartburn but no esophagitis (ENRD). However, a larger dose of omeprazole may be required for up to a quarter of patients.

R Grade A

The fourth study in primary care patients screened dyspeptic patients with the Carlsson–Dent questionnaire,[41] and those with a score suggestive of GERD were included in this study after initial endoscopy.[232] ENRD patients (48.5%) were randomized to placebo, omeprazole 10 mg or 20 mg od for 4 weeks. Patients with erosive esophagitis (51.5%) were randomized to omeprazole 10 mg or 20 mg od for 4 weeks (Table 2.8). Baseline heartburn was present in 83.5% of ENRD patients and in 95% of patients with erosive GERD. The benefit of treatment was greater in endoscopy positive than in endoscopy negative patients for all treatment arms. After the initial treatment phase, patients were followed for 6 months without therapy. Relapse rates were high (esophagitis 90%, ENRD 75 %) These results suggest that ENRD patients were more heterogeneous than those with endoscopically documented disease.

Patient QOL was evaluated in this study. Baseline PGWB scores were reduced in all patients prior to treatment and improved to a similar extent in all treatment arms. The GSRS reflux dimension improved significantly ($P < 0.01$) in ENRD patients after treatment with omeprazole and, in those with erosive disease, omeprazole 20 mg was superior to 10 mg.

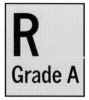

INTERMITTENT THERAPY AS A STRATEGY FOR LONG TERM MANAGEMENT OF MILD/MODERATE GERD

R Grade A

A group of 677 adults with moderate to severe heartburn (primary care practices, 31.3% ENRD, 68.7% mild to moderate esophagitis) were randomized to receive ranitidine 150 bid, or omeprazole 10 mg or 20 mg daily for 2 weeks (Table 2.8).[227,233] The proportion of patients completely free of heartburn at 2 weeks was higher in the omeprazole groups (ranitidine 26%, omeprazole 10 mg 40%, omeprazole 20 mg 55%). Patients on ranitidine or 10 mg omeprazole who remained symptomatic received double doses of their medications for a further 2 weeks, while those on 20 mg of omeprazole continued at this dose. At the end of 4 weeks, 74% of patients on ranitidine, and 82% in both omeprazole arms, had either mild or no symptoms. After the acute phase, patients were followed up for 12 months. During this period, a recurrence of symptoms was treated with the previously effective regimen for 2–4 weeks. This strategy was effective for most patients. These patients did not need drug treatment for about 7 months on average. Overall, symptoms were not adequately controlled in 22% of the patients, and the strategy of intermittent therapy for relapses was unacceptable for 9% of patients, who were then offered open label omeprazole (20 mg daily).

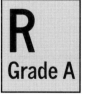

At baseline, PGWB scores of about 95 indicated impaired QOL compared to normal population values of 103.[227] Baseline GSRS scores indicated patient perception of their symptoms as being of moderate severity. With 4 weeks of treatment, PGWB scores had improved to a normal value of about 106, and the reflux dimension of GSRS scores also improved. In the follow-up period, relapses were accompanied by a fall in QOL to baseline levels, and with treatment, scores again improved. No differences in QOL scores were seen between patients with erosive esophagitis and ENRD at baseline, in response to therapy, at relapse or with subsequent treatment. This study provides important documentation that patients with ENRD, who are generally considered to have milder disease, are as impaired as those with erosive disease with respect to quality of life.

A prospective cost-effectiveness analysis of this study[234] indicated that the patients started on omeprazole 20 mg od had more symptom free days and days without medication compared to ranitidine and omeprazole tended to be the more cost-effective drug, although no statistically significant difference was demonstrated ($P = 0.1$).

SURGERY

Problems in interpreting surgical studies include the fact that outcomes are operator dependent and there may be a publication bias towards good results. The first factor is particularly evident for laparoscopic fundoplication, which has a well defined learning curve.[235,236] It is impossible to blind interventions and ideally, outcomes should be measured with the patient and the assessor unaware of the exact type of surgery performed. Most publications are observational case series or retrospective comparisons of old versus new techniques in single practices.[236,237] There is a dearth of randomized trials.

Comparison of laparoscopic and open fundoplication

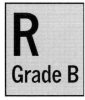

R Grade B

Retrospective comparisons of case series of open fundoplication with more recent laparoscopic fundoplication data have found similar outcomes.[236,237] Mean operating time and an intraoperative complication rate of 8% was the same in both groups.[236] Symptomatic improvement appears comparable, but the overall outcome depends on how symptoms are assessed. For example, patients may become completely asymptomatic only 40% of the time, but if success is measured as improvement, or patient satisfaction, or whether they would agree to have surgery again, 80–90% respond affirmatively.[237,238] Patients have greater satisfaction and symptom improvement 3 months after surgery, than they do at 1 month.[235,236]

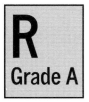

R Grade A

One randomized trial of open vs laparoscopic fundoplication[239] studied 110 patients, of whom five of 55 patients had to be converted to an open laparotomy. Of these, two were due to esophageal perforation (3.6%) and did not result in mortality. No difference in symptom relief was demonstrated between the two approaches and by 12 months, early symptoms of dysphagia and gas bloating had disappeared. All patients undergoing the laparoscopic surgery and 86% of the open group were satisfied with their results. This study supports the observational study results, which suggested that the laparoscopic approach produces results which are at least as good as the traditional approach.

R Grade A

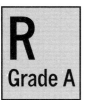

The major advantage for laparoscopic fundoplication is a significant reduction in hospital stay from 8–9 days for an open procedure to 2–5 days.[235,237,240] In a prospective case series of 61 patients the laparoscopic approach resulted in less time off work for the patient (laparoscopic 21.3 days, open surgery 38.2 days, $P = 0.02$).[235] Analysis of the short term direct and indirect costs, found that laparoscopic fundoplication was significantly less expensive than the open procedure.[235] QOL assessed by the PGWB instrument, normalized after both types of surgery. However, the GSRS showed some differences, with the laparoscopic group experiencing more indigestion and dyspeptic symptoms.[241] Validated instruments are recommended in the assessement of patients after surgery.

However, laparoscopic fundoplication is not without potential serious complications such as esophageal perforation, paraesopheageal herniations, pneumothorax, and splenic damage requiring splenectomy.[242] Postoperative dysphagia is often considered a complication of this type of surgery and may be more frequent with complete (Nissen) fundoplication.[243] However, one study reported that dysphagia improved in the majority of patients and only a small number reported worsening of dysphagia after surgery.[244]

Esophageal perforation is reported in as many as 2.2% of cases.[238] The laparoscopic approach may have fewer wound complications than open surgery.[236]

R Grade B

These data support the laparoscopic approach as the preferred method over open surgery. However, data on long term outcomes following laparoscopic surgery are lacking. One small follow-up study of open surgery patients after 20 years demonstrated that about 30% of the fundoplications were defective, and abnormal reflux on esophageal pH studies was also seen in about 30% of patients assessed.[245] Another study of 441 patients after a mean follow-up of 18 years following the Hill procedure for GERD, identified good and excellent subjective results in over 80% of patients.[246] Thus, it may be possible to attain durable results which are partly surgeon dependent.

The best laparoscopic procedure is still controversial. Two randomized trials have compared a partial (Toupet) versus a complete (Rosetti–Nissen) fundoplication.[243] The complete "wrap" results in higher LES pressures and this is also associated with more symptoms of dysphagia and gas-bloat.[243] The partial Toupet procedure may be associated with fewer short term adverse effects, but it is not known if the antireflux benefit is longlasting. The Toupet procedure was preferred in one study[243] and deemed to have no advantage in another.[247] In a series of 100 patients treated with a Toupet procedure, a 24h esophageal pH study at 22 months demonstrated abnormal reflux in 51% of patients, and nearly 60% of these patients were asymptomatic.[248] Although the Toupet procedure may be preferred for patients with impaired esophageal motility it is not recommended for other patients because it appears to be less effective for control of reflux.[248] The laparoscopic Nissen procedure has a reoperation rate of 1–7%, primarily due to mechanical complications.[249] The selection of the appropriate operation for the individual patient depends in part on the preoperative evaluation as well as on the intraoperative findings and associated technical limitations. There is no reason to refuse laparoscopic fundoplication for patients over the age of 65 years (range 65–79).[250]

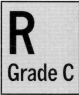

R Grade C

Medical vs surgical therapy

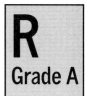

R Grade A

There are two prospective, randomized trials comparing antireflux surgery with medical therapy which have provided evidence that surgery is more effective.[251,252] Unfortunately, these studies are no longer relevant, since they do not take into account present day optimal medical therapy with proton pump inhibitors and laparoscopic surgery.

R Grade A

Three hundred and ten patients were randomized to receive open surgical fundoplication or continuous omeprazole therapy[253] and followed for 3 years. Only 11 of 155 patients randomized to surgery refused the treatment. Omeprazole treated patients were allowed dose increases to 40–60 mg daily to control symptoms. No significant differences in outcomes were demonstrated, and about 75% of patients remained free of treatment failure over 3 years. Quality of life assessments (PGWB and GSRS) improved in both groups. Thus, surgical therapy was as effective as continuous omeprazole therapy in this trial. The only weakness of this study is that laparoscopic fundoplication was not performed, and the results are available thus far in abstract form only.

Cost-effectiveness of medical vs surgical therapy

A Finnish study modeled the costs of antireflux surgery and medical therapy for GERD and concluded that the cost of surgery is about half that of lifelong daily acid suppressive therapy.[254] This study considered the financial loss due to fatal income with surgery. Thus, when projecting the costs over a lifetime, surgery may be more cost-effective, although this depends on a variety of assumptions and the country for which calculations are made.

An evaluation in the Netherlands of omeprazole and Nissen fundoplication concluded that the surgical approach is more cost-effective after 4 years.[255] If the surgery is laparoscopic fundoplication, the authors concluded that the breakeven point occurs at 1.4 years. However, the assumptions used in the analysis create limitations. The cost of medical therapy was "inflated" by repeated endoscopies for treatment failures, which are not always necessary. The maintenance of healing of esophagitis was the only outcome measure, and clinically important outcomes such as symptom relief and QOL assessments were not considered. Only direct medical costs were considered and costs due to surgical complications were not included.

Since laparoscopic surgery has become more widely available, there has been a renewed interest in surgery for GERD. Although patients may be well controlled on PPI, some patients are choosing laparoscopic surgery as an alternative to long term medical therapy.[244] With the relative ease and safety of laparoscopic surgery, it has become a reasonable alternative for selected patients. As with all surgery, patient selection has improved through objective testing with preoperative esophageal pH-metry and manometry. Even if cost-effectiveness modeling studies favor surgery, a decision to have surgery cannot be imposed upon a patient. Ultimately, the final decision rests with an informed patient.

BARRETT'S ESOPHAGUS

Barrett's esophagus has been defined as the replacement of the squamous lining of the distal esophagus by three or more centimeters of circumferential columnar epithelium in continuity with the gastric mucosa.[256] This length is arbitrary and this definition excludes tongues of columnar epithelium that are commonly seen at the gastroesophageal junction. Thus, some experts have argued that the definition should be based more appropriately on the histological changes rather than the length of the metaplastic segment.[257] The presence of specialized intestinal epithelium with goblet cells is necessary for the definition of Barrett's epithelium. The recent literature has increasingly used the term "short segment Barrett's esophagus" for patients who fail to fulfill the traditional definition.[257,258]

Barrett's esophagus is a strong risk factor for adenocarcinoma of the esophagus.[259–65] It is important to determine the true relationship and magnitude of the cancer risk to the defined histological abnormality. There is increasing evidence that adenocarcinoma can arise from very short segments of metaplastic epithelium.[261,262] Moreover, the risk appears to be related only to the presence of specialized intestinal epithelium and not to the junctional or cardia types of epithelium.[266,267]

Prevalence of Barrett's metaplasia

In 733 unselected autopsies, seven cases of Barrett's esophagus were found, for a prevalence of 9.5 per 1000.[268] In a prior clinical study, an age- and sex-adjusted prevalence rate of 22.6 cases of Barrett's esophagus per 100 000 population was found in

Olmstead County, MN. In the series of 226 autopsies from the same county, a much higher prevalence of Barrett's was found than was predicted from their prior clinical study. The estimated prevalence in autopsies was estimated to be 376 cases per 100 000, indicating that most cases of Barrett's go unrecognized.[268] In another study by the same authors of 51 311 patients undergoing upper GI endoscopy, the overall prevalence of Barrett's esophagus was 8.9 per 1000, and increased with age to plateau at the seventh decade.[269] However, the mean length of columnar epithelium did not increase with age, or during follow-up of disease over a mean of 7.3 years, and did not increase in the presence of esophagitis or decrease in the absence of esophagitis. The overall prevalence of 8.9 per 1000 in those who did not have carcinoma, was similar to the previous finding of 9.5 per 1000, ie approximately 1%. In a similar Italian study of 14 898 patients undergoing upper GI endoscopy, the prevalence of Barrett's was 7.4 per 1000.[270]

The prevalence of Barrett's metaplasia in patients with esophagitis is nearly 10-fold higher. In 1020 US patients with symptoms of gastroesophageal reflux disease the overall prevalence was 8%.[271] In a Canadian endoscopic study of 742 patients with symptoms of GERD, Barrett's was identified in 6.3% and no cases of esophageal cancer detected.[272]

The prevalence of short segment Barrett's mucosa has been reported to be 18–24% of patients undergoing endoscopy when hematoxylin and eosin (H&E) staining is used.[264,273] This may underestimate the presence of Barrett's mucosa, the prevalence increasing to 36% when alcian blue staining is used.[274]

Barrett's esophagus and GERD

Barrett's esophagus is considered to be the end result of the damaging effects of long standing exposure to acidic gastric juice.[275–7] In 97 subjects with symptoms of GERD, endoscopic biopsies identified Barrett's mucosa in 12.4% of patients.[277] Barrett's mucosa has been induced in the esophagus in dogs and rodents exposed to gastric refluxate, although these studies have been published only in abstract form.[278–81] Thus, despite popular belief, conclusive proof that GERD is the cause of Barrett's epithelium is lacking.

Barrett's esophagus and cancer

The incidence of adenocarcinoma has been evaluated in five studies. In a retrospective study of Mayo Clinic records, adenocarcinoma and Barrett's esophagus were diagnosed simultaneously in 18 of 122 cases.[282] In the remaining 104 patients with Barrett's epithelium esophageal adenocarcinoma developed in two patients over a period of 8.5 years.

At least four studies have been undertaken to determine the risk of progression of Barrett's esophagus to cancer.[282–85] These studies show that the median risk is about 1 in 100 patient years of follow-up (range 1:52 to 1:441 patient years).

Surveillance for dysplasia in Barrett's esophagus

Regular endoscopic surveillance of patients with Barrett's metaplasia has been advocated by working parties, based on the assumption that the detection of pre-neoplastic changes will result in a significant increase in survival.[286] However, this approach has been increasingly questioned with respect to the management strategy and the costs.[287–93]

ARGUMENTS IN SUPPORT OF A SURVEILLANCE STRATEGY

Adenocarcinoma found with Barrett's metaplasia does not appear to arise *de novo* but, rather, to evolve in the metaplastic tissue through initial dysplastic change, then through a dysplasia to carcinoma sequence. Evidence to support this progression comes from a number of histological[258,266,267,270,294–96] and surveillance studies.[297,298] These studies suggest that the development of adenocarcinoma from low-grade dysplasia took between 4 and 4.3 years with high-grade dysplasia being detected prior to the development of cancer. The time to cancer development in patients with high grade dysplasia was estimated to be 3.5 years.

However, in most cases, esophageal cancer is detected at the time of initial endoscopy and at an advanced stage, when the prognosis is very poor. In a study over 7 years from the Cleveland Clinic,[291] investigators found 72 cases of Barrett's esophagus and 10 had an adenocarcinoma at the time of initial diagnosis. Only one case developed in the remaining 62 patients during subsequent surveillance. Similarly Wright *et al* found that 47 patients of 348 had a coexisting adenocarcinoma at the time of initial diagnosis, and only six cancers developed in 166 patients over a subsequent 3-year surveillance period.[299]

R Grade B

Fifty-seven per cent of all esophageal tumors on the National Cancer database for 1988 were stage III or IV at the time of detection with poor 5-year disease specific survivals of 15% and 3% respectively.[300] It is argued that surveillance programs will detect cancers at an earlier stage when the outlook is much better. In stage I or II cases the 5-year disease specific survival rates were 42% and 29% respectively.[300]

R Grade B

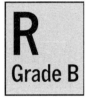

One study of 77 patients compared the staging of esophageal cancer in 58 patients diagnosed at initial endoscopy and the 19 patients with cancer detected during surveillance.[300] The group under surveillance was found to have significantly more patients with favorable grade 0–I tumors (58%) than those diagnosed with cancer at first endoscopy (17%). Moreover, these differences were accompanied by significantly better survival of 62% for those in surveillance compared to 20% for those with cancer at diagnosis. Further support for surveillance comes from a case control study of 166 patients with esophageal cancer in which lymph node involvement was present in only 17% of those who were in a surveillance program, compared to 52% in those who were not.[299]

ARGUMENTS AGAINST A SURVEILLANCE STRATEGY

There is evidence for a marked increase in incidence of adenocarcinoma of the esophagus, which now accounts for about half of all esophageal cancers.[301] However, the absolute numbers remain relatively low, with age adjusted rates for distal esophageal cancer and cancer of the gastroesophageal junction in 1990 of 2.5 and 3.4 per 100 000 respectively.[301,302]

Estimates of the incidence of adenocarcinoma in patients undergoing surveillance for Barrett's esophagus vary considerably. The highest estimates range from 1 in 52 to 1 in 55 patient-years in the studies reported by Hameeteman *et al*[298] and Ovaska *et al.*[303] The lowest estimates range from 1 in 208 to 1 in 441 patient years in the studies reported by Drewitz *et al*[284] and Cameron *et al*[282] respectively. The wide range in these estimates is considered to be due to the small number of cases in most series[293] since none reported more than six cancers and the number of patients studied ranged from 32 to 187. The incidence of adenocarcinoma during surveillance is low as reported by Achkar *et al*[291] at one in 62 and Wright *et al*[299] six in 166. Williamson *et al*,[283] found only five cases of adenocarcinoma in 176 patients under surveillance for some 16 years. This translates into a very low estimate of one cancer per 563 patient years.

R Grade B

These low incidence figures argue against the widespread institution of surveillance programs. Cameron *et al*[268] found the prevalence of Barrett's esophagus at autopsy was 20 times higher than the estimate from endoscopic diagnosis. Thus, for each case of Barrett's, another 20 cases go unrecognized. Considering that the true prevalence of Barrett's esophagus in the community is much higher than was previously thought, the observed incidence of adenocarcinoma of the esophagus is very small in relation to the community prevalence of Barrett's epithelium.[293]

R Grade B

R Grade B

R Grade B

One hundred and sixty-six patients with Barrett's esophagus who deliberately did not undergo a surveillance program were re-examined a mean of 9.3 years later.[304] The authors were able to obtain follow-up information in 93% of the patients comprising 1440 patient years. They determined that the incidence of esophageal cancer was 1 in 180 patient years, a 40-fold increased risk compared to an age and gender matched group from the general population. The tumors developed anywhere from 1 to 16 years after the initial diagnosis of Barrett's was made. Those that developed cancer had a significantly longer length of Barrett's epithelium (9.4 cm with cancer vs 6.6 cm without cancer, $P = 0.02$) and most had Barrett's ulcer at initial endoscopy. Barrett's ulcer was seen more frequently in patients with Barrett's epithelium longer than 10 cm. All eight patients with cancer were symptomatic and the cancer was detected at diagnostic endoscopy. Of interest is that only two of these patients died because of their esophageal cancer, one of postoperative complications and the other 4 years postoperatively with liver metastases. Three had successful surgery, and three died of unrelated illness (pancreatitis, myocardial infarction, asthma). During the follow-up period, there were 79 other unrelated deaths at a mean age of 75 years. The authors concluded that a surveillance program would have had marginal benefit, as so few actually died of esophageal cancer.[304] A Danish study[305] also found that only 1.3% of the patients had a diagnosis of Barrett's esophagus more than 1 year before cancer was identified and only 19% of their patients had Barrett's diagnosed at any time. Thus, most cancers were detected in patients who could not have entered into a surveillance program and this strategy would be unlikely to reduce the death rate from esophageal cancer in the general population.

Unfortunately, there are no randomized controlled trials of surveillance strategies. Cost-effectiveness studies based on a randomized trial would be an important adjunct to decision making.

At this time, the question of whether surveillance should be undertaken cannot be answered. In the absence of a definitive study, there are arguments to support both sides of the controversy. However, recognizing that Barrett's mucosa is a risk factor for esophageal adenocarcinoma, it is difficult to disregard present recommendations for surveillance endoscopy every 1 or 2 years[286,306] until evidence to the contrary is available.

Treatment of Barrett's esophagus

The symptoms of Barrett's oesophagus are typically those of reflux disease, most commonly heartburn and acid regurgitation. However, a small proportion of patients do not have reflux symptoms. This may be because of replacement of the normal squamous epithelium by acid resistant Barrett's epithelium.

The treatment of reflux symptoms is the same whether or not Barrett's esophagus is present. The most effective antisecretory drugs in the management of gastroesophageal reflux disease are the proton pump inhibitors, which have proved to be superior to H_2RAs as reviewed extensively in the previous sections.[187,307] It is clear that this is also true for those with Barrett's esophagus.[199,308,309] For example, treatment with the proton pump inhibitor lansoprazole was effective and safe in 27 patients with Barrett's esophagus treated over a 3-year period.[310] A long term omeprazole study with at least 4 years follow-up, included 32 patients with Barrett's esophagus of 91 patients followed and reported no regression or progression of Barrett's mucosa.[199] Control of symptoms by a proton pump inhibitor does not necessarily mean that intraesophageal acid exposure has been normalized, even when high doses of the drug are prescribed.[3116–14] There are no experimental data to clarify the significance of this observation.

There are some data suggesting that regression of Barrett's metaplasia occurs with continuous PPI therapy.[315,316] However, these data remain controversial. Even when intraesophageal acid exposure is normalized by high dose proton pump inhibition, others have not found regression of Barrett's metaplasia.[313,317] It seems more likely that there is an extension of squamous islands in the Barrett's metaplasia,[308,313,317,318] which overlies the columnar epithelium of Barrett's esophagus[266,319,320] to make it appear that the mucosa has normalized. Similar findings were reported in a small case series of 14 Barrett's patients treated with antireflux surgery and followed for up to 3 years.[321] In the immediate postoperative period, the length of Barrett's epithelium ranged from 2 to 12 cm. In the follow-up period, squamous islands were identified in 12 of 14 patients (ie partial regeneration) and in two patients, there appeared to be complete histological regression of Barrett's. Thus, the role of controlling esophageal acid exposure in the management of Barrett's remains controversial and will require a large RCT over a prolonged time period before definitive recommendations will be possible.

R Grade A

One randomized trial comparing medical therapy with antireflux surgery with follow-up for 1–11 years,[322] showed that while similar symptom relief was achieved, medically treated patients had more persistent inflammation and esophageal strictures. About 25% of the patients treated with surgery appeared to have some regression of Barrett's and three of 32 had upward progression. With medical therapy there was regression in 7.4% (2/27) and apparent progression in 41% (11/27). Mild dysplasia occurred in five patients in the medical group and high grade dysplasia was seen in one patient in each arm. This study suggested that surgery was the more effective intervention. This study is limited by the small sample size and also by the fact that omeprazole was included as medical therapy only in the last 2 years of follow-up.

R Grade B

A recent Swedish case–control study reported an odds ratio of 43.5 for the development of esophageal adenocarcinoma in patients with longstanding (duration >20 years) symptoms of GERD.[16] In contrast, such a history of GERD was associated with only a small increased risk of adenocarcinoma of the cardia (OR 4.4) and with no increase in risk of squamous cell carcinoma of the esophagus (OR 1.1). Cancers were associated with Barrett's esophagus in only 62% of cases and Barrett's did not influence the association between reflux symptoms and adenocarcinoma. The authors[16] concluded a "strong and probably causal relation between gastroesophageal reflux and esophageal adenocarcinoma". These results may lead to the recommendation that effective acid suppressive therapy be provided for all patients with more severe symptoms.

A contrasting Danish chart review found that reflux symptoms were present in only 22% of the 524 patients with esophageal adenocacinoma.[305] This is a much lower figure than in the Swedish study, where 60% of interviewed patients had reflux symptoms. The retrospective chart review data may have underestimated the prevalence of reflux symptoms.

Since there is no convincing evidence of regression of Barrett's metaplasia with high dose, long term proton pump inhibition, regeneration of Barrett's metaplasia in an acid reflux free environment after laser ablation has been studied.[318,323,324] In17 patients treated with long term PPI and 17 patients treated with antireflux surgery, there was some squamous regeneration in the tubular esophagus. However, some overlying of Barrett's glands and intestinal metaplasia by the apparently normal squamous mucosa also occurred.[323,324] This approach cannot be recommended at this time for patients with Barrett's esophagus until stronger evidence for effectiveness is available.

REFERENCES

1 Kitchin LI, Castell DO. Rationale and efficacy of conservative therapy for gastroesophageal reflux disease. *Arch Intern Med* 1991; **151**: 448–54.

2 Nebel OT, Forbes MF, Castell DO. Symptomatic gastroesophageal reflux: incidence and precipitating factors. *Am J Dig Dis* 1976; **21**(11): 953–6.

3 Thompson WG, Heaton KW. Heartburn and globus in apparently healthy people. *Can Med Assoc J* 1982; **126**: 46–8.

4 Anonymous. *Heartburn across America: A Gallup Organization national survey*. Princeton, NJ: Gallup Organization, 1988.

5 Isolauri J, Laippala P. Prevalence of symptoms suggestive of gastroesophageal reflux disease in an adult population. *Ann Med* 1995; **27**: 67–70.

6 Locke GR, Talley NJ, Fett SL *et al.* Prevalence and clinical spectrum of gastroesophageal reflux: a population-based study in Olmsted County, Minnesota. *Gastroenterology* 1997; **112**(5): 1448–56.

7 Wienbeck M, Barnert J. Epidemiology of reflux disease and reflux esophagitis. *Scand J Gastroenterol* Suppl. 1989; **156**: 7–13.

8 Graham DY, Smith JL, Patterson DJ. Why do apparently healthy people use antacid tablets? *Am J Gastroenterol* 1983; **78**(5): 257–60.

9 Brunnen PL, Karmody AM, Needham CD. Severe peptic oesophagitis. *Gut* 1969; **10**: 831–7.

10 Ben Rejeb M, Bouché O, Zeitoun P. Study of 47 consecutive patients with peptic esophageal stricture compared with 3880 cases of reflux esophagitis. *Dig Dis Sci* 1992; **37**(5): 733–6.

11 McDougall NI, Johnston BT, Kee F *et al.* Natural history of reflux oesophagitis: a 10 year follow up of its effect on patient symptomatology and quality of life. *Gut* 1996; **38**: 481–6.

12 Heading RC. Epidemiology of oesophageal reflux disease. *Scand J Gastroenterol* 1989; **24**(Suppl 168): 33–7.

13 Wienbeck M, Barnert J. Epidemiology of reflux disease and reflux esophagitis. *Scand J Gastroenterol* 1989; **24**(Suppl 156): 7–13.

14 Isolauri J, Luostarinen M, Isolauri E *et al.* Natural course of gastroesophageal reflux disease: 17–22 year follow-up of 60 patients. *Am J Gastroenterol* 1997; **92**(1): 37–41.

15 Ollyo JB, Monnier P, Fontolliet C *et al.* The natural history, prevalence and incidence of reflux oesophagitis. *Gullet* 1993; **3**(Suppl 3): 3–10.

16 Lagergren J, Bergstrom R, Lindgren A *et al.* Symptomatic gastroesophageal reflux as a risk factor for esophageal adenocarcinoma. *N Engl J Med* 1999; **340**(11): 825–31.

17 Dent J, Holloway RH, Toouli J *et al.* Mechanisms of lower oesophageal sphincter incompetence in patients with symptomatic gastro-oesophageal reflux. *Gut* 1988; **29**: 120–8.

18 Dent J. Recent views on the pathogenesis of gastro-oesophageal reflux disease. *Baillières Clin Gastroenterol* 1987; **1**(4): 727–5.

19 Holloway RH, Hongo M, Berger K *et al.* Gastric distension: a mechanism for postprandial gastroesophageal reflux. *Gastroenterology* 1985; **89**(4): 779–84.

20 Venables CW. Mucus, pepsin and peptic ulcer. *Gut* 1986; **27**: 233–8.

21 Goldberg HI, Dodds WJ, Gee S *et al.* Role of acid and pepsin in acute experimental esophagitis. *Gastroenterology* 1969; **56**(2): 223–30.

22 Mittal RK, Lange RC, McCallum RW. Identification and mechanism of delayed esophageal acid clearance in subjects with hiatus hernia. *Gastroenterology* 1987; **92**(1): 130–5.

23 Sloan S, Kahrilas PJ. Impairment of esophageal emptying with hiatal hernia. *Gastroenterology* 1991; **100**(3): 596–605.

24 Breen KJ, Whelan G. The diagnosis of reflux oesophagitis: an evaluation of five investigative procedures. *Aust NZ J Surg* 1978; **48**(2): 156–61.

25 Richter JE, Castell DO. Gastroesophageal reflux: pathogenesis, diagnosis, and therapy. *Ann Int Med* 1982; **97**: 93–103.

26 Wu WC. Ancillary tests in the diagnosis of gastroesophageal reflux disease. *Gastroenterol Clin North Am* 1990; **19**(3): 671–82.
27 Howard PJ, Maher L, Pryde A *et al*. Symptomatic gastro–oesophageal reflux, abnormal oesophageal acid exposure, and mucosal acid sensitivity are three separate, though related, aspects of gastro-oesophageal reflux disease. *Gut* 1991; **32**: 128–32.
28 Klauser AG, Schindlbeck NE, Müller–Lissner SA. Symptoms in gastro-oesophageal reflux disease. *Lancet* 1990; **335**: 205–8.
29 Johnsson F, Joelsson B, Gudmundsson K *et al*. Symptoms and endoscopic findings in the diagnosis of gastroesophageal relux disease. *Scand J Gastroenterol* 1987; **22**: 714–18.
30 Klauser AG, Heinrich C, Schindlbeck NE *et al*. Is long-term esophageal pH monitoring of clinical value? *Am J Gastroenterol* 1989; **84**(4): 362–6.
31 Talley NJ, Colin-Jones D, Koch KL *et al*. Functional dyspepsia: a classification with guidelines for diagnosis and management. *Gastroenterology Intl* 1991; **4**(4): 145–60.
32 Joelsson B, Johnsson F. Heartburn – the acid test. *Gut* 1989; 30: 1523–5.
33 Masclee AAM, De Best ACAM, De Graaf R *et al*. Ambulatory 24-hour pH-metry in the diagnosis of gastroesophageal reflux disease. Determination of criteria and relation to endoscopy. *Scand J Gastroenterol* 1990; **25**(3): 225–30.
34 Vitale GC, Cheadle WG, Sadek S *et al*. Computerized 24-hour ambulatory esophageal pH monitoring and esophagogastroduodenoscopy in the reflux patient. *Ann Surg* 1984; **200**(6): 724–8.
35 Venables TL, Newland RD, Patel AC *et al*. Omeprazole 10 milligrams once daily, omeprazole 20 milligrams once daily, or ranitidine 150 milligrams twice daily, evaluated as initial therapy for the relief of symptoms of gastro-oesophageal reflux disease in general practice. *Scand J Gastroenterol* 1997; **32**: 965–73.
36 DeMeester TR, Wang CI, Wernly JA *et al*. Technique, indications, and clinical use of 24 hour esophageal pH monitoring. *J Thorac Cardiovasc Surg* 1980; **79**: 656–70.
37 Galmiche JP, Bruley des Varannes S. Symptoms and disease severity in gastro-oesophageal reflux disease. *Scand J Gastroenterol* 1994; **29**(Suppl 201): 62–8.
38 Johannessen T, Petersen H, Kleveland PM *et al*. The predictive value of history in dyspepsia. *Scand J Gastroenterol* 1990; **25**: 689–97.
39 Johnsson F, Roth Y, Damgaard Pedersen NE *et al*. Cimetidine improves GERD symptoms in patients selected by a validated GERD questionnaire. *Aliment Pharmacol Ther* 1993; **7**: 81–6.
40 Tefera L, Fein M, Ritter MP.TR *et al*. Can the combination of symptoms and endoscopy confirm the presence of gastroesophageal reflux disease? *The American Surgeon* 1997; **63**: 933–6.
41 Carlsson R, Dent J, Bolling–Sternevald E *et al*. The usefulness of a structured questionnaire in the assessment of symptomatic gastroesophageal reflux disease. *Scand J Gastroenterol* 1998; **33**: 1023–9.
42 Kaul B, Petersen H, Grette K *et al*. Scintigraphy, pH measurement, and radiography in the evaluation of gastoesophageal reflux. *Scand J Gastroenterol* 1985; **20**: 289–94.
43 Kaul B, Petersen H, Myrvold HE. Hiatus hernia in gastroesophageal reflux disease. *Scand J Gastroenterol* 1986; **21**: 31–4.
44 Berstad A, Weberg R, Frøyshov Larsen I *et al*. Relationship of hiatus hernia to reflux esophagitis. A prospective study of coincidence, using endoscopy. *Scand J Gastroenterol* 1986; **21**: 55–8.
45 Smout AJPM, Geus WP, Mulder PGH. Gastro-oesophageal reflux disease in the Netherlands. Results of a multicentre pH study. *Scand J Gastroenterol* 1996; **31**(Suppl 218): 10–15.
46 Fuchs KH, DeMeester TR, Albertucci M. Specificity and sensitivity of objective diagnosis of gastroesophageal reflux disease. *Surgery* 1987; **102**(4): 575–80.
47 DeVault KR, Castell DO. Guidelines for the diagnosis and treatment of gastroesophageal reflux disease. *Arch Intern Med* 1995; **155**: 2165–73.
48 Sellar RJ, De Caestecker JS, Heading RC. Barium radiology: a sensitive test for gastro- oesophageal reflux. *Clin Radiology* 1987; **38**: 303–7.
49 Chen YM, Ott DJ, Gelfand DW *et al*. Multiphasic examination of the esophagogastric region for strictures, rings and hiatal hernia: evaluation of the individual techniques. *Gastrointestinal Radiology* 1985; **10**: 311–16.
50 Fransson SG, Sökjer H, Johansson KE *et al*. Radiologic diagnosis of gastro-oesophageal reflux. Comparison of barium and low-density contrast medium. *Acta Radiologica* 1987; **28**: 295–8.
51 Graziani L, De Nigris E, Pesaresi A *et al*. Reflux oesophagitis: radiographic-endoscopic correlation in 39 symptomatic cases. *Gastrointestinal Radiology* 1983; **8**: 1–6.
52 Pope CE. Pathophysiology and diagnosis of reflux esophagitis. *Gastroenterology* 1976; **70**: 445–54.
53 Ott DJ, Dodds WJ, Wu WC *et al*. Current status of radiology in evaluating for gastroesophageal

reflux disease. *J Clin Gastroenterol* 1982; **4**: 365–375.

54 Chen MY, Ott DJ, Sinclair JW *et al.* Gastroesophageal reflux disease: correlation of esophageal pH testing and radiographic findings. *Radiology* 1992; **185**(2): 483–6.

55 Jenkins AF, Cowan RJ, Richter JE. Gastroesophageal scintigaphy: is it a sensitive screening test for gastroesophageal reflux disease? *J Clin Gastroenterol* 1985; **7**(2): 127–31.

56 Spechler SJ. Epidemiology and natural history of gastro-oesophageal reflux disease. *Digestion* 1992; **51**(Suppl 1): 24–9.

57 Knuff TE, Benjamin SB, Worsham GF *et al.* Histologic examination of chronic gastro-esophageal relux: an evaluation of biopsy methods and diagnostic criteria. *Dig Dis Sci* 1984; **29**: 194–201.

58 Ismail–Beigi F, Pope CE. Distribution of the histological changes of gastroesophageal reflux in the distal esophagus of man. *Gastroenterology* 1974; **66**: 1109–13.

59 Schindlbeck NE, Wiebecke B, Klauser AG *et al.* Diagnostic value of histology in non erosive gastro-oesophageal reflux disease. *Gut* 1996; **39**: 151–4.

60 Berstad A, Hatlebakk JG. The predictive value of symptoms in gastro-oesophageal reflux disease. *Scand J Gastroenterol* 1995; **30**(Suppl 211): 1–4.

61 Hatlebakk JG, Berstad A. Endoscopic grading of reflux oesophagitis: what observations corelate with gastro-oesophageal reflux? *Scand J Gastroenterol* 1997; **32**: 760–5.

62 Armstrong D, Emde C, Inauen W *et al.* Diagnostic assessment of gastroesophageal reflux disease: what is possible vs what is practical? *Hepato-gastroenterology* 1992; **39**(Suppl 1): 3–13.

63 Armstrong D, Bennett JR, Blum AL *et al.* The endoscopic assessment of esophagitis: a progress report on observer agreement. *Gastroenterology* 1996; **111**(1): 85–92.

64 Bernstein LM, Baker LA. A clinical test for esophagitis. *Gastroenterology* 1958; **34**: 760–81.

65 Kaul B, Petersen H, Grette K *et al.* The acid perfusion test in gastroesophageal reflux disease. *Scand J Gastroenterol* 1986; **21**: 93–6.

66 Richter JE. Acid perfusion (Bernstein) test. Editors: Castell DO, Wu WC, Ott DJ. In: *Gastroesophageal reflux disease: pathogenesis, diagnosis and therapy.* London, England, Futura Publishing Co Inc. 1985, pp 139–48.

67 Rosen SN, Pope CE. Extended esophageal pH monitoring. An analysis of the literature and assessment of its role in the diagnosis and management of gastroesophageal reflux. *J Clin Gastroenterol* 1989; **11**(3): 260–70.

68 Schindlbeck NE, Heinrich C, König A *et al.* Optimal thresholds, sensitivity, and specificity of long-term pH-metry for the detection of gastroesophageal reflux disease. *Gastroenterology* 1987; **93**: 85–90.

69 Johnsson F, Joelsson B, Isberg PE. Ambulatory 24 hour intraesophgeal pH-monitoring in the diagnosis of gastroesophageal reflux disease. *Gut* 1987; **28**: 1145–50.

70 Jamieson JR, Stein HJ, DeMeester TR *et al.* Ambulatory 24h esophageal pH monitoring: normal values, optimal thresholds, specificity, and reproducibility. *Am J Gastroenterol* 1992; **87**(9): 1102–11.

71 Mattox HE, Richter JE. Prolonged ambulatory esophageal pH monitoring in the evaluation of gastroesophageal reflux disease. *Am J Med* 1990; **89**: 345–56.

72 Wyman JB, Dent J, Holloway RH. Changes in oesophageal pH associated with gastro-oesophageal reflux. Are traditional criteria sensitive for detection of reflux? *Scand J Gastroenterol* 1993; **28**(9): 827–32.

73 Mattioli S, Pilotti V, Spangaro M et al. Reliability of 24-hour home esophageal pH monitoring in diagnosis of gastroesophageal reflux. *Dig Dis Sci* 1989; **34**(1): 71–8.

74 Schlesinger PK, Donahue PE, Schmid B *et al.* Limitations of 24-hour intraesophageal pH monitoring in the hospital setting. *Gastroenterology* 1985; **89**(4): 797–804.

75 Watson RG, Tham TC, Johnston BT *et al.* Double blind cross-over placebo controlled study of omeprazole in the treatment of patients with reflux symptoms and physiological levels of acid reflux—the "sensitive oesophagus". *Gut* 1997; **40**(5): 587–90.

76 Schenk BE, Kuipers EJ, Klinkenberg Knol EC *et al.* Omeprazole as a diagnostic tool in gastroesophageal reflux disease. *Am J Gastroenterol* 1997; **92**(11): 1997–2000.

77 Ward BW, Wu WC, Richter JE *et al.* Ambulatory 24-hour esophageal pH monitoring: technology seaching for a clinical application. *J Clin Gastroenterol* 1986; **8**(Suppl 1): 59–67.

78 Wiener GJ, Richter JE, Copper JB *et al.* The symptom index: a clinically important parameter of ambulatory 24-hour esophageal pH monitoring. *Am J Gastroenterol* 1988; **83**(4): 358–61.

79 Trimble KC, Pryde A, Heading RC. Lowered oesophageal sensory thresholds in patients with symptomatic but not excess gastro-oesophageal reflux: evidence for a spectrum of visceral sensitivity in GORD. *Gut* 1995; **37**(1): 7–12.

80 Shi G, Bruley des Varannes S, Scarpignato C *et al.* Reflux related symptoms in patients with normal oesophageal exposure to acid. *Gut* 1995; **37**(4): 457–64.

81 Eriksen CA, Cullen PT, Sutton D *et al.* Abnormal esophageal transit in patients with typical reflux symptoms but normal endoscopic and pH profiles. *Am J Surg* 1991; **161**: 657–61.
82 Fiorucci S, Santucci L, Chiucchiú S *et al.* Gastric acidity and gastroesophageal reflux patterns in patients with esophagitis. *Gastroenterology* 1992; **103**(3): 855–61.
83 Johnsson F, Weywadt L, Solhaug JH *et al.* One-week omeprazole treatment in the diagnosis of gastro-oesophageal reflux disease. *Scand J Gastroenterol* 1998; **33**: 15–20.
84 Bate CM, Riley SA, Chapman RWG *et al.* Evaluation of omeprazole as a cost-effective diagnostic test foe gastro-oesophageal reflux disease. *Aliment Pharmacol Ther* 1999; **13**: 59–66.
85 Schindlbeck NE, Klauser AG, Voderholzer WA et al. Empiric therapy for gastroesophageal reflux disease. *Arch Intern Med* 1995; **155**: 1808–12.
86 Achem SR, Kolts BE, MacMath T *et al.* Effects of omeprazole versus placebo in treatment of noncardiac chest pain and gastro-esophageal reflux. *Dig Dis Sci* 1997; **42**(10): 2138–45.
87 Fass R, Fennerty MB, Ofman JJ *et al.*The clinical and economic value of a short course of omeprazole in patients with noncardiac chest pain. *Gastroenterology* 1998; **115**(1): 42–49.
88 Sonnenberg A, Delco F, El–Serag HB. Empirical therapy versus diagnostic tests in gastroesophageal reflux disease. A medical decision analysis. *Dig Dis Sci* 1998; **43**(5): 1001–8.
89 Harvey RF, Gordon PC, Hadley N *et al.* Effects of sleeping with the bed-head raised and of ranitidine in patients with severe peptic oesophagitis. *Lancet* 1987; **ii**: 1200–3.
90 Stanciu C, Bennett JR. Effects of posture on gastro-oesophageal reflux. *Digestion* 1977; **15**: 104–9.
91 Johnson LF, DeMeester TR. Evaluation of elevation of the head of the bed, bethanecol, and antacid foam tablets on gastroesophageal reflux. *Dig Dis Sci* 1981; **26**: 673–80.
92 Hamilton JW, Boisen RJ, Yamamoto DT *et al.* Sleeping on a wedge diminishes exposure of the esophagus to refluxed acid. *Dig Dis Sci* 1988; **33**(5): 518–22.
93 Becker DJ, Sinclair J, Castell DO *et al.* A comparison of high and low fat meals on postprandial esophageal acid exposure. *Am J Gastroenterol* 1989; **84**: 782–86.
94 Nebel OT, Castell DO. Lower esophageal sphincter pressure changes after food ingestion. *Gastroenterology* 1972; **63**(5): 778–83.
95 Murphy DW, Castell DO. Chocolate and heartburn: evidence of increased esophageal acid exposure after chocolate ingestion. *Am J Gastroenterol* 1988; **93**: 633–6.
96 Sigmund CJ, McNally EF. The action of a carminative on the lower esophageal sphincter. *Gastroenterology* 1969; **56**: 13–18.
97 Babka JC, Castell DO. On the genesis of heartburn. The effects of specific foods on the lower esophageal sphincter. *Am J Dig Dis* 1973; **18**(5): 391–7.
98 Allen ML, Mellow MH, Robinson MG *et al.* The effect of raw onions on acid reflux and reflux symptoms. *Am J Gastroenterol* 1990; **85**: 377–80.
99 Thomas FB, Steinbaugh JT, Fromkes JJ *et al.* Inhibitory effect of coffee on lower esophageal sphincter pressure. *Gastroenterology* 1980; **79**(6): 1262–6.
100 McArthur K, Hogan D, Isenberg JI. Relative stimulatory effects of commonly ingested beverages on gastric acid secretion in humans. *Gastroenterology* 1982; **83**(1 Pt 2): 199–203.
101 Vitale GC, Cheadle WG, Patel B *et al.* The effect of alcohol on nocturnal gastroesophageal reflux. *JAMA* 1987; **258**: 2077–9.
102 Price SF, Smithson KW, Castell DO. Food sensitivity in reflux esophagitis. *Gastroenterology* 1978; **75**(2): 240–3.
103 Waring JP, Eastwood TF, Austin JM *et al.* The immediate efects of cessation of cigarette smoking on gastroesophageal reflux. Am J *Gastroenterol* 1989; **84**: 1076–8.
104 Graham DY, Patterson DJ. Double–blind comparison of liquid antacid and placebo in the treatment of symptomatic reflux esophagitis. *Dig Dis Sci* 1983; **28**(6): 559–63.
105 Farup PG, Weberg R, Berstad A *et al.* Low-dose antacids versus 400 mg cimetidine twice daily for reflux oesophagitis. A comparative, placebo-controlled, multicentre study. *Scand J Gastroenterol* 1990; **25**: 315–20.
106 Grove O, Bekker C, Jeppe-Hansen MG *et al.* Ranitidine and high-dose antacid in reflux oesophagitis. A randomized, placebo-controlled trial. *Scand J Gastroenterol* 1985; **20**: 457–61.
107 Koelz HR. Treatment of reflux esophagitis with H_2-Blockers, antacids and prokinetic drugs. An analysis of randomized clinical trials. *Scand J Gastroenterol* 1989; **24**(Suppl 156): 25–36.
108 Poynard T, and a French Co-operative Study Group. Relapse rate of patients after healing of esophagitis – a prospective study of alginate as self-care treatment for 6 months. *Aliment Pharmacol Ther* 1993; **7**: 385–92.
109 Poynard T, Vernisse B, Agostini H, for a multicentre group. Randomized, multicentre comparison of sodium alginate and cisapride in the symptomatic treatment of uncomplicated gastro–oesophageal reflux. *Aliment Pharmacol Ther* 1998; **12**: 159–65.

110 Hunt RH. The relationship between the control of pH and healing and symptom relief in gastro-oesophageal reflux disease. *Aliment Pharmacol Ther* 1995; **9**(Suppl 1): 3–7.
111 Hatlebakk JG, Berstad A. Gastro-oesophageal reflux during 3 months of therapy with ranitidine in reflux oesophagitis. *Scand J Gastroenterol* 1996; **31**: 954–8.
112 Bell NJV, Burget D, Howden CW *et al.*Appropriate acid suppression for the management of gastro-oesophageal reflux disase. *Digestion* 1992; **51**(Suppl 1): 59–67.
113 Bell NJV, Hunt RH. Role of gastric acid suppression in the treatment of gastro-oesophageal reflux disease. *Gut* 1992; **33**: 118–24.
114 Bate CM, Green JR, Axon AT *et al.* Omeprazole is more effective than cimetidine for the relief of all grades of gastro-oesophageal reflux disease-associated heartburn, irrespective of the presence or absence of endoscopic oesophagitis. *Aliment Pharmacol Ther* 1997; **11**(4): 755–63.
115 Bate CM, Green JR, Axon AT *et al.* Omeprazole is more effective than cimetidine in the prevention of recurrence of GERD-associated heartburn and the occurrence of underlying oesophagitis. *Aliment Pharmacol Ther* 1998; **12**(1): 41–7.
116 Bianchi Porro G, Pace F, Sangaletti O *et al.* High-dose famotidine in the maintenance treatment of refractory esophagitis: results of a medium-term open study. *Am J Gastroenterol* 1991; **86**(11): 1585–7.
117 Carlsson R, Galmiche JP, Dent J *et al.* Prognostic factors influencing relapse of oesophagitis during maintenance therapy with antisecretory drugs: a meta-analysis of long-term omeprazole trials. *Aliment Pharmacol Ther* 1997; **11**: 473–82.
118 Chiba N, de Gara CJ, Wilkinson JM *et al.* Speed of healing and symptom relief in grade II to IV gastroesophageal reflux disease: a meta-analysis. *Gastroenterology* 1997; **112**(6): 1798–810.
119 Simon TJ, Berlin RG, Tipping R *et al.* Efficacy of twice daily doses of 40 or 20 milligrams famotidine or 150 milligrams ranitidine for treatment of patients with moderate to severe erosive esophagitis. Famotidine Erosive Esophagitis Study Group. *Scand J Gastroenterol* 1993; **28**: 375–80.
120 McCarty-Dawson D, Sue SO, Morrill B *et al.* Ranitidine versus cimetidine in the healing of erosive esophagitis. *Clin Ther* 1996; **18**(6): 1150–60.
121 Castell DO, Richter JE, Robinson M *et al.* Efficacy and safety of lansoprazole in the treatment of erosive reflux esophagitis. *Am J Gastroenterol* 1996; **91**(9): 1749–57.
122 Mulder CJ, Dekker W, Gerretsen M, on behalf of the Dutch Study Group. Lansoprazole 30mg versus omeprazole 40mg in the treatment of reflux oesophagitis grade II, III and IVa (a Dutch multicentre trial). *Eur J Gastroenterol Hepatol* 1996; **8**: 1101–6.
123 Dekkers CPM, Beker JA, Thjodleifsson B *et al.* Double-blind, placebo-controlled comparison of rabeprazole 20mg vs omeprazole 20mg in the treatment of erosive or ulcerative gastro-oesophageal reflux disease. *Aliment Pharmacol Ther* 1999; **13**: 49–57.
124 van Rensburg CJ, Honiball PJ, Grundling HD *et al.* Efficacy and tolerability of pantoprazole 40 mg versus 80 mg in patients with reflux oesophagitis. *Aliment Pharmacol Ther* 1996; **10**(3): 397–401.
125 Earnest DL, Dorsch E, Jones J *et al.* A placebo-controlled dose-ranging study of lansoprazole in the management of reflux esophagitis. *Am J Gastroenterol* 1998; **93**(2): 238–43.
126 Sontag SJ, Kogut DG, Fleischmann R *et al.* Lansoprazole heals erosive reflux esophagitis resistant to histamine H2-receptor antagonist therapy. *Am J Gastroenterol* 1997; **92**(3): 429–37.
127 Mulder CJ, Dekker W, Gerretsen M. Lansoprazole 30 mg versus omeprazole 40 mg in the treatment of reflux oesophagitis grade II, III and IVa (a Dutch multicentre trial). Dutch Study Group. *Eur J Gastroenterol Hepatol* 1996; **8**(11): 1101–6.
128 Mee AS, Rowley JL, & the Lansoprazole clinical research goup. Rapid symptom relief in reflux oesophagitis: a comparison of lansoprazole and omeprazole. *Aliment Pharmacol Ther* 1996; **10**: 757–63.
129 Hatlebakk JG, Berstad A, Carling L *et al.* Lansoprazole versus omeprazole in short-term treatment of reflux oesophagitis. Results of a Scandinavian multicentre trial. *Scand J Gastroenterol* 1993; **28**: 224–8.
130 Vcev A, Stimac D, Vceva A *at al.* Lansoprazole versus omeprazole in the treatment of reflux esophagitis. *Acta Med Croatica* 1997; **51**(3): 171–4.
131 Corinaldesi R, Valentini M, Belaiche J *et al.* Pantoprazole and omeprazole in the treatment of reflux oesophagitis: a European multicentre study. *Aliment Pharmacol Ther* 1995; **9**: 667–71.
132 Mossner J, Holscher AH, Herz R *et al.* A double-blind study of pantoprazole and omeprazole in the treatment of reflux oesophagitis: a multicentre trial. *Aliment Pharmacol Ther* 1995; **9**: 321–6.

133 Hunt RH. Habit, prejudice, power and politics: issues in the conversion of H2-receptor antagonists to over-the-counter use. *Can Med Assoc J* 1996; **154**(1): 49–53.
134 Gottlieb S, Decktor DL, Eckert JM *et al.* Efficacy and tolerability of famotidine in preventing heartburn and related symptoms of upper gastrointestinal discomfort. *Am J Therapeutics* 1995; **2**(5): 314–19.
135 Johannessen T, Kristensen P. On-demand therapy in gastroesophageal relux disease: a comparison of the early effects of single doses of fast-dissolving famotidine wafers and ranitidine tablets. *Clin Ther* 1997; **19**(1): 73–81.
136 Engzelius JM, Solhaug JH, Knapstad LJ *et al.* Ranitidine effervescent and famotidine wafer in the relief of episodic symptoms of gastro-oesophageal reflux disease. *Scand J Gastroenterol* 1997; **32**: 513–18.
137 Wilhelmsen I, Hatlebakk JG, Olaffson S *et al.* On demand therapy of reflux oesophagitis: a study of symptoms, patient satisfaction, and quality of life. *Gastroenterology* 1998; **114**(4): A331. (Abstract)
138 Euler AR, Murdock RH, Jr., Wilson TH *et al.* Ranitidine is effective therapy for erosive esophagitis. *Am J Gastroenterol* 1993; **88**(4): 520–4.
139 Roufail W, Belsito A, Robinson M *et al.* Ranitidine for erosive oesophagitis: a double-blind, placebo-controlled study. Glaxo Erosive Esophagitis Study Group. *Aliment Pharmacol Ther* 1992; **6**: 597–607.
140 Silver MT, Murdock RH, Jr., Morrill BB *et al.* Ranitidine 300mg twice daily and 150 mg four-times daily are efffective in healing erosive esophagitis. *Aliment Pharmacol Ther* 1996; **10**: 373–80.
141 Johnson NJ, Boyd EJS, Mills JG *et al.* Acute treatment of reflux oesophagitis: a multi-centre trial to compare 150 mg ranitidine b.d. with 300 mg ranitidine q.d.s. *Aliment Pharmacol Ther* 1989; **3**: 259–66.
142 Pace F, Maconi G, Molteni P *et al.* Meta-analysis of the effect of placebo on the outcome of medically treated reflux esophagitis. *Scand J Gastroenterol* 1995; **30**: 101–5.
143 Grande L, Lacima G, Ros E *et al.* Lack of effect of metoclopramide and domperidone on esophageal peristalsis and esophageal acid clearance in reflux esophagitis. A randomized, double–blind study. *Dig Dis Sci* 1992; **37**: 583–8.
144 Ceccatelli P, Janssens J, Vantrappen G *et al.* Cisapride restores the decreased lower oesophageal sphincter pressure in reflux patients. *Gut* 1988; **29**: 631–5.
145 Collins BJ, Spence RAJ, Ferguson R *et al.* Cisapride: Influence on oesophageal and gastric emptying and gastro-oesoghageal reflux in patients with reflux oesophagitis. *Hepato-gastroenterology* 1987; **34**: 113–16.
146 Robertson CS, Evans DF, Ledingham SJ *et al.* Cisapride in the treatment of gastro-oesophageal reflux disease. *Aliment Pharmacol Ther* 1993; **7**: 181–90.
147 Sekiguchi T, Nishioka T, Matsuzaki T *et al.* Comparative efficacy of acid inhibition by drug therapy in reflux esophagitis. *Gastroenterologia* 1991; **26**(2): 137–44.
148 Castell DO, Sigmund CJr, Patterson D *et al.* Cisapride 20mg b.i.d. provides symptomatic relief of heartburn and related symptoms of chronic mild to moderate gastroesophageal reflux disease. *Am J Gastroenterol* 1998; **93**(4): 547–52.
149 Richter JE, Long JF. Cisapride for gastroesophageal reflux disease: a placebo-controlled, double-blind study. *Am J Gastroenterol* 1995; **90**: 423–30.
150 Geldof H, Hazelhoff B, Otten MH. Two different dose regimens of cisapride in the treatment of reflux oesophagitis: a double-blind comparison with ranitidine. *Aliment Pharmacol Ther* 1993; **7**: 409–15.
151 Dakkak M, Jones BP, Scott MG *et al.* Comparing the efficacy of cisapride and ranitidine in oesophagitis: a double-blind, parallel group study in general practice. *Br J Clin Pract* 1994; **48**: 10–14.
152 Galmiche JP, Fraitag B, Filoche B *et al.* Double-blind comparison of cisapride and cimetidine in treatment of reflux esophagitis. *Dig Dis Sci* 1990; **35**(5): 649–55.
153 Janisch HD, Hüttemann W, Bouzo MH. Cisapride versus ranitidine in the treatment of reflux esophagitis. *Hepato-gastroenterology* 1988; **35**(3): 125–7.
154 Maleev A, Mendizova A, Popov P *et al.* Cisapride and cimetidine in the treatment of erosive esophagitis. *Hepato-gastroenterology* 1990; **37**(4): 403–7.
155 Arvanitakis C, Nikopoulos A, Theoharidis A *et al.* Cisapride and ranitidine in the treatment of gastro-oesophageal reflux disease – a comparative randomized double-blind trial. *Aliment Pharmacol Ther* 1993; **7**: 635–41.
156 Baldi F, Bianchi PG, Dobrilla G *et al.* Cisapride versus placebo in reflux esophagitis. A multicenter double–blind trial. *J Clin Gastroenterol* 1988; **10**(6): 614–18.
157 Lepoutre L, VanDerSpek P, Vanderlinden I *et al.* Healing of grade-II and III oesophagitis through motility stimulation with cisapride. *Digestion* 1990; **45**: 109–14.
158 Toussaint J, Gossuin A, Deruyttere M *et al.* Healing and prevention of relapse of reflux

oesophagitis by cisapride. *Gut* 1991; **32**: 1280–5.
159 Galmiche JP, Barthelemy P, Hamelin B. Treating the symptoms of gastro-oesophageal reflux disease: a double blind comparison of omeprazole and ciaspride. *Aliment Pharmacol Ther* 1997; **11**: 765–73.
160 Kimmig JM. Treatment and prevention of relapse of mild oesophagitis with omeprazole and cisapride: a comparison of two strategies. *Aliment Pharmacol Ther* 1995; **9**: 281–6.
161 McKenna CJ, Mills JG, Goodwin C *et al.* Combination of ranitidine and cisapride in the treatment of reflux oesophagitis. *Eur J Gastroenterol Hepatol* 1995; **7**: 817–22.
162 Blum AL, Adami B, Bouzo MH *et al.* Effect of cisapride on relapse of esophagitis. A multinational, placebo-controlled trial in patients healed with an antisecretory drug. The Italian Eurocis Trialists. *Dig Dis Sci* 1993; **38**: 551–60.
163 Hatlebakk JG, Johnsson F, Vilien M *et al.* The effect of cisapride in maintaining symptomatic remission in patients with gastro-oesophageal reflux disease. *Scand J Gastroenterol* 1997; **32**: 1100–6.
164 Vigneri S, Termini R, Leandro G *et al.* A comparison of five maintenance therapies for reflux esophagitis. *N Engl J Med* 1995; **333**(17): 1106–10.
165 Tytgat GN, Anker-Hansen O, Carling L *et al.* Effect of cisapride on relapse of reflux oesophagitis, healed with antisecretory drugs. *Scand J Gastroenterol* 1992; **27**: 175–83.
166 McDougall NI, Watson RGP, Collins JSA *et al.* Maintenance therapy with cisapride after healing of erosive oesophagitis: a double-blind placebo-controlled trial. *Aliment Pharmacol Ther* 1997; **11**: 487–95.
167 Wysowski DE, Bacsanyi J. Cisapride and fatal arrhythmia. *N Engl J Med* 1996; **335**: 290–1.
168 Hameeteman W, v.d.Boomgaard DM, Dekker W *et al.* Sucralfate versus cimetidine in reflux esophagitis. A single-blind multicentre study. *J Clin Gastroenterol* 1987; **9**(4): 390–4.
169 Chopra BK, Kazal HL, Mittal PK *et al.* A comparison of the clinical efficacy of ranitidine and sucralfate in reflux esophagitis. *J Assoc Physicians India* 1992; **40**: 439–41.
170 Bremner CG, Marks IN, Segal I *et al.* Reflux esophagitis therapy: Sucralfate versus ranitidine in a double blind multicenter trial. *Am J Med* 1991; **91**(2A): 119S–122S.
171 Simon B, Mueller P. Comparison of the effect of sucralfate and ranitidine in reflux esophagitis. *Am J Med* 1987; **83**(Suppl 3B): 43–7.
172 Schotborgh RH, Hameeteman W, Dekker W *et al.* Combination therapy of sucralfate and cimetidine, compared with sucralfate monotherapy, in patients with peptic reflux esophagitis. *Am J Med* 1989; **86**(Suppl 6A): 77–80.
173 Herrera JL, Shay SS, McCabe M *et al.* Sucralfate used as adjunctive therapy in patients with severe erosive peptic esophagitis resulting from gastroesophageal reflux. *Am J Gastroenterol* 1990; **85**: 1335–8.
174 Tytgat GNJ, Koelz HR, Vosmaer GDC, and the Sucralfate Investigational Working Team. Sucralfate maintenance therapy in reflux esophagitis. *Am J Gastroenterol* 1995; **90**(8): 1233–7.
175 Jorgensen F, Elsborg L. Sucralfate versus cimetidine in the treatment of reflux esophagitis, with special reference to the esophageal motor function. *Am J Med* 1991; **91**: 114S–118S.
176 Starlinger M, Appel WH, Schemper M *et al.* R. Long-term treatment of peptic esophageal stenosis with dilation and cimetidine: factors influencing clinical results. *Eur Surg Res* 1985; **17**: 207–14.
177 Ferguson R, Dronfield MW, Atkinson M. Cimetidine in treatment of reflux esophagitis with peptic stricture. *BMJ* 1979; **2**: 472–4.
178 Smith PM, Kerr GD, Cockel R *et al.* A comparison of omeprazole and ranitidine in the prevention of recurrence of benign esophageal stricture. The RESTORE Investigator Group. *Gastroenterology* 1994; 107(5): 1312–18.
179 Marks RD, Richter JE, Rizzo J *et al.* Omeprazole versus H2-receptor antagonists in treating patients with peptic stricture and esophagitis. *Gastroenterology* 1994; **106**: 907–15.
180 Swarbrick ET, Gough AL, Foster CS *et al.* Prevention of recurrence of oesophageal stricture, a comparison of lansoprazole and high-dose ranitidine. *Eur J Gastroenterol Hepatol* 1996; **8**(5): 431–8.
181 Jaspersen D, Diehl KL, Schoeppner H *et al.* A comparison of omeprazole, lansoprazole, and pantoprazole in the maintenance treatment of severe reflux oesophagitis. *Aliment Pharmacol Ther* 1998; **12**: 49–52.
182 Koelz HR, Birchler R, Bretholz A *et al.* Healing and relapse of reflux esophagitis during treatment with ranitidine. *Gastroenterology* 1986; **91**(5): 1198–1205.
183 Hetzel DJ, Dent J, Reed WD *et al.* Healing and relapse of severe peptic esophagitis after treatment with omeprazole. *Gastroenterology* 1988; **95**(4): 903–12.
184 Olbe L, Lundell L. Medical treatment of reflux esophagitis. *Hepato-gastroenterology* 1992; **39**(4): 322–4.
185 Klinkenberg–Knol EC, Jansen JBMJ, Lamers CBHW *et al.* Temporary cessation of long-term

maintenance treatment with omeprazole in patients with H_2-receptor-antagonist-resistant reflux oesophagitis. Effects on symptoms, endoscopy, serum gastrin, and gastric acid output. *Scand J Gastroenterol* 1990; **25**: 1144–50.
186 Sontag SJ, Kogut DG, Fleischmann R *et al.* Lansoprazole prevents recurrence of erosive reflux esophagitis previously resistant to H_2-RA therapy. *Am J Gastroenterol* 1996; **91**(9): 1758–65.
187 Chiba N. Proton pump inhibitors in acute healing and maintenance of erosive or worse esophagitis: a systematic overview. *Can J Gastroenterol* 1997; **11**(Suppl B): 66B–73B.
188 Lundell L, Backman L, Ekstrom P *et al.* Prevention of relapse of reflux esophagitis after endoscopic healing: the efficacy and safety of omeprazole compared with ranitidine. *Scand J Gastroenterol* 1991; **26**: 248–56.
189 Gough AL, Long RG, Cooper BT *et al.* Lansoprazole versus ranitidine in the maintenance treatment of reflux oesophagitis. *Aliment Pharmacol Ther* 1996; **10**: 529–39.
190 Carling L, Axelsson CK, Forssell H *et al.* Lansoprazole and omeprazole in the prevention of relapse of reflux oesophagitis: a long-term comparative study. *Aliment Pharmacol Ther* 1998; **12**(10): 985–90.
191 Simon TJ, Roberts WG, Berlin RG *et al.* Acid suppression by famotidine 20mg twice daily or 40mg twice daily in preventing relapse of endoscopic recurrence of erosive esophagitis. *Clin Ther* 1995; **17**(6): 1147–56.
192 Bardhan KD, Cherian P, Vaishnavi A *et al.* Erosive oesophagitis: outcome of repeated long term maintenance treatment with low dose omeprazole 10 mg or placebo. *Gut* 1998; **43**(4): 458–64.
193 Robinson M, Lanza F, Avner D *et al.* Effective maintenance treatment of reflux esophagitis with low-dose lansoprazole. A randomized, double-blind, placebo-controlled trial. *Ann Intern Med* 1996; **124**(10): 859–67.
194 Sontag SJ, Robinson M, Roufail W *et al.* Daily omeprazole surpasses intermittent dosing in preventing relapse of oesophagitis: a US multi-centre double-blind study. *Aliment Pharmacol Ther* 1997; **11**: 373–80.
195 Dent J, Yeomans ND, MacKinnon M *et al.* Omeprazole v ranitidine for prevention of relapse in reflux oesophagitis. A controlled double blind trial of their efficacy and safety. *Gut* 1994; **35**: 590–8.
196 Hallerback B, Unge P, Carling L *et al.* Omeprazole or ranitidine in long-term treatment of reflux esophagitis. The Scandinavian Clinics for United Research Group. *Gastroenterology* 1994; **107**(5): 1305–11.
197 Bate CM, Booth SN, Crowe JP *et al.* Omeprazole 10 mg or 20 mg once daily in the prevention of recurrence of reflux oesophagitis. *Gut* 1995; **36**: 492–8.
198 Hatlebakk JG, Berstad A. Lansoprazole 15 and 30 mg daily in maintaining healing and symptom relief in patients with reflux oesophagitis. *Aliment Pharmacol Ther* 1997; **11**: 365–72.
199 Klinkenberg-Knol EC, Festen HPM, Jansen JBMJ *et al.* Long-term treatment with omeprazole for refractory reflux esophagitis: efficacy and safety. *Ann Int Med* 1994; **121**(3): 161–7.
200 Klinkenberg-Knol EC, for the International Long-Term Omeprazole Study Group. Eleven years' experience of continuous maintenance treatment with omeprazole in GERD-patients. *Gastroenterology* 1998; **114**(4): A180(G0735). (Abstract)
201 Sridhar S, Huang JQ, O'Brien BJ *et al.* Clinical economics review: cost-effectiveness of treatment alternatives for gasto-oesophageal reflux disease. *Aliment Pharmacol Ther* 1996; **10**: 865–73.
202 Sadowski D, Champion M, Goeree R *et al.* Health economics of gastroesophageal reflux disease. *Can J Gastroenterol* 1997; **11**(Suppl B): 108B–112B.
203 Bate CM. Cost-effectiveness of omeprazole in the treatment of reflux oesophagitis. *Br J Med Econ* 1991; **1**: 53–61.
204 Bate CM, Richardson PDI. A one year model for the cost-effectiveness of treating reflux oesophagitis. *Br J Med Econ* 1992; **2**: 5–11.
205 Bate CM, Richardson PDI. Symptomatic assessment and cost effectiveness of treatments for reflux oesophagitis: comparisons of omperazole and histamine H_2-receptor antagonists. *Br J Med Econ* 1992; **2**: 37–48.
206 Bate CM. Omeprazole vs Ranitidine and cimetidine in reflux oesophagitis: The British perspective. *PharmacoEconomics* 1994; **5**(Suppl 3): 35–43.
207 Hillman AL, Bloom BS, Fendrick AM *et al.* Cost and quality effects of alternative treatments for persistent gastroesophageal reflux disease. *Arch Intern Med* 1992; **152**: 1467–72.
208 Bloom BS. Cost and quality effects of treating erosive esophagitis: a re-evaluation. *PharmacoEconomics* 1995; **8**: 139–46.
209 Jones RH, Bosanquet N, Johnson NJ *et al.* Cost-effective management strategies for acid-peptic disorders. *Br J Med Econ* 1994; **7**: 99–114.
210 Zagari M, Villa KF, Freston JW. Proton pump inhibitors versus H_2-receptor antagonists for the treatment of erosive gastroesophageal reflux

disease: a cost-comparative study. *Am J Man Care* 1995; **1**: 247–55.

211 O'Brien BJ, Goeree R, Hunt R *et al. Economic evaluation of alternative therapies in the long term management of peptic ulcer disease and gastroesophageal reflux disease. 1996*. McMaster University. Canadian Coordinating Office of Health Technology Assessment (CCOHTA) report 1996.

212 Jönsson B, Stålhammar NO. The cost-effectiveness of omeprazole and ranitidine in intermittent and maintenance treatment of reflux oesophagitis – the case of Sweden. *Br J Med Econ* 1993; **6**: 111–26.

213 Harris RA, Kuppermann M, Richter JE. Proton pump inhibitors or histamine-2 receptor antagonists for the prevention of recurrences of erosive reflux esophagitis: a cost-effectiveness analysis. *Am J Gastroenterol* 1997; **92**(12): 2179–87.

214 Harris RA, Kuppermann M, Richter JE. Prevention of recurrences of erosive reflux esophagitis: a cost-effectiveness analysis of maintenance proton pump inhibition. *Am J Med* 1997; **102**(1): 78–88.

215 Eggleston A, Wigerinck A, Huijghebaert S *et al.* Cost effectiveness of treatment for gastro-oesophageal reflux disease in clinical practice: a clinical database analysis. *Gut* 1998; **42**: 13–16.

216 Ware JEJ, Sherbourne CD. The MOS 36–item short–form health survey (SF–36). I. Conceptual framework and item selection. *Med Care* 1992; **30**(6): 473–83.

217 Dupuy HJ. The Psychological General Well–Being (PGWB) index. In: Wenger NK, Mattson ME, Furberg CF, Elinson J (eds). *Assessment of quality of life in clinical trials of cardiovascular therapies*, New York, Le Jacq Publishing Inc., 1984, pp 170–83.

218 Dimenas E, Glise H, Hallerback B *et al.* Well–being and gastrointestinal symptoms among patients referred to endoscopy owing to suspected duodenal ulcer. *Scand J Gastroenterol* 1995; **30**: 1046–52.

219 Lind T, Havelund T, Carlsson R *et al.* Heartburn without oesophagitis: efficacy of omeprazole therapy and features determining therapeutic response. *Scand J Gastroenterol* 1997; **32**: 974–9.

220 Revicki DA, Wood M, Wiklund I *et al.* Reliability and validity of the Gastrointestinal Symptom Rating Scale in patients with gastroesophageal reflux disease. *Qual Life Res* 1998; **7**(1): 75–83.

221 Wiklund IK, Junghard O, Grace E *et al.* Quality of life in reflux and dyspepsia patients. Psychometric documentation of a new disease-specific questionnaire (QOLRAD). *Eur J Surg* 1998; Suppl 583: 41–9.

222 Stewart AL, Greenfield S, Hays RD *et al.* Functional status and well-being of patients with chronic conditions: results from the medical outcomes study. *JAMA* 1989; **262**: 907–13.

223 Dimenas E. Methodological aspects of evaluation of quality of life in upper gastrointestinal disease. *Scand J Gastroenterol* 1993; **28**: 18–21.

224 Dimenas E, Glise H, Hallerback B *et al.* Quality of life in patients with upper gastrointestinal symptoms: an improved evaluation of treatment regimens? *Scand J Gastroenterol* 1993; **28**: 681–7.

225 Dimenas E, Carlsson R, Glise H *et al.* Relevance of norm values as part of the documentation of quality of life instruments for use in upper gastrointestinal diseases. *Scand J Gastroenterol* 1996; **31**(Suppl 221): 8–13.

226 Mathias SD, Castell DO, Elkin EP *et al.* Health-related quality of life of patients with acute erosive esophagitis. *Dig Dis Sci* 1996; **41**(11): 2123–9.

227 Wiklund I, Bardhan KD, Müller LS *et al.* Quality of life during acute and intermittent treatment of gastro-oesophageal reflux disease with omeprazole compared with ranitidine. Results from a multicentre clinical trial. The European Study Group. *Ital J Gastroenterol Hepatol* 1998; **30**(1): 19–27.

228 Dettmer A, Vogt R, Sielaff F *et al.* Pantoprazole 20 mg is effective for relief of symptoms and healing of lesions in mild reflux oesophagitis. *Aliment Pharmacol Ther* 1998; **12**(9): 865–72.

229 Hungin APS, Gunn SD, Bate CM *et al.* A comparison of the efficacy of omeprazole 20mg once daily with ranitidine 150mg bd in the relief of symptomatic gastro-oesophageal reflux disease in general practice. *Br J Clin Res* 1993; **4**: 73–88.

230 Rush DR, Stelmach WJ, Young TL *et al.* Clinical effectiveness and quality of life with ranitidine vs placebo in gastroesophageal reflux disease patients: a clinical experience network (CEN) study. *J Fam Pract* 1995; **41**(2): 126–36.

231 Venables TL, Newland RD, Patel AC *et al.* Maintenance treatment for gastro-oesophageal reflux disease. A placebo-controlled evaluation of 10 milligrams omeprazole once daily in general practice. *Scand J Gastroenterol* 1997; **32**: 627–32.

232 Carlsson R, Dent J, Watts R *et al.* and the International GORD Study Group. Gastro-oesophageal reflux disease in primary care: an international study of different treatment strategies with omeprazole. *Eur J Gastroenterol Hepatol* 1998; **10**: 119–24.

233 Bardhan KD, Müller-Lissner SA, Bigard MA *et al.* for the European Study Group. Symptomatic

gastroesophageal reflux disease (GERD): intermittent treatment (IT) with omeprazole (OM) and ranitidine (RAN) as a strategy for management. *Gastroenterology* 1997; **112**(4): A65 (abstract).

234 Bardhan KD, Müller-Lissner SA, Bigard MA et al. for the European Study Group. Cost-effectiveness (CE) of omeprazole (OM) and ranitidine (RAN) in intermittent treatment (IT) of symptomatic gastroesophageal reflux disease (GERD). *Gastroenterology* 1997; **112**(4): A65 (abstract).

235 Champault G, Volter F, Rizk N *et al.* Gastroesophageal reflux: conventional surgical treatment versus laparoscopy. A prospective study of 61 cases. *Surg Laparosc Endosc* 1996; **6**(6): 434–40.

236 Eshraghi N, Farahmand M, Soot SJ *et al.* Comparison of outcomes of open versus laparoscopic Nissen fundoplication performed in a single practice. *Am J Surg* 1998; **175**(5): 371–4.

237 Peters JH, Heimbucher J, Kauer WK, Incarbone R, Bremner CG, DeMeester TR. Clinical and physiologic comparison of laparoscopic and open Nissen fundoplication. *J Am Coll Surg* 1995; **180**(4): 385–93.

238 Jones R, Canal DF, Inman MM *et al.* Laparoscopic fundoplication: a three-year review. *Am Surg* 1996; **62**(8): 632–6.

239 Laine S, Rantala A, Gullichsen R *et al.* Laparoscopic vs conventional Nissen fundoplication. A prospective randomized study. *Surg Endosc* 1997; **11**(5): 441–4.

240 Blomqvist AM, Lönroth H, Dalenbäck J *et al.* Laparoscopic or open fundoplication? A complete cost analysis. *Surg Endosc* 1998; **12**(10): 1209–12.

241 Blomqvist A, Lönroth H, Dalenbäck J *et al.* Quality of life assessment after laparoscopic and open fundoplications. Results of a prospective, clinical study. *Scand J Gastroenterol* 1996; **31**(11): 1052–8.

242 Watson DI, Jamieson GG. Antireflux surgery in the laparoscopic era. *Br J Surg* 1998; **85**(9): 1173–84.

243 Bell RCW, Hanna P, Powers B *et al.* Clinical and manometric results of laparoscopic partial (Toupet) and complete (Rosetti–Nissen) fundoplication. *Surg Endosc* 1996; **10**(7): 724–8.

244 Anvari M, Allen CJ. Prospective evaluation of dysphagia before and after laparoscopic Nissen fundoplication without routine division of short gastrics. *Surg Laparosc Endosc* 1996; **6**(6): 424–9.

245 Luostarinen M, Isolauri J, Laitinen J *et al.* Fate of Nissen fundoplication after 20 years. A clinical, endoscopical, and functional analysis. *Gut* 1993; **34**(8): 1015–20.

246 Low DE, Anderson RP, Ilves R *et al.* Fifteen– to twenty-year results after the Hill antireflux operation. *J Thorac Cardiovasc Surg* 1989; **98**(3): 444–9.

247 Laws HL, Clements RH, Swillie CM. A randomized, prospective comparison of the Nissen fundoplication versus the Toupet fundoplication for gastroesophageal reflux disease. *Ann Surg* 1997; **225**(6): 647–53.

248 Jobe BA, Wallace J, Hansen PD *et al.* Evaluation of laparoscopic Toupet fundoplication as a primary repair for all patients with medically resistant gastroesophageal reflux. *Surg Endosc* 1997; **11**(11): 1080–3.

249 Watson A. Update: total versus partial laparoscopic fundoplication. *Dig Surg* 1998; **15**(2): 172–80.

250 Trus TL, Laycock WS, Wo JM *et al.* Laparoscopic antireflux surgery in the elderly. *Am J Gastroenterol* 1998; **93**(3): 351–3.

251 Behar J, Sheahan DG, Biancani P *et al.* Medical and surgical management of reflux esophagitis. A 38-month report of a prospective clinical trial. *N Engl J Med* 1975; **293**(6): 263–8.

252 Spechler SJ. Comparison of medical and surgical therapy for complicated gastroesophageal reflux disease in veterans. The Department of Veterans Affairs Gastroesophageal Reflux Disease Study Group. *N Engl J Med* 1992; **326**: 786–92.

253 Lundell L, Dalenbäck J, Hattlebakk J *et al.* Omeprazole (OME) or antireflux surgery (ARS) in the long term management of gastroesophageal reflux disease (GERD): results of a multicentre, randomized clinical trial. *Gastroenterology* 1998; **114**(4): A207(G0848). (Abstract)

254 Viljakka M, Nevalainen J, Isolauri J. Lifetime costs of surgical versus medical treatment of severe gastro-oesophageal reflux disease in Finland. *Scand J Gastroenterol* 1997; **32**(8): 766–72.

255 Van den Boom G, Go PMMYH, Hameeteman W *et al.* Cost effectiveness of medical versus surgical treatment in patients with severe or refractory gastroesophageal reflux disease in the Netherlands. *Scand J Gastroenterol* 1996; **31**: 1–9.

256 Stein HJ, Siewert JR. Barrett's esophagus: pathogenesis, epidemiology, functional abnormalities, malignant degeneration, and surgical management. *Dysphagia* 1993; **8**(3): 276–88.

257 Spechler SJ, Goyal RK. Barrett's esophagus. *N Engl J Med* 1986; **315**(6): 362–71.

258 Haggitt RC. Barrett's esophagus, dysplasia, and adenocarcinoma. *Hum Pathol* 1994; **25**(10): 982–93.

259 Gottfried MR, McClave SA, Boyce HW. Incomplete intestinal metaplasia in the

diagnosis of columnar lined esophagus (Barrett's esophagus). *Am J Clin Pathol* 1939; **92**(6): 741–6.

260 Pera M, Cameron AJ, Trastek VF *et al.* Increasing incidence of adenocarcinoma of the esophagus and esophagogastric junction. *Gastroenterology* 1993; **104**(2): 510–13.

261 Schnell TG, Sontag SJ, Chejfec G. Adenocarcinomas arising in tongues or short segments of Barrett's esophagus. *Dig Dis Sci* 1992; **37**(1): 137–43.

262 Cameron AJ, Lomboy CT, Pera M *et al.* Adenocarcinoma of the esophagogastric junction and Barrett's esophagus. *Gastroenterology* 1995; **109**(5): 1541–6.

263 Hamilton SR, Smith RR, Cameron JL. Prevalence and characteristics of Barrett esophagus in patients with adenocarcinoma of the esophagus or esophagogastric junction. *Hum Pathol* 1988; **19**(8): 942–8.

264 Clark GW, Smyrk TC, Burdiles P *et al.* Is Barrett's metaplasia the source of adenocarcinomas of the cardia? *Arch Surg* 1994; **129**(6): 609–14.

265 Thompson JJ, Zinsser KR, Enterline HT. Barrett's metaplasia and adenocarcinoma of the esophagus and gastroesophageal junction. *Hum Pathol* 1983; **14**(1): 42–61.

266 Skinner DB, Walther BC, Riddell RH *et al.* Barrett's esophagus. Comparison of benign and malignant cases. *Ann Surg* 1983; **198**(4): 554–65.

267 Hamilton SR, Smith RR. The relationship between columnar epithelial dysplasia and invasive adenocarcinoma arising in Barrett's esophagus. *Am J Clin Pathol* 1987; **87**(3): 301–12.

268 Cameron AJ, Zinsmeister AR, Ballard DJ *et al.* Prevalence of columnar-lined (Barrett's) esophagus. Comparison of population-based clinical and autopsy findings. *Gastroenterology* 1990; **99**(4): 918–22.

269 Cameron AJ, Lomboy CT. Barrett's esophagus: age, prevalence, and extent of columnar epithelium. *Gastroenterology* 1992; **103**(4): 1241–5.

270 Gruppo Operativo per lo Studio delle Precancerosi dell'Esofago (GOSPE). Barrett's esophagus: epidemiological and clinical results of a multicentric survey. *Int J Cancer* 1991; **48**(3): 364–8.

271 Sarr MG, Hamilton SR, Marrone GC et al. Barrett's esophagus: its prevalence and association with adenocarcinoma in patients with symptoms of gastroesophageal reflux. *Am J Surg* 1985; **149**(1): 187–93.

272 Blustein PK, Beck PL, Meddings JB *et al.* The utility of endoscopy in the management of patients with gastroesophageal reflux symptoms. *Am J Gastroenterol* 1998; **93**(12): 2508–12.

273 Spechler SJ, Zeroogian JM, Antonioli DA *et al.* Prevalence of metaplasia at the gastro-oesophageal junction. *Lancet* 1994; **344**(8936): 1533–6.

274 Nandurkar S, Talley NJ, Martin CJ *et al.* Short segment Barrett's oesophagus: prevalence, diagnosis and associations. *Gut* 1997; **40**(6): 710–15.

275 DeMeester TR, Attwood SE, Smyrk TC *et al.* Surgical therapy in Barrett's esophagus. *Ann Surg* 1990; **212**(4): 528–40.

276 Bozymski EM, Herlihy KJ, Orlando RC. Barrett's esophagus. *Ann Intern Med* 1982; **97**(1): 103–7.

277 Winters CJ, Spurling TJ, Chobanian SJ *et al.* Barrett's esophagus. A prevalent, occult complication of gastroesophageal reflux disease. *Gastroenterology* 1987; **92**(1): 118–24.

278 Fink MA, Martin CJ, Ewing HP *et al.* A longitudinal study of the development of experimental Barrett's esophagus in the dog. *Gastroenterology* 1991; **100**(5): A825. (Abstract)

279 Pollness CM, Martin CJ, Ewing HP *et al.* Bile affects the pattern of metaplasia in experimental columnar lined esophagus (CLE). *Gastroenterology* 1993; **104**(4): A173. (Abstract)

280 Martin CJ, Shaw ME, Ewing HP *et al.* Pancreatic reflux produces intestinal metaplasia in experimental columnar lined oesophagus. *Aust NZ J Surg* 1995; **65**: A422. (Abstract)

281 Nakano K, Sato H, Kimura T *et al.* An experimental model of Barrett's esophagus by jejunoesophageal reflux. *Gastroenterology* 1996; **110**(4): A206. (Abstract)

282 Cameron AJ, Ott BJ, Payne WS. The incidence of adenocarcinoma in columnar-lined (Barrett's) esophagus. *N Engl J Med* 1985; **313**(14): 857–9.

283 Williamson WA, Ellis FHJ, Gibb SP *et al.* Barrett's esophagus. Prevalence and incidence of adenocarcinoma. *Arch Intern Med* 1991; **151**(11): 2212–16.

284 Drewitz DJ, Sampliner RE, Garewal HS. The incidence of adenocarcinoma in Barrett's esophagus: a prospective study of 170 patients followed 4.8 years. *Am J Gastroenterol* 1997; **92**(2): 212–15.

285 Van der Veen AH, Dees J, Blankensteijn JD *et al.* Adenocarcinoma in Barrett's oesophagus: an overrated risk. *Gut* 1989; **30**(1): 14–18.

286 Dent J, Bremner CG, Collen MJ *et al.* Barrett's oesophagus. *J Gastroenterol Hepatol* 1991; **6**(1): 1–22.

287 Cameron AJ. Barrett's esophagus: does the incidence of adenocarcinoma matter? *Am J Gastroenterol* 1997; **92**(2): 193–4.

288 Kahrilas PJ. It's not the American way—yet. *Am J Gastroenterol* 1994; **89**(5): 657–8.

289 Spechler SJ. Endoscopic surveillance for patients with Barrett esophagus: does the cancer risk justify the practice? *Ann Intern Med* 1987; **106**(6): 902–4.
290 Streitz JMJ, Andrews CWJ, Ellis FHJ. Endoscopic surveillance of Barrett's esophagus. Does it help? *J Thorac Cardiovasc Surg* 1993; **105**(3): 383–7.
291 Achkar E, Carey W. The cost of surveillance for adenocarcinoma complicating Barrett's esophagus. *Am J Gastroenterol* 1988; **83**(3): 291–4.
292 Provenzale D, Kemp JA, Arora S *et al*. A guide for surveillance of patients with Barrett's esophagus. *Am J Gastroenterol* 1994; **89**(5): 670–80.
293 Nandurkar S, Talley NJ. Barrett's esophagus: the long and the short of it. *Am J Gastroenterol* 1999; **94**(1): 30–40.
294 Reid BJ, Sanchez CA, Blount PL *et al*. Barrett's esophagus: cell cycle abnormalities in advancing stages of neoplastic progression. *Gastroenterology* 1993; **105**(1): 119–29.
295 Reid BJ, Barrett MT, Galipeau PC *et al*. Barrett's esophagus: ordering the events that lead to cancer. *Eur J Cancer Prev* 1996; **5** (Suppl 2): 57–65.
296 McArdle JE, Lewin KJ, Randall G *et al*. Distribution of dysplasias and early invasive carcinoma in Barrett's esophagus. *Hum Pathol* 1992; **23**(5): 479–82.
297 Miros M, Kerlin P, Walker N. Only patients with dysplasia progress to adenocarcinoma in Barrett's oesophagus. *Gut* 1991; **32**(12): 1441–6.
298 Hameeteman W, Tytgat GN, Houthoff HJ *et al*. Barrett's esophagus: development of dysplasia and adenocarcinoma. *Gastroenterolgy* 1989; **96**(5): 1249–56.
299 Wright TA, Gray MR, Morris AI *et al*. Cost effectiveness of detecting Barrett's cancer. *Gut* 1996; **39**(4): 574–9.
300 Daly JM, Karnell LH, Menck HR. National Cancer Data Base report on esophageal carcinoma. *Cancer* 1996; **78**(8): 1820–8.
301 Blot WJ, Devesa SS, Kneller RW *et al*. Rising incidence of adenocarcinoma of the esophagus and gastric cardia. *JAMA* 1991; **265**(10): 1287–9.
302 Blot WJ, Devesa SS, Fraumeni JFJ. Continuing climb in rates of esophageal adenocarcinoma: an update. *JAMA* 1993; **270**(11): 1320.
303 Ovaska J, Miettinen M, Kivilaakso E. Adenocarcinoma arising in Barrett's esophagus. *Dig Dis Sci* 1989; **34**(9): 1336–9.
304 van der Burgh A, Dees J, Hop WCJ *et al*. Oesophageal cancer is an uncommon cause of death in patients with Barrett's oesophagus. *Gut* 1996; **39**: 5–8.
305 Bytzer P, Christensen PB, Damkier P *et al*. Adenocarcinoma of the esophagus and Barrett's esophagus: a population-based study. *Am J Gastroenterol* 1999; **94**(1): 86–91.
306 Beck IT, Champion MC, Lemire S *et al*. The Second Canadian Consensus Conference on the Management of Patients with Gastroesophageal Reflux Disease. *Can J Gastroenterol* 1997; **11**(Suppl B): 7B–20B.
307 Hunt RH. Importance of pH control in the management of GERD. *Arch Intern Med* 1999; **159**: 649–57.
308 Neumann CS, Iqbal TH, Cooper BT. Long term continuous omeprazole treatment of patients with Barrett's oesophagus. *Aliment Pharmacol Ther* 1995; **9**(4): 451–4.
309 Sontag SJ, Schnell TG, Chejfec G *et al*. Lansoprazole heals erosive reflux oesophagitis in patients with Barrett's oesophagus. *Aliment Pharmacol Ther* 1997; **11**(1): 147–56.
310 Sampliner RE. Effect of up to 3 years of high-dose lansoprazole on Barrett's esophagus. *Am J Gastroenterol* 1994; **89**(10): 1844–8.
311 Lamers CB. The changing role of H2-receptor antagonists in acid-related diseases. *Eur J Gastroenterol Hepatol* 1996; **8** Suppl 1: S3–S7.
312 Katzka DA, Castell DO. Successful elimination of reflux symptoms does not insure adequate control of acid reflux in patients with Barrett' s esophagus. *Am J Gastroenterol* 1994; **89**(7): 989–991.
313 Sharma P, Sampliner RE, Camargo E. Normalization of esophageal pH with high-dose proton pump inhibitor therapy does not result in regression of Barrett's esophagus. *Am J Gastroenterology* 1997; **92**(4): 582–585.
314 Ouatu Lascar R., Triadafilopoulos G. Complete elimination of reflux symptoms does not guarantee normalization of intraesophageal acid reflux in patients with Barrett's esophagus. *Am J Gastroenterol* 1998; **93**(5): 711–716.
315 Gore S, Healey CJ, Sutton R *et al*. Regression of columnar lined (Barrett's) oesophagus with continuous omeprazole therapy. *Aliment Pharmacol Ther* 1993; **7**(6): 623–628.
316 Deviere J, Buset M, Dumonceau JM *et al*. Regression of Barrett's epithelium with omeprazole. *N Engl J Med* 1989; **320**(22): 1497–8.
317 Sampliner RE, Garewal HS, Fennerty MB *et al*. Lack of impact of therapy on extent of Barrett's esophagus in 67 patients. *Dig Dis Sci* 1990; **35**(1): 93–6.
318 Sampliner RE, Hixson LJ, Fennerty MB *et al*. Regression of Barrett's esophagus by laser ablation in an antacid environment. *Dig Dis Sci* 1993; **38**(2): 365–8.

319 Sampliner RE, Steinbronn K, Garewal HS *et al.* Squamous mucosa overlying columnar epithelium in Barrett' s esophagus in the absence of anti-reflux surgery. *Am J Gastroenterol* 1988; **83**(5): 510–12.
320 Riddell RH. The biopsy diagnosis of gastroesophageal reflux disease, "carditis," and Barrett's esophagus, and sequelae of therapy. *Am J Surg Pathol* 1996; **20**(Suppl 1): S31–S50.
321 Low DE, Levine DS, Dail DH *et al.* Histological and anatomic changes in Barrett's esophagus after antireflux surgery. *Am J Gastroenterol* 1999; **94**(1): 80–5.
322 Ortiz A, Martinez de Haro LF, Parrilla P *et al.* Conservative treatment versus antireflux surgery in Barrett' s oesophagus: long-term results of a prospective study. *Br J Surg* 1996; **83**(2): 274 8.
323 Barham CP, Jones RL, Biddlestone LR *et al.* Photothermal laser ablation of Barrett's oesophagus: endoscopic and histological evidence of squamous re-epithelialisation. *Gut* 1997; **41**(3): 281–4.
324 Salo JA, Salminen JT, Kiviluoto TA *et al.* SP. Treatment of Barrett's esophagus by endoscopic laser ablation and antireflux surgery. *Ann Surg* 1998; **227**(1): 40–4.

3 Ulcer disease and *Helicobacter pylori* infection: etiology and treatment

NAOKI CHIBA, RICHARD H HUNT

INTRODUCTION

Peptic ulcer disease, particularly duodenal ulcer disease, has long been thought to result from gastric acid hypersecretion and pepsin damage. Indeed Schwarz's dictum,[1] "no acid, no ulcer" is still relevant. Peptic ulcers were thought to be caused by a variety of factors, such as smoking, stress, and non-steroidal anti-inflammatory drugs (NSAIDs), including aspirin. Therapy was directed primarily against lowering acid production in the stomach to permit healing of ulceration. However, the discovery and characterization of intragastric infection with *Helicobacter pylori* has revolutionized our concepts of pathogenesis and ulcer therapy. As duodenal ulcer has long been thought to result from an imbalance between protective and aggressive factors in the mucosa, *H. pylori* can be considered an "aggressive" factor which may tip the balance toward mucosal damage and result in ulceration. Thus, the assignment of an etiological role to *H. pylori* does not contradict the traditional concepts, but rather extends them.

Warren and Marshall's seminal paper in 1983[2] first identified the spiral bacterium that is now known as *Helicobacter pylori*, associated with active chronic gastritis. Their subsequent paper[3] determined an association between the gastric infection and peptic ulcer, particularly duodenal ulcers, in which 100% of their patients had *H. pylori* present in antral biopsies.

Initial skepticism to the general acceptance of this infection as an important pathogen has been dispelled with increasing evidence. This chapter reviews and presents the evidence for the etiological role of *H. pylori* in peptic ulcer disease and summarizes the evidence for effective treatments for ulcer disease based on the approach of eradication of the infection. To accomplish this, individual studies and published reviews and summaries were identified through electronic searching of Medline and recursive searching of journal articles. References are mainly to published papers, but relevant data from recent studies presented in abstracts are also presented.

APPROACH TO THIS PROBLEM

What is the evidence for the role of *H. pylori* in peptic ulcer disease? One approach would be to determine whether "Koch's postulates" to link this infectious agent with disease(s) are fulfilled. The postulates state that the "agent (1) must be found in patients with the disease only, (2) must be grown outside of the body, (3) when inoculated into a susceptible animal, must cause the same disease, and (4) must be grown from the lesions observed".[4]

Many of the organisms currently accepted as pathogens do not necessarily fit all of Koch's postulates. Furthermore, there is limited applicability to chronic disease such as that caused by *H. pylori* infection.[5] A more applicable approach is to use the criteria for assessing epidemiological evidence, as outlined by Hill.[6]

An early methodological review[5] concluded that there was insufficient evidence in 1990 to establish *H. pylori* as a cause of duodenal ulcer. Since then, much new evidence has accumulated and is summarized in Table 3.1 below.

ASSOCIATION OF *H. PYLORI* WITH ULCER DISEASE (STRENGTH, CONSISTENCY, AND SPECIFICITY)

Here we consider the prevalence of *H. pylori* in both duodenal (DU) and gastric (GU) ulcer patients.

Duodenal ulcer

The prevalence of *H. pylori* in ulcer disease has been well reviewed by Kuipers *et al*,[7] who identified relevant studies published since the discovery of *H. pylori* in 1983. In the decade to 1993 they found that infection with *H. pylori* was present in 94.9% (95% CI, 94–96%) of 1695 DU patients studied. Borody *et al* found *H. pylori* in 94% of 302 DU patients in Australia.[8] Of the 14 patients who were negative for *H. pylori* at the time of endoscopy, 4 had taken antibiotics shortly before endoscopy and may have had false negative results, and 8 had NSAID induced ulcers. Overall, only 1 of 302 patients had no cause for DU identified. Thus, almost all DU which are not caused by NSAIDs are attributable to *H. pylori*. There are relatively few reports of *H. pylori* negative DU.[8–11] A summary rate of up to 6% has been suggested.[12] However, there is recent evidence to suggest that the prevalence of *H. pylori* negative DU may be increasing.[13–16] One American study identified *H. pylori* infection in only 62% of DU and 44% of GU patients.[16] No reason for these low *H. pylori* prevalence rates was offered. Most DU recurrences after eradication of *H. pylori* are related to NSAIDs[17] but a smaller number may be related to high acid output.[18]

A strong association by itself, does not prove causality.[4,5] While the association of *H. pylori* with DU is strong and consistent, it is not specific, since *H. pylori* is also found in many patients without ulcer disease. The reasons why *H. pylori* causes disease in a minority of patients infected with the organism are not yet known. This question is the subject of intense ongoing research.

Gastric ulcer

There are fewer studies on the role of *H. pylori* in GU and NSAIDs play an important role in their etiology. *H. pylori* infection is diagnosed in 60–100% of GU patients (mean about 70%).[7,19]. As Thijs *et al* point out,[19] many of the earlier studies suffered methodological problems that probably led to an underestimate of the prevalence of *H. pylori* in GU disease. Most GU are associated with *H. pylori* related active chronic gastritis whether or not NSAIDs are involved.[19–21] However, up to 11% may have no identifiable cause.[21] The

Table 3.1 Evidence for role of *H. pylori* in peptic ulcer dise (PUD) according to Hill's criteria

Association (strength, consistency, specificity) of *H. pylori* with PUD
prevalence of *H. pylori* in DU ~90%, GU ~80%
strength and *consistency* of association is high
specificity is low as *H. pylori* seen in many without ulcers
overall, data are supportive

Temporal relationship: does *H. pylori* infection precede PUD?
self administration of *H. pylori* shown to cause active chronic gastritis – fulfills one of Koch's postulates
but, no direct evidence that PUD is caused
case–control study (Nomura[22]) shows preceding *H. pylori* infection increases risk of DU, GU, and gastric cancer
cohort study (Sipponen[25]) >10% *H. pylori* positives developed DU over 10 years but <1% if *H. pylori* negative
thus, data are supportive

Biological gradient
no consistent data to support correlation of higher levels of bacterial load with PUD

Biological plausibility
numerous plausible pathophysiological alterations (see text) that include:
vacA causing epithelial cell damage – not consistent
cagA associations with disease states such as DU, gastric cancer, and MALTomas – not consistent or universally seen
elevated gastrin and acid secretion that revert to normal after *H. pylori* eradication
numerous alterations in mucosal cytokines
thus, data are supportive

Effects of interventions: outcomes following *H. pylori* eradication
alterations in natural history of PUD disease with *H. pylori* eradication provides strongest evidence that *H. pylori* is a true pathogen. RCT data of *H. pylori* eradication shows:
DU and GU relapse effectively prevented
DU and GU heal with eradication of *H. pylori* infection alone without ulcer healing drugs
DU heal faster when *H. pylori* eradicated than with ulcer healing drugs alone
DU refractory to ulcer healing drugs can heal if *H. pylori* eradicated
re-bleeding from ulcers can be prevented
thus, data are strongly supportive

Coherence of *H. pylori* data with previous epidemiological data
consistent historical correlations between presumed *H. pylori* prevalence, ulcer disease prevalences, death rates and perforations from ulcer disease
improvements in hygiene and sanitation in industrialized nations have resulted in declining prevalence of both *H. pylori* and ulcer disease
prevalence of *H. pylori* infection and ulcer disease have become the same in males/females
thus, data are supportive

study by Nomura[22] also showed that prior infection with *H. pylori* increased the risk that the patient may develop GU subsequently.

Thus, overall, *H. pylori* is present in more than 90% of DU and 80% of GU.[23] *H. pylori* negative ulcers are commonly caused by NSAIDs.[19] Furthermore, the proportion of *H. pylori* negative ulcers increases as the overall prevalence of *H. pylori* infection falls.[15,16]

TEMPORAL RELATIONSHIP

Whether *H. pylori* infection precedes the development of ulcer disease cannot be assessed by retrospective, point prevalence studies, since it is impossible to assess retrospectively when these patients were infected.[5]

Marshall[24] described three "self-administration" experiments in humans. In these cases active chronic gastritis ensued, fulfilling one of Koch's postulates for at least the first step in the development of peptic ulceration, although actual ulcer disease did not develop.

The temporal relationship between infection with *H. pylori* and the development of DU has been best proven in a cohort study reported by Sipponen *et al.*[25] Of the 321 patients with *H. pylori* at study entry, 34 developed a DU over the next 10 years while only 1 of 133 *H. pylori* negative patients developed an ulcer.

An IgG serological nested case–control study of a group of 5443 Japanese-American men with stored sera obtained between 1967 and 1970 demonstrated that pre-existing *H. pylori* infection increased the subsequent risk of developing either DU or GU disease over a surveillance period of greater than 20 years.[22] The odds ratio for development of ulcer was 4.0 (95% CI 1.1–14.2) for DU and 3.2 (CI 1.6–6.5) for GU. The relationship was statistically significant even when the ulcer diagnosis was first made 10 or more years after the serum sample had been obtained. A further analysis of this Hawaiian cohort[26] identified that *H. pylori* infected men of higher birth order had an increased risk of GU (OR 1.64) but not DU. Those *H. pylori* infected men from larger sibships (OR 2.06) and higher birth order (OR 1.67) were at increased risk of developing gastric cancer. These data are consistent with the hypothesis that early infection with *H. pylori* increases the risk of developing gastric ulcer and cancer.

BIOLOGICAL GRADIENT

Showing a higher bacterial load in the stomach of patients with ulcers vs those without an ulcer would be good evidence supporting a causative role.[4] In biopsy studies, there has been insufficient gastric mucosal sampling to assess whether there was a biological gradient present.[5] It is problematical to rely on biopsy specimens due to sampling error. A test such as a urea breath test (UBT) may be more useful in this regard. Ingested urea is digested by bacterial urease activity with the labeled CO_2 breakdown product being excreted in the breath. Significant correlation has been observed between labeled CO_2 excretion in the breath and intragastric bacterial load[27,28] and mucosal inflammation.[27–29] However, there has not been consistent correlation with endoscopic findings.[27] Most of the available literature did not find a correlation of endoscopic findings with higher UBT values, and authors did not report whether the finding of higher test results predicted the finding of a duodenal ulcer.[30–32] Thus, data supporting a relationship between a higher load of *H. pylori* and ulcer development are limited.

BIOLOGICAL PLAUSIBILITY

H. pylori is an unique bacterium that has evolved ecologically to survive and persist in the harsh acidic environment of the stomach. Bacterial urease, flagellar motility, and surface adhesins appear necessary for colonization.[33] Despite its high prevalence of infection, not all infected persons develop disease, and most remain asymptomatic. Are there more virulent strains that predispose to disease states? The vacuolating cytotoxin (*vacA*) which causes surface epithelial cell damage and vacuolation of epithelial cells has not been found consistently to correlate with disease states.[33] The *cagA* protein is a marker of the *cag* pathogenicity island of *H. pylori* and several studies have determined that in developed countries, DU, intestinal metaplasia, gastric carcinoma, and mucosa-associated lymphoid tissue (MALT) lymphoma are more commonly seen in patients infected with a *cagA* positive strains.[33] However, this relationship is not universally seen in all ethnic origins.

If *H. pylori* is primarily an *intragastric* infection, how does it cause ulcers in the duodenal bulb? Observations prior to and after the discovery of *H. pylori* identified that patients with DU had gastric metaplasia in the duodenal bulb.[34–39] This change is thought to arise as a result of hypersecretion of acid as observed in DU patients. The gastric metaplasia may[40–42] or may not[43] improve after *H. pylori* eradication. Patients infected with *H. pylori* have increased basal and stimulated gastrin release irrespective of whether they have DU disease or not.[44–46] The elevated gastric acid secretion also results in increased postprandial duodenal acid load.[47] Furthermore, *H. pylori* eradication[48,49] or suppression[50] results in normalization of these gastrin levels in most subjects, with lowering of acid secretion.[44,48] However, a subset of patients with recurrent duodenal ulcer have persistently high acid secretion despite *H. pylori* eradication.[51] Once gastric metaplasia occurs, *H. pylori* can colonize islands of gastric metaplasia in the duodenum. Numerous toxigenic factors have been identified by which *H. pylori* might cause mucosal damage, although there is no one pathophysiological factor accepted as being pathognomonic. Adhesion of *H. pylori* to epithelial cells results in elevated levels of mucosal cytokines such as IL-8 which is increased in the mucosa of *H. pylori* infected patients.[52] Of interest is the observation that *cagA* positive strains are associated with higher levels of TNF-α, IL-1β, IL-6, IL-8, and corresponding inflammation (active chronic gastritis) in the gastric mucosa.[53] A T-helper subtype 1 (Th1) proinflammatory cytokine response may predominate in ulcer disease whereas a mixed Th1/Th2 pattern predominates in those with chronic gastritis but no ulcer.[54] There may be a link between increased IL-8 and gastrin release that is potentiated by *H. pylori* sonicates.[55] Thus, there are mutifactorial plausible mechanisms by which *H. pylori* may cause pathogenic effects.

EFFECT OF INTERVENTIONS ON ULCER HEALING AND *H. PYLORI* ERADICATION

Healing of duodenal ulcer with acid suppressive therapy

Treatment of duodenal ulcer in the era before *H. pylori* was revolutionized by H_2-receptor antagonists, and subsequently, proton pump inhibitors (PPI) whose effects were proven in placebo controlled trials. Numerous methodologically sound, double-blind randomized controlled trials using comparative healing rates of endoscopically proven ulcers as the outcome measure have established that PPI heal ulcers faster than H_2-blockers and also provide more rapid symptom relief.[56–62]

R
Grade A

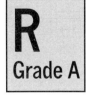

For this chapter the literature was reviewed and summary results of the systematic review of 21 such randomized controlled trials is presented in Table 3.2.[56–76] PPI heal more completely and faster than an H_2-blocker at both 2 and 4 weeks (Table 3.2).

Table 3.2 Systematic review of duodenal ulcer healing proportions at 2 and 4 weeks from comparative trials of a proton pump inhibitor (PPI) vs H_2-receptor antagonist (H_2RA)

Assessment of healing	Ulcers healed with PPI (%)	Ulcers healed with H_2RA (%)	% ARR (95% CI)	NNT
2 weeks	67.1	47.2	19.9 (15.6–24.2)	5
4 weeks	91.9	81.4	10.4 (7.7–3.1)	10

Systematic review of 21 trials in which PPI (omeprazole, lansoprazole, pantoprazole) were directly compared against an H_2-receptor antagonist (cimetidine, ranitidine, famotidine) in standard doses.

Table 3.3 Benefits of maintenance therapy with H_2-receptor antagonists

Ulcer recurrence once healed

With no maintenance therapy – 6 month recurrence 56%, 12 month >74%[83,84]
With H_2-receptor antagonist maintenance therapy – between 20 and 30% ulcer recurrence[82,86,87]
Ranitidine 300 mg hs approximately twice as effective as 150 mg hs, especially in smokers[89]

Prevention of recurrent ulcer hemorrhage

Cohort study: In a 9-year follow-up, ulcer hemorrhage seen in <2% with maintenance ranitidine compared to >12% in those without maintenance therapy[83]
RCT data: 9% rebleeding with ranitidine vs 36% with placebo over 61-week follow-up[128]

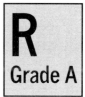

R
Grade A

There is no proven difference in ulcer healing rates and safety between different PPI.[77–79] A meta-analysis[80] has shown a close linear relationship between the degree of suppression of intragastric acidity and DU healing. A more complex meta-analysis of this relationship between the duration of acid suppression and healing led to the definition of three primary determinants of the benefits of antisecretory drugs: (a) the degree of suppression of acidity; (b) the duration of suppression of acidity over the 24 hour period; and (c) the duration of the treatment.[81] For DU, the duration of time the intragastric acidity can be maintained at or above pH 3.0 is the most important factor. This model identified that maintaining intragastric pH at or above the threshold pH of 3.0 for 18–20 hours of the day predicts a 100% healing of DU.[81] Lesser degrees of acid suppression were found to prolong the duration of time needed to achieve optimal healing. Thus, these models of degree of acid suppression help to explain the results of controlled healing trials.

Prevention of duodenal ulcer recurrence

R
Grade A

Although ulcers were healed effectively by acid suppressive therapy, ulcer recurrence was almost inevitable, with about 80% recurrence at 1 year once treatment was stopped.[58,71,72,82–84] Thus, in an effort to prevent recurrent ulcer, patients were given maintenance therapy with H_2-receptor antagonists (Table 3.3). In a large ($n = 399$) 2 year maintenance study of ranitidine 150 mg daily vs placebo, ulcer symptoms remained controlled in only about half the patients but ulcer recurrence was prevented in 83% of patients.[85] This study also identified significantly ($P < 0.002$) more complications, such as bleeding, in the placebo arm. After a long term follow-up of

R Grade A

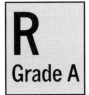

464 patients on maintenance ranitidine, 81% remained free of symptomatic DU recurrence over 9 years.[83] A 1-year relapse rate of between 20 and 30% has been identified consistently through meta-analyses[86,87] and reviews.[82] Most of the maintenance studies used suboptimal half doses of the H_2-receptor antagonists, and full ulcer healing doses were more effective in preventing relapse.[82,88,89] Treatment of ulcers with tri-potassium di-citrato bismuthate appeared to prolong remission beyond that seen with H_2-antagonists. It has since been suggested that this effect is, in part, due to the suppressive effects of bismuth on *H. pylori* infection and its ability as a single agent to eradicate *H. pylori* in around 20% of patients.[90]

Eradication of *H. pylori* infection

PREVENTION OF DUODENAL ULCER RECURRENCE

The identification of *H. pylori* infection and its higher prevalence in ulcer disease has provided an opportunity to change the natural history of ulcer disease. The most clinically relevant evidence for the role of *H. pylori* comes from intervention trials in which *H. pylori* is eradicated and recurrence of ulcer disease prevented.

R Grade A

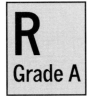

The first reported randomized trial in 1987[91] showed that the risk of recurrent DU could be reduced to virtually zero when *H. pylori* eradication therapy was given. In 1988, Marshall *et al*[92] reported a double-blind trial of DU patients in which more ulcers healed and fewer ulcers recurred over 12 months with *H. pylori* eradication therapy. Other important early contributions supported these observations.[93–97]

R Grade A

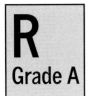

Reviews of studies from 1987 to 1994 agree that the recurrence rate for DU at 1 year ranges from 0 to 9% when *H. pylori* infection is successfully eradicated.[19,98,99] There are fewer data on ulcer recurrence after periods longer than 1 year after *H. pylori* eradication, but reported recurrence rates range from 0 to 18%.[99] Labenz reported that at 1 year, infection with *H. pylori* recurred in 2.4%, while DU recurred in only 0.8%.[100] Longer follow-up showed no *H. pylori* or ulcer recurrence at 3 and 4 years.[100] Another study reported that 92% of patients remained free of *H. pylori* after 7 years of follow-up while those who were *H. pylori* positive remained persistently positive.[11] In 15 comparative studies of patients with *H. pylori* eradication versus no eradication, the ulcer recurrence rate was 7% in those in whom *H. pylori* was eradicated vs 67% in those who remained infected.[99] A systematic overview[101] has shown that the median 12-month DU recurrence rate is 67% if *H. pylori* infection persists but is reduced to 6% if *H. pylori* is eradicated. Comparable results for GU recurrence are 59% vs 4%.

HEALING OF DUODENAL ULCER

R Grade A

The interval to reassessment after *H. pylori* eradication therapy is completed may influence ulcer healing data. In a cohort study of patients given *H. pylori* eradication therapy it was observed that at 1 month, 22/212 (10.4%) had persistent DU. These patients were followed for another 2 months without additional ulcer healing treatment, and ultimately only three ulcers remained unhealed, for a total healing success rate of 98.1%.[102]

Furthermore, DU heal faster when *H. pylori* infection is eradicated than with acid suppressive therapy alone using either H_2-receptor antagonists[92,95,97] or omeprazole.[103]

Ulcers refractory to healing with conventional acid suppressive therapy may heal with *H. pylori* eradication therapy[93,104–107] and remain healed over a 4-year follow-up period.[100] In the pre-*H. pylori* era, it was shown that ulcers could be healed with antibiotics alone.[108–111] Similar results have been shown in subsequent studies that aimed to heal ulcers with *H. pylori* eradication treatment alone without the need for additional ulcer healing drugs.[111–113] These findings further emphasize the important role of *H. pylori* as a bacterial pathogen.

Healing of gastric ulcer with acid suppressive therapy

Gastric ulcer (GU) healing rates in the pre-*H. pylori* era with H_2-receptor antagonists were 3–43% at 2 weeks, 54–70% at 4 weeks, 82–92% at 8 weeks, and 89–94% at 12 weeks.[114] Thus GU take 4–8 weeks longer to heal than DU. There are no important differences in healing rate between various H_2-receptor antagonists (H_2-RA). However, PPI have been shown to produce higher healing rates than H_2-RA in several randomized trials.[114–17] Grade A An early meta-analysis[114] demonstrated that the most important determinant of healing was duration of treatment. A later meta-analysis, comparing omeprazole and ranitidine in healing GU demonstrated more rapid and complete healing with more potent acid suppression.[114] Another meta-analysis of the rates of GU healing, expressed as ulcers healed per week, showed that PPI (represented by omeprazole) healed GU 24% faster than other agents.[118] Grade A

Prevention of recurrence of gastric ulcer

For GU, maintenance H_2-receptor antagonists (cimetidine, ranitidine, famotidine, nizatidine) in half standard dose at night, can reduce the risk of 1-year symptomatic recurrence to 6.7–36% when compared to 49–76% without therapy.[82] A PPI (omeprazole, lansoprazole, pantoprazole) in standard dose daily reduced GU recurrence to only 4.5% over 6 months.[119]

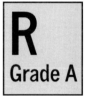

R
Grade A

Eradication of *H. pylori*

HEALING OF GASTRIC ULCER

Eradication of *H. pylori* speeds gastric ulcer healing with a 6-week healing rate of 84.9% compared with 60% in patients with persistent *H. pylori* infection (P = 0.0148).[120] Grade A

PREVENTION OF RECURRENCE OF GASTRIC ULCER

Curing *H. pylori* infection has been shown in randomized controlled trials to reduce the recurrence rate of GU, although there are fewer available data than is the case for DU.[19,96,99,121–124] The study by Sung *et al*[123] is particularly noteworthy, as GU were healed by *H. pylori* eradication therapy alone without an antisecretory drug, ie conventional ulcer healing therapy. *H. pylori* eradication almost eliminates GU recurrence while persistently infected patients have a relapse rate of about 50%.[98,99]. Labenz reported that at 1 year, *H.*

R
Grade A

pylori recurrence was 3.4% while GU recurrence was not seen.[100] Longer follow-up showed no *H. pylori* infection or ulcer recurrence at 3 and 4 years.[100]

DUODENAL ULCER COMPLICATIONS AND EFFECTS OF *H. PYLORI*

Gastroduodenal ulcer disease causes serious complications such as bleeding in 15–20% of patients, perforation in about 5%, and obstruction in about 2%.[125] A natural history study of duodenal ulcer before the *H. pylori* era provided interesting data from 2119 patients.[126] Of these patients, 13.5% presented with hemorrhage as the first indication of ulcer disease. The overall mortality was 4.5% in those patients who bled and only 1% in those without bleeding. Most of the deaths which were not due to bleeding were due to perforation. The re-bleeding rate was 13% overall versus 2% for patients who continued on therapy.

R Grade A

As the rate of recurrent bleeding in the past was high, strategies for prevention of re-bleeding have been considered necessary. Two randomized, placebo controlled trials have evaluated a maintenance dose of ranitidine 150 mg. One trial did not show that ranitidine reduced re-bleeding. However, the study lacked statistical power.[127] The other trial[128] showed a significantly reduced risk of re-bleeding (ranitidine 9%, placebo 36%, ARR 27%, NNT 4). However, the maintenance H_2-blocker arm still carried a re-bleeding risk of nearly 10%, and half the episodes were asymptomatic. The risk of re-bleeding did not diminish over time. Those patients on placebo were at continuous risk of re-bleeding over the 3-year follow-up period.

The prevalence of *H. pylori* infection in bleeding duodenal ulcers appears to be lower than in non-bleeding ulcers.[129] For bleeding gastric ulcers, 10% of patients were neither infected with *H. pylori* nor taking NSAIDs.[125]

Currently it is accepted that eradication of *H. pylori* leads to a reduction in ulcer recurrence, and hence prevents recurrent bleeding. In open and cohort studies, patients with *H. pylori* eradication had a re-bleeding rate of less than 3.5% per year, while those with persistent *H. pylori* infection exhibited re-bleeding rates of 50% at 1 year[130] Grade B to 82% at 4 years.[131] Grade A There is also evidence from randomized, placebo controlled trials that eradication of *H. pylori* prevents the risk of recurrent DU bleeding. In patients with a bleeding DU and persistent *H. pylori* infection, the rate of ulcer re-bleeding ranged from 27 to 37% per year. However, if *H. pylori* is eradicated, the re-bleeding risk is virtually zero (Table 3.4).

R Grade A/B

There are three controlled trials which compare *H. pylori* eradication with maintenance acid suppressive therapy. In one of these the allocation of patients to the two interventions was not randomized;[132] the other two were randomized trials.[133,134] Although these comparative trials were generally better designed than the placebo controlled trials, and included larger numbers of patients, the re-bleeding rates were nevertheless low in all studies, and statistically significant differences were not shown between the treatment groups. There is the possibility of a type II error. However, all studies agreed that if *H. pylori* infection was eradicated, recurrent bleeding was not seen even without the need for maintenance therapy. The pooled re-bleeding rate in the ranitidine arms of the three trials was 5.6%.[132–134]

There are few data available concerning the role of *H. pylori* infection in other complications such as ulcer perforation. A controlled trial involving 60 patients undergoing simple closure of perforated duodenal ulcer demonstrated a significant ($P < 0.05$) benefit for decreasing complications of peptic ulcer disease with postoperative

Table 3.4 Summary of *H. pylori* eradication and ulcer bleeding recurrence rates

Bleeding ulcer recurrence rate (%) after *H. pylori* eradication vs no maintenance therapy

Study	*H. pylori* eradication	No therapy	FU (mth)	*P*	ARR (%)	NNT
Open/cohort studies						
Jaspersen, 1995[130]	3.4 ($n = 29$)	50 ($n = 4$)[a]	12	–	47	2
Macri, 1998[131]	0 ($n = 21$)	81.8 ($n = 11$)[b]	48	<0.002	82	1
Randomized controlled trials						
Graham, 1993[217]	0 ($n = 17$)	28.6 ($n = 14$)	12	0.031	29	3
Jaspersen, 1995[218]	0 ($n = 29$)	27.3 ($n = 22$)	12	<0.01	27	3
Labenz, 1994[219]	0 ($n = 42$)	37.5 ($n = 24$)	12	0.01	38	3
Rokkas, 1995[220]	0 ($n = 16$)	33.0 ($n = 15$)	12	0.018	33	3

Bleeding ulcer recurrence rate after *H. pylori* eradication vs ranitidine maintenance therapy

Study	*H. pylori* eradication	RM[c]	FU (mth)	*P*
Non-randomized controlled trial				
Santander, 1996[132]	2.3 ($n = 84$)[d]	12.1 ($n = 41$)	12	<0.001
Randomized controlled trials				
Riemann, 1997[133]	4.2 ($n = 47$)[e]	8.3($n = 48$)	24	0.29
Sung, 1997[134]	0 ($n = 97$)	3.0 ($n = 99$)	12	0.08

FU, follow-up; RM, ranitidine maintenance.

[a] Open study with one rebleed after successful eradication and 50% rebleeding with persistent infection.

[b] Cohort study of patients given eradication therapy, then *H. pylori* positive and negative followed for 48 months.

[c] Maintenance therapy with ranitidine 150 mg daily.

[d] These two patients who rebled were reinfected with *H. pylori*.

[e] Both patients that rebled were *H. pylori* negative but were on NSAIDs.

cimetidine treatment.[135] This study did not consider the role of *H. pylori* infection. NSAID use increases the risk of ulcer perforation by a factor of 5–8.[136] Separate relative risks for duodenal and gastric ulcers are not known. In 80 patients presenting with acute perforated duodenal ulcer, the prevalence of *H. pylori* infection was only about 50%, approximately equal to that in a control group, and NSAIDs were frequently the cause of the perforation.[137] There is very little literature to support a role for *H. pylori* as an important cause of perforation. However, *H. pylori* is an important cause of ulcer. Therefore, it is rational to eradicate *H. pylori* in patients who have suffered from perforated ulcer, and thus eliminate an important risk factor.

R
Grade C

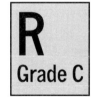

COHERENCE OF THE DATA WITH EARLIER EPIDEMIOLOGICAL INFORMATION

The presumed prevalence of *H. pylori* infection parallels data showing that there was a peak in ulcer disease at the end of the last century.[4] This is consistent with epidemiological data that shows that the death rate of DU patients was highest in those born around 1890.[138] Comparable findings of highest ulcer perforation risks were identified in a cohort of men born between 1900 and 1920.[139] This is also the generation with the highest *H. pylori* prevalence in an *H. pylori* seropositivity study performed in the UK.[140] This relationship is consistent with the hypothesis that *H. pylori* plays an important role in ulcer complications.

Improvements in hygiene and sanitation are associated with a declining risk of infection, as is the case today in industrialized nations compared to less developed countries which still endure a poor socioeconomic status. The number of admissions for ulcer disease has steadily declined since the middle of this century, which infers a declining severity and prevalence of DU.[141] This decline parallels a declining prevalence of *H. pylori* infection.

While DU disease has long been thought to be a disease of men, more recent data since 1979 have shown that the prevalence of DU and the death rate for men and women have become similar.[142] This is consistent with the prevalence of *H. pylori* infection, which is the same in both sexes.[143]

These epidemiological data are consistent with the other kinds of evidence which establish the role of *H. pylori* in ulcer disease.

H. PYLORI ERADICATION THERAPY

Antibiotic regimens

The evolution of *H. pylori* eradication treatment has been rapid. It was determined early on that this infection was easy to suppress but difficult to cure. Thus, if the patient were tested too early following completion of a course of an eradication treatment, the organism would be "cleared" but be falsely identified as having been eradicated. A time interval of at least 4 weeks after the end of eradication treatment was identified as the minimum necessary to define eradication.[90,144]

Triple and quadruple bismuth based therapies

The first meta-analysis of *H. pylori* eradication regimens[90] Grade A established that single antimicrobial agents were insufficient to eradicate *H. pylori*. A later review identified clarithromycin as a drug that can eradicate *H. pylori* infection in up to 54% of patients when given alone. However, resistance can rapidly develop, and its use as a single agent is not recommended.[145] Combinations of two antimicrobials were found to result in improved eradication rates and the best regimens were "bismuth triple therapies".[90] The best regimen in 1992 was triple therapy with bismuth, metronidazole, and tetracycline (BMT), which was superior to triple therapy with bismuth, metronidazole, and amoxicillin.[90,99,146] Grade A However, the large number of pills required and relatively long 2-week duration of treatment affected compliance adversely. Poor compliance (<60% of pills) led to only 69% eradication success compared to 96% in patients who take >60% of pills.[147] Later meta-analyses demonstrated that 1 week of therapy was as effective as 2 weeks of treatment.[99,146,148] Grade A The greater number of adverse effects suffered with bismuth triple therapies leads to more treatment discontinuation than is observed with PPI triple therapies (to be discussed below).[146] In patients who harbor a metronidazole resistant *H. pylori* infection, eradication efficacy was reduced to 58% compared to 86% for metronidazole sensitive strains.[146]

R Grade A

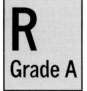

Proton pump inhibitors (PPIs) have been used in combination with the traditional bismuth triple therapy. This quadruple regimen has high pooled eradication rates (80–90%) with 1 week of treatment[146,148–50] and is superior to bismuth triple therapy without a PPI. Only omeprazole[151,152] and lansoprazole[153] have been evaluated. This may be an effective regimen for treatment failures, and even metronidazole resistant strains may be successfully eradicated, although definitive studies are required before drawing firm conclusions.[154] However, the major drawback of this regimen is that it requires four times daily dosing with a total of 18 pills. Adverse effects are generally mild, but frequent enough that they may impair compliance. Most patients can complete the treatment if counselled about possible adverse effects.

PPI based combination therapies

COMBINATIONS WITH ONE ANTIBIOTIC

Further advances in treatment have been dominated by combinations of a proton pump inhibitor (PPI) with either one or two antimicrobial drugs. The PPI are potent acid suppressing agents that effectively heal duodenal and gastric ulcers and provide prompt symptom relief. They may have a synergistic effect with antimicrobials by providing an optimal intragastric pH milieu.[155,156] They also have some direct suppressive effects on *H. pylori*. Thus, there is a good rationale to use these agents as part of an *H. pylori* eradication regimen.

PPI PLUS AMOXICILLIN DUAL THERAPY

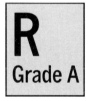

R Grade A

Dual therapy with omeprazole and amoxicillin (OA) enjoyed a brief period of popularity. Overall efficacy in several reviews and meta-analyses was in the order of 60% and results were not consistent. Therefore this regimen is not recommended.[99,145,146,148,157–9]

PPI PLUS CLARITHROMYCIN DUAL THERAPY

R Grade A

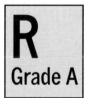

With the identification of clarithromycin as the most effective single therapy,[160] it came to be used as dual therapy with omeprazole. This combination gave more consistent and reliable results than OA dual therapy. However, the eradication rate with this regimen is still only around 70%.[146,148,157] Two weeks of therapy with relatively high doses of clarithromycin 500 mg bid to tid were required. The increased cost of this regimen detracted from its usefulness.[146]

COMBINATIONS OF PPI WITH TWO ANTIBIOTICS (TRIPLE THERAPY, SEE TABLE 3.5)

R Grade A

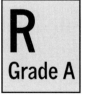

Better eradication rates were achieved with regimens that combined a PPI with two antimicrobials. The first regimen, known as the Bazzoli regimen,[161] used omeprazole 20 mg od, clarithromycin 250 mg bid, and tinidazole 500 mg bid for 1 week and achieved 100% efficacy. A meta-analysis of such treatments suggested that this was the most effective therapy overall.[146] Many subsequent trials using omeprazole, lansoprazole or pantoprazole have demonstrated that the PPI based triple therapies are consistently superior to dual therapies.[146] Limited data with a fourth PPI, rabeprazole, shows similar efficacy.[162] Unfortunately, most of the early studies with these PPI based regimens were methodologically weaker, open evaluations with small sample sizes.

The first large randomized placebo controlled trial was the MACH I study.[163] While this study was criticized for having only one test of *H. pylori* eradication after treatment,

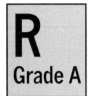

R Grade A

R Grade A

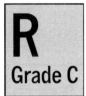

R Grade C

R Grade A

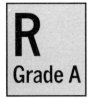

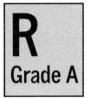

the regimens identified as being the most effective have stood the test of time and are recommended by most consensus conferences.[164–7] The most effective 1-week, twice daily regimens of the MACH-1 study were: (a) omeprazole 20 mg, clarithromycin 500 mg, and amoxicillin 1 g; or (b) omeprazole 20 mg, clarithromycin 250 mg, and metronidazole 400 mg. Studies with similar efficacy were reported using lansoprazole[14,168–75] or pantoprazole based triple therapies.[146,176–9] The MACH-1 omeprazole triple therapies have now been evaluated in both active duodenal[180] and gastric ulcer[181] disease patients with consistent results. Furthermore, the MACH-2 study carefully evaluated antibiotic resistance and determined that baseline metronidazole resistance reduced the efficacy of the OCM (omeprazole, clarithromycin, metonidazole) triple therapy from 95% to 76%.[182,183] A similar reduction in efficacy of about 15% was reported in a lansoprazole study.[175] Importantly, the MACH-2 study also showed that the addition of omeprazole, with its potent acid suppression, helped partially to overcome metronidazole resistance. When baseline metronidazole resistance was present, clarithromycin and metronidazole alone was successful in only 30% of cases, but with the addition of omeprazole the efficacy was improved to 76%. In the MACH studies, the dosage of metronidazole was 400 mg bid, slightly lower than the 500 mg bid available in Canada and other countries. However, a meta-analysis has shown these two doses to be similarly effective.[184] The higher metronidazole dose may be better on theoretical grounds, since higher doses may be more effective against resistant *H. pylori* strains.[185]

Based on these individual studies, as well as reviews[145,186–8] and meta-analyses as summarized in Table 3.5, numerous worldwide *H. pylori* consensus conferences have all consistently advocated as first line therapy, the regimens of PPI with clarithromycin and amoxicillin (PCA) or metronidazole (PCM, or tinidazole where available) all twice daily for 1 week.[164,165,189,190] These twice daily, 1-week regimens are well tolerated with few drop-outs due to drug intolerance. A randomized trial did not show a difference in efficacy between a lower dose of clarithromycin (250 mg bid) vs the conventional 500 mg bid dose

Table 3.5 Summary from reviews of PPI plus two antibiotics for 1 week

Study	Analysis	PPI + C + NI Overall MER % (95% CI)	PPI + C + A Overall MER % (95% CI)
Unge, 1996[158]	ITT	87 (83–90)	85 (82–89)
Van der Hulst, 1996[188]	APT	88 (85.5–90.5)	88.7 (86.8–90.5)
Huang, 1997[150]	ITT	87 (85–90) for PPI-CM[a] 88 (84–93) for PPI-CT[a]	83 (75–92)
Penston, 1997[146]	APT	81 (77–85) for OCM[a] 93 (87–99) for LCM[a] 86 (77–95) for PCM[a] 90 (88–92) for OCT[a]	86 (83–90) for OCA[b] 86 (79–93) for LCA[b]
Chiba,[c] 1999[148]	PP	88.6 (86.4–90.8)	86.8 (79.4–94.2)

C, clarithromycin; NI, nitroimidazole (metronidazole or tinidazole); A, amoxicillin; MER, mean eradication rate; ITT, intention to treat; APT, all patients treated; PP, per protocol.

[a]Data reported separately for various proton pump inhibitors (PPI): omeprazole (O) or lansoprazole (L) or pantoprazole (P), clarithromycin (C) and metronidazole (M) or tinidazole (T).

[b]Data reported separately for various PPI: omeprazole (O) or lansoprazole (L), clarithromycin (C) and amoxicillin (A).

[c]Meta-analysis to 1995.

in combination with pantoprazole 40 mg bid and metronidazole 500 mg bid. Patients treated with the lower dose had only half the incidence of adverse effects.[191] While the smaller dose of clarithromycin may be adequate for many patients, consensus groups have advocated the 500 mg bid dose for consistency and to avoid possible confusion and prescribing errors.

R Grade A

Amoxicillin allergy is common and this is a contraindication to use of the PCA regimen. Since this regimen does not contain metronidazole, there is rationale for using it in patients with suspected or documented metronidazole resistant strains.[192]

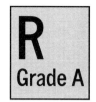

PPI – a necessary component of eradication treatment regimens

There is evidence to support the view that the PPI is a necessary component of PPI triple therapies to achieve optimal eradication rates.[183,193,194] In one such study, all patients were given 1 week clarithromycin 250 mg and tinidazole 500 mg bid and were randomized to receive either no omeprazole, omeprazole 20 mg once daily, or omeprazole 20 mg bid. The eradication rates were higher in the omeprazole groups (omeprazole once daily 88%, twice daily 89%, placebo 64%, ARR for twice daily omeprazole vs antibiotics alone = 0.25, NNT = 4).[193] In the omeprazole groups, 22 patients who harbored metronidazole resistant strains of *H. pylori* were cured by the omeprazole regimen, providing further evidence that the addition of the PPI may help overcome metronidazole resistance.

R Grade A

Duration of acid suppressive therapy

There is good evidence[112,195–8] that uncomplicated, active duodenal ulcers heal without the need to continue ulcer healing drugs beyond the duration of eradication therapy. The best study design was the study by Labenz.[196] In this study, all patients received a 1-week course of omeprazole, clarithromycin, and metronidazole, following which patients were randomized to receive either omeprazole 20 mg daily for 3 more weeks or an identical placebo. At 2 weeks, ulcer healing was 91% in the omeprazole arm and 76% in the placebo arm ($P = 0.14$) and at 4 weeks all ulcers had healed in both arms. This approach reduces the cost of treatment.

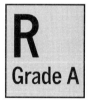

R Grade A

Ranitidine bismuth citrate regimens

Ranitidine bismuth citrate (RBC) is a new chemical entity, which incorporates bismuth into the ranitidine molecule and was specifically developed for *H. pylori* eradication. When combined with clarithromycin, eradication rates range from 74 to 98% by per protocol (PP) analysis, with eradication rates of 55–96% by intention to treat (ITT) analysis.[199–206] A criticism of these studies is that data were often reported as confusing "observed" intention to treat, an unfamiliar term not previously used in reporting study data. For all intents and purposes, "observed" appears to be an analysis slightly more conservative than "per protocol" and less so than "intention to treat". This was problematical in some studies in which the intention to treat data were not clearly presented.[207] In a large randomized controlled trial, RBC for 4 weeks with clarithromycin 500 mg bid for 2 weeks was as effective as RBC with clarithromycin 500 mg tid in

H. pylori eradication and DU healing.[202] Clarithromycin doses of 500 mg bid and 250 mg qid were found to be equally effective.[205,207] Grade A However, in two studies, there was a trend towards the bid regimen being more effective than the same total dose given on a qid regimen.[205,207] Although the bid regimen is convenient, the longer 2-week therapy makes this treatment the most costly of currently available regimens. A randomized trial comparing 1 week and 2 weeks of therapy with RBC did not show a statistically significant difference in effectiveness between these regimens. However, the eradication rates (ITT analysis) were only between 75% (1 week) and 80% (2 weeks).[209] Grade A The dual combination of RBC with clarithromycin may[209] or may not bc cffcctivc against clarithromycin resistant *H. pylori*.[210]

Randomized trials comparing 1-week[199,206] and 2-week[205] RBC triple therapies with 2- week RBC and clarithromycin dual therapy did not show statistically significant differences in effectiveness. Grade A However, in these trials, triple therapy was not superior to dual therapy as may have been anticipated.

Randomized trials of a variety of RBC triple regimens have shown *H. pylori* eradication rates (ITT analysis) of between 61% and 94% as shown in Table 3.6. Grade A

A trial which compared RBC 400 mg bid versus omeprazole 20 mg bid in combination with amoxicillin 1 g bid and clarithromycin 500 mg did not show a statistically significant difference in eradication rates (RAC 94%, OAC 87.5%) or ulcer healing (RAC 90%, OAC 89.6%), suggesting that RBC may be successfully used in place of a PPI.[211] Grade A Five additional randomized trials whose results are still in abstract form have not shown differences in effectiveness between RBC and PPI based triple therapies.[212]

RBC *in vitro* appears to act synergistically in combination with other antibiotics against metronidazole[213,214] and clarithromycin resistant *H. pylori* strains.[215] In addition, RBC may decrease the emergence of metronidazole resistance.[213] In clinical trials of RBC, clarithromycin and metronidazole,[216] and RBC, clarithromycin, and amoxicillin,[199] baseline metronidazole resistance did not appear to impair treatment efficacy. However, RBC, tetracycline, and metronidazole triple therapy was significantly less effective in eradicating *H. pylori* when metronidazole resistance was present (eradication rate: metronidazole sensitive 97%, metronidazole resistant 57%).[199] These are important observations that require further objective study to determine the appropriate role of RBC regimens in patients with resistant infections.

Table 3.6 Summary of RBC triple therapies

Regimen	Range of ITT eradication (%)	Study (reference number)
RBC + clarithromycin + metronidazole or tinidazole	77–94	205, 206, 221–223
RBC + clarithromycin + amoxicillin	71–92	166,199,222,223
RBC + tetracycline + metronidazole	80–86	166,199
RBC + clarithromycin + tetracycline	90	224
RBC + amoxicillin + tinidazole	61	223

SUMMARY

H. pylori can now be accepted as a definite pathogen which fulfills almost all of Hill's criteria for causation. *H. pylori* eradication results in cure of ulcer disease and markedly reduces ulcer recurrence and ulcer complications such as bleeding. Eradication of *H. pylori* heals ulcers without the need to continue ulcer healing drugs, heals refractory ulcers, and also results in faster ulcer healing than occurs with traditional acid suppressive therapy. Effective therapies to eradicate *H. pylori* are now available. Further recommendations on optimal treatments for treatment failures and antibiotic resistant infections require more definitive data.

Recommended *H. pylori* eradication therapy

Recommended first line therapy in 1999

Proton-pump inhibitor (PPI) *Either* Omeprazole 20 mg bid or lansoprazole 30 mg bid or pantoprazole 40 mg bid *Or* Ranitidine bismuth citrate (RBC) 400 mg bid	+	Clarithromycin 500 mg bid bid	+	Amoxicillin 1 g bid or metronidazole 500 mg bid or tinidazole 500 mg bid

- Treatment for 1 week is adequate in most
- Longer 10–14 day treatment may be needed in some areas (e.g. USA)
- More data available for PPI triple therapies
- PPI is a necessary part of treatment and helps partially to overcome *H. pylori* metronidazole resistance, however, with PPI + clarithromycin and metronidazole, metronidazole resistance does reduce eradication efficacy by about 15%
- With metronidazole or tinidazole, clarithromycin dose may suffice at 250 mg bid
- With RBC triple therapies, data about antibiotic resistance is evolving

Recommended for treatment failures

- Lack evidence based recommendations from RCTs
- Suggest using a different first line regimen with at least one different antibiotic
- Consider PPI bid plus bismuth triple therapy (colloidal bismuth citrate or bismuth subsalicylate 2 tabs qid, metronidazole 250–500 mg qid, tetracycline 500 mg qid) for 7–14 days

REFERENCES

1 Schwarz K. Uber penetrierende Magen- und Jejunalgeschwure. *Beitr Klin Chir* 1910; **67**: 96–128.

2 Warren JR, Marshall BJ. Unidentified curved bacillus on gastric epithelium in active chronic gastritis. *Lancet* 1983; **i**: 1273–5.

3 Marshall BJ, Warren JR. Unidentified curved bacilli in the stomach of patients with gastritis and peptic ulceration. *Lancet* 1984; 16 June: 1311–15.

4 Mégraud F, Lamouliatte H. *Helicobacter pylori* and duodenal ulcer. Evidence suggesting causation. *Dig Dis Sci* 1992; **37**: 769–72.

5 Rabeneck L, Ransohoff DF. Is *Helicobacter pylori* a cause of duodenal ulcer? A methodologic critique of current evidence. *Am J Med* 1991; **91**: 566–72.

6 Hill BA. The environment and disease: association or causation? *Proc R Soc Med* 1965; **58**: 295–300.

7 Kuipers EJ, Thijs JC, Festen HPM. The prevalence of *Helicobacter pylori* in peptic ulcer disease. *Aliment Pharmacol Ther* 1995; **9**(Suppl 2): 59–69.
8 Borody TJ, George LL, Brandl S *et al.* *Helicobacter pylori* negative duodenal ulcer. *Am J Gastroenterol* 1991; **86:** 1154–7.
9 Nensey YW, Schubert TT, Bologna SD *et al.* *Helicobacter pylori* negative duodenal ulcer. *Am J Med* 1991; **91:** 15–18.
10 McColl KEL, El-Nujumi AM, Chittajallu RS *et al.* A study of the pathogenesis of *Helicobacter pylori* negative chronic duodenal ulceration. *Gut* 1993; **34:** 762–8.
11 Forbes GM, Glaser ME, Cullen DJE *et al.* Duodenal ulcer treated with *Helicobacter pylori* eradication: Seven year follow-up. *Lancet* 1994; **343:** 258–60.
12 Neil GA, Suchower LJ, Johnson E *et al.* *Helicobacter pylori* eradication as a surrogate marker for the reduction of duodenal ulcer recurrence. *Aliment Pharmacol Ther* 1998; **12**(7): 619–33.
13 Peterson WL, Ciociola AA, Sykes DL *et al.* Ranitidine bismuth citrate plus clarithromycin is effective for healing duodenal ulcers, eradicating *H. pylori* and reducing ulcer recurrence. RBC *H. pylori* Study Group. *Aliment Pharmacol Ther* 1996; **10**(3): 251–61.
14 Schwartz H, Krause R, Sahba B *et al.* Triple versus dual therapy for eradicating *Helicobacter pylori* and preventing ulcer recurrence: a randomized, double-blind, multicenter study of lansoprazole, clarithromycin, and/or amoxicillin in different dosing regimens. *Am J Gastroenterol* 1998; **93**(4): 584–90.
15 Jyotheeswaran S, Shah AN, Jin HO *et al.* Prevalence of *Helicobacter pylori* in peptic ulcer patients in greater Rochester, NY: is empirical triple therapy justified? *Am J Gastroenterol* 1998; **93**(4): 574–8.
16 Cloud ML, Enas N, Humphries TJ and the Rabeprazole Study Group. Rabeprazole in treatment of acid peptic diseases. Results of three placebo-controlled dose–response clinical trials in duodenal ulcer, gastric ulcer, and gastroesophageal reflux disease. *Dig Dis Sci* 1998; **43:** 993–1000.
17 Hyvärinen H, Salmenkylä S, Sipponen P. *Helicobacter pylori*-negative duodenal and pyloric ulcer: role of NSAIDs. *Digestion* 1996; **57:** 305–9.
18 Harris AW, Gummett PA, Phull PS *et al.* Recurrence of duodenal ulcer after *Helicobacter pylori* eradication is related to high acid output. *Aliment Pharmacol Ther* 1997; **11:** 331–4.
19 Thijs JC, Kuipers EJ, van ZA *et al.* Treatment of *Helicobacter pylori* infections. *Q J Med* 1995; **88:** 369–89.
20 Rauws EAJ, Langenberg W, Houthoff HJ *et al.* *Campylobacter pyloridis*-associated chronic active antral gastritis. *Gastroenterology* 99 1988; **94:** 33–40.
21 Borody TJ, Brandl S, Andrews P *et al.* *Helicobacter pylori* negative gastric ulcer. *Am J Gastroenterol* 1992; **87:** 1403–6.
22 Nomura A, Stemmerman GN, Chyou P-H *et al.* *Helicobacter pylori* infection and the risk for duodenal and gastric ulceration. *Ann Intern Med* 1994; **120:** 977–81.
23 Walsh JH, Peterson WL. The treatment of *Helicobacter pylori* infection in the management of peptic ulcer disease. *N Engl J Med* 1995; **333:** 984–91.
24 Marshall BJ. *Helicobacter pylori* in peptic ulcer: have Koch's postulates been fulfilled? *Ann Med* 1995; **27:** 565–8.
25 Sipponen P, Varis K, Fraki O *et al.* Cumulative 10-year risk of symptomatic duodenal and gastric ulcer disease in people with or without chronic gastritis: a clinical follow-up study of 454 outpatients. *Scand J Gastroenterol* 1990; **25:** 966–73.
26 Blaser MJ, Chyou P-H, Nomura A. Age at establishment of *Helicobacter pylori* infection and gastric carcinoma, gastric ulcer, and duodenal ulcer risk. *Cancer Res* 1995; **55:** 562–5.
27 Perri F, Clemente R, Pastore M. The ^{13}C-urea breath test as a predictor of intragastric bacterial load and severity of *Helicobacter pylori* gastritis. *Scand J Clin Lab. Invest* 1998; **58:** 19–27.
28 Labenz J, Börsch G, Peitz U *et al.* Validity of a novel biopsy urease test (HUT) and a simplified ^{13}C-urea breath test for diagnosis of *Helicobacter pylori* infection and estimation of the severity of gastritis. *Digestion* 1996; **57**(6): 391–7.
29 Hilker E, Domschke W, Stoll R. ^{13}C-urea breath test for detection of *Helicobacter pylori* and its correlation with endoscopic and histologic findings. *J Physiol Pharmacol* 1996; **47:** 79–90.
30 Moshkowitz M, Konikoff FM, Peled Y *et al.* High *Helicobacter pylori* numbers are associated with low eradication rate after triple therapy. *Gut* 1995; **36:** 845–7.
31 Sharma TK, Prasad VM, Cutler AF. Quantitative noninvasive testing for *Helicobacter pylori* does not predict gastroduodenal ulcer disease. *Gastrointest Endosc* 1996; **44:** 679–82.
32 Lewis JD, Kroser J, Bevan J *et al.* Urease-based tests for *Helicobacter pylori* gastritis. Accurate for diagnosis but poor correlation with disease severity. *J Clin Gastroenterol* 1997; **25:** 415–20.
33 Moran AP, Wadström T. Pathogenesis of *Helicobacter pylori*. *Curr Opin Gastroenterol* 1998; **14**(Suppl 1): S9–S14.

34 Yang H, Dixon MF, Zuo J *et al.* *Helicobacter pylori* infection and gastric metaplasia in the duodenum in China. *J Clin Gastroenterol* 1995; **20:** 110–12.
35 Harris AW, Gummett PA, Walker MM *et al.* Relation between gastric acid output, *Helicobacter pylori*, and gastric metaplasia in the duodenal bulb. *Gut* 1996; **39:** 513–20.
36 Walker MM, Dixon MF. Gastric metaplasia: its role in duodenal ulceration. *Aliment Pharmacol Ther* 1996; **10** (Suppl 1): 119–28.
37 Madsen JE, Vetvik K, Aase S. *Helicobacter*-associated duodenitis and gastric metaplasia in duodenal ulcer patients. *APMIS* 1991; **99:** 997–1000.
38 Steer HW. Surface morphology of the gastroduodenal mucosa in duodenal ulceration. *Gut* 1984; **25:** 1203–10.
39 Carrick J, Lee A, Hazell S *et al.* *Campylobacter pylori*, duodenal ulcer, and gastric metaplasia: possible role of functional heterotopic tissue in ulcerogenesis. *Gut* 1989; **30:** 790–7.
40 Khulusi S, Mendall MA, Badve S *et al.* Effect of *Helicobacter pylori* eradication on gastric metaplasia of the duodenum. *Gut* 1995; **36:** 193–7.
41 Rudnicka L, Bobrzynski A, Stachura J. Short-term eradication therapy for *Helicobacter pylori* does not reduce the incidence of gastric metaplasia in duodenal ulcer patients. *Pol J Pathol* 1997; **48:** 103–6.
42 Khulusi S, Badve S, Patel P *et al.* Pathogenesis of gastric metaplasia of the human duodenum: role of *Helicobacter pylori*, gastric acid, and ulceration. *Gastroenterology* 1996; **110:** 452–8.
43 Urakami Y, Kimura M, Seki H. Gastric metaplasia and *Helicobacter pylori*. *Am J Gastroenterol* 1997; **92:** 795–9.
44 el-Omar E, Penman I, Dorrian CA *et al.* Eradicating *Helicobacter pylori* infection lowers gastrin mediated acid secretion by two thirds in patients with duodenal ulcer. *Gut* 1993; **34:** 1060–5.
45 Gillen D, el-Omar EM, Wirz AA *et al.* The acid response to gastrin distinguishes duodenal ulcer patients from *Helicobacter pylori*-infected healthy subjects. *Gastroenterology* 1998; **114:** 50–7.
46 Graham DY, Opekun A, Lew GM *et al.* *Helicobacter pylori*-associated exaggerated gastrin release in duodenal ulcer patients. The effect of bombesin infusion and urea ingestion. *Gastroenterology* 1991; **100:** 1571–5.
47 Hamlet A, Olbe L. The influence of *Helicobacter pylori* infection on postprandial duodenal acid load and duodenal bulb pH in humans. *Gastroenterology* 1996; **111:** 391–400.
48 el Omar EM, Penman ID, Ardill JE *et al.* *Helicobacter pylori* infection and abnormalities of acid secretion in patients with duodenal ulcer disease. *Gastroenterology* 1995; **109:** 681–91.
49 Harris AW, Gummett PA, Misiewicz JJ *et al.* Eradication of *Helicobacter pylori* in patients with duodenal ulcers lowers basal and peak acid outputs in response to gastrin releasing peptide and pentagastrin. *Gut* 1996; **38:** 663–7.
50 Beardshall K, Moss S, Gill J *et al.* Suppression of *Helicobacter pylori* reduces gastrin releasing peptide stimulated gastrin release in duodenal ulcer patients. *Gut* 1992; **33:** 601–3.
51 Harris AW, Gummett PA, Phull PS. Recurrence of duodenal ulcer after *Helicobacter pylori* eradication is related to high acid output. *Aliment Pharmacol Ther* 1997; **11:** 331–4.
52 Rieder G, Hatz RA, Moran AP *et al.* Role of adherence in interleukin-8 induction in *Helicobacter pylori*-associated gastritis. *Infect Immunol* 1997; **65:** 3622–30.
53 Yamaoka Y, Kita M, Kodama T *et al.* Induction of various cytokines and development of severe mucosal inflammation by *cagA* gene positive *Helicobacter pylori* strains. *Gut* 1997; **41:** 442–51.
54 D'Elios MM, Manghetti M, Almerigogna F *et al.* Different cytokine profile and antigen-specificity repertoire in *Helicobacter pylori*-specific T cell clones from the antrum of chronic gastritis patients with or without peptic ulcer. *Eur J Immunol* 1997; **27:** 1751–5.
55 Beales I, Blaser MJ, Srinivasan S *et al.* Effect of *Helicobacter pylori* products and recombinant cytokines on gastrin release from cultured canine G cells. *Gastroenterol* 1997; **113:** 465–71.
56 Wilairatana S, Kurathong S, Atthapaisalsarudee C *et al.* Omeprazole or cimetidine once daily for the treatment of duodenal ulcers? *J Gastroenterol Hepatol* 1989; **4**(Suppl 2): 45–52.
57 Archambault AP, Pare P, Bailey RJ *et al.* Omeprazole (20 mg daily) versus cimetidine (1200 mg daily) in duodenal ulcer healing and pain relief. *Gastroenterology* 1988; **94:** 1130–4.
58 Bardhan KD, Bianchi Porro G, Bose K *et al.* A comparison of two different doses of omeprazole versus ranitidine in treatment of duodenal ulcers. *J Clin Gastroenterol* 1986; **8:** 408–13.
59 Hawkey CJ, Long RG, Bardhan KD *et al.* Improved symptom relief and duodenal ulcer healing with lansoprazole, a new proton pump inhibitor, compared with ranitidine. *Gut* 1993; **34:** 1458–62.
60 Judmaier G, Koelz HR and the Pantopazole–Duodenal Ulcer Study Group. Comparison of pantoprazole and ranitidine in the treatment of acute duodenal ulcer. *Aliment Pharmacol Ther* 1994; **8:** 81–6.

61 McFarland RJ, Bateson MC, Green JRB *et al.* Omeprazole provides quicker symptom relief and duodenal ulcer healing than ranitidine. *Gastroenterol* 1990; **98:** 278–83.
62 van Rensburg CJ, van Eeden PJ, Marks I *et al.* Improved duodenal ulcer healing with pantoprazole compared with ranitidine: a multicentre study. *Eur J Gastroenterol Hepatol* 1994; **6:** 739–43.
63 Arber N, Avni Y, Eliakim R *et al.* A multicenter, double-blind, randomized controlled study of omeprazole versus ranitidine in the treatment of duodenal ulcer in Israel. *Isr J Med Sci* 1994; **30:** 757–61.
64 Barbara L, Blasi A, Cheli R *et al.* Omeprazole vs. ranitidine in the short-term treatment of duodenal ulcer: an Italian Multicenter study. *Hepatogastroenterology* 1987; **34:** 229–32.
65 Classen M, Dammann HG, Domschke W *et al.* Omeprazole heals duodenal, but not gastric ulcers more rapidly than ranitidine. Results of two German multicentre trials. *Hepatogastroenterology* 1985; **32:** 243–5.
66 Cremer M, Lambert R, Lamers CBHW *et al* and the European Pantoprazole Study Group. A double–blind study of pantoprazole and ranitidine in treatment of acute duodenal ulcer. A multicentre study. *Dig Dis Sci* 1995; **40:** 1360–4.
67 Crowe JP, Wilkinson SP, Bate CM *et al* and the OPUS (Omeprazole Peptic Ulcer Study) Research Group. Symptom relief and duodenal ulcer healing with omeprazole or cimetidine. *Aliment Pharmacol Ther* 1989; **3:** 83–91.
68 Hui WM, Lam SK, Lau WY *et al.* Omeprazole and ranitidine in duodenal ulcer healing and subsequent relapse: a randomized double-blind study with weekly endoscopic assessment. *J Gastroenterol Hepatol* 1989; **4**(Suppl 2): 35–43.
69 Hotz J, Kleiner R, Grymbowski T *et al.* Lansoprazole versus famotidine: efficacy and tolerance in the acute management of duodenal ulceration. *Aliment Pharmacol Ther* 1992; **6:** 87–95.
70 Lanza F, Goff J, Scowcroft C *et al.* Double-blind comparison of lansoprazole, ranitidine, and placebo in the treatment of acute duodenal ulcer. Lansoprazole Study Group. *Am J Gastroenterol* 1994; **89:** 1191–200.
71 Londong W, Barth H, Dammann WHG *et al.* Dose-related healing of duodenal ulcer with the proton pump inhibitor lansoprazole. *Aliment Pharmacol Ther* 1991; **5:** 245–54.
72 Misra SC, Dasarathy S, Sharma MP. Omeprazole versus famotidine in the healing and relapse of duodenal ulcer. *Aliment Pharmacol Ther* 1993; **7:** 443–9.
73 Mulder CJJ, Tijtgat GNJ, Cluysenaer OJJ *et al.* Omeprazole (20 mg o.m.) versus ranitidine (150 mg b.d.) in duodenal ulcer healing and pain relief. *Aliment Pharmacol Ther* 1989; **3:** 445–51.
74 Schepp W, Classen M. Pantoprazole and ranitidine in the treatment of acute duodenal ulcer. A multicentre study. *Scand J Gastroenterol* 1995; **30:** 511–14.
75 Wang CY, Wang TH, Lai KH *et al.* Alimentary tract and pancreas. Double-blind comparison of omeprazole 20 mg OM and ranitidine 300 mg NOCTE in duodenal ulcer: a Taiwan multi–centre study. *J Gastroenterol Hepatol* 1992; **7:** 572–6.
76 Valenzuela JE, Berlin RG, Snape WJ *et al.* U.S. experience with omeprazole in duodenal ulcer. Multicenter double-blind comparative study with ranitidine. *Dig Dis Sci* 1991; **36:** 761–8.
77 Ekstrom P, Carling L, Unge P *et al.* Lansoprazole versus omeprazole in active duodenal ulcer. A double-blind, randomized, comparative study. *Scand J Gastroenterol* 1995; **30:** 210–15.
78 Beker J, Bianchi Porro G, Bigard M *et al.* Double-blind comparison of pantoprazole and omeprazole for the treatment of acute duodenal ulcer. *Eur J Gastroenterol Hepatol* 1995; **7:** 407–10.
79 Rehner M, Rohner HG, Schepp W. Comparison of pantoprazole versus omeprazole in the treatment of acute duodenal ulceration – a multicentre study. *Aliment Pharmacol Ther* 1995; **9:** 411-16.
80 Jones DB, Howden CW, Burget DW *et al.* Acid suppression in duodenal ulcer: a meta-analysis to define optimal dosing with antisecretory drugs. *Gut* 1987; **28:** 1120–7.
81 Burget DW, Chiverton SG, Hunt RH. Is there an optimal degree of acid suppression for healing of duodenal ulcers? A model of the relationship between ulcer healing and acid suppression. *Gastroenterol* 1990; **99:** 345–51.
82 Dammann HG, Walter TA. Efficacy of continuous therapy for peptic ulcer in controlled clinical trials. *Aliment Pharmacol Ther* 1993; **7**(Suppl 2): 17–25.
83 Penston JG, Wormsley KG. Nine years of maintenance treatment with ranitidine for patients with duodenal ulcer disease. *Aliment Pharmacol Ther* 1992; **6:** 629–45.
84 O'Brien BJ, Goeree R, Hunt R *et al.* Economic evaluation of alternative therapies in the long term management of peptic ulcer disease and gastroesophageal relux disease. McMaster University. Canadian Coordinating Office of Health Technology Assessment (CCOHTA) report. 1996.
85 Ruszniewski Ph, Slama A, Pappo M *et al.* and GEMUD. Two year maintenance treatment of duodenal ulcer disease with ranitidine 150 mg: a prospective multicentre randomised study. *Gut* 1993; **34:** 1662–5.

86 Palmer RH, Frank WO, Karlstadt R. Maintenance therapy of duodenal ulcer with H_2-receptor antagonists – a meta-analysis. *Aliment Pharmacol Ther* 1990; **4:** 283–94.

87 Kurata JH, Koch GG, Nogawa AN. Comparison of ranitidine and cimetidine ulcer maintenace therapy. *J Clin Gastroenterol* 1987; **9:** 644–50.

88 Penston JG, Wormsley KG. Review article: maintenance treatment with H_2-receptor antagonists for peptic ulcer disease. *Aliment Pharmacol Ther* 1992; **6:** 3–29.

89 Lee FI, Hardman M, Jaderberg ME. Maintenance treatment of duodenal ulceration: ranitidine 300 mg at night is better than 150 mg in cigarette smokers. *Gut* 1991; **32:** 151–3.

90 Chiba N, Rao BV, Rademaker JW *et al.* Meta-analysis of the efficacy of antibiotic therapy in eradicating *Helicobacter pylori*. *Am J Gastroenterol* 1992; **87:** 1716–27.

91 Coghlan JG, Humphries H, Dooley C *et al.* *Campylobacter pylori* and recurrence of duodenal ulcer – a 12 month follow up study. *Lancet* 1987; **ii:** 1109–11.

92 Marshall BJ, Goodwin CS, Warren JR *et al.* Prospective double-blind trial of duodenal ulcer relapse after eradication of *Campylobacter pylori*. *Lancet* 1988; **ii:** 1437–42.

93 Rauws EAJ, Tytgat GNJ. Cure of duodenal ulcer associated with eradication of *Helicobacter pylori*. *Lancet* 1990; **335:** 1233–5.

94 George LL, Borody TJ, Andrews P *et al.* Cure of duodenal ulcer after eradication of *Helicobacter pylori*. *Med J Aust* 1990; **153:** 145–9.

95 Graham DY, Lem GM, Evans DG *et al.* Effect of triple therapy (antibiotics plus bismuth) on duodenal ulcer healing. A randomized controlled trial. *Ann Intern Med* 1991; **115:** 266–9.

96 Graham DY, Lew GM, Klein PD *et al.* Effect of treatment of *Helicobacter pylori* infection on the long-term recurrence of gastric or duodenal ulcer. A randomized, controlled study. *Ann Intern Med* 1992; **116:** 705–8.

97 Hentschel E, Brandstatter G, Dragosics B *et al.* Effect of ranitidine and amoxicillin plus metronidazole on the eradication of *Helicobacter pylori* and the recurrence of duodenal ulcer. *N Engl J Med* 1993; **328:** 308–12.

98 Tytgat GNJ. Review article: treatments that impact favourably upon the eradication of *Helicobacter pylori* and ulcer recurrence. *Aliment Pharmacol Ther* 1994; **8:** 359–68.

99 Penston JG. *Helicobacter pylori* eradication – understandable caution but no excuse for inertia. *Aliment Pharmacol Ther* 1994; **8:** 369–89.

100 Labenz J, Börsch G. Highly significant change of the clinical course of relapsing and complicated peptic ulcer disease after cure of *Helicobacter pylori* infection. *Am J Gastroenterol* 1994; **89:** 1785–8.

101 Hopkins RJ, Girardi LS, Turney EA. Relationship between *Helicobacter pylori* eradication and reduced duodenal and gastric ulcer recurrence: a review. *Gastroenterol* 1997; **110:** 1244–52.

102 Gisbert JP, Boixeda D, Martín De Argila C *et al.* Unhealed duodenal ulcers despite *Helicobacter pylori* eradication. *Scand J Gastroenterol* 1997; **32:** 643–50.

103 Hosking SW, Ling TK, Yung MY *et al.* Randomised controlled trial of short term treatment to eradicate *Helicobacter pylori* in patients with duodenal ulcer. *Br Med J* 1992; **305**(6852): 502–4.

104 Avsar E, Kalayci C, Tözün N *et al.* Refractory duodenal ulcer healing and relapse: comparison of omeprazole with *Helicobacter pylori* eradication. *Eur J Gastroenterol Hepatol* 1996; **8:** 449–52.

105 Bianchi Porro G, Parente F, Lazzaroni M. Short and long term outcome of *Helicobacter pylori* positive resistant duodenal ulcers treated with colloidal bismuth subcitrate plus antibiotics or sucralphate alone. *Gut* 1993; **34:** 466–9.

106 Mantzaris GJ, Hatzis A, Tamvakologos G *et al.* Prospective, randomized, investigator-blind trial of *Helicobacter pylori* infection treatment in patients with refractory duodenal ulcers. Healing and long-term relapse rates. *Dig Dis Sci* 1993; **38:** 1132–6.

107 Wagner S, Gebel M, Haruma K *et al.* Bismuth subsalicylate in the treatment of H_2-blocker resistant duodenal ulcers: role of *Helicbacter pylori*. *Gut* 1992; **33:** 179–83.

108 Zheng ZT, Wang ZY, Chu YX *et al.* Double-blind short-term trial of furazolidone in peptic ulcer. *Lancet* 1985; **i:** 1048–9.

109 Zhao HY, Li G, Guo J *et al.* Furazolidone in peptic ulcer. *Lancet* 1985; **ii:** 276–7.

110 Quintero Diaz M, Sotto Eschobar A. Metronidazole versus cimetidine in the treatment of gastroduodenal ulcer. *Lancet* 1986; **i:** 907.

111 Lam SK, Ching CK, Lai KC *et al.* Does treatment of *Helicobacter pylori* with antibiotics alone heal duodenal ulcer? A randomised double blind placebo controlled study. *Gut* 1997; **41:** 43–8.

112 Hosking SW, Ling TKW, Chung SCS *et al.* Duodenal ulcer healing by eradication of *Helicobacter pylori* without anti-acid treatment: randomized controlled trial. *Lancet* 1994; **343:** 508–10.

113 Logan RPH, Gummett PA, Misiewicz JJ *et al.* One week's anti-*Helicobacter pylori* treatment for duodenal ulcer. *Gut* 1994; **35:** 15–18.

114 Howden CW, Jones DB, Peace KE *et al.* The treatment of gastric ulcer with antisecretory drugs. Relationship of pharmacological

effect to healing rates. *Dig Dis Sci* 1988; **33:** 619–24.

115 Holt S, Howden CW. Omeprazole: overview and opinion. *Dig Dis Sci* 1991; **36:** 385–93.

116 Howden CW, Hunt RH. The relationship between suppression of acidity and gastric ulcer healing rates. *Aliment Pharmacol Ther* 1990; **4:** 25–33.

117 Howden CW, Burget DW, Hunt RH. A meta-analysis to predict gastric ulcer healing from acid suppression. *Gastroenterology* 1991; **100:** A13. (Abstract)

118 Howden CW, Burget DW, Hunt RH. A comparison of different drug classes with respect to rapidity of healing of gastric ulcer (GU). *Gastroenterology* 1993; **104:** A105. (Abstract)

119 Pilotto A, Di Mario F, Battaglia G *et al.* The efficacy of two doses of omeprazole for short-and long-term peptic ulcer treatment in the elderly. *Clin Ther* 1994; **16:** 935–41.

120 Labenz J, Börsch G. Evidence for the essential role of *Helicobacter pylori* in gastric ulcer disease. *Gut* 1994; **35:** 19–22.

121 Tatsuta M, Ishikawa H, Iishi H *et al.* Reduction of gastric ulcer recurrence after suppression of *Helicobacter pylori* by cefixime. *Gut* 1990; **31:** 973–6.

122 Asaka M, Ohtaki T, Kato M. Causal role of *Helicobacter pylori* in peptic ulcer relapse. *J Gastroenterol* 1994; **29**(Suppl 7): 134–8.

123 Sung JJY, Chung SCS, Ling TKW *et al.* Antibacterial treatment of gastric ulcers associated with *Helicobacter pylori*. *N Engl J Med* 1995; **332:** 139–42.

124 Bayerdörffer E, Miehlke S, Lehn N *et al.* Cure of gastric ulcer disease after cure of *Helicobacter pylori* infection – German Gastric Ulcer Study. *Eur J Gastroenterol Hepatol* 1996; **8:** 343–9.

125 Laine L. *Helicobacter pylori* and complicated ulcer disease. *Am J Med* 1996; **100:** 52S–59S.

126 Bardhan KD, Nayyar AK, Royston C. The outcome of bleeding duodenal ulcer in the era of H_2 receptor antagonist therapy. *Q J Med* 1998; **91:** 231–7.

127 Murray WR, Cooper G, Laferla G *et al.* Maintenance ranitidine treatment after haemorrhage from a duodenal ulcer: a 3 year follow up study. *Scand J Gastroenterol* 1988; **23:** 183–7.

128 Jensen DM, Cheng S, Kovacs TOG *et al.* A controlled study of ranitidine for the prevention of recurrent hemorrhage from duodenal ulcer. *N Engl J Med* 1994; **330:** 382–6.

129 Hosking SW, Yung MY, Chung SC *et al.* Differing prevalence of *Helicobacter* in bleeding and nonbleeding ulcers. *Gastroenterology* 1992; **102:** A85 (Abstract).

130 Jaspersen D, Körner T, Schorr W *et al.* Omeprazole–amoxycillin therapy for eradication of *Helicobacter pylori* in duodenal ulcer bleeding: preliminary results of a pilot study. *J Gastroenterol* 1995; **30:** 319–21.

131 Macri G, Milani S, Surrenti E *et al.* Eradication of *Helicobacter pylori* reduces the rate of duodenal ulcer rebleeding: a long-term follow-up study. *Am J Gastroenterol* 1998; **93:** 925–7.

132 Santander C, Grávalos RG, Gómez–Cedenilla A *et al.* Antimicrobial therapy for *Helicobacter pylori* infection versus long-term maintenance antisecretion treatment in the prevention of recurrent hemorrhage from peptic ulcer: prospective nonrandomized trial on 125 patients. *Am J Gastroenterol* 1996; **91:** 1549–52.

133 Riemann JF, Schilling D, Schauwecker P *et al.* Cure with omeprazole plus amoxicillin versus long-term ranitidine therapy in *Helicobacter pylori*-associated peptic ulcer bleeding. *Gastrointest Endosc* 1997; **46:** 299–304.

134 Sung JJY, Leung WK, Suen R *et al.* One-week antibiotics versus maintenance acid suppression therapy for *Helicobacter pylori*-associated peptic ulcer bleeding. *Dig Dis Sci* 1997; **42:** 2524–8.

135 Simpson CJ, Lamont G, Macdonald I *et al.* Effect of cimetidine on prognosis after simple closure of perforated duodenal ulcer. *Br J Surg* 1987; **74:** 104–5.

136 Svanes C, Øvrebø K, Søreide O. Ulcer bleeding and perforation: non-steroidal anti-inflammatory drugs or *Helicobacter pylori*. *Scand J Gastroenterol* 1996; **31**(Suppl 220): 128–31.

137 Reinbach DH, Cruickshank G, McColl KE. Acute perforated duodenal ulcer is not associated with *Helicobacter pylori* infection. *Gut* 1993; **34:** 1344–7.

138 Susser M. Civilization and peptic ulcer. *Lancet* 1962; **1:** 115–19.

139 Svanes C, Lie RT, Kvåle G *et al.* Incidence of perforated ulcer in Western Norway 1935–1990: cohort or period dependent time trends? *Am J Epidemiol* 1995; **141:** 836–44.

140 Banatvala N, Mayo K, Mégraud F *et al.* The cohort effect and *Helicobacter pylori*. *J Infect Dis* 1993; **168:** 219–21.

141 Coggon D, Lambert P, Langman MJS. 20 years of hospital admissions for peptic ulcer in England and Wales. *Lancet* 1981; **i:** 1302–4.

142 Kurata JH. Ulcer epidemiology: an overview and proposed research framework. *Gastroenterology* 1989; **96:** 569–80.

143 Mégraud F, Brassens-Rabbé MP, Denis F *et al.* Seroepidemiology of *Campylobacter pylori* in various populations. *J Clin Microbiol* 1989; **27:** 1870–3.

144 Hopkins RJ, Girardi LS, Turney EA. *Helicobacter pylori* eradication as a surrogate for reduced

peptic ulcer recurrence: a literature-based meta-analysis. *Gut* 1995; **37**(Suppl 1): A46(181) (Abstract).

145 Huang JQ, Hunt RH. Review: eradication of *Helicobacter pylori*. Problems and recommendations. *J Gastroenterol Hepatol* 1997; **12:** 590–8.

146 Penston JG, McColl KEL. Eradication of *Helicobacter pylori*: an objective assessment of current therapies. *Br J Clin Pharmacol* 1997; **43:** 223–43.

147 Graham DY, Lew GM, Malaty HM *et al.* Factors influencing the eradication of *Helicobacter pylori* with triple therapy. *Gastroenterology* 1992; **102:** 493–6.

148 Chiba N, Hunt RH. Drug therapy of *H. pylori* infection: a meta-analyss. In: Bianchi Porro G, Scarpignato, C (eds). *Clinical pharmacology and therapy of H. pylori infection. Progress in basic and clinical pharmacology.* 1999 (in press).

149 Chiba N, Hunt RH. Bismuth, metronidazole and tetracycline (BMT) ± acid suppression in *H. pylori* eradication: a meta-analysis. *Gut* 1996; **39**(Suppl 2): A36(4A: 27). (Abstract)

150 Huang JQ, Chiba N, Wilkinson J *et al.* Attempt by meta-analysis to define the optimal treatment regimen for eradicating *Helicobacter pylori (H. pylori)* infection. *Can J Gastroenterol* 1997; **11**(Suppl A): 44A(S14) (Abstract).

151 de Boer W, Driessen W, Jansz A *et al.* Effect of acid suppression on efficacy of treatment for *Helicobacter pylori* infection. *Lancet* 1995; **345:** 817–20.

152 De Boer WA, Driessen WMM, Potters HVPJ *et al.* Randomized study comparing 1 with 2 weeks of quadruple therapy for eradicating *Helicobacter pylori. Am J Gastroenterol* 1994; **89:** 1993–7.

153 De Boer WA, van Etten RJXM, Lai JYL *et al.* Effectiveness of quadruple therapy using lansoprazole, instead of omeprazole, in curing *Helicobacter pylori* infection. *Helicobacter* 1996; **1:** 145–50.

154 Tytgat GNJ. Aspects of anti-*Helicobacter pylori* eradication therapy. In: Hunt RH, Tytgat GNJ (eds) *Helicobacter pylori: basic mechanisms to clinical cure.* Lancaster: Kluwer Academic Publishers, 1996, pp. 340–7.

155 Hunt RH. Hp and pH: implications for the eradication of *Helicobacter pylori. Scand J Gastroenterol* (Suppl): 1993; **196:** 12–16.

156 Hunt RH. pH and Hp-gastric acid secretion and *Helicobacter pylori*: implications for ulcer healing and eradication of the organism. *Am J Gastroenterol* 1993; **88:** 481–3.

157 Chiba N, Wilkinson JM, Hunt RH. Clarithromycin (C) or amoxicillin (A) dual and triple therapies in *H. pylori (Hp)* eradication: A meta-analysis. *Gut* 1995; **37**(Suppl 2): A31(T124) (Abstract).

158 Unge P, Berstad A. Pooled analysis of anti-*Helicobacter pylori* treatment regimens. *Scand J Gastroenterol* 1996; **31**(Suppl 220): 27–40.

159 Unge P. What other regimens are under investigation to treat *Helicobacter pylori* infection? *Gastroenterol* 1997; **113**(6 Suppl): S131–S148.

160 Peterson WL, Graham DY, Marshall BJ *et al.* Clarithromycin as monotherapy for eradication of *Helicobacter pylori*: a randomized, double-blind trial. *Am J Gastroenterol.* 1993; **88:** 1860–4.

161 Bazzoli F, Zagari RM, Fossi S *et al.* Efficacy and tolerability of a short term, low dose triple therapy for eradication of *Helicobacter pylori. Gastroenterology* 1993; **104:** A40 (Abstract).

162 Prakash A, Faulds D. Rabeprazole. *Drugs* 1998; **55:** 261–7.

163 Lind T, Veldhuyzen van Zanten SJO, Unge P *et al.* Eradication of *Helicobacter pylori* using one week triple therapies combining omeprazole with two antimicrobials – the *MACH* 1 study. *Helicobacter* 1996; **1:** 138–4.

164 Malfertheiner P, on behalf of the European *Helicobacter Pylori* Study Group (EHPSG). Current European concepts in the management of *Helicobacter pylori* infection. The Mäastricht Consensus report. *Gut* 1997; **41:** 8–13.

165 Hunt R, Thomson ABR, Consensus Conference participants. Canadian *Helicobacter pylori* Consensus Conference. *Can J Gastroenterol* 1998; **12:** 31–41.

166 Peura DA. The Report of the Digestive Health Initiative^{SM} International Update Conference on *Helicobacter pylori. Gastroenterology* 1997; **113**(Suppl): S4–S8.

167 Lam SK, Talley NJ. Report of the 1997 Asia Pacific Consensus Conference on the management of *Helicobacter pylori* infection. *J Gastroenterol Hepatol* 1998; **13:** 1–12.

168 Lamouliatte H, Cayla R, Zerbib F *et al.* Dual therapy using a double dose of lansoprazole with amoxicillin versus triple therapy using a double dose of lansoprazole, amoxicillin, and clarithromycin to eradicate *Helicobacter pylori* infection: results of a prospective randomized open study. *Am J Gastroenterol* 1998; **93:** 1531–4.

169 Spinzi GC, Bierti L, Bortoli A *et al.* Comparison of omeprazole and lansoprazole in short-term triple therapy for *Helicobacter pylori* infection. *Aliment Pharmacol Ther* 1998; **12:** 433–8.

170 Fennerty MB, Kovacs TO, Krause R. A comparison of 10 and 14 days of lansoprazole triple therapy for eradication of *Helicobacter pylori. Arch Intern Med* 1998; **158:** 1651–6.

171 Cammarota G, Tursi A, Papa A *et al. Helicobacter pylori* eradication using one-week low-dose lansoprazole plus amoxycillin and either clarithromycin or azithromycin. *Aliment Pharmacol Ther* 1996; **10:** 997–1000.

172 Takimoto T, Satoh K, Taniguchi Y *et al.* The efficacy and safety of one-week triple therapy with lansoprazole, clarithromycin, and metronidazole for the treatment of *Helicobacter pylori* infection in Japanese patients. *Helicobacter* 1997; **2:** 86–91.
173 Lazzaroni M, Bargiggia S, Porro GB. Triple therapy with ranitidine or lansoprazole in the treatment of *Helicobacter pylori*-associated duodenal ulcer. *Am J Gastroenterol* 1997; **92:** 649–52.
174 Chey WD, Fisher L, Elta GH *et al.* Bismuth subsalicylate instead of metronidazole with lansoprazole and clarithromycin for *Helicobacter pylori* infection: a randomized trial. *Am J Gastroenterol* 1997; **92:** 1483–6.
175 Misiewicz JJ, Harris AW, Bardhan KD *et al.* One week triple therapy for *Helicobacter pylori*: a multicentre comparative study. Lansoprazole *Helicobacter* Study Group. *Gut* 1997; **41:** 735–9.
176 Frevel M, Daake H, Janisch HD *et al.* Pantoprazole plus clarithromycin and metronidazole versus pantoprazole plus clarithromycin and amoxycillin for therapy of *H. pylori* infection. *Gastroenterology* 1997; **112:** A119 (Abstract).
177 Adamek RJ, Szymanski C, Pfaffenbach B. Pantoprazole vs omeprazole in one-week low-dose triple therapy for cure of *H. pylori* infection. *Gastroenterology* 1997; **112:** A53 (Abstract).
178 Adamek RJ, Pfaffenbach B, Szymanski Ch. Does pre-treatment with pantoprazole affect the efficacy of a modern triple therapy in *HP* cure? *Gut* 1997; **41**(Suppl 3): A211 (Abstract).
179 Labenz J, Tillenburg B, Weismüller J *et al.* Efficacy and tolerability of a one-week triple therapy consisting of pantoprazole, clarithromycin and amoxycillin for cure of *Helicobacter pylori* infection in patients with duodenal ulcer. *Aliment Pharmacol Ther* 1997; **11:** 95–100.
180 Veldhuyzen van Zanten SJO, Bradette M, Farley A *et al.* The DU–MACH study: eradication of *Helicobacter pylori*, ulcer healing and relapse in duodenal ulcer patients. Omeprazole and clarithromycin in combination with either amoxicillin or metronidazole. *Gut* 1997; **41**(Suppl 1): A103(09/381) (Abstract).
181 Malfertheiner P, Bayerdörffer E, Diete U *et al.* The GU–MACH study: eradication of *Helicobacter pylori*, ulcer healing and relapse in gastric ulcer patients. Omeprazole and clarithromycin in combination with either amoxicillin or metronidazole. *Gut* 1997; **41**(Suppl 1): A97(09/356) (Abstract).
182 Lind T, Bardhan KD, Bayerdörffer E *et al.* The MACH 2 study: optimal *Helicobacter pylori* therapy needs omeprazole and can be reliably assessed by UBT. *Gastroenterology* 1997; **112:** A200 (Abstract).
183 Megraud F, Lehn N, Lind T *et al.* The MACH 2 study. *Helicobacter pylori* resistance to antimicrobial agents and its influence on clinical outcome. *Gastroenterology* 1997; **112:** A216 (Abstract).
184 Chiba N, Sinclair P. Metronidazole 500 mg is as effective as metronidazole 400 mg in the MACH 1 regimen for *H. pylori* eradication: a meta-analysis. *Can J Gastroenterol* 1998; **12**(Suppl A): 91A (Abstract).
185 Bardhan KD, Bayerdorffer E, Delchier JP *et al* on behalf of the HOMER investigators in Canada FGS & UK. *H. pylori (Hp)* eradication with omeprazole (O), metronidazole (M) and amoxicillin (A): the impact of drug dosing and resistance on efficacy – the HOMER story. *Gastroenterology* 1998; **114:** A65(G0264) (Abstract).
186 Tytgat GNJ. Current indications for *Helicobacter pylori* eradication therapy. *Scand J Gastroenterol* 1996; **31**(Suppl 215): 70-3.
187 Unge P. Review of *Helicobacter pylori* eradication regimens. *Scand J Gastroenterol* 1996; 31 (Suppl 215): 74–81.
188 van der Hulst RWM, Keller JJ, Rauws EAJ *et al.* Treatment of *Helicobacter pylori* infection: a review of the world literature. *Helicobacter* 1996; **1:** 6–19.
189 Consensus conference. Ulcer and gastritis at the time of *Helicobacter pylori*. *Gastroenterol Clin Biol* 1996; **20** (1 Pt 2): S1–S165.
190 Kang JY, Fock KM, Ng HS *et al.* Working Party report of the Gastroenterological Society of Singapore. Part I—*Helicobacter pylori* and peptic ulcer disease in Singapore. *Singapore Med J* 1996; **37:** 304–6.
191 Ellenrieder V, Fensterer H, Waurick M *et al.* Influence of clarithromycin dosage on pantoprazole combined triple therapy for eradication of *Helicobacter pylori*. *Aliment Pharmacol Ther* 1998; **12:** 613–18.
192 Lerang F, Moum B, Haug JB *et al.* Highly effective triple therapy with omeprazole, amoxicillin and clarithromycin in previous *H. pylori* treatment failures. *Gut* 1996; **39**(Suppl 2): A36 (4A: 25) (Abstract).
193 Moayyedi P, Sahay P, Tompkins DS *et al.* Efficacy and optimum dose of omeprazole in a new 1-week triple therapy regimen to eradicate *Helicobacter pylori*. *Eur J Gastroenterol Hepatol* 1995; **7:** 835–40.
194 Bazzoli F, Zagari M, Pozzato P *et al.* Evaluation of short-term low-dose triple therapy for the eradication of *Helicobacter pylori* by factorial design in a randomized, double-blind, controlled study. *Aliment Pharmacol Ther* 1998; **12:** 439–45.
195 Misiewicz JJ, Harris AW, Bardhan KD *et al.* One week low-dose *H. pylori* eradication therapy

heals 90% of duodenal ulcers. *Gut* 1996; **39** (Suppl 2): A34(4A: 15) (Abstract).

196 Labenz J, Idstrom JP, Tillenburg B *et al.* One-week low-dose triple therapy for *Helicobacter pylori* is sufficient for relief from symptoms and healing of duodenal ulcers. *Aliment Pharmacol Ther* 1997; **11:** 89–93.

197 Goh KL, Navaratnam P, Peh SC *et al. Helicobacter pylori* eradication with short–term therapy leads to duodenal ulcer healing without the need for continued acid suppression therapy. *Eur J Gastroenterol Hepatol* 1996; **8:** 421–3.

198 Gisbert JP, Boixeda D, Martín DA *et al.* New one-week triple therapies with metronidazole for the eradication of *Helicobacter pylori*: clarithromycin or amoxycillin as the second antibiotic. *Med Clin (Barc.)* 1998; **110:** 1–5.

199 De Boer WA, Haeck PW, Otten MH *et al.* Optimal treatment of *Helicobacter pylori* with ranitidine bismuth citrate (RBC): a randomized comparison between two 7-day triple therapies and a 14-day dual therapy. *Am J Gastroenterol* 1998; **93:** 1101–7.

200 Pounder RE, Wyeth JW, Duggan AE *et al.* Ranitidine bismuth citrate with clarithromycin for the eradication of *Helicobacter pylori* and for ulcer healing. *Helicobacter* 1997; **2:** 132–9.

201 Kolkman JJ, Tan TG, Oudkerk Pool M *et al.* Ranitidine bismuth citrate with clarithromycin versus omeprazole with amoxycillin in the cure of *Helicobacter pylori* infection. *Aliment Pharmacol Ther* 1997; **11:** 1123–9.

202 Dobrilla G, Di Matteo G, Dodero M *et al.* Ranitidine bismuth citrate with either clarithromycin 1 g/day or 1.5 g/day is equally effective in the eradication of *H. pylori* and healing of duodenal ulcer. *Aliment Pharmacol Ther* 1998; **12:** 63–8.

203 Peterson WL, Ciociola AA, Sykes DL *et al* and the RBC *H. pylori* ulcer group. Ranitidine bismuth citrate plus clarithromycin is effective for healing duodenal ulcers, eradicating *H. pylori* and reducing ulcer recurrence. *Aliment Pharmacol Ther* 1996; **10:** 251–61.

204 Pare P, Romaozinho J, Bardhan KD *et al.* Ranitidine bismuth citrate (RBC) is more effective than omeprazole in the eradication of *H. pylori* when co-prescribed with clarithromycin. *Gastroenterol* 1997; **112:** A251 (Abstract).

205 Bardhan KD, Wurzer H, Marcelino M *et al.* Ranitidine bismuth citrate with clarithromycin given twice daily effectively eradicates *Helicobacter pylori* and heals duodenal ulcers. *Am J Gastroenterol* 1998; **93:** 380–5.

206 van der Wouden EJ, Thijs JC, Van Zwet AA *et al.* One-week triple therapy with ranitidine bismuth citrate, clarithromycin and metronidazole versus two-week dual therapy with ranitidine bismuth citrate and clarithromycin for *Helicobacter pylori* infection: a randomized, clinical trial. *Am J Gastroenterol* 1998; **93:** 1228–31.

207 Axon ATR, Ireland A, Lancaster-Smith MJ *et al.* Ranitidine bismuth citrate and clarithromycin twice daily in the eradication of *Helicobacter pylori. Aliment Pharmacol Ther* 1997; **11:** 81–7.

208 Pozzato P, Zagari M, Cardelli A *et al.* Ranitidine bismuth citrate plus clarithromycin 7-day regimen is effective in eradicating *Helicobacter pylori* in patients with duodenal ulcer. *Aliment Pharmacol Ther* 1998; **12:** 447–51.

209 Megrand F, Pichavant R, Palegry D *et al.* Ranitidise bismuth citrate (RBC) co-prescribed with clarithromycin is more effective in the eradication of *Helicobacter pylori* than omeprazole with clarithromycin. *Gut* 1997: **41** (Suppl 1): A92 (09/337) (Abstract).

210 Perschy TB, McSorley DJ, Sorrells SC *et al.* Ranitidine bismuth citrate in combination with clarithromycin is effective against *H. pylori* strains with susceptible or intermediate clarithromycin sensitivity. *Gastroenterology* 1997; **112:** A257 (Abstract).

211 Sung JJY, Leung WK, Ling TKW *et al.* One-week use of ranitidine bismuth citrate, amoxycillin and clarithromycin for the treatment of *Helicobacter pylori*-related duodenal ulcer. *Aliment Pharmacol Ther* 1998; **12:** 725–30.

212 Pipkin GA, Williamson R, Wood JR. Review article: one-week clarithromycin triple therapy regimens for eradication of *Helicobacter pylori. Aliment Pharmacol Ther* 1998; **12:** 823–37.

213 McLaren A, Donnelly C, McDowell S *et al.* The role of ranitidine bismuth citrate in significantly reducing the emergence of *Helicobacter pylori* strains resistant to antibiotics. *Helicobacter* 1997; 2(1):21–6.

214 López–Brea M, Domingo D, Sánchez I *et al.* Synergism study of ranitidine bismuth citrate and metronidazole against metronidazole resistant *H. pylori* clinical isolates. *Gastroenterology* 1997; **112:** A201 (Abstract).

215 Osato MS, Graham DY. Ranitidine bismuth citrate enhances clarithromycin activity against clinical isolates of *H. pylori. Gastroenterology* 1997; **112:** A1057 (Abstract).

216 vd Wouden EJ, Thijs JC, Van Zwet AA *et al.* Metronidazole resistance does not influence the efficacy of triple therapy with ranitidine bismuth citrate (RBC), clarithromycin (CLA) and metronidazole (MET) for *H. pylori (Hp)* infection. *Gastroenterology* 1998; **114:** A323(G1321) (Abstract).

217 Graham DY, Hepps KS, Ramirez FC *et al.* Treatment of *Helicobacter pylori* reduces the rate of rebleeding in peptic ulcer disease. *Scand J Gastroenterol* 1993; **28:** 939–42.

218 Jaspersen D, Koerner T, Schorr W *et al. Helicobacter pylori* eradication reduces the rate of

rebleeding in ulcer hemorrhage. *Gastrointest Endosc* 1995; **41:** 5–7.

219 Labenz J, Borsch G. Role of *Helicobacter pylori* eradication in the prevention of peptic ulcer bleeding relapse. *Digestion* 1994; **55:** 19–23.

220 Rokkas T, Karameris A, Mavrogeorgis A *et al.* Eradication of *Helicobacter pylori* reduces the possibility of rebleeding in peptic ulcer disease. *Gastrointest Endosc* 1995; **41:** 1–4.

221 Savarino V, Mansi C, Mele MR *et al.* A new 1-week therapy for *Helicobacter pylori* eradication: ranitidine bismuth citrate plus two antibiotics. *Aliment Pharmacol Ther* 1997; **11:** 699–703.

222 Cammarota G, Cannizzaro O, Tursi A *et al.* One-week therapy for *Helicobacter pylori* eradication: ranitidine bismuth citrate plus medium-dose clarithromycin and either tinidazole or amoxycillin. *Aliment Pharmacol Ther* 1998; **12:** 539–43.

223 Ricciardiello L, Cannizzaro O, D'Angelo A *et al.* Efficacy and safety of three 7-day *Helicobacter pylori* eradication regimens containing ranitidine bismuth citrate. *Aliment Pharmacol Ther* 1998; **12:** 533–7.

224 Williams MP, Hamilton MR, Sercombe JC *et al.* Seven-day treatment for *Helicobacter pylori* infection: ranitidine bismuth citrate plus clarithromycin and tetracycline hydrochloride. *Aliment Pharmacol Ther* 1997; **11:** 705–10.

Ulcer disease and non-steroidal anti-inflammatory drugs: etiology and treatment

4

ALAA ROSTOM, ANDREAS MAETZEL, PETER TUGWELL, GEORGE WELLS

BACKGROUND

Non-steroidal anti-inflammatory drugs (NSAIDs) including aspirin are important agents in the management of patients with a variety of arthritic and inflammatory conditions.[1] Additionally, aspirin has gained importance in the treatment and prevention of both myocardial infarction and stroke.[2–5] The efficacy of these agents is well described, making NSAIDs among the most frequently used medications, with an estimated world market in excess of $6 billion annually.[6]

NSAIDs including aspirin (ASA) cause a variety of gastrointestinal toxicities, which are associated with excess utilization of health care resources at a substantial cost.[7] Minor adverse effects such as nausea and dyspepsia are relatively common, but these clinical symptoms correlate poorly with serious adverse gastrointestinal events.[8,9] Although, endoscopic ulcers, occurring with or without symptoms, can be documented in as many as 40% of chronic NSAID users,[10] serious NSAID induced gastrointestinal toxicities are much less common.[9] Due to the vast numbers of individuals using these drugs, however, they have been linked directly to over 70 000 hospitalizations and over 7000 deaths annually in the United States alone.[11] NSAID use can also add significantly to the morbidity and mortality of chronic arthritic conditions. Among rheumatoid arthritis patients who are chronically using NSAIDs, the chance of hospitalization or death due to a gastrointestinal event is about 1.3–1.6% per year,[11] accounting for about 2600 deaths and 20 000 hospitalizations each year.[1] These figures have led some to the suggestion that NSAID toxicity is among the "deadliest" of rheumatic disorders.[11]

The serious gastrointestinal complications such as hemorrhage, perforation, or death occur collectively with an incidence of about 2% per year in an average patient population.[9] The relative risk of upper gastrointestinal hemorrhage or perforation with NSAID use varies in the literature from 4.7 in hospital based case–control studies to 2.0 in cohort studies.[12–14] Gabriel *et al* in a meta-analysis of 16 studies found that non-ASA NSAIDs were associated with a 2.7-fold increased risk of serious gastrointestinal events resulting in hospitalization.[15] Similarly, Langman *et al* found that ASA and non-ASA NSAID use increased the risk of bleeding peptic ulcer 3.1-fold and 3.5-fold respectively.[16] In a recent large prospective cohort study of 126 000 patients conducted over three years, MacDonald *et al* found that NSAIDs increased the risk of any adverse gastrointestinal event 3.9-fold, similar to the findings above. However, NSAIDs appeared to raise the risk 8.0-fold, when only hemorrhage or perforation were considered,[17] a level which is sufficiently high as to imply causation. Armstrong *et al* found that 60% of 235 consecutive

Box 4.1 Risk factors for NSAID gastrointestinal toxicity
Age >60
Previous peptic ulcer disease
Underlying medical conditions
Concomitant corticosteroid use
Concomitant anticoagulant therapy or ASA
High dose of NSAID or multiple NSAIDs
Type of NSAID
Duration of NSAID use/compliance
Helicobacter pylori? see text

patients presenting with a significant peptic ulcer complication were taking NSAIDs, and nearly 80% of all ulcer related deaths occurred in NSAIDs users.[18]

NSAIDs have also been linked to a variety of other gastrointestinal toxicities, including pyloric stenosis, small bowel ulcerations, strictures, lower gastrointestinal bleeds, and the exacerbation of colitis.[6,19–21] Some experts suggest that the most effective means to prevent NSAID induced gastrointestinal toxicity is to discontinue the use of the NSAID, or to substitute a non-gastrointestinal toxic analgesic in its stead.[22] However, this approach is clearly not always feasible since a large proportion of NSAID users rely heavily on these medications, and a delicate balance exists between the therapeutic benefits and the risks of these drugs.[23]

The focus of this chapter will be to review the current evidence for the treatment and prevention of NSAID induced upper gastrointestinal toxicity. We will discuss the risk factors for NSAID induced gastrointestinal toxicity, including the current evidence for the role of *Helicobacter pylori* as a possible coexistent risk factor. The issues surrounding the use of surrogate outcomes and their relationship to true clinical events in the interpretation of clinical trials in this area will be discussed. This chapter will also be supplemented by findings from our Cochrane collaborative systematic review of the same subject.

RISK FACTORS FOR NSAID RELATED GASTROINTESTINAL TOXICITY

Several studies, meta-analyses, and reviews have addressed the issue of risk factors for NSAID induced gastrointestinal toxicity. Increasing age (>65), previous peptic ulcer disease with or without previous hemorrhage, and co-morbid medical illnesses, particularly heart disease, have been consistently shown to increase the risk of an adverse gastrointestinal event among patients on long term NSAID therapy.[9,11,13,15,24–28] Using multiple logistic regression to adjusts for risk factors simultaneously, Silverstein *et al* found that among patients on chronic NSAIDs with none of these risk factors, only 0.4% developed a serious adverse gastrointestinal event at 6 months, whereas 9% of patients with all three risk factors experienced such an event.[9] Other risk factors have also been identified (Box 4.1). High doses of NSAIDs and the use of multiple NSAIDs increase the risk of adverse outcomes, as do the combined use of NSAIDs with corticosteroids, ASA, or warfarin.[27,29] Specific NSAIDs (Table 4.1), and in some studies female gender, are also associated with an increased risk of gastrointestinal toxicity.[25–27,30–33] The newer COX-2

Table 4.1 Individual NSAIDs and the risk of gastrointestinal events (relative to ibuprofen)

Drug	Relative risk
Azopropazone	4.07
Fenoprofen	3.08
Piroxicam	2.82
Flurbiprophen	2.31
All others	1.91
Mefenamic acid	1.81
Diclofenac retard	1.68
Naproxen	1.44
Diclofenac	1.35
Ketoprofen	1.29
Indomethacin	1.25
Ibuprofen	1.00
Fenbuten	0.50
Nabumetone	0.37
Dose:	
Low	1.00
Medium	1.25
High	1.39

Adapted from MacDonald *et al.*[17]

specific NSAIDS with reportedly lower gastrointestinal toxicity will be discussed at the end of this chapter.

The duration of NSAID use has been reported as a risk factor for gastrointestinal toxicity with most studies suggesting that the risk is highest within the first month of use.[12,16,31,34,35] However there is increasing evidence to suggest that the risk of significant NSAID toxicity does not diminish with prolonged use beyond 1 month. Silverstein *et al*, in their prospective study of misoprostol for the prevention of serious NSAID related gastrointestinal events, did not find a decreased risk with continued NSAID use.[9] Furthermore, in a large prospective cohort study of NSAID related gastrointestinal toxicity, MacDonald *et al.* found that there was a four-fold relative risk increase associated with the use of NSAIDs and that this risk was nearly constant over the 3-year follow-up period.[17] Additionally these investigators found that a two-fold relative risk of gastrointestinal toxicity persisted for at least 1 year after the last exposure to NSAIDs.

Compliance with NSAID use also appears to be a risk factor for gastrointestinal toxicity. Wynne *et al*, in a study of patient awareness of adverse effects and symptoms associated with NSAIDs, found that patients suffering an adverse gastrointestinal event had a higher rate of compliance (96%) with their NSAID use than those not suffering an event (70%).[36] Similarly, Griffin *et al* found that patients suffering a terminal NSAID related gastrointestinal event were more likely to have filed a prescription for an NSAID in the preceding month.[12] Symptoms, however, correlate quite poorly with the occurrence of endoscopic ulceration and adverse gastrointestinal events, and thus cannot be considered predictors of adverse gastrointestinal events.[8,9,18,29,37]

The role of *Helicobacter pylori* infection as a risk factor for NSAID related gastrointestinal toxicity is controversial and is discussed later below.

DO ENDOSCOPIC ULCERS PREDICT CLINICAL EVENTS?

Gastrointestinal ulcers are established as the pathophysiological correlate of clinical gastrointestinal events resulting from the chronic use of NSAIDs. For this reason endoscopically confirmed ulcers have been used as surrogate outcomes for clinical gastrointestinal events resulting from NSAID use. Endoscopic definitions of gastroduodenal ulcers are controversial,[38] and do not equate with the pathological definition, which defines an ulcer as a loss of mucosal surface of sufficient depth to penetrate the muscularis mucosa.[39] In most clinical trials of NSAID prophylaxis, an endoscopic ulcer is defined as a break in the mucosal surface, usually greater than 3 mm in diameter with some appreciable depth. The strictness of these criteria has varied from study to study, with some authors requiring the use of an endoscopic measuring tool, or an estimation based on the size of an open biopsy forceps to measure the ulcer diameter. Formal estimates of inter-observer variability among the endoscopists are often not presented, particularly in the larger multicenter trials. Some authors define an ulcer as the loss of mucosal surface of 5 mm or greater in diameter to better differentiate them from erosions and to achieving closer agreement with clinical events.[38] Varying definitions of endoscopic ulcers and the occasional use of composite endpoints all complicate comparison of results across studies.

Unfortunately, endoscopic ulcers are not ideal surrogate outcomes for clinical gastrointestinal events such as bleeding or perforation of an ulcer. In fact, the proportion of endoscopic ulcers that never become clinically symptomatic, is estimated to be as high as 85%.[9,40] Furthermore, with the publication of a large randomized controlled trial that used actual clinical endpoints to measure the efficacy of misoprostol,[9] it became possible to compare the reduction in clinical events with that of the reduction in endoscopic ulcers from previous studies of misoprostol. Some authors argue that the relative risk reduction of 40% observed on clinical events with misoprostol is similar to that observed for the reduction of endoscopic ulcers.[9,41,42] However, we have found, in our own review of the literature, that the relative risk reduction in endoscopic ulcers with misoprostol is closer to 80%. Unfortunately Silverstein's study is the only RCT using clinical gastrointestinal events as the primary outcome measure, but it was not designed to look at the relationship of clinical events to endoscopic ulcers.[9]

From a theoretical perspective, Wittes *et al*[43] point out that, if a surrogate (in this case an endoscopic ulcer) is a marker for a variety of processes, then an intervention that alters the risk of the surrogate by a mechanism unrelated to the risk of the real endpoint (clinical gastrointestinal event) will appear effective in a surrogate endpoint trial, but will not be effective in practice (see Figure 4.1). This point should be kept in mind when assessing trials of NSAID ulcer prophylaxis. At most the current evidence would limit this extrapolation to endoscopic studies of misoprostol or to other prostaglandin analogues. Since there are currently no prospective studies of the effects of H_2-receptor antagonists or H^+ pump inhibitors on clinical gastrointestinal events among chronic NSAID users, extrapolation of the misoprostol data across drug classes to these other agents is purely speculative at this point. A study of one of these agents showing a reduction in clinical events similar to that seen with misoprostol would be required to finally put to rest this controversy over the use of endoscopic ulcers as surrogates and in the extrapolation of these data across drug classes.

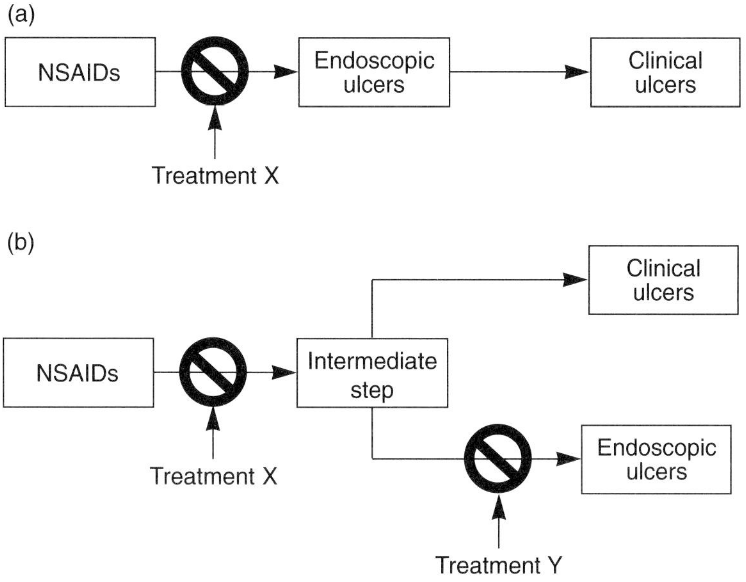

Figure 4.1 If the mechanism of clinical ulcers goes through endoscopic ulcers, then treatment X will prevent both endoscopic and clinical ulcers (a). However, if NSAIDs cause endoscopic ulcers and clinical ulcers by two different mechanisms, then treatment X will still be effective in preventing both, but treatment Y will only be effective in preventing endoscopic ulcers (b)

THE ROLE OF *HELICOBACTER PYLORI* IN NSAID ASSOCIATED ULCERS

The causal role of *Helicobacter pylori* (Hp) in the development of gastroduodenal ulcers has added a new perspective to the management of patients with gastrointestinal complaints.[44–46] NSAIDs are now thought to cause approximately 25% of gastroduodenal ulcers,[47] and do so in the absence of Hp.[48–51] The detection of any possible interaction between Hp and NSAIDs is complicated by the fact that NSAID use is most frequent among elderly patients, the same group with the highest Hp prevalence in Western populations.[52,53] Additionally, when an ulcer is found in the presence of both factors, it can be difficult to determine if it is an NSAID ulcer with incidental Hp, an Hp ulcer with incidental NSAIDs, or an Hp ulcer exacerbated by NSAIDs.[54,55] Despite this, an interaction between Hp and NSAIDs seems unlikely based on several retrospective epidemiological studies.[47,56–59] Unfortunately the only prospective study of NSAID induced clinical gastrointestinal events did not consider Hp status and thus does not shed any light on this controversy.[9] The studies described below describe our current understanding of the role of Hp in NSAID related upper gastrointestinal toxicity.

Retrospective case–control studies

Although gastric ulcers predominate over duodenal ulcers among chronic NSAID users, NSAID related ulcer complications appear to occur with equal frequency at both sites, leading some experts to speculate that clinically important events, such as hemorrhage or perforation, are the result of NSAIDs exacerbating pre-existing Hp related ulcers.[60–62] Heresbach *et al* assessed the prevalence of Hp and the severity of gastropathy in 66 chronic NSAID users and 45 controls. There was no difference in the prevalence of Hp between NSAID users and controls, but among patients taking NSAIDs, a significantly higher incidence of Hp was found among those patients with the most severe gastropathy.[63] Taha *et al* likewise found that NSAID users who were Hp positive and had gastric erosions were more likely to develop ulcers with continued NSAID use.[64] Publig *et al* found that 83% of 42 chronic NSAID users with peptic ulcers were Hp positive as opposed to 45% in a control group of 38 chronic NSAID users without ulcers ($P < 0.001$).[65] However, other investigators have found that Hp is relatively under-represented among patients presenting with upper gastrointestinal bleeds, suggesting that NSAIDs alone were responsible for this complication.[50]

Conflicting evidence for interaction between Hp and NSAIDs

That an interaction between Hp and NSAIDs leads to a lower risk of ulcers is also theoretically possible if one factor antagonizes the action of the other. Hawkey *et al* found that omeprazole and ranitidine were more effective at both healing and preventing ulcers in Hp positive than in Hp negative subjects.[66,67] Since relapse in these studies was defined as a composite of three endpoints, it is difficult to determine which endpoint was most responsible for this apparent difference. However, in support of Hawkey's findings, Labenz *et al* found that the presence of Hp enhanced the ability of omeprazole to raise gastric pH among patients with duodenal ulcer.[68] Additionally, Hp blunts the NSAID induced reduction of gastric mucosal prostaglandin E_2 production,[59,69,70] and reduces early NSAID induced mucosal damage.[70] However, Konturek *et al.*[70] found that at 2 weeks, Hp negative subjects had significantly lower endoscopic severity scores and mucosal micro-bleeding rates than Hp positive subjects. On the other hand, at 4 weeks, Laine *et al*[59] found no difference in endoscopic gastroduodenal injury scores between Hp positive and negative subjects on continuous NSAID therapy. Konturek *et al*[70] also found that the presence of Hp blunted mucosal adaptation to a 2 week course of aspirin therapy, while Lipscomb *et al* found that the adaptation to naproxen at 1 month was independent of Hp status.[71]

Randomized controlled trials of Hp eradication

Two randomized trials assessed the efficacy of Hp eradication therapy on subsequent NSAID ulcer development.[72,73] Bianchi Porro *et al* studied the effect of Hp eradication on ulcer healing and recurrence in 100 chronic NSAID users with peptic ulcers.[72] Of the 70 Hp positive patients, 34 were randomized to omeprazole alone 20 mg twice daily for 4–8 weeks, and 36 to receive the omeprazole regimen plus a 2 week course of amoxycillin (1 g twice daily). The 30 Hp negative patients were treated with omeprazole alone, 20 mg twice daily for 4–8 weeks. The presence of Hp did not statistically affect the healing rates at either 4 or 8 weeks. The 62 patients with healed ulcers were divided into three groups for a study of the relationship of Hp status to recurrence. Of these patients 19 were Hp negative, 29 Hp persistent, and 14 had Hp infection eradicated. The 6-month cumulative recurrence rates were: 27% (Hp negative), 46% (Hp positive), and 31% (Hp successfully eradicated). The differences among these recurrence rates were not statistically significant, although the study probably lacked adequate power to detect a clinically meaningful difference.

R Grade A

In a recent study, Chan *et al* recruited NSAID naive patients with musculoskeletal complaints in a single-blind randomized trial.[73] Of 202 patients screened, 100 Hp positive patients who were free of ulcers at a screening endoscopy were randomized to receive naproxen alone or Hp eradication (bismuth, tetracycline, and metronidazole) followed by naproxen. At 8 weeks, 12 of the 47 patients (26%) in the naproxen alone group developed ulcers (9 gastric, 2 duodenal, 1 both), whereas, 3 of 45 (7%) in the triple therapy group developed gastric ulcers ($P = 0.01$), for a 74% relative risk reduction with Hp eradication. The difference in ulcer frequencies was also statistically significant when analysed on an intention to treat basis. This is the first study to prospectively assess the effect of Hp eradication for the primary prophylaxis against NSAID ulcer development This study included mostly "high" risk older patients, with coexistent medical problems, so these results may not be generalizable to other patient groups.

R Grade A

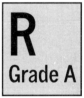

Based on this preliminary evidence, it is reasonable to eradicate Hp if it is present in chronic NSAID users who present with an ulcer, since it is difficult to determine which factor was most responsible.[61,74] There is no evidence, however, to suggest that Hp eradication alone is adequate for secondary ulcer prophylaxis in those who require continued NSAID therapy. There is insufficient evidence to support a recommendation for the eradication of Hp as primary prophylaxis in all chronic NSAID users. However, in a subset of high risk, older Hp positive patients, Hp eradication appears to reduce the incidence of endoscopic ulcers. The impact of this practice on clinical gastrointestinal events and its cost effectiveness remain to be determined.

MISOPROSTOL

Misoprostol is a synthetic prostaglandin E_1 analogue.[75–78] It reduces basal and stimulated gastric acid secretion through a direct effect on parietal cells,[78] and reduces gastric damage caused by a variety of aggressive factors including bile salts and NSAIDs.[79] Misoprostol's protective effects are felt to be related to its ability to stimulate gastric bicarbonate and mucus secretion, and to maintain mucosal blood flow and the mucosal permeability barrier. Misoprostol also promotes epithelial proliferation in response to injury.[75] It appears that at doses of misoprostol sufficient to protect gastric mucosa, suppression of acid secretion also occurs.[77] However, since standard doses of H_2-receptor antagonists inhibit gastric acid secretion at least as effectively as misoprostol, and yet have not been shown to protect the gastric mucosa against NSAID induced ulceration (see next section), it is likely that mechanisms other than acid suppression are important for the prevention of gastric ulcers. Additionally, misoprostol has recently been shown to be superior to even 40 mg of omeprazole daily for both the healing and prevention of gastroduodenal erosions.[80]

Misoprostol appears to be effective in preventing acute gastroduodenal injury induced by short courses of ASA and NSAIDs as measured by mucosal, or fecal blood loss, and by endoscopic injury scores.[81–85] However the clinical relevance of this effect is unclear, given the adaptation of gastroduodenal mucosa to acute injury with continued NSAID use.[71,86,87]

Definition of terms

In the discussion that follows, we use the relative risk (RR) to indicate the likelihood of an outcome receiving the active treatment as compared to those on placebo or control medication.[88,89] For example a RR of 0.25, means that the treatment is associated with only 25% of the risk of the outcome as compared to placebo. Conversely, a RR of 0.25 means that the treatment reduces the "risk" of an event by 75% relative to the placebo or other control (1 − 0.25 = 0.75 or 75%). This relative risk reduction differs from the absolute risk reduction (ARR), which is the arithmetic difference in the proportion of patients with the outcome between the control and treatment groups.

Prevention of endoscopically defined ulcers

We found 19 studies that assessed the long term effect of misoprostol for the prevention of NSAID induced ulcers.[9,80,90–106] The dose of misoprostol varied from 200 μg to 800 μg daily, and follow-up period ranged between 4 to 48 weeks. Although these studies considered erosions and ulcers in their analysis, the data we present below refer only to endoscopic ulcers >3 mm in diameter.

Nine studies with 3329 patients compared the incidence of endoscopically defined ulcers, after at least 3 months of misoprostol to that observed with placebo.[80,91,92,95,96,99,102,103,106] In these trials the proportions of patients receiving placebo medication who developed gastric and duodenal ulcers were 12%, and 6%, respectively.

GASTRIC ULCERS

R Grade A

R Grade A

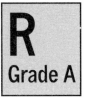

R Grade A

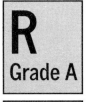

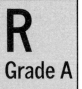

Four studies showed a statistically significant reduction in endoscopically defined gastric ulcers with misoprostol when compared to placebo.[91,92,96,106] Both Raskin[92] and Graham[96] showed a nearly identical 76% relative risk reduction in endoscopic ulcers with misoprostol (RR = 0.24), whereas Graham[106] showed a relative risk reduction of 93% with misoprostol (RR = 0.07). This discrepancy in the observed effect between these studies likely stems from the unique characteristics of the Graham[106] study, in which 25% of the patients had documented ulcers at study onset, and entered a healing phase prior to enrolment into the prophylaxis phase. The ulcer rate of 21% in patients randomized to placebo, was nearly double that seen in the other two studies. Two studies, by Roth *et al* and Verdickt *et al*, failed to show a significant reduction in gastric ulcers with misoprostol.[99,102] The Roth study included only 113 patients, whereas the Verdickt study had an unusually low placebo ulcer rate of 3% due to the inclusion of younger patients at lower risk. Our meta-analysis showed a pooled relative risk of 0.17 (95% CI 0.10–0.29) in favour of misoprostol 800 μg daily, indicating that the use of misoprostol is associated with an 83% relative risk reduction in endoscopically defined gastric ulcers among chronic NSAID users evaluated at 3 months when compared to placebo. This corresponds to a 10% absolute risk reduction (from 11.7% to 1.9%). The NNT, the number of patients needed to treat with misoprostol to prevent one endoscopically defined ulcer at 3 months, is 10.

DUODENAL ULCERS

Five studies evaluated the efficacy of misoprostol for prevention of endoscopically defined duodenal ulcers at 3 months.[91,92,96,99,102] Three studies showed a significant reduction in duodenal ulcer rates with misoprostol prophylaxis.[92,96,102] Grade A The pooled risk reduction of 84% with misoprostol 800 μg daily (RR = 0.16, 95% CI 0.07–0.37) is nearly identical to that observed for prevention of gastric ulcers. When both gastric and duodenal ulcers were considered together, among a total of 1647 patients, misoprostol reduced the risk of NSAID induced endoscopically defined ulcers by 71% (RR = 0.29, 95% CI 0.21–0.41) when compared to placebo, which corresponds to a 10% absolute risk reduction (from 12.0% to 2.1%). Grade A

Dose response

The meta analysis also demonstrated a dose–response relationship for endoscopically defined gastric ulcers. Five studies with 2371 patients used misoprostol 400 μg.[80,91,92,102,106] One study with 928 patients used 600 μg daily,[92] and six with 2155 patients used 800 μg daily.[92,95,96,99,103,106] The highest dose of misoprostol was associated with the lowest risk of gastric ulcers when compared to placebo (RR = 0.18, 95% CI 0.11–0.28), whereas low dose misoprostol (400 μg daily) was associated with a relative risk of 0.38 (95% CI 0.30–0.49). This difference, which corresponds to an 12.8% absolute risk reduction with 800 μg of misoprostol daily, was statistically significant ($P = 0.0055$). Grade A However, the relative risk associated with the intermediate misoprostol dose (600 μg daily) was not significantly different from either the low or high dose (RR = 0.24, 95% CI 0.13–0.44). The pooled relative risk reduction of 78% (a 4.7% absolute risk reduction) for duodenal ulcers with misoprostol 800 μg daily (RR = 0.22, 95% CI 0.09–0.53) was not significantly different from that associated with lower daily misoprostol dosages, again suggesting a pathophysiological difference between gastric and duodenal ulcers. Grade A

One-month studies

R Grade A

The analyses presented above all used the occurrence of ulcer after 3 months of therapy as the outcome measure. Seven studies, with 1634 patients, compared the rates of endoscopically defined ulcers with misoprostol to placebo after only 1 month.[94,95,97,98,100,104,105] Meta-analysis revealed an 87% relative risk reduction of gastric ulcers with misoprostol (RR = 0.13) and an 84% relative risk reduction of duodenal ulcers (RR = 0.16).

Overall, these studies show that misoprostol is of clear benefit for the prevention of both endoscopically defined gastric and duodenal ulcers, with a relative risk reduction of over 70%, and an absolute risk reduction of nearly 10%, compared to placebo. It also appears that higher doses of misoprostol are more effective than lower doses. However these studies do not provide any clear evidence with regards to the efficacy of misoprostol in the prevention of clinically significant adverse upper gastrointestinal events such as hemorrhage or perforation.

NSAID induced clinical events

Silverstein *et al*, in 1995, published the landmark MUCOSA study, the first prospective study to evaluate the efficacy of misoprostol for the prevention of clinically important

Box 4.2 Definite gastrointestinal events: Silverstein et al[9]
Surgery proven perforated ulcer
Endoscopy proven gastric outlet obstruction caused by ulceration and stricture
Hematemesis, with endoscopically proven gastric or duodenal ulcer or erosion
Active or recent visualized bleeding from endoscopically proven ulceration or erosion
Melena with endoscopically proven ulceration or erosion
Heme-positive stool with endoscopically proven ulceration or erosion, plus either a decrease hematocrit or an orthostatic change in blood pressure or pulse
Hematemesis without endoscopically proven ulceration or erosion
Melena, with heme-positive stool and without endoscopically proven ulceration or erosion

NSAID induced adverse upper gastrointestinal events.[9] In this 6-month study, 8843 rheumatoid arthritis patients with a mean age of 68 who were receiving continuous NSAID therapy were randomized to receive misoprostol, 800 μg daily (4404 patients), or placebo (4439). The patients were followed for the development of any suspicious gastrointestinal events. These events were reviewed by a blinded external committee and categorized as definite gastrointestinal complications if they fell into one of eight criteria (Box 4.2). As well, three other criteria were defined, such as melena without other supporting evidence, which were classified as suggestive of possible or previous but not active bleeding. Of a total of 242 suspected gastrointestinal events, 67 were identified as definite, as defined by categories 1–8, with 49 patients having "serious" gastrointestinal events (categories 1–6). Overall there was a combined event incidence of 0.76% over 6 months or about 1.5% per year. Considering all definite gastrointestinal events, 25 of 4404 (0.57%) of patients receiving misoprostol had events, compared to 42 of 4439 (0.95%) patients receiving the placebo (OR 0.60, representing an RR of 40%, $P = 0.049$). Grade A The absolute risk difference was 0.38% (from 0.95% to 0.57%). However, if only perforation or obstruction (categories 1–2) were considered, then 1 of 4404 receiving misoprostol compared to 10 of 4439 who received placebo suffered an event, for an odds ratio of 0.101 or a 90% RR in these events ($P = 0.012$). However, the observed difference in occurrence of endoscopically proven gastrointestinal hemorrhage (categories 3–6) was not statistically significant (placebo, 23 of 4439, misoprostol 15 of 4404, $P > 0.20$). Grade A

The wealth of data provided in this study has allowed clinicians and researchers alike to choose among the categories they feel are important. This opportunity has resulted in widely differing estimates of the risk reductions associated with misoprostol therapy. For example, Maiden and Madhok in an editorial,[107] calculated that the NNT for prevention of gastric outlet obstruction is 1480. Grade A However, these authors chose the rarest event and expressed the results based on a 6-month observation period. The NNT calculated for prevention of obstruction or perforation (categories 1–2) for 1 year is 264. Grade A If any definite gastrointestinal complication is chosen as the outcome measure (categories 1–8), the NNT is 132. Clearly these choices would have considerable impact on the interpretation of the results of this study, and on the calculated cost effectiveness of this therapy.

Adverse effects

The most frequently reported adverse effects with misoprostol therapy are diarrhea and abdominal pain. Additionally, misoprostol is an abortifacient and it must be used

Table 4.2 Meta-analysis of adverse effects observed in randomized placebo controlled trials of misoprostol for prevention of NSAID induced ulcer

Dose	Outcome	RR	95% CI	Risk difference (%)	Heterogeneity
All	D/O adverse effects overall	1.41*	1.31–1.51	7.0	No
	D/O nausea	1.26*	1.07–1.48	1.1	No
	D/O diarrhea	2.36*	2.01–2.77	4.6	No
400 µg/ day	D/O adverse effects overall	1.15	0.89–1.49	1.2	No
	D/O diarrhea	1.38	0.67–2.84	0.6	No
	D/O abdominal pain	1.53	0.90–2.59	1.3	No
	Diarrhea	1.92*	1.64–2.26	0.6	No
800 µg/ day	D/O adverse effect overall	1.14	0.31–1.51	7.1	No
	D/O diarrhea	2.45*	2.09–2.88	5.2	No
	D/O abdominal pain	1.38*	1.17–1.63	1.7	No
	Diarrhea	3.05*†	2.42–3.83	5.2	No

D/O, drop-outs due to the outcome stated.
*Statistically significant difference from placebo.
†Statistically significant difference from lower dose.

cautiously in women of childbearing age. In the study by Silverstein *et al* 732 out of 4404 patients on misoprostol experienced diarrhea or abdominal pain, compared to 399 out of 4439 on placebo for a relative risk of 1.82 associated with misoprostol ($P < 0.001$). Overall 27% of patients on misoprostol experienced one or more adverse effects.[9] Table 4.2 summarizes our review of the misoprostol trials which showed that misoprostol was associated with a small but statistically significant 1.4-fold excess risk of drop-out due to drug induced adverse effects, and an excess risk of drop outs due to nausea (RR = 1.26), and diarrhea (RR = 2.36). When analysed by dose, misoprostol 800 µg daily showed a statistically significant excess risk of drop-outs due to diarrhea (RR = 2.45) and abdominal pain (RR = 1.38). Both misoprostol doses were associated with a statistically significant risk of diarrhea. However, the risk of diarrhea with 800 µg/day (RR = 3.05) was significantly higher than that seen with 400 µg/day (RR = 1.92) ($P = 0.0012$).

Cost-effectiveness

The cost-effectiveness of misoprostol for the prophylaxis of NSAID related endoscopically defined ulcers has been evaluated in eight studies.[108–115] Misoprostol was found to be either cost-saving or cost-effective when calculations were based on the estimate of 80% for prevention of endoscopically defined ulcers. Misoprostol was later shown to reduce clinically serious gastrointestinal events by only 40%.[9] By relying on studies with endoscopically defined ulcers as the outcomes, authors of earlier economic evaluations overestimated the reduction in downstream events, such as outpatient endoscopy and hospitalizations. Furthermore, the MUCOSA study also showed that approximately 85% of endoscopic ulcers are asymptomatic and never get investigated.[40] A revision of the cost-effectiveness of misoprostol, based on this new evidence, showed that misoprostol is not cost-effective when prescribed to all patients, but becomes cost-effective when specifically selecting patients who are at higher risk of a clinically serious gastrointestinal event,[40] such as older patients and those with a positive history of peptic ulcer disease.

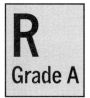

R Grade A

In conclusion, misoprostol prophylaxis significantly reduces the risk of ulcers as well as serious gastrointestinal events in patients on long term NSAID therapy. The use of misoprostol, particularly at higher doses, is associated with more frequent gastrointestinal adverse effects, often resulting in the patient discontinuing the medication, which is an important consideration, considering the symptoms associated with NSAID use alone. The effectiveness outside of clinical trials of misoprostol for prevention of ulcer may be lower than figures which have been presented above. However, since misoprostol is the only agent that has been directly shown to reduce serious NSAID related gastrointestinal complications, it should be considered the first line agent in the primary prophylaxis of NSAID complications, particularly in high risk groups.

H_2-RECEPTOR ANTAGONISTS

Treatment of NSAID induced ulcers

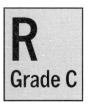

R Grade C

The efficacy of H_2-receptor antagonists for the treatment and prevention of NSAID related upper gastrointestinal toxicity has been exclusively evaluated in studies in which ulcers were defined endoscopically. In several early open label studies of cimetidine for healing of ulcers associated with the use of NSAIDs, it was shown that greater than 75% of gastric and duodenal ulcers could be healed with 12 weeks of therapy despite continued use of NSAIDs.[116–120] There was a trend toward improved efficacy with higher doses. However, in a randomized trial in which patients with NSAID induced ulcers were randomized to receive standard dose ranitidine, or the more potent acid suppressor omeprazole, omeprazole was nearly twice as effective,[121] although ranitidine was still effective.[121,122] O'Laughlin *et al* found that ulcer size correlated inversely with healing rates. At 8 weeks, ulcers with a diameter <5 mm were healed in greater than 90% of patients compared to 35% healing for ulcers >5 mm.[123] Hudson *et al* reported similar observations.[41] The potency of acid suppression and initial ulcer size are important determinants of the rapidity of ulcer healing, and that continued use of NSAIDs in the presence of gastric acid may slow ulcer healing.

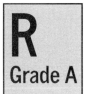

R Grade A

Prevention of NSAID induced ulcers

STANDARD DOSES

R Grade A

Standard doses of H_2-receptor antagonists have been consistently shown to be effective for prevention of endoscopically defined duodenal ulcers, but not of gastric ulcers.[42,90,124–132] Koch *et al*[133] in a meta-analysis of randomized trials which employed standard doses of H_2-receptor antagonists[124–127,129,130] and Stalnikowicz *et al*[10] were also unable to show a benefit for the prevention of gastric ulcers. Similarly, our meta-analysis of the standard dose H_2-receptor antagonist trials confirms that there is no overall reduction in the relative risk of endoscopically defined gastric ulcers with these agents (RR = 0.70, 95% CI –0.39 to 1.24), whereas there is a significant reduction in endoscopic duodenal ulcers (RR = 0.24, 95% CI –0.10 to 0.57). Grade A The use of these agents presumably in standard doses, in an observational cohort of 1921 patients with rheumatoid arthritis, did not reduce the risk of serious gastrointestinal complications. Patients on H_2-receptor antagonists or antacids who were asymptomatic had a significantly greater risk of serious gastrointestinal complications.[134] Grade B

HIGHER DOSES

Although achlorhydria has been reported not to prevent early NSAID induced gastric lesions,[135] there is accumulating evidence that profound acid suppression can reduce acute NSAID and ASA induced gastric mucosal injury.[136–138] Based on these observations, several investigators have tested the hypothesis that higher doses of H_2-receptor antagonists may achieve more consistent acid suppression and may therefore be effective for prevention of gastric ulcer in chronic NSAID users. Hudson *et al*, in a two phase study, assessed the efficacy of famotidine for the healing and prevention of NSAID induced ulcers.[41] Of 389 patients who agreed to participate, 285 were free of ulcers at a screening endoscopy and were entered into the primary prevention study discussed below. The 104 patients with ulcers (76 gastric, 42 duodenal, 14 both) were entered into the open label healing phase study and received famotidine 40 mg twice daily. An ulcer was defined as an excavated mucosal break >3 mm, and endoscopic assessments of healing were made at 4 and 12 weeks. The cumulative healing rates at 4 weeks for those who continued and discontinued NSAIDs were 65.9% and 81.3%, respectively. At 12 weeks the healing rates were 89% and 100%. The apparent trend towards somewhat lower ulcer healing rates in those who continued NSAIDs was not statistically significant at either time period; however, only 16 out of 104 patients agreed to stop their NSAID use. Therefore, there is a strong possibility of a type II error. The proportion of ulcers healed was significantly and inversely correlated with ulcer size, but not with the presence of Hp infection. Among those patients who continued to use NSAIDs, ulcer healing at 4 and 12 weeks was not statistically different for patients with gastric or duodenal ulcers.

R
Grade C

In the maintenance, secondary prophylaxis phase, the 78 patients who had their ulcers healed and continued to use NSAIDs were randomized in a double blind fashion to either famotidine 40 mg twice daily or placebo.[41] Over 24 weeks the cumulative incidence of gastroduodenal ulcer was 53.5 % in placebo patients and 26.0% in famotidine treated patients (P = 0.011). Famotidine also seemed to be effective for the prevention of gastric ulcers (placebo 41.4%, famotidine, P = 0.026). The placebo ulcer rates in this study are relatively high. In our review of all the misoprostol studies the pooled placebo gastric and duodenal ulcer rates were 12% and 6% respectively in primary prophylaxis studies. A history of previous peptic ulcer is associated with increased risk of NSAID induced gastrointestinal complications (OR 2.29).[9] Whether the inclusion of such high risk patients included in the prophylaxis phase of this trial is enough to explain such a high placebo ulcer rate among NSAID users is not known.

R
Grade C

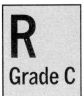

In a companion study to Hudson's, Taha *et al* performed a randomized double-blind placebo controlled trial of famotidine for the primary prevention of NSAID induced ulceration.[42] The 285 patients on chronic NSAIDs who were free of ulcers at the initial endoscopic screening were randomized to receive either famotidine 40 mg twice daily, 20 mg twice daily, or placebo. The higher dose of famotidine was effective for prevention of duodenal ulcer (famotidine 2%, placebo 14%, P = 0.01, NNT = 8) and gastric ulcer

R Grade A

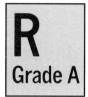

(famotidine 8%, placebo 20%, $P = 0.03$, NNT = 8). As expected, however, standard dose famotidine was effective for prevention of duodenal ulcer (famotidine 4%, placebo 13%, $P = 0.04$), but not for prevention of gastric ulcer.

The presence of duodenal erosions or submucosal hemorrhages at the baseline endoscopy, was associated with an increased risk of subsequent ulceration (hazard rate ratio, 2.9; 95% CI 1.2–6.9). However, only a trend towards an increased risk of ulceration could be documented for the presence of *H. pylori* (hazard rate ratio, 1.7; 95% CI 0.8–3.5).[42]

The efficacy of other H_2-receptor antagonists in this setting has also has also been assessed. Wolde *et al* randomized 20 patients with rheumatoid arthritis and a history of previous peptic ulceration who continued on NSAIDs, to receive high dose ranitidine (300 mg twice daily) or placebo.[139] At 12 months, duodenal ulcers occurred in four of 10 patients on placebo, but in none on ranitidine ($P = 0.04$, one-tailed test). However, this difference is not statistically significant if a more appropriate two-tailed statistical test is used. Gastric ulcers occurred in six and three patients on placebo and ranitidine respectively ($P = 0.18$). Unfortunately this study was terminated early due to slow patient recruitment, and there is a high probability of a type 2 error.

R Grade A

Simon *et al* randomized 269 arthritic patients on chronic NSAIDs with peptic ulcers to nizatidine 150 mg daily, 150 mg twice daily, or 300 mg twice daily.[132] At 8 weeks over 90% of gastric and duodenal ulcers were healed with all three nizatidine doses, though there was a trend towards higher healing rates with higher doses. In the maintenance phase, 221 patients with healed ulcers who continued to use NSAIDs were randomized to receive nizatidine 150 mg daily or 150 mg twice daily for 6 months. The observed difference in cumulative ulcer relapse rates (150 mg 5.8%, 300 mg, 1.8%) was not statistically significant. These rates are much lower than those reported by Hudson, in an apparently similar arthritic population, and the absence of a placebo group further complicates the interpretation of this study.

R Grade A

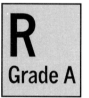

Levine *et al*, randomized 498 dyspeptic patients with osteoarthritis treated with daily NSAIDs, to receive nizatidine 150 mg twice daily, or placebo. At 12 weeks 24 patients on nizatidine and 34 on placebo developed a gastric and/or duodenal ulcer.[127] A statistically significant benefit was only observed for patients older than age 65 or with a past history of peptic ulcers, though correction for multiple comparisons were not performed.

H_2-receptor antagonists were generally quite well tolerated in the presented studies. Standard doses of these agents appear to be effective for preventing NSAID induced duodenal but not gastric ulcers. However, higher doses of H_2-receptor antagonists appear to be effective for healing and prevention of both gastric and duodenal ulcers in patients taking NSAIDs chronically. The clinical use of this class of drugs for the prevention of gastroduodenal ulceration may be questioned for several reasons. In the randomized trials of famotidine, the ulcer rates in the placebo groups are higher than are generally reported. Furthermore, since continued use of H_2-receptor antagonists is associated with tolerance to their acid suppression effects,[140–142] the long term efficacy of these drugs must be questioned. Finally, even if effective for ulcer prevention, there is no economic or therapeutic advantage to using double doses of these drugs rather than standard doses of proton pump inhibitors which produce more potent and reliable acid suppression.

PROTON PUMP INHIBITORS

Proton pump inhibitors (PPIs) block the final step of gastric acid secretion by inhibiting parietal cell H^+-K^+-ATPase. Direct evidence for the efficacy of PPIs in the primary or secondary prevention of clinically important NSAID induced upper gastrointestinal toxicity is lacking. Several factors have prompted interest in the use of PPIs for prophylaxis against NSAID induced ulcers:

1 dissatisfaction with the adverse effects of misoprostol;
2 the apparent efficacy of PPIs in healing NSAID ulcers;
3 the proven efficacy of PPIs in other acid-peptic disorders;
4 early evidence from published reports;
5 extrapolation of results from the high dose H_2-receptor antagonists studies;
6 high cost of double dose H^2-receptor antagonists.

Omeprazole and lansoprazole appear to be effective for the prevention of early NSAID induced upper gastrointestinal injury assessed either endoscopically or through the detection of mucosal blood loss, in healthy volunteers given aspirin or naproxen.[136–138,143] However, as discussed previously the clinical relevance of these early lesions is in question.

Healing of ulcers with continued NSAID use

Omeprazole has been shown to heal both gastric and duodenal ulcers irrespective of continued NSAID use.[67,80,121,144–146] Walan *et al*, in a double-blind trial, assessed the healing rates of benign gastric and prepyloric ulcers in 602 patients randomized to receive either omeprazole (40 mg or 20 mg) or ranitidine (150 mg) bid.[121] In a subset of 58 patients with endoscopically documented ulcers who continued to take NSAIDs, the proportions of patients whose ulcers healed at 8 weeks were: omeprazole 40 mg, 95% (similar to results for patients with non-NSAID ulcers), omeprazole 20 mg, 82%, and ranitidine 53% (P <0.05). These data suggest that selected patients with endoscopically documented NSAID ulcers can experience ulcer healing with omeprazole despite continued NSAID use. However, caution should be exercised in extrapolating these results to patients presenting with NSAID induced upper gastrointestinal hemorrhage. In these patients the decision to continue the NSAID must be individualized, since the safety and efficacy of omeprazole in this setting has not been assessed.

R
Grade A

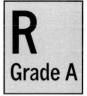

Healing of ulcers and prevention of ulcer recurrence

Recently two large randomized controlled trials have addressed the efficacy of omeprazole in the healing and subsequent prevention of NSAID related gastroduodenal ulceration among chronic NSAID users: the OMNIUM and ASTRONAUT studies.[67,80] These two trials were of nearly identical design, and included an 8-week healing phase, followed by a 26-week secondary prophylaxis phase. The results of the healing phase will be addressed first.

HEALING PHASE

Patients were eligible for entry into the healing phase of these studies if they: (i) were between the ages of 18 and 85; (ii) had any condition requiring continuous NSAID therapy; and (iii) were willing to consent to a screening endoscopy. If patients were found to have an ulcer with a diameter >3 mm with an appreciable depth or greater than 10 erosions in the stomach or duodenum, they were enrolled in the study. A total of 935 patients with a mean age of 62 were enrolled into the OMNIUM study.[80] Thirty five percent

R Grade A

of these patients had erosions only, 40% had gastric ulcers, 20% had duodenal ulcers, with the remainder having combinations of these lesions. The patients were randomized to receive omeprazole 20 mg daily (n = 308), omeprazole 40 mg daily (n = 315), or misoprostol 800 µg daily (n = 298). Overall treatment success was defined as ulcer healing, the presence of less than five erosions and the presence of not more than mild dyspeptic symptoms. At 8 weeks the healing rates for gastric ulcers were 87%, 80%, and 73%, for the omeprazole 20 mg, omeprazole 40 mg, and the misoprostol groups, respectively. The difference between the omeprazole 20 mg and misoprostol groups was statistically significant (P – 0.004). Duodenal ulcer healing rates were significantly higher with omeprazole 20 mg (93%) and 40 mg (89%) than with misoprostol (77%) (P <0.001). In contrast, misoprostol produced significantly higher healing rates of gastroduodenal erosions than either omeprazole doses (87% vs 77% and 79%, respectively, P = 0.01). The authors identified that the presence of duodenal ulcer, or erosions in contrast to gastric ulcers, and the presence of Hp were significant favorable prognostic factors predicting ulcer healing.

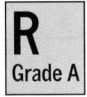

R Grade A

R Grade A

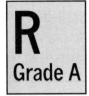

In the healing phase of the ASTRONAUT study 541 slightly younger patients (mean age of 57) were randomized to receive omeprazole 20 mg (n = 174), omeprazole 40 mg (n = 187) or ranitidine 150 mg bid (n = 174) for 8 weeks.[67] The baseline characteristics and ulcer distributions were similar to those of the OMNIUM study. Omeprazole at either dose was more effective than ranitidine for healing of gastric ulcer (omeprazole 20 mg 84%, omeprazole 40 mg 87%, ranitidine 64%, P <0.001). Omeprazole was also more effective than ranitidine for healing duodenal ulcer (omeprazole 20 mg 92%, omeprazole 40 mg 88%, ranitidine 81%, P = 0.03 for comparison of omeprazole 20 mg and ranitidine). Both doses of omeprazole were more effective than ranitidine for healing erosions (omeprazole 20 mg 89%, omeprazole 40 mg 86%, ranitidine 77%, P = 0.008 for the comparison of omeprazole 20 mg and ranitidine). At 4 weeks but not at 8 weeks omeprazole 20 mg daily was superior to ranitidine for the relief of moderate to severe dyspeptic symptoms. The same favorable prognostic factors identified in the OMNIUM study were found.

PREVENTION OF ULCER RECURRENCE (SECONDARY PROPHYLAXIS)

Patients who experienced healing of their ulcers during the initial phase of these two studies were re-randomized to maintenance treatment without consideration for the treatment they initially received for purposes of ulcer healing. The patients were followed for a total of 6 months with endoscopic evaluations made at 1, 3, and 6 months or if troublesome symptoms arose. Patients were considered to be in remission if they were free of ulcers, had less than 10 gastric or duodenal erosions, and had not more than mild dyspeptic symptoms.

R Grade A

The OMNIUM maintenance study randomized 732 chronic NSAID users whose ulcer/erosions were healed during the healing phase study, to receive maintenance therapy with omeprazole 20 mg daily, misoprostol 200 µg twice daily, or placebo.[80] At 6 months 61%, 48%, and 27% of patients were in remission as defined above for the omeprazole, misoprostol, and placebo groups respectively. The results reached statistical significance for omeprazole vs misoprostol (P = 0.001) and for omeprazole vs placebo (P <0.001). When only erosions were considered, fewer patients relapsed on misoprostol than on omeprazole or placebo (7% vs 12% and 14% respectively).

The ASTRONAUT maintenance study randomized 432 patients who achieved treatment success during the healing phase study.[67] This study compared maintenance omeprazole

20 mg daily to standard dose ranitidine (150 mg twice daily). At 6 months 72% of patients on omeprazole vs 59% on ranitidine were in remission ($P = 0.004$). Again, in both these maintenance phase studies the presence of Hp was associated with a significantly higher likelihood of remaining in remission. It would have been interesting to see if omeprazole would have fared as well against higher doses of misoprostol or double dose ranitidine. Clearly, the investigators chose a dose of misoprostol which they felt would be most tolerable. However, it is clear, as discussed in the previous sections, that standard doses of H_2-receptor antagonists are ineffective at preventing NSAID induced gastric ulcers.

R Grade A

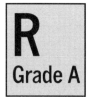

In a randomized double-blind Nordic multicenter study, Ekstrom *et al* compared omeprazole 20 mg daily to placebo for the primary prophylaxis of 175 predominately osteoarthritic, chronic NSAIDs users with a mean age of 60 years.[147] The authors used the same composite outcome of the proportion of patients in remission as defined above for the OMNIUM and ASTRONAUT maintenance studies. At 3 months, peptic ulcers were detected in 4.7% (4/85) of the omeprazole group and 16.7% (15/90) of the control group. Interestingly this nearly four-fold reduction in ulcer risk with omeprazole was irrespective of Hp status or peptic ulcer history. In the control group these two factors were associated with a four-fold and five-fold increased risk of ulcers respectively. Greater than mild dyspeptic symptoms were experienced by 8.2% (7/85) of patients in the omeprazole group vs 20.0% (18/90) in the control group. The number of patients found to have more than 10 erosions was similar between the two groups. In total 24.7% (21/85) vs 50.0% (45/90) experienced any of the outcomes for the omeprazole and control groups respectively ($P < 0.001$).

R Grade A

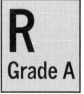

Cullen *et al*, in a study published only in abstract form, randomized 168 patients to receive omeprazole 20 mg daily or placebo.[148] The patients were enrolled after a 6-month period of NSAID usage. A clinical evaluation and endoscopy upon entry were used to verify the absence of the same three study endpoints used in the previous studies above, and were repeated at 1, 3, and 6 months post randomization. At 6 months 86% of patients in the omeprazole group and 60% in the control group were free of endoscopic ulcers or erosions ($P < 0.01$). Endoscopic ulcers alone were present in 3.6% and 16.5% of patients on omeprazole and placebo respectively. When all three endpoints were considered (symptoms, ulcers, and erosions), 78% of patients on omeprazole vs 53% on placebo were in "remission" ($P < 0.01$).

R Grade A

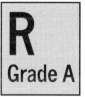

The use of a composite endpoint in all these studies to define remission makes it difficult to appreciate the individual causes of relapse. However, when we pooled the results of ulcer occurrences alone, omeprazole significantly reduced the risk of gastric (RR = 0.37, 95% CI 0.27–0.51) and duodenal (RR = 0.19, 95% CI 0.09–0.40) ulcers. Omeprazole is associated with significantly less NSAID induced dyspeptic symptoms (RR = 0.50, 95% CI 0.30–0.82), and appears to be associated with significantly less diarrhea and abdominal cramps than misoprostol.

Summary

Collectively these studies demonstrate that omeprazole and presumably other H^+ pump inhibitors are effective for healing both gastric and duodenal NSAID induced ulcers irrespective of continued NSAID use or *H. pylori* status. These agents also appear to be effective for the prevention of endoscopically diagnosed NSAID induced ulcers. However, their efficacy for the prevention of serious NSAID related gastrointestinal complications is unknown. Therefore, omeprazole is not currently recommended in preference to

Table 4.3 Rank order of COX-1 inhibitory potency among NSAIDs with reported COX-2 selectivity

Rank	COX-2 NSAID
Highest COX-1 potency	DuP 697
	SC-558451
	Celecoxib
	Meloxicam
	SC-57666
	SC-58125
	Flosulide
	Etodolac
	L-745,337
Lowest COX-1 potency	DFU-T-614

Adapted from Reindeau *et al.*[163]

misoprostol as first line therapy for the primary prophylaxis of NSAID related clinical events. However, it is reasonable to recommend its use in patients who are intolerant of misoprostol, or for whom it is contraindicated. Interestingly, misoprostol appears to be more effective than omeprazole for both the healing and prevention of gastroduodenal erosions. The clinical significance of this effect, if any, is not known. It may prove to be important, for example in the prevention of NSAID induced occult blood loss.

The appropriate choice of therapy for secondary prophylaxis against NSAID ulcer recurrence among chronic NSAID users is unclear. Currently the only agent indicated for the prevention of NSAID ulcers is misoprostol, which is also the only agent that has been of proven benefit in the prevention of NSAID induced clinical events. However, in reality most clinicians will prescribe a PPI to heal NSAID induced ulcers, and will continue this agent for secondary prophylaxis. Given the results of the OMNIUM and ASTRONAUT studies, this may be appropriate, but a degree of caution is indicated given the limitations of these studies, and the absence of direct evidence of omeprazole's effectiveness against clinical gastrointestinal events. The cost-effectiveness of omeprazole or other PPIs for the primary or secondary prophylaxis against NSAID induced upper gastrointestinal toxicity has not been established.

THE NEWER NSAIDS

It is felt that NSAIDs exert their therapeutic anti-inflammatory and analgesic effects through the inhibition of inducible cyclo-oxygenase-2 (COX-2), whereas their gastric and renal toxicities arise from the inhibition of the constitutive COX-1 isoform.[149,150] It has been recognized for some time that different NSAIDs have differing propensities toward gastroduodenal toxicity,[16,17] and recently it has been proposed that those NSAIDs with the greatest affinity for COX-1 are associated with the highest risk of gastrointestinal toxicity. As a result of these observations, there has been a rapid development of new NSAIDs with increasing COX-2 selectivity, with claims of retained anti-inflammatory and analgesic activity, but with little gastrointestinal toxicity. Table 4.3 summarizes the relative COX-1 inhibitory activity of various COX-2 selective NSAIDs.

The literature relating to these selective COX-2 inhibitors is only beginning to accumulate, and there are several ongoing trials that are likely to influence our understanding of these agents. Early evidence suggests that COX-2 selective NSAIDs have lower gastrointestinal toxicity. Singh *et al*, in an article published in abstract form, reviewed the data of eight ARAMIS (Arthritis, Rheumatism, and Aging Medical Information System) centers' experience with serious NSAID related gastrointestinal events among consecutively diagnosed rheumatoid arthritis patients.[151] Sixteen NSAIDs were studied for a total 19 289 patient years. No serious events occurred with the COX-2 selective nabumetone or etodolac whereas indomethacin and meclofenamate were associated with 2.96 and 3.53 events per year respectively. Salsalate, diclofenac, and ibuprofen were also associated with significantly lower yearly event rates when compared to indomethacin and meclofenamate, but were not statistically different from nabumetone or etodolac.[151] In a meta-analysis of endoscopic studies comparing the rates of ulcerations or erosions with low risk NSAIDs with those of "any" other NSAIDs, Ferraz *et al* found that nabumetone, etodolac, and salsalate were associated with an overall 87% relative risk reduction of endoscopic ulcers or erosions when compared to "any" NSAID.[152] Similarly, Distel *et al*, in a systematic review of the safety of meloxicam, found that the most common non-serious gastrointestinal effects of both meloxicam and standard NSAIDs were dyspepsia, nausea, abdominal pain, and diarrhea. However, discontinuation of therapy due to these adverse effects was significantly less common with meloxicam.[153] Serious gastrointestinal events such as perforation, ulcers, or bleeds were also significantly less common with meloxicam or diclofenac then with naproxen or piroxicam.[153] Selective COX-2 inhibitors also appear to be effective analgesic/anti-inflammatory agents, as reported in several trials among patients with rheumatoid arthritis and osteoarthritis.[154–157]

Recently, two kinds of data were presented in abstract form. Goldstein *et al*[158] presented the results of a meta-analysis of 14 randomized controlled trials which included 11 007 rheumatoid and osteoarthritis patients who received either placebo (n = 1864), celecoxib (n = 6376) in doses ranging from 25 to 400 mg bid, or an NSAID (n = 2768) (naproxen 500 mg bid, diclofenac 50–75 mg bid, or ibuprofen 800 mg tid) for 2–24 weeks. These studies assessed clinically important gastrointestinal adverse events in a protocol similar to that used in the MUCOSA trial. NSAIDs were associated with a 1.48% excess risk of clinically significant upper gastrointestinal events (95% CI 0.35%–2.62%) compared to celecoxib, while no excess risk was observed with celecoxib compared to placebo (95% CI −0.08% to 0.47%). Overall, nine clinically important events occurred in the NSAID group, while two occurred with celecoxib, for a relative risk of 0.12 (95% CI 0.03–0.54). This can be compared to a relative risk of 0.60 observed with misoprostol in the MUCOSA study.

R
Grade A

Laine *et al*[159] using endoscopic endpoints, randomized 1516 osteoarthritis patients with no ulcer at baseline endoscopy to receive placebo, rofecoxib (25 mg or 50 mg qid), or ibuprofen 800 mg tid in two identical trials. At 12 weeks, 47 of 733 patients who received rofecoxib, and 101 of 354 who received ibuprofen developed ulcers, for a relative risk of 0.22 (95% CI 0.16–0.31). From our meta-analysis, misoprostol was approximately twice as effective for reducing the risk of endoscopically defined ulcers as it was for preventing clinically important events. However, this pattern does not seem to hold for the COX-2 inhibitors, based on these two trials. This apparent difference may be clarified when these results are published in full.

R
Grade A

Other NSAID derivatives are also actively being studied. The unique linking of a standard NSAID with a nitric oxide releasing component appears to be particularly promising. Experimentally these agents may be characterized by enhanced anti-platelet

Table 4.4 Evidence for efficacy

Drug class	NSAID ulcer healing	Clinical events prevention	Gastric ulcers prevention	Duodenal ulcers prevention
Prostaglandin analogues	X	X	X	X
H_2–receptor antagonists standard dose	X			X
H_2–receptor antagonists double dose	X		X	X
Proton pump inhibitors	X		X	X

activity when linked to aspirin, with reduced gastrointestinal toxicity.[160] Additionally, early animal studies suggests that these agents, unlike COX-2 selective NSAIDs, can actually accelerate gastric ulcer healing.[161,162]

The early evidence from such studies provides some promise of truly safe agents which may move our focus away from concurrent preventive therapy towards the use of single agents that retain anti-inflammatory/analgesic activity, while exhibiting low gastrointestinal toxicity. However, these agents are not the first NSAIDs to promise low gastrointestinal toxicity. Hopefully, the ongoing trials of the safety and effectiveness of these agents will shed light on the remaining questions, such as their safety and effectiveness when potentially high doses are used outside the context of randomized controlled trials, their effects on pre-existing ulcers which may contain the inducible COX-2 isoform, and their effects on other gastrointestinal conditions such as inflammatory bowel disease.

R Grade B

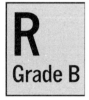

The available evidence suggests that the least toxic NSAID in the lowest effective dose should be used whenever possible to limit the toxicity of these agents. The combination of NSAIDs with other anti-inflammatory agents, including aspirin, corticosteroids, and with oral anticoagulants is associated with an increased risk of serious adverse gastrointestinal events, and again should be avoided when possible. Patients with different risk characteristics can have drastically different rates of adverse gastrointestinal events when treated with NSAIDs long term. Therefore, the addition of a second agent for the prevention of NSAID induced adverse gastrointestinal events should likely be reserved for high risk patients, particularly older patients with previous peptic ulcer disease and concomitant coronary artery disease. Misoprostol at 800 μg daily is the only agent thus far that has been directly shown to reduce the occurrence of significant adverse NSAID related gastrointestinal events. Lower doses of misoprostol are associated with a lower incidence of diarrhea and cramps, but also appear to be slightly less effective for preventing endoscopically defined gastric ulcers. The effects of low doses of misoprostol on clinical gastrointestinal events are unknown, and the use of lower doses may be associated with a significant clinical tradeoff. Higher doses of potent H_2-receptor antagonists and standard doses of proton pump inhibitors appear to be effective for prevention of endoscopically defined duodenal and gastric ulcers and NSAID related dyspepsia and they are significantly better tolerated than misoprostol. However, the effectiveness of these agents for the prevention of clinical gastrointestinal events is unknown, as is their cost-effectiveness. Finally, all these agents appear to be effective at healing NSAID induced ulcers despite continued NSAID use. However, the more potent acid suppression afforded by PPIs and potent H_2-receptor antagonists appears to be more effective than misoprostol for this purpose (Table 4.4).

R
Grade A

REFERENCES

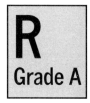

1 Fries JF, Miller SR, Spitz PW *et al.* Identification of patients at risk for gastropathy associated with NSAID use. *J Rheumatol* 1990; **20** (Suppl): 12–19.
2 Patrono O. Aspirin as an antiplatelet drug. *N Engl J Med* 1994; **330**(18): 1287–94.
3 Stroke prevention in atrial fibrillation investigators. Stroke prevention in atrial fibrillation study: final results. *Circulation* 1991; **84**: 527–39.
4 Anonymous. Steering Committee of the physicians' health study research group: final report on the aspirin component of the ongoing physician's health study. *N Engl J Med* 1989; **321**: 129–35.
5 The SALT collaborative study group. Swedish aspirin low-dose trial of 75 mg aspirin as secondary prophylaxis after cerebrovascular ischemic events. *Lancet 1991*; **338**: 1345–9.
6 Wallace JL. Nonsteroidal anti-inflammatory drugs and gastroenteropathy: the second hundred years [review]. *Gastroenterology* 1997; **112**: 1000–16.
7 Smalley WE, Griffin MR, Fought RL *et al.* Excess costs from gastrointestinal disease associated with nonsteroidal anti-inflammatory drugs. *J Gen Intern Med* 1996; **11**: 461–9.
8 Larkai EN, Smith JI, Lidsky MD. Gastroduodenal mucosa and dyspeptic symptoms in arthritic patients during chronic non-steroidal anti-inflammatory drug use. *Am J Gastroenterol* 1987; **82**: 1153–8.
9 Silverstein FE, Graham DY, Senior JR *et al.* Misoprostol reduces serious gastrointestinal complications in patients with rheumatoid arthritis receiving nonsteroidal anti-inflammatory drugs. A randomized, double-blind, placebo-controlled trial [see comments]. *Ann Intern Med* 1995; **123**: 241–9.
10 Stalnikowicz R, Rachmilewitz D. NSAID-induced gastroduodenal damage: is prevention needed? A review and metaanalysis. *J Clin Gastroenterol* 1993; **17**: 238–43.
11 Fries JF. NSAID gastropathy: the second most deadly rheumatic disease? Epidemiology and risk appraisal. *J Rheumatol* 1991; **28** (Suppl): 6–10.
12 Griffin MR, Ray WA, Schaffner W. Nonsteroidal anti-inflammatory drug use and death from peptic ulcer in elderly persons. *Ann Intern Med* 1988; **109**: 359–63.
13 Bollini P, Rodriguez G, Gutthann S. The impact of research quality and study design on epidemiologic estimates of the effect of nonsteroidal anti-inflammatory drugs on upper gastrointestinal tract disease. *Arch Intern Med* 1992; **152**: 1289–95.
14 McMahon AD, Evans JM, White G *et al.* A cohort study (with re-sampled comparator groups) to measure the association between new NSAID prescribing and upper gastrointestinal hemorrhage and perforation. *J Clin Epidemiol* 1997; **50**: 351–6.
15 Gabriel SE, Jaakkimainen L, Bombardier C. Risk for serious gastrointestinal complications related to use of non-steroidal anti-inflammatory drugs: A meta-analysis. *Ann Intern Med* 1991; **115**: 787–96.
16 Langman MJ, Weil J, Wainwright P *et al.* Risks of bleeding peptic ulcer associated with individual non-steroidal anti-inflammatory drugs [see comments] [published erratum appears in *Lancet* 1994; **343**: 1302]. *Lancet* 1994; **343**: 1075–8.
17 MacDonald TM, Morant SV, Robinson GC. Association of upper gastrointestinal toxicity of non-steroidal anti-inflammatory drugs with continued exposure: Cohort Study. *Br Med J* 1997; **315**: 1333–7.
18 Armstrong CP, Blower AL. Nonsteroidal antiinflammatory drugs and life threatening complications of peptic ulceration. *Gut* 1987; **28**: 527–32.
19 Kaufmann HJ, Taubin HL. Nonsteroidal anti-inflammatory drugs activate quiescent inflammatory bowel disease. *Ann Intern Med* 1987; **107**: 513–16.
20 Wallace JL. NSAID gastroenteropathy: past, present and future [review]. *Can J Gastroenterol* 1996; **10**: 451–9.
21 Matsuhashi N, Yamada A, Hiraishi M *et al.* Multiple strictures of the small intestine after long-term nonsteroidal anti-inflammatory drug therapy. *Am J Gastroenterol* 1992; **87**: 1183–6.
22 Tannenbaum H, Davis P, Russell AS *et al.* An evidence-based approach to prescribing

NSAIDs in musculoskeletal disease: a Canadian consensus. Canadian NSAID Consensus Participants [see comments] [review]. *Can Med Assoc J* 1996; **155**: 77–88.
23 Lichtenstein DR, Syngal S, Wolfe MM. Nonsteroidal antiinflammatory drugs and the gastrointestinal tract. The double-edged sword [review]. *Arth Rheum* 1995; **38**: 5–18.
24 Hallas J, Lauritsen J, Villadsen HD *et al.* Nonsteroidal anti-inflammatory drugs and upper gastrointestinal bleeding, identifying high risk groups by excess risk estimates. *Scand J Gastroenterol* 1995; **30**: 438–44.
25 Hansen JM, Hallas J, Lauritsen JM *et al.* Non-steroidal anti-inflammatory drugs and ulcer complications: a risk factor analysis for clinical decision-making. *Scand J Gastroenterol* 1996; **31**: 126–30.
26 Laporte JR, Carne X, Vidal X *et al.* Upper gastrointestinal bleeding in relation to previous use of analgesics and non-steroidal anti-inflammatory drugs. *Lancet* 1991; **337**: 85–9.
27 Rodriguez LA. Nonsteroidal anti-inflammatory drugs, ulcers and risks. A collaborative meta-analysis. *Semin Arth Rheum* 1997; **26**: 16–20.
28 Hochain P, Berkelmans I, Czernichow P *et al.* Which patients taking non-aspirin non-steroidal anti-inflammatory drugs bleed? A case-control study. *Eur J Gastroenterol Hepatol* 1995; **7**: 419–26.
29 Scheiman JM. Nsaids, gastrointestinal injury, and cytoprotection. *Gastroenterol Clin North Am* 1998; **25**: 270–98.
30 Gutthann SP, Garcia RL, Raiford DS. Individual nonsteroidal antiinflammatory drugs and other risk factors for upper gastrointestinal bleeding and perforation. *Epidemiology* 1997; **8**: 18–24.
31 Henry D, Dobson A, Turner C. Variability in the risk of major gastrointestinal complications from nonaspirin nonsteroidal anti-inflammatory drugs. *Gastroenterology* 1993; **105**: 1078–88.
32 Henry D, Lim LL, Garcia RL *et al.* Variability in risk of gastrointestinal complications with individual non-steroidal anti-inflammatory drugs: results of a collaborative meta-analysis [see comments]. *Br Med J* 1996; **312**: 1563–16.
33 Smalley WE, Griffin MR. The risks and costs of upper gastrointestinal disease attributable to NSAIDs [review]. *Gastroenterol Clin North Am* 1996; **25**: 373–96.
34 Carson JL, Strom BL, Morse ML *et al.* The relative gastrointestinal toxicity of the non-steroidal anti-inflammatory drugs. *Arch Intern Med* 1987; **147**: 1054–9.
35 Griffin MR, Piper JM, Daughtery JR *et al.* Non-steroidal anti-inflammatory drug use and increased risk for peptic ulcer disease in elderly persons. *Ann Intern Med* 1991; **114**: 257–63.
36 Wynne HA, Long A. Patient awareness of the adverse effects of non-steroidal anti-inflammatory drugs (NSAIDs). *Br J Clin Pharmacol* 1996; **42**: 253–6.
37 Jorde R, Burhol PG. Asymptomatic peptic ulcer disease. *Scand J Gastroenterol* 1987; **22**: 129–34.
38 Graham DY. High-dose famotidine for prevention of NSAID ulcers? [editorial; comment]. *Gastroenterology* 1997; **112**: 2143–5.
39 Robbins SL, Cotran RS, Kumar V. *Pathologic basis of disease*, 3rd edn. Philadelphia: WB Saunders, 1984.
40 Maetzel A, Ferraz MB, Bombardier C. The cost-effectiveness of misoprostol in preventing serious gastrointestinal events associated with the use of nonsteroidal antiinflammatory drugs. *Arth Rheum* 1998; **41**: 16–25.
41 Hudson N, Taha AS, Russell RI *et al.* Famotidine for healing and maintenance in nonsteroidal anti-inflammatory drug-associated gastro-duodenal ulceration [see comments]. *Gastroenterology* 1997; **112**: 1817–22.
42 Taha AS, Hudson N, Hawkey CJ *et al.* Famotidine for the prevention of gastric and duodenal ulcers caused by nonsteroidal antiinflammatory drugs [see comments]. *N Engl J Med* 1996; **334**: 1435–9.
43 Wittes J, Lakatos E, Prosbstfeild J. Surrogate endpoints in clinical trial: cardiovascular diseases. *Stat Med* 1989; **8**: 415–25.
44 Van Der Hulst R, Rauws E *et al.* Recurrence after eradication of *Helicobacter pylori*: a prospective long-term follow-up study. *Gastroenterology* 1997; **113**: 1082–6.
45 Rauws EJ, Tytgat GN. *Helicobacter pylori* in duodenal and gastric ulcer disease [review]. *Baillières Clin Gastroenterol* 1995; **9**: 529–47.
46 Veldhuyzen van Zanten SJ, Sherman PM. *Helicobacter pylori* infection as a cause of gastritis, duodenal ulcer, gastric cancer and nonulcer dyspepsia: a systematic overview [see comments] [review]. *Can Med Assoc J* 1994; **150**: 177–85.
47 Kurata JH, Nogawa AN. Meta-analysis of risk factors for peptic ulcer. Nonsteroidal antiinflammatory drugs, *Helicobacter pylori*, and smoking. *J Clin Gastroenterol* 1997; **24**: 2–17.
48 Veldhuyzen van Zanten S. Ulcers, *H. pylori*, NSAIDs, and dyspepsia. *Gastroenterology* 1997; **113**(6): S90–S92.

49 Borody TJ, George LL, Brandl S. *Helicobacter pylori* negative duodenal ulcer. *Am J Gastroenterol* 1991; **86**: 1154–7.

50 Laine L, Martin-Sorensen M, Weinstein W. NSAID-associated gastric ulcers do not require H.pylori for their development. *Am J Gastroenterol* 1992; **87**: 1398–402.

51 McColl K, El-Nujumi A, Chittajullu R. A study of the pathogenesis of *Helicobacter pylori*-negative duodenal ulceration. *Gut* 1993; **34**: 762–8.

52 Dooley CP, Cohen H, Fitzgibbon P. Prevalence of *Helicobacter pylori* infection and histologic gastritis in asymptomatic persons. *N Engl J Med* 1989; **321**: 1562–6.

53 Graham DY, Lidsky MD, Cox AM *et al.* Long-term nonsteroidal antiinflammatory drug use and *Helicobacter pylori* infection. *Gastroenterology* 1991; **100**: 1653–7.

54 Sontag SJ. Guilty as charged: bugs and drugs in gastric ulcer [review]. *Am J Gastroenterol* 1997; **92**: 1255–61.

55 Graham DY. Nonsteroidal anti-inflammatory drugs, *Helicobacter pylori*, and ulcers: where we stand [review]. *Am J Gastroenterol* 1996; **91**: 2080–6.

56 Goggin PM, Collins DA, Jazrawi RP *et al.* Prevalence of *Helicobacter pylori* infection and its effect on symptoms and non-steroidal anti-inflammatory drug induced gastrointestinal damage in patients with rheumatoid arthritis. *Gut* 1993; **34**: 1677–80.

57 Schubert TT, Bologna SD, Nensey Y *et al.* Ulcer risk factors: interactions between *Helicobacter pylori* infection, nonsteroidal use, and age. *Am J Med* 1993; **94**: 413–18.

58 Pilotto A, Leandro G, Di MF *et al.* Role of *Helicobacter pylori* infection on upper gastrointestinal bleeding in the elderly: a case-control study. *Dig Dis Sci* 1997; **42**: 586–91.

59 Laine L, Cominelli F, Sloane R *et al.* Interaction of NSAIDs and *Helicobacter pylori* on gastrointestinal injury and prostaglandin production: a controlled double-blind trial. *Aliment Pharmacol Ther* 1995; **9**: 127–35.

60 Soll AH. Pathogenesis of peptic ulcer and implications for therapy. *N Engl J Med* 1990; **322**: 909–16.

61 Soll AH. Consensus conference. Medical treatment of peptic ulcer disease. Practice guidelines. Practice Parameters Committee of the American College of Gastroenterology [review] [published erratum appears in JAMA 1996; **275**: 1314] *JAMA* 1996; **275**: 622–9.

62 Somerville K, Faulkner G, Langman M. Non-steroidal anti-inflammatory drugs and bleeding peptic ulcer. *Lancet* 1986; **i**: 462–4.

63 Heresbach D, Raoul JL, Bretagne JF *et al.* *Helicobacter pylori*: a risk and severity factor of non-steroidal anti-inflammatory drug induced gastropathy. *Gut* 1992; **33**: 1608–11.

64 Taha AS, Sturrock RD, Russell RI. Mucosal erosions in longterm non-steroidal anti-inflammatory drug users: predisposition to ulceration and relation to *Helicobacter pylori*. *Gut* 1995; **36**: 334–6.

65 Publig W, Wustinger C, Zandl C. Non-steroidal anti-inflammatory drugs (NSAID) cause gastrointestinal ulcers mainly in *Helicobacter pylori* carriers. *Wien Klin Wochenschr* 1994; **106**: 276–9.

66 Hawkey CJ, Swannell AJ, Yeomans ND. Increased effectiveness of omeprazole compared to ranitidine in non steroidal anti inflammatory drug (NSAID) users with reference to *H. pylori* status. *Gut* 1996; **39**: A33.

67 Yeomans ND, Tulassay Z, Juhasz L *et al.* A comparison of omeprazole with ranitidine for ulcers associated with nonsteroidal antiinflammatory drugs. *N Engl J Med* 1998; **338**: 719–26.

68 Labenz J, Tillenburg B, Peitz U *et al.* *Helicobacter pylori* augments the ph-increasing effect of omeprazole in patients with duodenal ulcer. *Gastroenterology* 1996; **110**: 725–32.

69 Hudson N, Balsitis M, Filipowicz S. Effect of *Helicobacter pylori* colonization on gastric mucosal eicosanoid synthesis in patients taking NSAIDs. *Gut* 1993; **34**: 748–51.

70 Konturek J, Dembinski A, Konturek SJ. Infection of *Helicobacter pylori* and gastric adaptation to continued administration of aspirin in humans. *Gastroenterology* 1998; **114**: 245–55.

71 Lipscomb GR, Wallis N, Armstrong G *et al.* Influence of *Helicobacter pylori* on gastric mucosal adaptation to naproxen in man. *Dig Dis Sci* 1996; **41**: 1583–8.

72 Porro GB, Parente F, Imbesi V. Role of *Helicobacter pylori* in ulcer healing and recurrence of gastric and duodenal ulcers in long term NSAID users: response to omeprazole dual therapy. *Gut* 1996; **39**: 22–6.

73 Chan FK, Sung JJ, Chung SC *et al.* Randomised trial of eradication of *Helicobacter pylori* before non-steroidal anti-inflammatory drug therapy to prevent peptic ulcers. *Lancet* 1997; **350**: 975–9.

74 Thijs JC, Kuipers EJ, van ZA *et al.* Treatment of *Helicobacter pylori* infections [review]. *Q J Med* 1995; **88**: 369–89.

75 Levi S, Goodlad RA, Lee CY *et al.* Inhibitory effect of non-steroidal anti-inflammatory drugs on mucosal cell proliferation associated with gastric ulcer healing [see comments]. *Lancet* 1990; **336**: 840–3.

76 Smedfors B, Johansson C. Stimulation of dudenal bicarbonate secretion by misoprostol. *Dig Dis Sci* 1998; **31**: 96–100.

77 Walt RP. Misoprostol for the treatment of peptic ulcer and antiinflammatory drug induced gastroduodenal ulceration. *N Engl J Med* 1992; **327**: 1575–80.

78 Wilson DE, Quadros E, Rajapaksa T *et al.* Effects of misoprostol on gastric acid and mucus secretion in man. *Dig Dis Sci* 1986; **31**: 126–9.

79 Collins PW. Misoprostol: discovery, development, and clinical applications. *Med Res Rev* 1990; **10**: 149–72.

80 Hawkey CJ, Karrasch JA, Szczepanski L *et al.* Omeprazole compared to misoprostol for ulcers associated with nonsteroidal antiinflammatory drugs. *N Engl J Med* 1998; **338**: 727–34.

81 Cohen MM, Clark L, Armstrong L *et al.* Reduction of aspirin-induced fecal blood loss with low-dose misoprostol tablets in man. *Dig Dis Sci* 1985; **30**: 605–11.

82 Lanza FL, Fakouhi D, Rubin A *et al.* A double-blind placebo-controlled comparison of the efficacy and safety of 50, 100, and 200 micrograms of misoprostol QID in the prevention of ibuprofen-induced gastric and duodenal mucosal lesions and symptoms. *Am J Gastroenterol* 1989; **84**: 633–6.

83 Ryan JR, Vargas R, Clay GA *et al.* Role of misoprostol in reducing aspirin-induced gastrointestinal blood loss in arthritic patients. *Am J Med* 1987; **83**: 41–6.

84 Silverstein FE, Kimmey MB, Saunders DR *et al.* Gastric protection by misoprostol against 1300 mg of aspirin. An endoscopic study. *Dig Dis Sci* 1986; **31**: 137S–141S.

85 Hunt JN, Smith JI, Jiang CL *et al.* Effect of synthetic prostaglandin E1 analogue on aspirin induced gastric bleeding and secretion. *Dig Dis Sci* 1983; **28**: 897–902.

86 Konturek JW, Dembinski A, Stoll R *et al.* Mucosal adaptation to aspirin induced gastric damage in humans. Studies on blood flow, gastric mucosal growth, and neutrophil activation. *Gut* 1994; **35**: 1197–204.

87 Konturek JW, Dembinski A, Konturek SJ *et al.* *Helicobacter pylori* and gastric adaptation to repeated aspirin administration in humans. *J Phys Pharmacol* 1997; **48**: 383–91.

88 Fletcher RH, Fletcher SW, Wagner EH. *Clinical epidemiology: the essentials*, 2nd edn. Baltimore: Williams & Wilkins, 1988.

89 Sackett DL, Haynes RB Guyatt GH *et al. Clinical epidemiology: a basic science for clinical medicine*, 2nd edn. Boston: Little, Brown, 1998.

90 Raskin JB, White RH, Jaszewski R *et al.* Misoprostol and ranitidine in the prevention of NSAID-induced ulcers: a prospective, double-blind, multicenter study. *Am J Gastroenterol* 1996; **91**: 223–7.

91 Agrawal NM, Van KH, Erhardt LJ *et al.* Misoprostol coadministered with diclofenac for prevention of gastroduodenal ulcers. A one-year study. *Dig Dis Sci* 1995; **40**: 1125–31.

92 Raskin JB, White RH, Jackson JE *et al.* Misoprostol dosage in the prevention of nonsteroidal anti-inflammatory drug-induced gastric and duodenal ulcers: a comparison of three regimens. *Ann Intern Med* 1995; **123: 344–50.**

93 Valentini M, Cannizzaro R, Poletti M *et al.* Nonsteroidal antiinflammatory drugs for cancer pain: comparison between misoprostol and ranitidine in prevention of upper gastrointestinal damage. *J Clin Oncol* 1995; **13**: 2637–42.

94 Delmas PD, Lambert R, Capron MH. Misoprostol in the prevention of gastric erosions caused by nonsteroidal anti-inflammatory agents [in French]. *Rev Rhumatisme* 1994; pp.126–31.

95 Elliott SL, Yeomans ND, Buchanan RR *et al.* Efficacy of 12 months' misoprostol as prophylaxis against NSAID-induced gastric ulcers. A placebo-controlled trial. *Scand J Rheumatol* 1994; **23**: 171–6.

96 Graham DY, White RH, Moreland LW *et al.* Duodenal and gastric ulcer prevention with misoprostol in arthritis patients taking NSAIDs. Misoprostol Study Group [see comments]. *Ann Intern Med* 1993; **119**: 257–62.

97 Henriksson K, Uribe A, Sandstedt B *et al.* *Helicobacter pylori* infection, ABO blood group, and effect of misoprostol on gastroduodenal mucosa in NSAID-treated patients with rheumatoid arthritis. *Dig Dis Sci* 1993; **38**: 1688–96.

98 Melo GA, Roth SH, Zeeh J *et al.* Double-blind comparison of efficacy and gastroduodenal safety of diclofenac/misoprostol, piroxicam, and naproxen in the treatment of osteoarthritis. *Ann Rheum Dis* 1993; **52**: 881–5.

99 Roth SH, Tindall EA, Jain AK *et al.* A controlled study comparing the effects of nabumetone, ibuprofen, and ibuprofen plus misoprostol on the upper gastrointestinal tract mucosa. *Arch Intern Med* 1993; **153**: 2565–71.

100 Bolten W, Gomes JA, Stead H *et al.* The gastroduodenal safety and efficacy of the fixed combination of diclofenac and misoprostol in the treatment of osteoarthritis. *Br J Rheumatol* 1992; **31**: 753–8.

101 Geis G, Stead MWC, Nicholson P. Prevalence of mucosal lesions in the stomach and duodenum due to chronic use of NSAID in patients with

rheumatoid arthritis or osteoarthritis, and interim report on prevention by misoprostol of diclofenac associated lesions. *J Rheumatol* 1991; **18**: 114.

102 Verdickt W, Moran C, Hantzschel H *et al.* A double-blind comparison of the gastroduodenal safety and efficacy of diclofenac and a fixed dose combination of diclofenac and misoprostol in the treatment of rheumatoid arthritis. *Scand J Rheumatol* 1992; **21**: 85–91.

103 Agrawal NM, Roth S, Graham DY *et al.* Misoprostol compared with sucralfate in the prevention of nonsteroidal anti-inflammatory drug-induced gastric ulcer. A randomized, controlled trial [see comments]. *Ann Intern Med* 1991; **115**: 195–200.

104 Chandrasekaran AN, Sambandam PR, Lal HM *et al.* Double blind, placebo controlled trial on the cytoprotective effect of misoprostol in subjects with rheumatoid arthritis, osteoarthritis and seronegative spondarthropathy on NSAIDs [see comments]. *J Assoc Phys India* 1991; **39**: 919–21.

105 Saggioro A, Alvisi V, Blasi A *et al.* Misoprostol prevents NSAID-induced gastroduodenal lesions in patients with osteoarthritis and rheumatoid arthritis [published erratum appears in *Ital J Gastroenterol* 1991; **23(5)**: 273]. *Ital J Gastroenterol* 1991; **23**: 119–23.

106 Graham DY, Agrawal NM, Roth SH. Prevention of NSAID-induced gastric ulcer with misoprostol: multicentre, double-blind, placebo-controlled trial. *Lancet* 1988; **ii**: 1277–80.

107 Maiden N, Madhok R. Misoprostol in patients taking non-steroidal anti-inflammatory drugs [editorial] [see comments]. *Br Med J* 1995; **311**: 1518–19.

108 Jonsson B, Haglund U. Cost-effectiveness of misoprostol in Sweden. *Int J Technol Assessment Hlth Care* 1992; **8**: 234–44.

109 Knill–Jones R, Drummond M, Kohli H *et al.* Economic evaluation of gastric ulcer prophylaxis in patients with arthritis receiving non-steroidal anti-inflammatory drugs. *Postgrad Med J* 1990; **66**: 639–46.

110 De PG, Bader JP. Cost-effectiveness of preventive treatment with misoprostol in non-steroidal anti-inflammatory agents related gastric ulcers [in French]. *Gastroenterol Clin Biol* 1991; **15**: 399–404.

111 Gabriel SE, Campion ME, O'Fallon WM. A cost-utility analysis of misoprostol prophylaxis for rheumatoid arthritis patients receiving nonsteroidal antiinflammatory drugs. *Arth Rheum* 1994; **37**: 333–41.

112 Gabriel SE, Jaakkimainen RL, Bombardier C. The cost-effectiveness of misoprostol for nonsteroidal antiinflammatory drug-associated adverse gastrointestinal events. *Arth Rheum* 1993; **36**: 447–59.

113 Hillman AL, Bloom BS. Economic effects of prophylactic use of misoprostol to prevent gastric ulcer in patients taking nonsteroidal anti-inflammatory drugs. *Arch Intern Med* 1989; **149**: 2061–5.

114 Edelson JT, Tosteson AN, Sax P. Cost-effectiveness of misoprostol for prophylaxis against nonsteroidal anti-inflammatory drug-induced gastrointestinal tract bleeding [see comments]. *JAMA* 1990; **264**: 41–7.

115 Carrin GJ, Torfs KE. Economic evaluation of prophylactic treatment with misoprostol in osteoarthritic patients treated with NSAIDs. The case of Belgium. *Rev Epidemiol Sante Publ* 1990; **38**: 187–99.

116 Bijlsma JW. Treatment of NSAID-induced gastrointestinal lesions with cimetidine: an international multicenter collaborative study. *Aliment Pharmacol Ther* 1988; **2** (Suppl 1): 85–95.

117 Croker JR, Cotton PB, Boyle AC *et al.* Cimetidine for peptic ulcer in patients with arthritis. *Ann Rheum Dis* 1980; **39**: 275–8.

118 Farah D, Sturrock RD, Russell RI. Peptic ulcer in rheumatoid arthritis [see comments]. *Ann Rheum Dis* 1988; **47**: 478–80.

119 LoIudice TA, Saleem T, Lang JA. Cimetidine in the treatment of gastric ulcer induced by steroidal and nonsteroidal anti-inflammatory agents. *Am J Gastroenterol* 1981; **75**: 104–10.

120 O'Laughlin JC, Silvoso GR, Ivey KJ. Healing of aspirin-associated peptic ulcer disease despite continued salicylate ingestion. *Arch Intern Med* 1981; **141**: 781–3.

121 Walan A, Bader JP, Classen M *et al.* Effect of omeprazole and ranitidine on ulcer healing and relapse rates in patients with benign gastric ulcers. *N Engl J Med* 1989; **320**: 69–75.

122 Mani V. Ranitidine in NSAID ulcers. *Natl Med J India* 1992; **5**: 69.

123 O'Laughlin JC, Silvoso GK, Ivey KJ. Resistance to medical therapy of gastric ulcers in rheumatic disease patients taking aspirin. A double-blind study with cimetidine and follow-up. *Dig Dis Sci* 1982; **27**: 976–80.

124 Ehsanullah RS, Page MC, Tildesley G *et al.* Prevention of gastroduodenal damage induced by non-steroidal anti-inflammatory drugs: controlled trial of ranitidine. *Br Med J* 1988; **297**: 1017–21.

125 Robinson MG, Griffin JJ, Bowers J *et al.* Effect of ranitidine on gastroduodenal mucosal damage induced by nonsteroidal antiinflammatory drugs. *Dig Dis Sci* 1989; **34**: 424–8.

126 Robinson M, Mills RJ, Euler AR. Ranitidine prevents duodenal ulcers associated with non-

steroidal anti-inflammatory drug therapy. *Aliment Pharmacol Ther* 1991; **5**: 143–50.
127 Levine LR, Cloud ML, Enas NH. Nizatidine prevents peptic ulceration in high-risk patients taking nonsteroidal anti-inflammatory drugs [see comments]. *Arch Intern Med* 1993; **153**: 2449–54.
128 Roth SH, Bennett RE, Mitchell CS *et al.* Cimetidine therapy in nonsteroidal anti-inflammatory drug gastropathy. Double-blind long-term evaluation. *Arch Intern Med* 1987; **147**: 1798–801.
129 Bianchi Porro G., Pace F, Caruso I. Why are non-steroidal anti-inflammatory drugs important in peptic ulceration? [review]. *Aliment Pharmacol Ther* 1987; **1** (Suppl): 547S.
130 Berkowitz JM, Rogenes PR, Sharp JT *et al.* Ranitidine protects against gastroduodenal mucosal damage associated with chronic aspirin therapy. *Arch Intern Med* 1987; **147**: 2137–9.
131 Simon B, Bergdolt H, Dammann H *et al.* Ranitidine in the therapy and prevention of NSAR-induced (non-steroidal anti-rheumatic agents) gastroduodenal lesions in patients with rheumatism [in German]. *Zeitschr Gastroenterol* 1991; **29**: 217–21.
132 Simon B, Muller P. Nizatidine in therapy and prevention of non-steroidal anti-inflammatory drug-induced gastroduodenal ulcer in rheumatic patients. *Scand J Gastroenterol* 1994; **206** (Suppl): 25–8.
133 Koch M, Dezi A, Ferrario F *et al.* Prevention of nonsteroidal anti-inflammatory drug-induced gastrointestinal mucosal injury. A meta-analysis of randomized controlled clinical trials [see comments]. *Arch Intern Med* 1996; **156**: 2321–32.
134 Singh G, Ramey DR, Morfeld D *et al.* Gastrointestinal tract complications of nonsteroidal anti-inflammatory drug treatment in rheumatoid arthritis. A prospective observational cohort study. *Arch Intern Med* 1996; **156**: 1530–6.
135 Janssen M, Dijkmans BA, Vandenbroucke JP *et al.* Achlorhydria does not protect against benign upper gastrointestinal ulcers during NSAID use. *Dig Dis Sci* 1994; **39**: 362–5.
136 Daneshmend TK, Stein AG, Bhaskar NK *et al.* Abolition by omeprazole of aspirin induced gastric mucosal injury in man. *Gut* 1990; **31**: 514–17.
137 Scheiman JM, Behler EM, Loeffler KM *et al.* Omeprazole ameliorates aspirin-induced gastroduodenal injury. *Dig Dis Sci* 1994; **39**: 97–103.
138 Bergmann JF, Chassany O, Simoneau ML. Protection against aspirin induced gastric lesions by lansoprazole: simultaneous evaluation of functional and morphologic responces. *Clin Pharmacol Ther* 1992; **52**: 413–16.
139 Wolde S, Dijkmans BA, Janssen M *et al.* High-dose ranitidine for the prevention of recurrent peptic ulcer disease in rheumatoid arthritis patients taking NSAIDs. *Aliment Pharmacol Ther* 1996; **10**: 347–51.
140 Nwokolo CU, Prewett EJ, Sawyerr AM *et al.* Tolerance during 5 months of dosing with ranitidine, 150 mg nightly: a placebo-controlled, double-blind study. *Gastroenterology* 1991; **101**: 948–53.
141 Smith JT, Gavey C, Nwokolo CU *et al.* Tolerance during 8 days of high-dose H_2-blockade: placebo-controlled studies of 24-hour acidity and gastrin. *Aliment Pharmacol Ther* 1990; **4** (Suppl); 63.
142 Nwokolo CU, Smith JT, Gavey C *et al.* Tolerance during 29 days of conventional dosing with cimetidine, nizatidine, famotidine or ranitidine. *Aliment Pharmacol Ther* 1990; **4** (Suppl): 45.
143 Oddsson E, Gudjonsson H, Thjodleifsson B. Comparison between ranitidine and omeprazole for protection against gastroduodenal damage caused by naproxen. *Scand J Gastroenterol* 1992; **27**: 1045–8.
144 Lauritsen K, Rutgersson K, Bolling E. Omeprazole 20 or 40 mg daily for healing of duodenal ulcer? A double blind comparative study. *Eur J Gastroenterol Hepatol* 1992; **4**: 995–1000.
145 Hawkey CJ, Swannell AJ, Eriksson S. Benefits of omeprazole over misoprostol in healing NSAID associated ulcers. *Gastroenterology* 1996; **110**: A131.
146 Hawkey CJ, Foren I, Langstrom G. Omeprazole vs misoprostol: different effectiveness in healing gastric and duodenal ulcers vs erosions in NSAID users: The Omnium study. *Gut* 1997; **40**: A1.
147 Ekstrom P, Carling L, Wetterhus S *et al.* Prevention of peptic ulcer and dyspeptic symptoms with omeprazole in patients receiving continuous non-steroidal anti-inflammatory drug therapy. A Nordic multicentre study [see comments]. *Scand J Gastroenterol* 1996; **31**: 753–8.
148 Cullen D, Bardhan KD, Eisner M. Primary gastroduodenal prophylaxis with omeprazole for NSAID users. *Gastroenterol* 1996; **110**: A86.
149 Dvornik DM. Tissue selective inhibition of prostaglandin biosynthesis by etodolac [review]. *J Rheumatol* 1997; **47** (Suppl): 40–7.
150 Robinson DR. Regulation of prostaglandin synthesis by anti-inflammatory drugs. *J Rheumatol* 1997; **24**: 32–9.

151 Singh G, Terry R, Ramey DR *et al.* Comparative toxicity of NSAIDs. *Arth Rheum* 1997; A507–S115.

152 Ferraz MB, Maetzel A, Bombardier C. Meta-analysis comparing the effects of low risk non-steroidal antiinflammatory drugs (NSAIDs) on the gastric and duodenal mucosa. *Arth Rheum* 1995; **38**: A647–S261.

153 Distel M, Mueller C, Bluhmki E *et al.* Safety of meloxicam: a global analysis of clinical trials. *Br J Rheumatol* 1996; **35** (Suppl): 77.

154 Engelhardt G, Homma D, Schlegel K *et al.* Anti-inflammatory, analgesic, antipyretic and related properties of meloxicam, a new non-steroidal anti-inflammatory agent with favourable gastrointestinal tolerance. *Inflamm Res* 1995; **44**: 423–33.

155 Hosie J, Distel M, Bluhmki E. Meloxicam in osteoarthritis: a 6-month, double-blind comparison with diclofenac sodium. *Br J Rheumatol* 1996; **35** (Suppl): 43.

156 Wojtulewski JA, Schattenkirchner M, Barcelo P *et al.* A six-month double-blind trial to compare the efficacy and safety of meloxicam 7.5 mg daily and naproxen 750 mg daily in patients with rheumatoid arthritis. *Br J Rheumatol* 1996; **35** (Suppl): 8.

157 Reginster JY, Distel M, Bluhmki E. A double-blind, three-week study to compare the efficacy and safety of meloxicam 7.5 mg and meloxicam 15 mg in patients with rheumatoid arthritis. *Br J Rheumatol* 1996; **35** (Suppl): 21.

158 Goldstein J, Agrawal NM, Silverstein F *et al.* Celecoxib is associated with a significantly lower incidence of clinically significant upper gastrointestinal (UGI) events in osteoarthritis (OA) and rheumatoid arthritis (RA) patients as compared to NSAIDs. *Gastroenterology* 1999; **116: A174.**

159 Laine L, Hawkey C, Harper S *et al.* Effect of the COX-2 specific inhibitor (C-2SI) rofecoxib on ulcer formation. A double-blind comparison with ibuprofen and placebo. *Gastroenterology* 1999; **116**: A229.

160 Wallace JL, McKnight W, Del SP *et al.* Anti-thrombotic effects of a nitric oxide-releasing, gastric-sparing aspirin derivative. *J Clin Invest* 1995; **96**: 2711–18.

161 Elliott SN, McKnight W, Cirino G *et al.* A nitric oxide-releasing nonsteroidal anti-inflammatory drug accelerates gastric ulcer healing in rats [see comments]. *Gastroenterology* 1995; **109**: 524–30.

162 Wallace JL, Reuter B, Cicala C *et al.* Novel nonsteroidal anti-inflammatory drug derivatives with markedly reduced ulcerogenic properties in the rat. *Gastroenterology* 1994; **107**: 173–9.

163 Reindeau D, Charleson S, Cromlish W. Comparison of the cyclooxygenase-1 inhibitory properties of non steroidal anti-inflamatory drugs (NSAIDs) and selective COX-2 inhibitors, using sensitive microsomal and platelet assays. *Can J Physiol Pharmacol* 1997; **75**: 1088–95.

5 Acute non-variceal gastrointestinal hemorrhage: treatment

NICHOLAS CHURCH, KELVIN PALMER

INTRODUCTION

Peptic ulcer is the commonest cause of acute non-variceal bleeding, accounting for approximately half of the cases.[1] Other major causes such as gastroduodenal erosions, gastritis, esophagitis, Mallory–Weiss tears, and vascular malformations are not usually life threatening and respond to conservative therapy.

Approximately 80% of cases pursue a benign course without rebleeding in hospital and specific intervention is not required. The remaining 20% have severe bleeding due to erosion of a major artery. Most deaths from bleeding arise from this subgroup. The crude death rate from gastrointestinal bleeding has not significantly improved over five decades. Avery Jones in 1957 reported a hospital mortality of 16%[2] whilst a large audit of acute gastrointestinal bleeding performed in England in 1997 reported a very similar mortality of 11%.[3] This disappointing observation must, however, be tempered by the fact that the case mix of patients now admitted is very different to that of previous decades. For example, less that 2% of patients admitted with acute bleeding in 1947 were aged over 80 years whilst approximately a quarter of patients currently admitted are octogenarians. There is a close relationship between increasing age and hospital mortality: increasing age is inevitably associated with a high prevalence of chronic disease, rendering patients susceptible to complications following major hemorrhage.

The risk of death following admission to hospital for gastrointestinal bleeding has been quantified by Rockall *et al*[4] (Table 5.1). Independent factors associated with a poor prognosis were identified from data derived from a large population of patients whose clinical course was observed following hospital admission. Whilst the Rockall risk scoring system performed well when tested in a cohort of patients subsequently managed in the same geographical area, it has not been widely validated elsewhere. Recently the Rockall score has been shown to correlate well with observed mortality, but not rebleeding, in a Dutch population.[5]

As shown in Table 5.2, Rockall *et al* showed a good correlation between the risk score, rebleeding and hospital mortality. Deaths following admission to hospital because of acute gastrointestinal bleeding are rarely due to exsanguination. They are usually a consequence of postoperative complications when an urgent operation is undertaken, or of deterioration of comorbid conditions.

Over the past 10 years the treatment of choice for appropriate bleeding patients has been endoscopic therapy, and surgical intervention has been reserved for the failure of therapeutic endoscopy. Nevertheless, optimum management still relies very much on a team approach with appropriate use of drug therapy, endoscopic intervention, and

Table 5.1 The Rockall scoring system for risk of rebleeding and death after admission to hospital for acute gastrointestinal bleeding

Variable	**Score** 0	1	2	3
Age	<60 yr	60–79 yr	≥80 yr	
Shock	*No shock* Systolic BP >100	*Tachycardia* Systolic BP >100	*Hypotension* Systolic BP <100	
Pulse	<100	>100		
Comorbidity	Nil major		Cardiac failure, ischemic heart disease, any major comorbidity	Renal failure, liver failure, disseminated malignancy
Diagnosis	Mallory–Weiss tear, no lesion and no SRH	All other diagnoses	Malignancy of upper GI tract	
Major SRH	None, or dark spot		Blood in upper GI tract, adherent clot, visible or spurting vessel	

SRH, Stigmata of recent hemorrhage.
Source: Rockall *et al.*[4]

Table 5.2 Correlation between Rockall score and rebleeding and mortality

Risk score	*n*	Rebleed (%)	Mortality (%)
0	144	7(5)	0(0)
1	281	9(3)	0(0)
2	337	18(5)	1(0.2)
3	444	50(11)	13(3)
4	528	76(14)	28(5)
5	455	83(24)	49(11)
6	312	102(33)	54(17)
7	267	113(44)	72(27)
8+	190	101(42)	78(41)

surgery. Despite much evidence from randomized trials, the management of an individual patient still depends on clinical judgement concerning the probability that attempts at endoscopic intervention are likely to be fruitless and that surgery is inevitable. Management may be best undertaken in a specialized "bleeding unit" in which the patient is treated using agreed protocols and guidelines with endoscopy undertaken once appropriate resuscitation has been achieved and with management decisions based upon endoscopic and surgical opinions. Relatively weak evidence derived from comparison of results in case series with historical controls suggests that this approach may achieve lower hospital mortality and more efficient use of resources than management by generalists working in conventional medical or surgical units.[6,7]

SPECIFIC THERAPY

For the 80% of patients who have relatively minor bleeding and who do not have major endoscopic stigmata of bleeding, supportive therapy including use of intravenous fluid and the management of comorbidity (particularly cardiorespiratory disease) is sufficient.

Patients who present with clinical shock and who at endoscopy have an actively bleeding peptic ulcer have an 80% risk of continuing to bleed or rebleed in hospital.[8] Those who have a non-bleeding visible vessel have a 50% risk of further hemorrhage.[9] The "visible vessel" represents a pseudoaneurysm of the involved artery, or adherent blood clot, plugging the arterial defect.[10] Patients who are found to have an adherent blood clot over the ulcer usually have an underlying high risk lesion and should also be regarded as being at considerable risk of further hemorrhage in hospital. Patients who at endoscopy have a clean ulcer base or who have black or red spots are at very little risk of rebleeding.

It follows from these observations that patients with major endoscopic stigmata should be considered for specific hemostatic treatment and only such patients should be included in clinical trials of therapy for gastrointestinal bleeding. This review will only consider those studies that exclusively include patients having either a non-bleeding visible vessel, active hemorrhage, or adherent blood clot as entry criteria.

The specific non-surgical approaches to hemostasis are drug therapy and endoscopic therapy.

DRUG THERAPY

There are three principles underlying the use of drugs as agents which might stop active hemorrhage and prevent rebleeding. The first of these is that the stability of a blood clot is poor in an acid environment. Thus agents that suppress acid secretion, including H_2-receptor antagonists (H_2RA) and proton pump inhibitor (PPI) drugs might reduce rebleeding.[11] The second is that blood clot may be stabilized by decreasing fibrinolytic mechanisms using agents such as tranexamic acid. The third approach is that, since major gastrointestinal bleeding is due to arterial erosion, reduction of arterial blood flow by agents such as somatostatin and octreotide could achieve hemostasis and prevent rebleeding.

Acid suppressing drugs

The efficacy of H_2RA in the management of acute upper gastrointestinal bleeding has been assessed in randomized trials.[12,13] Unfortunately, no trial has shown benefit in terms of reduction of rebleeding incidence or mortality.

Experience involving the use of PPIs is inconsistent. The largest trial involved 1147 patients who were randomized to receive intravenous, then oral omeprazole or placebo.[14] No significant difference in hospital mortality, operation rate or rebleeding was demonstrated (Table 5.3). The study was not restricted to the high risk patients who had

Table 5.3 Omeprazole vs placebo for acute upper gastrointestinal bleeding

Outcome	Omeprazole	Placebo
All patients		
n	578	569
Rebleed (%)	77 (15)	91 (17)
Operation (%)	56 (11)	57 (11)
Death (%)	35 (7)	29 (6)
Gastric ulcer		
n	97	93
Rebleed (%)	26 (27)	23 (25)
Operation (%)	18 (19)	16 (17)
Death (%)	7 (7)	5 (5)
Duodenal ulcer		
n	149	164
Rebleed (%)	32 (21)	47 (29)
Operation (%)	27 (18)	34 (21)
Death (%)	16 (11)	8 (5)

Source: Daneshmend *et al.*[14]

Table 5.4 Omeprazole vs placebo for bleeding peptic ulcer

Outcome	Omeprazole (*n* = 110)	Placebo (*n* = 110)	*P* value
Rebleed (%)	12 (11)	40 (36)	<0.001
Surgery (%)	8 (8)	26 (23)	<0.001
Transfusion (mean units)	2.3	4.1	<0.001
Death	2	6	NS

Source: Khuroo *et al.*[15]

endoscopic stigmata of recent hemorrhage. Accordingly, event rates were rather low in the placebo group, and this may have limited the power of the study to show a difference.

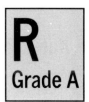

R Grade A

Khuroo *et al* randomized 220 bleeding ulcer patients who had major endoscopic stigmata to receive high dose oral omeprazole or placebo.[15] Rebleeding, the need for urgent surgery, blood transfusion, and mortality were all reduced in the actively treated group of patients (Table 5.4). The number of patients needed to treat with omeprazole to prevent one death was 25, and to prevent one operation was 7. This trial has been criticized because it included relatively young patients with relatively little comorbidity and, more importantly, because endoscopic therapy was not administered to any patient.

R Grade A

In a third study, 274 patients presenting with peptic ulcer and major endoscopic stigmata were randomized to receive omeprazole or a placebo.[16] Endoscopic intervention was administered to most patients. In this study outcome tended to be better in the group receiving active drug, although no statistically significant differences in transfusion requirement, rates of surgery, or mortality at day 3, 21, and 35 were demonstrated (Table 5.5).

Although omeprazole may be effective in the management of peptic ulcer hemorrhage it appears that any effect on rebleeding, surgery and death is modest, at best. The studies also suggest that benefit is least likely in the most severe cases. Indeed it is perhaps a little optimistic to expect that a drug that suppresses acid will have a major primary hemostatic effect in patients actively bleeding from a large defect within an eroded major artery. Nevertheless, there may be some merit in the routine use of high dose oral omeprazole, not least since this starts the ulcer healing process at an early stage, and we should advocate this in all ulcer bleeding patients. Proton pump inhibitors have few adverse effects and their cost in the context of an acutely bleeding patient is relatively modest.

Tranexamic acid

R Grade A

A meta-analysis of six controlled trials, which included 1267 patients, did not show a significant reduction in the rate of rebleeding, but did show a reduction in the need for surgery and in mortality which did reach statistical significance[17] (Table 5.6). This meta-analysis included trials in which many patients did not have major endoscopic stigmata of bleeding. Therefore, the results may not be applicable to patient populations at greatest risk.

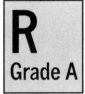

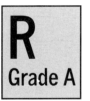

R Grade A

The largest study was undertaken by the Nottingham group.[18] Seven hundred and seventy-five patients presenting to hospital because of acute gastrointestinal bleeding were randomized to receive oral cimetidine, tranexamic acid or placebo. No significant difference in bleeding or operation rates was demonstrated, but there was a rather surprising large difference in mortality. Mortality was 11% in cimetidine treated patients, 10% in tranexamic acid treated patients, and 20% in placebo. The mortality rate of 20% in the placebo treated group is approximately twice that expected for conservatively treated patients based on the results of other studies. Furthermore, other studies do not demonstrate benefit from the use of cimetidine. It is possible that more high risk patients were inadvertently randomized to the placebo group in this study.

Table 5.5 Omeprazole vs placebo for bleeding peptic ulcer treated with endoscopic therapy

Outcome	Omeprazole (n = 134)	Placebo (n = 140)
Additional endoscopic Rx	3	10
Transfusion >3 units	16	25
Surgery	6	15
Death	2	0

Source: Schaffalitzky de Muckadell *et al.*[16]

Table 5.6 Tranexamic acid for gastrointestinal bleeding – a meta-analysis

Outcome	POR	95% CI	*P* value
Rebleeding	0.80	0.61–1.10	0.13
Operation	0.72	0.52–1.00	0.047
Death	0.60	0.40–0.89	0.01

Source: Henry and O'Connell.[17]

Somatostatin and octreotide

Somatostatin and its analogs have two actions which are theoretically valuable in the management of ulcer bleeding, namely inhibition of acid secretion and reduction of splanchnic blood flow. Mesenteric blood flow falls dramatically during infusions of somatostatin but it is not clear whether this is principally due to vasoconstriction of major blood vessels or peripheral arterioles.

There have been 14 controlled trials of somatostatin versus other therapy in the management of patients presenting with acute gastrointestinal bleeding.[19–32] Two meta-analyses suggest that somatostatin but not octreotide has a primary hemostatic role and reduces the need for surgical intervention.[33,34] However, scrutiny of the relevant trials reveals many problems. Many of the studies were small and inclusion criteria varied widely from gastritis to major active bleeding.

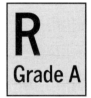

R
Grade A

The largest trial was reported by Sommerville *et al* in 1985[19] (Table 5.7). Six hundred and thirty of 779 potentially eligible actively bleeding patients were randomized to receive somatostatin (a bolus of 250 μg followed by 250 mg hourly for 72 hours) or a placebo. No significant differences in rebleeding, operation rate, and mortality were demonstrated between the treatment groups. The authors also reported the subgroup analysis of patients who had bled from gastric or duodenal ulcers. There were similar numbers of these in both active and placebo arms. Unfortunately the presence or absence of major stigmata of bleeding were not reported. The operation rate, mortality, and rebleeding rates were similar in the two groups. However, a statistically significant difference in mortality in duodenal ulcer patients was demonstrated, with more actively bleeding patients dying. Although this is a large study, and patients were randomized early, the possible efficacy of somatostatin may have been difficult to demonstrate because of the inclusion of many patients whose prognosis was excellent because they had relatively trivial bleeding or, at the other end of the spectrum, inclusion of patients in whom operation and possibly death was inevitable because bleeding was so severe.

R
Grade A

Table 5.7 Somatostatin vs placebo for acute gastrointestinal bleeding

Subgroup	Somatostatin	Placebo
All patients		
n	315	315
Rebleed (%)	70 (22)	89 (28)
Operation (%)	35 (11)	34 (11)
Death (%)	31 (10)	25 (8)
Gastric ulcer		
n	57	57
Rebleed (%)	18 (32)	21 (37)
Operation (%)	10 (18)	5 (9)
Death (%)	4 (7)	7 (12)
Duodenal ulcer		
n	77	81
Rebleed (%)	21 (27)	31 (38)
Operation (%)	13 (17)	18 (22)
Death (%)	15 (19)	5* (6)

Source: Sommerville *et al*.[19]
$^*P < 0.02$.

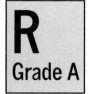

R
Grade A

A smaller study with contrasting results was reported by Magnusson *et al*[20] (Table 5.8). This trial only included patients who were in shock and actively bleeding, from peptic ulcers in almost all cases. Patients were randomized to receive somatostatin or placebo infusion. Uncontrolled hemorrhage and need for surgical operation were commoner in placebo then somatostatin treated patients. However, the mortality rate was not improved. Rebleeding was equally common in both groups and the apparent difference in transfusion requirements was not statistically significant. This small study lacked the power to demonstrate a significant difference in mortality should a true difference exist.

Currently, the evidence for routine use of somatostatin is weak and further studies are needed before this agent can be recommended as routine therapy for non-variceal acute gastrointestinal bleeding.

ENDOSCOPIC THERAPY

Many therapeutic endoscopic treatments have been used to try to stop active ulcer bleeding and prevent rebleeding. These can be classified into three basic endoscopic approaches (Table 5.9).

Table 5.8 Somatostatin vs placebo for acute gastrointestinal bleeding

	Somatostatin	Placebo
n	46	49
Peptic ulcer bleeding	36	42
Stigmata of major bleeding	38	41
Continued bleeding	8	16
Operation	5	14
Rebleeding	6	5
Median transfused units	5.8	7.2
Death	4	1

Source: Magnusson *et al*.[20]

Table 5.9 Endoscopic therapy

Modality	Type
Thermal	Argon laser
	Nd-YAG laser
	Heater probe
	Electrocoagulation
	Argon plasma coagulation
Injection	Adrenaline
	Sclerosants
	Alcohol
	Thrombin
	Fibrin glue
Mechanical	Hemoclips
	Staples
	Sutures

Thermal approaches involving laser, the heater probe and electrocoagulation by monopolar or bipolar probes attempt to induce thermocoagulation with thrombosis of the bleeding point. In experimental bleeding ulcers these approaches are more effective than injection treatments.[35] However, there is no good model of acute peptic ulcer bleeding. Experiments in animals are based upon observation following superficial mucosal injury, which is different from erosion of arteries by chronic or acute peptic ulcer. Injection therapy may produce tamponade by the injection of a relatively large volume of fluid into a rigid compartment, compressing the bleeding artery. Vasoconstriction induced by dilute adrenaline, endarteritis induced by sclerosants, dehydration following absolute alcohol injection or a direct effect upon blood clot formation following injection of thrombin or fibrin glue are other putative mechanisms. Mechanical clips, staples, and sewing attempt to produce hemostasis by clamping the bleeding arterial lesion.

Many clinical trials of endoscopic therapy for non-variceal bleeding have been published. The quality of these trials varies greatly. In general, the number of patients randomized in any one study is small and clinicians managing the patients have not been blinded to the type of endoscopic therapy. No trials have included a placebo control intervention for endoscopic therapy.

Thermal methods

LASER PHOTOCOAGULATION

Lasers were the first endoscopic therapeutic modality shown to be effective in managing acute non-variceal gastrointestinal bleeding. Initial experience involved the use of argon lasers but it became subsequently clear that the tissue characteristics of thermal injury achieved by Nd-YAG were more appropriate. In fact, clinical trials showed little difference in outcome in series involving argon or Nd-YAG laser treatment.

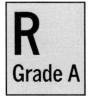

R Grade A

There have been three randomized trials comparing argon laser therapy and conservative therapy for bleeding peptic ulcer[36–38] and a further nine trials of Nd-YAG laser treatment[39–47] (Table 5.10). Most of these studies show that laser treatment significantly reduced the rates of rebleeding, transfusion requirement, and operation rate. One trial showed significant improvement in hospital mortality.[39] However, experience has not been universally positive with laser treatment. It is revealing to compare the best performed study with a large American multicenter study, published in the *New England Journal of Medicine*. Swain *et al*[39] randomized 138 patients to laser treatment or conservative therapy. He personally undertook all endoscopic examinations and treatments and was responsible for the clinical management of the treated subjects. His study revealed significant reduction in rebleeding, need for emergency surgery, and mortality in laser treated patients. In contrast Krejs *et al*[40] randomized a similar number of patients to laser therapy or to conservative treatment. Patients treated by laser tended to have a poor outcome compared to control patients. It was apparent in this study that endoscopic therapy was undertaken by a large number of endoscopists who varied in their expertise. Of all therapeutic endoscopic modalities, laser therapy is the most difficult to use. Even in Swain's hands up to 17% of ulcers could not be treated. The method is a "no touch" one and an awkwardly placed duodenal ulcer within a deformed duodenum may be extremely difficult to adequately treat. Thus the results in the hands of relatively inexperienced therapeutic endoscopists, each performing few procedures, was likely to have been variable. Furthermore, the patients included in this trial were managed in many units, rather than by a single "bleeding team".

R Grade A

Table 5.10 Nd–YAG trials for bleeding peptic ulcer

Study	Group	*n*	Rebleed (%)	Surgery (%)	Mortality (%)
Swain, 1986[39]	Laser	70	7 (10)	7 (10)	1 (1.4)
	Control	68	27 (40)	24 (35)	8 (12)
Krejs, 1987[40]	Laser	85	19 (22)	14 (16)	1 (1.2)
	Control	89	18 (20)	15 (17)	1 (1.1)
Rhode, 1980[41]	Laser	62	37 (59)	8 (13)	24 (39)
	Control	43	24 (57)	18 (41)	27 (63)
Rutgeerts, 1982[42]	Group 2: L	46	3 (7)	1 (2)	6 (13)
	Group 2: C	40	6 (15)[a]	5 (13)	6 (15)
	Group 3: L	17	3 (18)	2 (12)	2 (12)
	Group 3: C	26	8 (31)	6 (23)	4 (15)
MacLeod, 1983[43]	Laser	21	6 (29)	5 (24)	1 (5)
	Control	24	8 (33)	8 (33)	2 (8)
Homer, 1985[44]	Laser	17	3 (18)	—	0 (0)
	Control	25	8 (32)	—	2 (8)
Trudeau, 1985[45]	Laser	18	2 (11)	1 (5)	2 (11)
	Control	15	6 (40)	4 (26)	5 (33)
Buset, 1988[46]	Laser	42	10 (24)	3 (7)	1 (2)
	Control	46	17 (37)	2 (4)	2 (4)
Matthewson, 1990[47]	Laser	44	9 (20)	9 (20)	1 (2)
	Heater probe	57	16 (28)	13 (22)	6 (10)
	Control	42	18 (43)	13 (30)	4 (9)

[a]6 of 31 where bleeding stopped.
Rutgeerts group 2: active non-spurting bleeding.
Rutgeerts group 3: inactive bleeding with stigmata of recent hemorrhage.

Table 5.11 Heater probe for gastrointestinal bleeding

Study	Group	Rebleed (%)	Surgery (%)	Mortality (%)
Fullarton, 1989[48]	HP ($n = 20$)	0	0	0
	Sham ($n = 23$)	22*	13**	0
Jensen, 1988[49]	BICAP	44	22	3
	HP	22	3	3***
	Nil	72	41	9
	n (total) = 94			

*$P = 0.05$.
**P not stated.
***$P < 0.05$.
HP, heater probe; BICAP, bipolar electrocoagulation.

Endoscopic laser therapy has been found to be relatively safe with few complications; in particular, gastrointestinal perforation has been rare. However, since the technique is difficult, relatively expensive and because other approaches are at least as effective, laser therapy for peptic ulcer bleeding is no longer used.

HEATER PROBE

The heater probe transmits preset amounts of energy to the bleeding point via a Teflon tipped catheter. A powerful water jet is used to clean the ulcer base, help visualize the bleeding point and also to prevent the probe sticking to the bleeding point. Hemostasis is achieved both by tamponade and by application of heat. Best results are achieved using large sized probes.

There have been two trials in which the heater probe has been compared to conservative therapy.[48,49] Both showed significant benefit in terms of further bleeding, surgery and transfusion requirements, and one published only in abstract form[49] demonstrated a significant reduction in mortality (Table 5.11).

R
Grade A

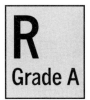

The heater probe is "user friendly". Its capacity to apply thermal energy by tangential application and its powerful water jet are particular advantages. Perforations have occurred following treatment, although these are unusual. Questions remain concerning the amount of energy that should be applied. In general, medium power settings (20 watts) are used but it is not possible to be prescriptive concerning the total amount of energy that should be given. Most authorities consider that treatment should be continued until active hemorrhage is stopped and until the treated area is charred.

ELECTROCOAGULATION

Monopolar electrocoagulation uses a metal ball-tipped probe. An electrical circuit is completed by a plate attached to the patient. Application of energy is rather haphazard and perforations and a death were reported in early series. Consequently this device is no longer used.

Bipolar electrocoagulation is based upon transmission of electrical energy between adjacent electrodes. The BICAP has eight separate electrodes over its surface. Early studies from the United Kingdom involving small numbers of patients showed no benefit for active treatment compared to conservative therapy. Subsequently however, trials from the United Kingdom and the USA showed that primary hemostasis, rebleeding, the need for surgery

Table 5.12 Electrocoagulation for gastrointestinal bleeding

Study	Group	*n*	Rebleed (%)	Surgery (%)	Mean units transfused
O'Brien, 1987[50]	Bipolar probe	101	17 (17)*	7 (7)	4.6**
	Nil	103	34 (33)	10 (10)	7.3
[a]Laine,1987,[51]	MPEC	21	—	3 (14)***	2.4†
	Sham	23	—	10 (43)	5.4
Brearley, 1987[52]	Bipolar probe	20	6 (30)	—	—
	Nil	21	8 (38)	—	—
[b]Laine, 1988[53]	MPEC	37	7 (19)‡	3 (8)	1.6‡
	Sham	37	15 (41)	11 (30)	3.0

*$P = 0.01$.
**$P = 0.13$.
***$P = 0.049$.
†$P = 0.002$.
‡$P<0.05$.
MPEC, monopolar electrocoagulation.
[a]Study included ulcers, Mallory–Weiss tears, and vascular malformations.
[b]Study was restricted to ulcers with non-bleeding visible vessels. See also Jensen,[49] Table 5.11.

and transfusion requirements were all improved by bipolar electrocoagulation compared to conventionally treated patients.[49–53] Grade A (Table 5.12). The efficacy of the heater probe and BICAP are comparable with similar low complication rates.[49,54]

ARGON PLASMA COAGULATION

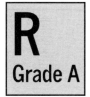

R Grade A

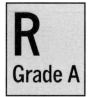

This procedure is based upon coagulation through a jet of argon gas. Relatively superficial thermal damage is achieved. The method is particularly applicable to mucosal and superficial bleeding lesions and its final role may be in dealing with vascular malformations such as gastric antral vascular ectasia. One trial has shown that argon beam coagulation is comparable in efficacy to heater probe therapy for ulcer hemostasis.[55] Nevertheless the tissue damage characteristics of argon plasma coagulation are less than ideal for managing arterial bleeding, and it will probably prove to be less appropriate for managing peptic ulcer bleeding than contact methods.

CONCLUSIONS

R Grade A

Thermal methods of hemostasis were shown to be superior to conservative management in two meta-analyses. In the study of Cook *et al*[57] the odds ratio for prevention of rebleeding was 0.48 (95% CI 0.32–0.76); and for avoidance of surgery was 0.47 (95% CI 0.27–0.80). Similarly, in the study of Henry and White,[56] the odds ratio for prevention of bleeding was 0.32 (95% CI 0.22–0.41) and for the avoidance of surgery was 0.31 (95% CI 0.19–0.43). Thermal contact methods (heater probe and bipolar coagulation) are technically easier to undertake than laser techniques. There are insufficient data to determine whether the heater probe is better than the BICAP.

The safety profile of thermal modalities is generally very good. Perforations are unusual and treatment induced exacerbation of bleeding is not usually clinically important.

Injection therapy

Injection treatment is simple to perform and is the cheapest available hemostatic modality. A large range of injection materials have been studied and it is difficult to prove that any of these is superior to others.

DILUTE ADRENALINE

In 1988 Chung *et al* reported a controlled trial in which patients with active ulcer bleeding were randomized to receive endoscopic injection with 1 : 10 000 adrenaline or were

Table 5.13 Adrenaline for gastrointestinal bleeding

Outcome	Adrenaline $n = 34$	Conservative $n = 34$
Primary hemostasis (%)	34 (100)	—[a]
Surgery (%)	5 (15)	14 (41)
Mortality (%)	3 (9)	2 (6)

Source: Chung *et al*.[58]
[a]20 patients stopped bleeding spontaneously.

Table 5.14 Adrenaline plus sclerosants for gastrointestinal bleeding

Study	Group	*n*	Rebleed (%)	Surgery (%)	Mortality (%)
Panès, 1987[59]	Adr + Pol + Cim	55	3 (5)	3 (5)	2 (4)
	Cim	58	25 (43)	20 (34)	4 (7)
Rajgopal, 1991[60]	Adr + Eth	56	7 (13)	6 (11)	2 (4)
	Nil	53	25 (47)	13 (25)	3 (6)
Balanzo, 1988[61]	Adr + Pol	36	7 (19)	7 (19)	—
	Nil	36	15 (42)	15 (42)	—
Oxner, 1992[62]	Adr + Eth	48	8 (17)	4 (8)	4 (8)
	Nil	45	21 (47)	8 (18)	9 (20)

Adr, adrenaline; Pol, polidocanol; Eth, ethanolamine; Cim, cimetidine.

treated conservatively.[58] Primary hemostasis was achieved in all injected patients and the need for subsequent urgent surgery was significantly reduced (Table 5.13). Rebleeding occurred in 24% of injected patients, suggesting that although dilute adrenaline did stop active bleeding, its vasoconstrictor effects were temporary.

R
Grade A

It seemed logical to combine an injection of adrenaline with that of an agent which might cause permanent sealing of the bleeding arterial defect. For this reason a series of trials were undertaken in which adrenaline injection was combined with a range of sclerosants.

The results of trials in which a combination of adrenaline plus sclerosants were compared to conservative therapy are summarized in Table 5.14.[59–62] All showed that active bleeding stopped more rapidly in treated patients, that rebleeding rates were less and that the need for a surgical operation was reduced. No single trial, however, was powerful enough to determine whether mortality was affected. A subsequent meta-analysis, involving thermal contact devices, laser and injection therapy performed by Cook *et al*,[57] did show a modest reduction in mortality, although this only achieved statistical significance for laser therapy.

R
Grade A

SCLEROSANTS

The sclerosants that have been studied are polidocanol, 5% ethanolamine oleate, and 3% sodium tetradecyl sulphate. There are no controlled trials in which outcome has been assessed in patients randomized to sclerosants versus conservative (no injection) therapy. Several trials compared the efficacy of sclerosants with other endoscopic therapies. Benedetti *et al*[63] showed similar efficacy for polidocanol and thrombin injection in patients presenting with a range of bleeding lesions. Strohm *et al*[64] randomized patients to one of four treatment arms (fibrin glue, 1% polidocanol, dilute adrenaline or adrenaline plus polidocanol) and showed no advantage for any one approach. Rutgeerts *et al* showed no difference in outcome for patients treated by polidocanol or Nd-YAG laser therapy.[65] In general these studies suffer from the problem of small sample size, and they probably lacked statistical power.

A series of case reports documented complications of injection by sclerosant,[66,67] particularly perforation and necrosis of the upper gastrointestinal tract. These complications did not occur following adrenaline injection and indeed the latter seems remarkably safe. Fears concerning the possible systemic affects of circulating adrenaline have not translated into cardiovascular mishaps. Since complications are mainly due to

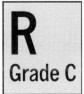

R
Grade C

Table 5.15 Adrenaline vs adrenaline plus sclerosant in gastrointestinal bleeding

Study	Group	*n*	Primary hemostasis	Rebleed	Surgery	Transfusion (units +/− range)	Mortality
Chung, 1993[69]	Adr + Alc	79	75	6	9	2 (0–23)	7
	Adr	81	79	9	12	3 (0–20)	4
Choudari, 1994[70]	Adr + Eth	52	—	7	4	8	0
	Adr	55	—	8	4	9	1
Villanueva, 1993[71]	Adr + Pol	33	32	7	5	2.03	1
	Adr	30	29	3	4	1.9	2

Adr, adrenaline; Alc, alcohol; Eth, ethanolamine; Pol, polidocanol.

Table 5.16 Alcohol vs conservative therapy for gastrointestinal bleeding

Study	Group	*n*	Rebleeding (%)	Surgery (%)	Mortality (%)
Pascu, 1989[72]	Alcohol	41	1 (2)*	1 (2)	1 (2)
	Conservative	39	5 (13)	14 (36)	6 (15)
Lazo, 1992[73]	Alcohol	25	2 (8)**	1 (4)*	—
	Conservative	14	8 (57)	7 (50)	—
Chiozzini, 1989[74]	Alcohol	16	2 (13)	—	—
	Adrenaline	19	5 (26)	—	—

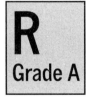

*$P < 0.05$.
**$P < 0.001$.

sclerosant injection, it was important to confirm the importance of combining the sclerosant with the adrenaline injection. Whilst the logic of attempting to induce endarteritis using sclerosants was reasonable, experiments in animals did not demonstrate that this could be achieved by injection using ethanolamine or absolute alcohol.[68] Three trials compared the efficacy of injection by adrenaline alone versus a combination of adrenaline plus a sclerosant.[69–71] As shown in Table 5.15, these three studies did not show that combination treatment was superior to injection by adrenaline alone. No study has directly compared outcome in patients randomized to dilute adrenaline or to a sclerosant.

R Grade A

Since the addition of sclerosants to an injection of adrenaline offers no proven advantage over injecting adrenaline alone, and because sclerosants have the potential to cause significant local complications following injection, they should no longer be employed as part of the injection treatment regimen.

ALCOHOL

The efficacy of injecting absolute alcohol into bleeding ulcers has been examined in several clinical trials. Three of these[72–74] (Table 5.16) randomized patients to alcohol injection or to conservative therapy and showed benefit in terms of reduction in rebleeding rates and need for surgical intervention.

In a prospective randomized comparative trial, Lin *et al*[75] reported that alcohol injection stopped active bleeding and prevented rebleeding in 86% of patients whose ulcers were injected, and this result was similar to the proportion of bleeding ulcers responding to injection with 3% sodium chloride, 50% dextrose, or normal saline. Only one small study[74] has attempted to compare the efficacy of alcohol with dilute adrenaline injection but this lacked statistical power to demonstrate differences in the effects of these interventions, should any exist.

The evidence that alcohol stops active bleeding and prevents rebleeding is stronger than that for the sclerosants. Unfortunately,the potential for adverse effects is probably higher for alcohol than for adrenaline. Deep ulcers commonly follow sclerotherapy for esophageal varices in man and a case report describes an ulcer perforation following alcohol injection.

Whilst alcohol injection is an effective hemostatic therapy, current evidence suggests that the magnitude of its effect is probably similar to that achieved by injection with adrenaline alone; because of its propensity for causing adverse effects, alcohol injection is not recommended as treatment for ulcer bleeding.

FIBRIN GLUE AND THROMBIN

The most attractive endoscopic approach is to directly cause blood clot formation by injecting thrombogenic substances. In the 1980s small trials examined the efficacy of bovine thrombin and showed little benefit compared to other modalities.

In 1996 Kubba *et al*[76] reported a comparison of endoscopic injection therapy using a combination of adrenaline plus human thrombin with dilute adrenaline injection alone (Table 5.17). A proportion of randomized patients had active bleeding at the time of

Table 5.17 Adrenaline plus thrombin vs adrenaline alone for gastrointestinal bleeding

Outcome	Adr + Throm *n* = 70	Adr alone *n* = 70
Rebleed	3	14*
Transfusion (units)	7	5
Surgery	3	5
Mortality	0	7**

Adr, adrenaline; Throm, thrombin.
*P <0.005.
**P <0.013.
Source: Kubba *et al.*[76]

Table 5.18 Adrenaline plus fibrin glue vs adrenaline plus polidocanol for gastrointestinal bleeding

Outcome	Adr + rep FG *n* = 284	Adr + single FG *n* = 285	Adr + Pol *n* = 281
Rebleed	43	55	64*
Transfusion (units)	3.7	3.2	3.3
Surgery	9	14	14
Perforation	2	2	3
Mortality (30 day)	12	15	13

*P <0.036.
Adr, adrenaline; FG, fibrin glue; Pol, polidocanol.
Source: Rutgeerts *et al.*[77]

R Grade A

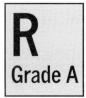

randomization, while the remainder had non-bleeding visible vessels. Rebleeding and mortality were significantly reduced in the group receiving combination therapy compared to patients receiving adrenaline alone. The number of patients needed to be treated with combination therapy rather than adrenaline alone to prevent one death is approximately 14. Paradoxically, no statistically significant differences in the need for surgical operation and the overall rate of hemostasis were demonstrated. Indeed, deaths in this study all occurred, as is usually the case, in patients who had significant comorbidity. Complications in this study were minimal. Although this was not a direct comparison of adrenaline versus thrombin, it did strongly suggest that human thrombin is an effective modality.

R Grade A

In a large multicenter European study[77] (Table 5.18) 850 patients were randomized to endoscopic injection with dilute adrenaline plus a single injection of fibrin glue, to adrenaline and repeated injection of fibrin glue given at daily intervals according to the discretion of the endoscopists, or to adrenaline plus 1% polidocanol. Fibrin glue is a mixture of fibrinogen and thrombin which is injected through a double-channelled endoscopy needle. Rebleeding rates were lowest in patients treated by repeated injection and serious rebleeding, requiring major blood transfusion or surgical operation, was significantly reduced in patients receiving repeated injections of glue compared to the polidocanol treated group. A total of seven perforations occurred in this study and these were distributed equally amongst the treated modalities.

Finally, a small study[78] which compared a combination of adrenaline plus fibrin glue with adrenaline plus Nd-YAG laser therapy did not show a difference in outcome, but this study probably lacked statistical power.

Although no direct comparisons have been made of injection therapy using thrombin alone versus other single agents, the impression gained from the trial evidence is that the use of thrombogenic agents confers significant benefit in terms of the usual endpoints. Acute complications occur infrequently. Although thrombin has been derived from pooled plasma, viral transmission has not been reported. Furthermore, no adverse effects have been apparent in terms of systemic coagulation.

Human thrombin is not currently commercially available. It is relatively inexpensive at £35 per vial, although more costly than adrenaline at £1 per vial.

CONCLUSION

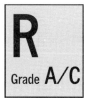

R Grade A/C

Injection therapy is effective and safe. The optimum injection regimen should probably include dilute adrenaline, which stops active hemorrhage. Rebleeding rates are reduced by the addition of agents such as thrombin or a thrombin–fibrinogen mixture. Sclerosants and alcohol should not be used since there is no evidence that they are beneficial and they increase the risk of serious complications.

Comparison of injection and thermal treatments

R Grade A

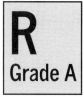

A number of small trials have compared injection with thermal therapies, and as in most studies in this field, numbers are small. In general, the two modalities appear to have equivalent efficacy.

Six trials have compared heater probe with injection[79–84] (Table 5.19). The two trials reported by Lin *et al*[79,80] showed that heater probe treatment was more effective in achieving primary hemostasis. These authors noted the heater probe to be better when ulcers were difficult to approach as it can be applied tangentially. They also found the water jet to be useful in spurting bleeding. It may be argued that alcohol is a less appropriate injection therapy than adrenaline, which may account for the apparent superiority of the heater probe in these studies. This view was supported by the findings of Chung *et al*[81]. They concluded that heater probe and adrenaline were equally effective, but that initial hemostasis was more easily achieved with adrenaline. Choudari[82] compared the heater probe with adrenaline plus ethanolamine and found no differences between the modalities. The remaining two trials by Saeed *et al*[83] and Llach *et al*[84] support this conclusion. Laine[85] showed that electrocoagulation and injection with ethanol were equivalent, although the size of this trial was suboptimal.

Two trials involved the Nd-YAG laser. Carter *et al* [86] compared laser with adrenaline and Pulanic *et al*,[87] in a much larger trial, compared laser with polidocanol. Neither showed a difference in outcome.

Current evidence does not allow a conclusion to be drawn on whether injection or thermal treatment is superior. We advocate the heater probe as the thermal method of choice. Some situations, particularly those involving awkwardly placed posterior duodenal ulcers, lend themselves better to use of the heater probe than to injection therapy.

Combination of injection and thermal treatments

The mechanisms leading to hemostasis associated with thermal treatment and injection therapy may differ, providing a rationale for combining a thermal modality and injection treatment. Currently, no study has shown overall benefit from use of such a combination. The only encouraging trend relates to a finding within a study reported by Chung *et al.*[88] This

Table 5.19 Comparison of heater probe with injection therapy

Study	Group	*n*	Primary hemostasis (%)	Rebleed (%)	Surgery (%)	Mortality (%)
Lin, 1988,[79]	HP	42	42 (100)	5 (12)	—	—
	PA	36	29 (81)	6 (22)	—	—
Lin, 1990[80]	HP	45	44 (98)*	8 (18)	3 (7)**	1 (2)†
	PA	46	31 (67)	2 (7)	2 (4)	0
	Control	46	—	—	12 (26)	7 (15)
Chung, 1991[81]	HP	64	53 (83)‡	6/53 (11)	14 (22)	4 (6)
	Adr	68	65 (96)	11 (17)	14 (21)	2 (3)
Choudari, 1992[82]	HP	60	—	9 (15)	7 (12)	3 (5)
	Adr + Eth	60	—	8 (13)	7 (12)	2 (3)
Saeed, 1993[83]	HP	39	35 (90)	4 (10)	—	—
	Ethanol	41	33 (81)	5 (12)	—	—
Llach, 1996[84]	HP	53	—	3 (6)	2 (4)	1 (2)
	Adr + Pol	51	—	2 (4)	2 (4)	1 (2)

*$P = 0.0004$.
**$P = 0.0024$ ($P = 0.027$ between control and HP; $P = 0.012$ between PA and HP).
†$P = 0.002$ ($P = 0.031$ between control and HP; $P = 0.018$ between control and PA).
‡$P < 0.05$.
HP, heater probe; PA, pure alcohol; Adr, adrenaline; Eth, ethanolamine; Pol, polidocanol.

Table 5.20 Adrenaline plus heater probe vs adrenaline alone for gastrointestinal bleeding

Outcome	Adr + HP	Adr alone
Overall	*n* = 136	*n* = 134
Primary hemostasis	135	131
Rebleed	5	12
Transfusion (units)	3	2
Surgery	8	14
Mortality	8	7
Subgroup with spurting hemorrhage	*n* = 32	*n* = 28
Primary hemostasis	31	25
Rebleed	2	6
Transfusion (units)	4	5
Surgery	2	8*
Mortality	Not stated	Not stated

*$P = 0.03$.
Adr, adrenaline; HP, heater probe.
Source: Cheung *et al.*[88]

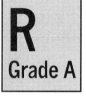

R Grade A

study involved randomization of appropriate ulcer bleeding patients to injection therapy using 1: 10 000 adrenaline or to a combination of adrenaline plus the heater probe (Table 5.20). Although there was no overall difference in outcome between patients randomized to either arm, a *post hoc* subgroup analysis did reveal positive findings. Sixty patients had active spurting hemorrhage from large ulcers, and within this group the primary hemostatic effect of both treatments was similar. However, the need for operation was significantly reduced in the group treated by heater probe and injection. The number of endpoints was small and this observation from subgroup analysis requires confirmation in further trials.

Failure of endoscopic therapy

It may be argued that endoscopists can adversely affect outcome in patients who fail endoscopic therapy. Repeated unsuccessful therapeutic endoscopy, large blood transfusion, and delayed surgical operation in those who ultimately fail attempted endoscopic hemostasis all increase the risk of death. Unfortunately, we cannot predict who will fail and who will respond to endoscopic therapy. Two analyses[89,90] both showed that the presence of active bleeding, large ulcer size, and an ulcer situated in the posterior duodenum were significantly more common in failures of therapy. There is a trend that patients who are in shock at presentation also fare worse. Finally, the lack of second look endoscopy with repeated endoscopic treatment if appropriate is associated with poor outcome. However, even in the highest risk group of patients, who present with active spurting hemorrhage from large posterior duodenal ulcers, Choudari *et al* showed that endoscopic hemostasis can be achieved in approximately 70% of patients.[90] Currently it is not possible to accurately define the subgroup of patients in whom endoscopic therapy should not be attempted. What is clear, however, is that patients who have actively bleeding, large posterior duodenal ulcers should be considered to be at very high risk of requiring urgent operation and that endoscopic therapy is repeated until the patient's condition stabilizes and the endoscopic appearance becomes satisfactory.

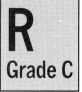

R Grade C

Table 5.21 Repeat endoscopic therapy vs surgery for patients who rebleed

Outcome	Endoscopic therapy $n = 48$	Surgery $n = 44$
Transfusion (units)	8	7
Complications (no. of pts)	7	16*
Mortality (30-day)	5	8

*$P = 0.03$.
Source: Lau *et al.*[91]

Policy concerning rebleeding after failed endoscopic therapy has been recently examined by Lau *et al.*[91] Of 3473 patients admitted with bleeding peptic ulcers, 1169 underwent endoscopic therapy in an attempt to achieve hemostasis. Primary hemostasis was achieved in a remarkable 98.5% of patients. One hundred of these rebled after endoscopic therapy and 92 were randomized to endoscopic retreatment or to emergency surgery. The characteristics of the two groups of patients were similar, including the median transfusion requirements before randomization. Endoscopic retreatment consisted of a combination of adrenaline injection plus the heater probe. Overall, more complications occurred in the group randomized to surgery and there was no significant difference in 30-day mortality between the two groups (Table 5.21). This paper suggests that endoscopic retreatment rather than immediate, urgent operative surgery, should be undertaken in patients who rebleed after endoscopic hemostatic therapy.

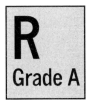

R
Grade A

Mechanical clips

Mechanical devices such as hemoclip have been developed. These can be applied to bleeding lesions although the technique is demanding. One study has compared outcome in patients randomized to hemoclip, endoscopic injection or a combination of these approaches.[92] Rebleeding tended to be least in patients treated by hemoclip alone. This is likely to be the first of many comparisons. Larger trials are necessary and currently the role of mechanical hemostatic devices is not proven.

Endoscopic therapy: summary

Endoscopic therapy for non-variceal hemorrhage is safe and effective, and should be used in the 20% of patients who have major endoscopic stigmata of recent hemorrhage. It is probable, but not proven, that combination of a thermal agent with injection is the best option. Thermal hemostasis is effective using either the heat probe or multipolar electrocoagulation. The best injection material is probably either fibrin glue or thrombin, which causes formation of a stable blood clot at the site of the arterial defect. Rebleeding should be treated first by further endoscopic intervention, although clinical judgement should dictate when urgent surgery is required for specific high risk cases.

The role of drug treatment in addition to endoscopic therapy is unclear. It is reasonable to administer a proton pump inhibitor drug at presentation, although the evidence for improved outcome is relatively weak. There is no evidence currently that other drug therapies are effective.

REFERENCES

1 Fleischen D. Etiology and prevalence of severe persistent upper gastrointestinal bleeding. *Gastroenterology* 1983; **84**: 538–43.

2 Avery Jones F. Haematemesis and melaena with special reference to bleeding peptic ulcer. *Br Med J* 1947; **ii**: 441–6.

3 Rockall TA, Logan RFA, Devlin HB *et al.* Incidence of and mortality from acute upper gastrointestinal haemorrhage in the United Kingdom. *Br Med J* 1995; **311**: 222–6.

4 Rockall TA, Logan RFA, Devlin HB *et al.* Risk assessment after acute upper gastrointestinal haemorrhage. *Gut* 1996; **38**: 316–21.

5 Vreeburg EM, Terwee CB, Snel P *et al.* Validation of the Rockall risk scoring system in upper gastrointestinal bleeding. *Gut* 1999; **44**: 331–5.

6 Holman RAE, Davis M, Gough KR *et al.* Value of centralised approach in the management of haematemesis and melaena: Experience in a district general hospital. *Gut* 1990; **31**: 504–8.

7 Sanderson JD, Taylor RFH, Pugh S *et al.* Specialised gastrointestinal units for the management of upper gastrointestinal bleeding. *Postgrad Med J* 1990; **66**: 654–6.

8 Bornman PC, Theodorou N, Shuttleworth RD *et al.* Importance of hypovolaemic shock and endoscopic signs in predicting recurrent haemorrhage from peptic ulceration: a prospective evaluation. *Br Med J* 1985; **291**: 245–7.

9 Griffiths WJ, Neumann DA, Welsh DA. The visible vessels as an indicator of uncontrolled or recurrent gastrointestinal haemorrhage. *N Engl J Med* 1979; **300**: 1411–13.

10 Swain CP, Storey DW, Bown SG. Nature of the bleeding vessel in recurrently bleeding gastric ulcers. *Gastroenterology* 1986; **90**: 595–606.

11 Patchett SE, Enright, Afdhal N *et al.* Clot lysis by gastric juice: an in vitro study. *Gut* 1989; **30**: 1704–7.

12 Walt RP, Cottrell J, Mann SG *et al.* Continuous intravenous famotidine for haemorrhage from peptic ulcer. *Lancet* 1992; **340**: 1058–62.

13 Collins R, Langman M. Treatment with histamine H_2 antagonists in acute upper gastrointestinal haemorrhage: implications of randomised trials. *N Engl J Med* 1985; **313**: 660–6.

14 Daneshmend TK, Hawkey CJ, Langman MJS *et al.* Omeprazole versus placebo for acute upper gastrointestinal bleeding: randomised double blind controlled trial. *Br Med J* 1992; **304**: 143–7.

15 Khuroo MS, Yattoo GN, Javid G *et al.* A comparison of omeprazole and placebo for bleeding peptic ulcer. *N Engl J Med* 1997; **336**: 1054–8.

16 Schaffalitzky de Muckadell OB, Havelund T, Harling H *et al.* *J Gastroenterol* 1997; **32**(4): 320–7.

17 Henry DA, O'Connell DL. Effect of fibrinolytic inhibitors on mortality from upper gastrointestinal haemorrhage. *Br Med J* 1989; **298**: 1142–6.

18 Barer D, Ogilvie A, Henry D *et al.* Cimetidine and tranexamic acid in the treatment of acute upper-gastrointestinal-tract bleeding. *N Engl J Med* 1983; **308**(26): 1571–5.

19 Sommerville KW, Henry DA, Davies JG *et al.*. Somatostatin in treatment of haematemesis and melaena. *Lancet* 1985; **i**: 130–2.

20 Magnusson I, Ihre T, Johansson C *et al.* Randomised double blind trial of somatostatin in the treatment of massive upper gastrointestinal haemorrhage. *Gut* 1985; **26**: 221–6.

21 Basso N, Bagarani M, Bracci F *et al.* Ranitidine and somatostatin. Their effects on bleeding from the upper gastrointestinal tract. *Arch Surg* 1986; **121**: 833–5.

22 Corraggio F, Scarpato P, Spina M *et al.* Somatostatin and ranitidine in the control of iatrogenic haemorrhage of the upper gastrointestinal tract. *Br Med J* 1984; **289**: 224.

23 Corraggio F, Bertini G, Catalona A *et al.* Clinical controlled trial of somatostatin with ranitidine and placebo in the control of peptic haemorrhage of the upper gastrointestinal tract. *Digestion* 1989; **43**: 190–5.

24 Galmiche JP, Cassigneul J, Faivre J *et al.* Somatostatin in peptic ulcer bleeding. Results of a double blind controlled trial. *Int J Clin Pharmacol Res* 1983; **III**: 379–87.

25 Saperas E, Pique JM, Perez-Ayuso R *et al.* Somatostatin compared with cimetidine in the treatment of bleeding peptic ulcer without visible vessel. *Aliment Pharmacol Ther* 1988; **2**: 153–9.

26 Kayasseh L, Gyr K, Keller U *et al.* Somatostatin and cimetidine in peptic ulcer haemorrhage. A randomised controlled trial. *Lancet* 1980; **i**: 844–6.

27 Antonioli A, Gandolfo M, Rigo GP *et al.* Somatostatin and cimetidine in the control of acute upper gastrointestinal bleeding. A controlled multicentre study. *Hepatogastroenterol* 1986; **33**: 71–4.

28 Tulassay Z, Gupta R, Papp J *et al.* Somatostatin versus cimetidine in the treatment of actively bleeding duodenal ulcer: a prospective, randomised, controlled trial. *Am J Gastroenterol* 1989; **84**: 6–9.

29 Torres AJ, Landa I, Hernandez F *et al.* Somatostatin in the treatment of severe upper

gastrointestinal bleeding: a multicentre controlled trial. *Br J Surg* 1986; **73**: 786–9.

30 Wagner PK, Rothmund M, Gronniger J. Secretin and somatostatin in treatment of acute upper gastrointestinal haemorrhage: a randomised trial. *Klin Wochenschr* 1983; **61**: 285–9.

31 Goletti O, Sidoti F, Lippolis PV *et al.* Omeprazole versus ranitidine and somatostatin in the treatment of acute severe gastroduodenal haemorrhage. *Br J Surg* 1992; **79** (Suppl): S123.

32 Christiansen J, Ottenjann R, Von Arx F. Placebo-controlled trial with the somatostatin analogue sms 201–995 in peptic ulcer bleeding. *Gastroenterology* 1989; **97**: 568–74.

33 Jenkins SA, Poulianos G, Coraggio F *et al.* Somatostatin in the treatment of non-variceal upper gastrointestinal bleeding. *Dig Dis Sci* 1998; **16**: 214–24.

34 Imperiale TF, Birgisson S. Somatostatin or octreotide compares with H_2 antagonists and placebo in the management of acute non-variceal upper gastrointestinal haemorrhage: a meta-analysis. *Ann Intern Med* 1997; **127**: 1062–71.

35 Rutgeerts P, Geboes K, Vantrappen G. Experimental studies of injection therapy for severe nonvariceal bleeding in dogs. *Gastroenterology* 1989; **97**: 601–21.

36 Vallon AG, Cotton PB, Laurence BH *et al.* Randomised trial of endoscopic argon laser photocoagulation in bleeding peptic ulcers. *Gut* 1981; **22**: 228–33.

37 Swain CP, Bown SG, Storey DW *et al.* Controlled trial of argon laser photocoagulation in bleeding peptic ulcer. *Lancet* 1981; **ii**: 1313–16.

38 Jensen DM, Machicado GA, Tapia JL *et al.* Controlled trial of endoscopic argon laser for severe ulcer haemorrhage. *Gastroenterology* 1984; **86**: 1125.

39 Swain CP, Salmon PR, Kirkham JS. Controlled trial of Nd-YAG laser photocoagulation in bleeding peptic ulcers. *Lancet* 1986; **i**: 1113–17.

40 Krejs GJ, Little KH, Westergaard H. Laser photocoagulation for the treatment of acute peptic ulcer bleeding. *N Engl J Med* 1987; **316**: 1618–21.

41 Rhode H, Thon K, Fischer M. Results of a defined concept of endoscopic Nd-YAG laser therapy in patients with upper gastrointestinal bleeding. *Br J Surg* 1980; **67**: 360.

42 Rutgeerts P, Vantrappen G, Broeckhaert. Controlled trial of YAG laser treatment of upper digestive haemorrhage. *Gastroenterology* 1982; **83**: 410–16.

43 Macleod I, Mills PR, Mackenzie JF. Neodymium yttrium aluminium garnet laser photocoagulation for major haemorrhage from peptic ulcers and single vessels. *Br Med J* 1983; **286**: 345–58.

44 Homer AC, Powell S, Vacary FR. Is Nd-YAG laser treatment for upper gastrointestinal bleeds of benefit in a district general hospital? *Postgrad Med J* 1985; **61**: 19–22

45 Trudeau W, Siepler JK, Ross K *et al.* Endoscopic Nd-YAG laser photocoagulation of bleeding ulcers with visible vessels. *Gastrointest Endosc* 1985; **31**: 138.

46 Buset M, Des Marez B, Vandermeeran A. Laser therapy for non bleeding visible vessel in peptic ulcer haemorrhage: a prospective randomised study. *Gastrointest Endosc* 1988; **34**: 173.

47 Matthewson K, Swain CP, Bland M *et al.* Randomised comparison of Nd-YAG laser, heater probe and no endoscopic therapy for bleeding peptic ulcers. *Gastroenterology* 1990; **98**: 1234–44.

48 Fullarton GM, Birnie GG, MacDonald A *et al.* Controlled trial of heater probe treatment in bleeding peptic ulcers. *Br J Surg* 1989; **76**: 541–4.

49 Jensen DM, Machicado GA, Kovacs TOG. Controlled randomised study of heater probe and BICAP for haemostasis of severe ulcer bleeding. *Gastroenterology* 1988; **94**: A208.

50 O'Brien JD, Day SJ, Burnham WR. Controlled trial of small bipolar probes in bleeding peptic ulcers. *Lancet* 1986; **i**: 464–8.

51 Laine L. Multipolar electrocoagulation in the treatment of active upper gastrointestinal tract haemorrhage. A prospective controlled trial. *N Engl J Med* 1987; **316**: 1613–17.

52 Brearley S, Hawker PC, Dykes PW *et al.* Peri-endoscopic bipolar diathermy coagulation of visible vessels using a 3.2 mm probe – a randomised clinical trial. *Endoscopy* 1987; **19**: 160–3.

53 Laine L. Multipolar electrocoagulation for the treatment of ulcers with non bleeding visible vessels: a prospective, controlled trial. *Gastroenterology* 1988; **94**: A246.

54 Pap JP. Heat probe versus BICAP in the treatment of upper gastrointestinal bleeding. *Am J Gastroenterol* 1987; **82**: 619–21.

55 Cipolletta L, Bianco MA, Rotondano G *et al.* Prospective comparison of argon plasma coagulator and heater probe in the endoscopic treatment of major peptic ulcer bleeding. *Gastrointest Endosc* 1998; **48**(2): 191–5.

56 Henry DA, White I. Endoscopic coagulation for gastrointestinal bleeding. *N Engl J Med* 1988; **318**: 186–7.

57 Cook DJ, Gayatt GH, Salena BJ *et al.* Endoscopic therapy for acute non-variceal haemorrhage: a meta-analysis. *Gastroenterology* 1992; **102**: 139–48.

58 Chung SCS, Leung JWC, Steele RJC. Endoscopic injection of adrenaline for actively bleeding

ulcers: a randomised trial. *Br Med J* 1988; **296**: 1631–3.

59 Panes J, Viver J, Forne M *et al.* Controlled trial of endoscopic sclerosis in bleeding peptic ulcers. *Lancet* 1987; 1292–4.

60 Rajgopal C, Palmer KR. Endoscopic injection sclerosis: effective treatment for bleeding peptic ulcer. *Gut* 1991; **32**: 727–9.

61 Balanzo J, Sainz S, Such J. Endoscopic haemostasis by local injection of epinephrine in bleeding ulcers. A prospective randomised trial. *Endoscopy* 1988; **20**: 289–91.

62 Oxner RBG, Simmonds NJ, Gertner DJ *et al.* Controlled trial of endoscopic injection treatment for bleeding peptic ulcers with visible vessels. *Lancet* 1992; **339**: 966–8.

63 Beneditti G, Sablich R, Lacchin T. Endoscopic injection sclerotherapy in non-variceal upper gastrointestinal bleeding. A comparative study of epinephrine and thrombin. *Endoscopy* 1990; **22**: 157–9.

64 Strohm WD, Rommele UE, Barton E *et al.*. Injection therapy of bleeding ulcers with fibrin or polidocanol. *Dtsch Med Wochenschr* 1994; **119**: 249–56.

65 Rutgeerts P, Vantrappen G, Brockaert L *et al.* Comparison of endoscopic polidocanol injection and YAG laser for bleeding peptic ulcers. *Lancet* 1989; **i**: 1164–7.

66 Levy J, Khakoo S, Barton R *et al.* Fatal injection sclerotherapy of a bleeding peptic ulcer. *Lancet* 1991; **337**: 504 (letter).

67 Loperfido S, Patelli G, La Torre L. Extensive necrosis of gastric mucosa following injection therapy of a bleeding peptic ulcer. *Endoscopy* 1990; **22**: 785–6 (letter).

68 Rajgopal C, Lessles AM, Palmer KR. Mechanisms of action of injection therapy for bleeding peptic ulcer. *Br J Surg* 1992; **79**: 782–4.

69 Chung SCS, Leung JWC, Leoug HT *et al.* Adding a sclerosant to endoscopic epinephrine injection in actively bleeding ulcers: randomised trial. *Gastrointest Endosc* 1993; **39**: 611–15.

70 Choudari CP, Palmer KR. Endoscopic injection therapy for bleeding peptic ulcer: a comparison of adrenaline alone with adrenaline plus ethanolamine oleate. *Gut* 1994; **35**: 608–10.

71 Villanueva C, Balanzo C, Espinos JC. Endoscopic injection therapy of bleeding ulcer: a prospective and randomised comparison of adrenaline alone or with polidocanol. *J Clin Gastroenterol* 1993; **17**: 195–200.

72 Pascu O, Draghici A, Acalovschi I. The effect of endoscopic haemostasis with alcohol on the mortality rate of non-variceal upper gastrointestinal haemorrhage: a randomised prospective study. *Endoscopy* 1989; **21**: 53–5.

73 Lazo MD, Andrade R, Medina MC *et al.* Effect of injection sclerosis with alcohol on the rebleeding rate of gastroduodenal peptic ulcers with nonbleeding visible vessels: a prospective, controlled trial. *Am J Gastroenterol* 1992; **87**(7): 843–6.

74 Chiozzini G, Bortoluzzi F, Pallini P *et al.* Controlled trial of absolute ethanol *vs* epinephrine as injection agent in gastroduodenal bleeding. *Gastroenterology* 1989; **96**: A86.

75 Lin HJ, Perng CL, Lee FY. Endoscopic injection for the arrest of peptic ulcer haemorrhage: final results of a prospective, randomised, comparative trial. *Gastrointest Endosc* 1993; **39**: 15–19.

76 Kubba AK, Murphy W, Palmer KR. Endoscopic injection for bleeding peptic ulcer: a comparison of adrenaline with adrenaline plus human thrombin. *Gastroenterology* 1996; **111**: 623–8.

77 Rutgeerts P, Rauws E, Wara P *et al.* Randomised trial of single and repeated fibrin glue compared with injection of polidocanol in treatment of bleeding peptic ulcer. *Lancet* 1997; **350**: 692–6.

78 Heldwein W, Avenhaus W, Schonekas H *et al.* Injection of fibrin tissue adhesive versus laser photocoagulation in the treatment of high risk bleeding peptic ulcers: a controlled randomised study. *Endoscopy* 1996; **28**(9): 756–60.

79 Lin HJ, Tsai YT, Lee SD *et al.* A prospectively randomised trial of heat probe thermocoagulation *versus* pure alcohol injection in nonvariceal peptic ulcer haemorrhage. *Am J Gastroenterol* 1988; **83**(3): 283–6.

80 Lin HJ, Lee FY, Kang WM *et al.* Heat probe thermocoagulation and pure alcohol injection in massive peptic ulcer haemorrhage: a prospective, randomised controlled trial. *Gut* 1990; **31**: 753–7.

81 Chung SCS, Leung JWC, Sung JY *et al.* Injection or heat probe for bleeding ulcer? *Gastroenterology* 1991; **100**: 33–7.

82 Choudari CP, Rajgopal C, Palmer KR. Comparison of endoscopic injection therapy versus the heater probe in major peptic ulcer haemorrhage. *Gut* 1992; **33**(9): 1159–61.

83 Saeed ZA, Winchester CB, Michaletz PA *et al.* A scoring system to predict rebleeding after endoscopic therapy of nonvariceal upper gastrointestinal haemorrhage, with a comparison of heat probe and ethanol injection. *Am J Gastroenterol* 1993; **88**(11): 1842–9.

84 Llach J, Bordas JM, Salmeron JM *et al.* A prospective randomised trial of heater probe thermocoagulation versus injection therapy in peptic ulcer haemorrhage. *Gastrointest Endosc* 1996; **43**(2 Pt 1): 117–20.

85 Laine L. Multipolar electrocoagulation versus injection therapy in the treatment of bleeding peptic ulcers. *Gastroenterology* 1990; **99**: 1303–6.

86 Carter R, Anderson JR. Randomised trial of adrenaline injection and laser photocoagulation in the control of haemorrhage from peptic ulcer. *Br J Surg* 1994; **81**: 869–71.
87 Pulanic R, Vucelic B, Rosandic M *et al.* Comparison of injection sclerotherapy and laser photocoagulation for bleeding peptic ulcers. *Endoscopy* 1995; **27**(4): 291–7.
88 Chung SCS, Lau JY, Sung JJ. Randomised comparison between adrenaline injection alone and adrenaline injection plus heat probe treatment for actively bleeding peptic ulcers. *Br Med J* 1997; **314**: 1307–11.
89 Villanueva C, Balanzo J, Espinos JC. Prediction of therapeutic failure in patients with bleeding peptic ulcer treated with endoscopic injection. *Dig Dis Sci* 1993; **38**: 2062–70.
90 Choudari CP, Rajgopal C, Elton RA *et al.* Failures of endoscopic therapy for bleeding peptic ulcers: an analysis of risk factors. *Am J Gastroenterol* 1994; **89**: 1968–72.
91 Lau JYW, Sung JJY, Lam Y *et al.* Endoscopic retreatment compared with surgery in patients with recurrent bleeding after initial endoscopic control of bleeding ulcers. *N Engl J Med* 1999; **340**: 751–6.
92 Chung IK, Ham JS, Kim HS *et al.* Comparison of the hemostatic efficacy of the endoscopic hemoclip method with hypertonic saline-epinephrine injection and a combination of the two for the management of bleeding peptic ulcers. *Gastrointest Endosc* 1999; **49**: 13–18.

6 Functional dyspepsia: diagnosis and treatment

SANDER JO VELDHUYZEN VAN ZANTEN

INTRODUCTION

In this chapter the diagnosis of functional dyspepsia and efficacy of therapeutic interventions will be evaluated. Functional dyspepsia, often referred to as non-ulcer dyspepsia, is an important health problem with a very high prevalence in the general population. In data from Sweden and Canada 5–7% of all consultations in primary care are for the symptom of dyspepsia.[1,2] In Sweden, up to 98% of patients receive a prescription if they consult a physician for dyspepsia.[1] Consequently, for the health care system the cost of medications, which are often prescribed for long periods of time, adds significantly to the already substantial expenditures for consultations and diagnostic investigations. The following topics will be reviewed: definition of functional dyspepsia, evaluation and diagnostic tests, trial methodology, and pharmacological treatments including antacids, H_2-receptor antagonists, proton pump inhibitors, prokinetic agents, and anti-helicobacter therapy. The treatment of functional dyspepsia was recently reviewed by the author with conclusions similar to those presented in this chapter.[3]

DEFINITION OF FUNCTIONAL DYSPEPSIA

There is agreement that the cardinal feature of functional dyspepsia is *unexplained pain or discomfort centered in the upper part of the abdomen*. Epigastric pain or discomfort may be accompanied by other symptoms such as excessive burping or belching, nausea, bloating, postprandial fullness, early satiety, or burning sensations. Increasingly, investigators have accepted the definition of the Rome Working Party.[4,5] In 1999 the Rome criteria for functional dyspepsia will be updated, and it is likely that the amended recommendations will be adopted by researchers who are active in this area. The criteria imply that pain or discomfort in the central upper abdomen must be the predominant complaint if the patient is to be labeled as having dyspepsia. This helps to differentiate dyspepsia from gastroesophageal reflux disease (GERD), where the predominant complaint is typically heartburn or acid regurgitation. Heartburn is not included in the Rome criteria for diagnosis of dyspepsia. In practice, however, most physicians do consider heartburn to be part of the syndrome of dyspepsia. Dyspepsia is a symptom of several entities including duodenal and gastric ulcers, GERD, and functional dyspepsia.

DIAGNOSIS OF FUNCTIONAL DYSPEPSIA

There is consensus that there is so much overlap in symptoms among duodenal and gastric ulcers, GERD, and functional dyspepsia that it is impossible to make a definitive diagnosis based on symptoms alone. The exception to this consensus is GERD, which will be discussed below. In essence, functional dyspepsia is a diagnosis of exclusion and in the setting of clinical trials generally requires that an upper gastrointestinal endoscopy be performed to exclude other diseases. In practice physicians often decide on a trial of empiric therapy for patients presenting with the symptom of dyspepsia without worrying about a definitive diagnosis of a particular disease. This strategy is often attractive given that the treatment for duodenal and gastric ulcers, GERD, and functional dyspepsia is similar. Either acid suppressive therapy or less frequently prokinetic agents are usually prescribed. Therefore, subclassification into separate diseases is not always necessary and in primary care may not be feasible. The decision whether or not to refer a patient for further investigation, usually either an upper gastrointestinal endoscopy or a barium study, is based on the severity of the presenting symptoms, age of the patient and on the presence or absence of "alarm symptoms" such as weight loss, evidence of bleeding or anemia, dysphagia, and vomiting.

DYSPEPSIA SUBGROUPS AND OVERLAP WITH GERD

The description of dyspepsia subgroups has become popular despite evidence of the existence of considerable overlap among them. The four recognized subgroups are: ulcer-like dyspepsia, reflux-like dyspepsia, dysmotility-like dyspepsia, and unclassified dyspepsia.[5–7] These subgroups are attractive because they coincide with current concepts about pathophysiological disturbances which explain specific symptoms. However, a study by Talley *et al* demonstrated considerable overlap among the different subgroups.[7] With the exception of reflux-like dyspepsia, subclassification into dyspepsia subgroups is not recommended.

Increasingly endoscopy negative GERD is now recognized as a distinct entity. This is a difficult issue in functional dyspepsia trial methodology. Solely relying on an endoscopy, which does not reveal macroscopic esophagitis, is probably insufficient if one wants to exclude all GERD patients. An example is the study by Klauser *et al*, in which 17% of patients referred for dyspepsia were diagnosed with esophagitis after an initial work-up.[8] However, a further 10% of patients were revealed to have endoscopy negative GERD after an extended work-up, which included 24 hour pH monitoring and scintigraphy. In practice it seems impossible to exclude all GERD patients in functional dyspepsia trials. A practical solution is to exclude patients who have heartburn as their dominant symptom, but allow patients who have both epigastric pain and heartburn to enrol as long as the epigastric pain is the predominant symptom.

DIAGNOSTIC INVESTIGATION: ENDOSCOPY OR X-RAY?

Referral for endoscopy is indicated in older patients presenting with new-onset dyspepsia. The recommendations formerly were to use age >45 years as an indication for investigations,[9] but it seems likely that this age can be increased to 50 years or perhaps even higher.[10,11] This cutoff age is largely driven by the incidence of gastric cancer in the population where one practices.[10,11] In family practice, upper gastrointestinal barium studies are still commonly used to rule out peptic ulcer disease and esophageal or gastric cancer in patients with dyspepsia. The technical review of the American Gastroenterology Association on Dyspepsia summarizes the consistent evidence of the superiority of upper gastrointestinal endoscopy for detection of structural abnormalities.[9] X-rays are still frequently used because of their lower cost, wider availability in the community, and the speed with which the test can be obtained. Often there is a significant waiting time before patients can be seen after they are referred to a gastroenterologist. "Open access endoscopy" is one method by which delay in diagnostic endoscopy can be shortened.

The AGA technical review assessed whether patients with new onset of symptoms should be investigated or treated empirically and came to the conclusion that the evidence is equivocal.[9] For example, in the study by Bytzer *et al*, empiric treatment was compared to direct endoscopy in patients presenting with dyspepsia.[12] Patients in the endoscopy arm were more satisfied, and subsequent health care costs were significantly lower in this group. However, a recommendation that endoscopy should be performed in all or most patients presenting with dyspepsia would probably be too costly for traditional health care systems. A more rational approach therefore seems to be to stratify patients according to their risk of having serious underlying disease. Factors that can be considered are age of the patient, background prevalence of serious disease, especially of esophageal and gastric cancer, and the presence or absence of alarm symptoms.

METHODOLOGICAL PROBLEMS IN FUNCTIONAL DYSPEPSIA TRIALS

In order to determine whether a treatment does more good than harm, valid and reliable outcome measures must be used in clinical trials. In the case of functional dyspepsia the lack of definite structural or pathophysiological abnormalities which explain the origin of functional dyspepsia symptoms[13–15] has hampered the development of such measures. Clinical trials must use outcome measures which rely on the recording of symptoms and their severity, as is the case in other functional gastrointestinal disorders. A recent systematic review of drug treatment of functional dyspepsia evaluated the quality of clinical trials in this field.[16] Few studies used validated outcome measures and methodological weaknesses were apparent in several trials. Problems included a lack of definition of functional dyspepsia, unclear inclusion and exclusion criteria, suboptimal study design, and short duration of treatment.

The most important problem in randomized controlled trials for interventions for functional dyspepsia studies is the lack of consensus on outcome measures. Only a small number of outcome measures have been validated. In the systematic review of functional dyspepsia studies, only 5 of 52 studies used a validated outcome measure.[16] Subjective endpoints, such as recording of symptoms and their severity, used to measure a clinical outcome in a trial should fulfill four requirements.[17]

1 The range of symptoms included should be important to, and representative of, the disease process.
2 The measurements should be reproducible (producing consistent results when repeated in subjects who have not changed).
3 The measurements should be responsive (able to detect change).
4 Changes in the measurement should reflect a real change in general health status.

Ideally, a separate study is required to demonstrate that an instrument meets these requirements, prior to its use in a randomized controlled trial. Currently several studies are in progress to develop disease specific quality-of-life questionnaires for functional dyspepsia, and a few have been published recently. These include: (a) the DIBS scale (measures the duration and intensity of epigastric pain), which is a multidimensional instrument that only focusses on the assessment of epigastric pain;[18] (b) the GSRS (the Gastrointestinal Symptom Rating Scale), an instrument which measures the severity of 15 upper and lower gastrointestinal symptoms;[19] (c) the Canadian Dyspepsia Score, which measures the severity of eight gastrointestinal symptoms common in functional dyspepsia;[20] (d) the Glasgow Dyspepsia Severity Score (GDSS), which includes severity of symptoms, and number of investigations, doctor visits and treatments over the previous 6 months;[21] and (e) the "Dublin" Dyspepsia Score, which measures severity, frequency, and duration of four upper gastrointestinal symptoms.[22] None of these scales has been sufficiently validated to be unequivocally recommended for general use in functional dyspepsia trials.

Another important weakness of many functional dyspepsia trials has been the relatively short duration of treatment. The duration of treatment was 4 weeks or less in 44 trials evaluated in the systematic review of 52 studies.[16] It was 8 weeks or longer in only four studies. Only seven studies had a follow-up period (varying from 3 to 52 weeks) after treatment was discontinued. The short duration of treatment is surprising given the known chronicity of functional dyspepsia symptoms. Therefore, studies that concluded that the intervention was beneficial for the duration of the study, do not provide evidence for any continued efficacy.

The placebo response rate is high in clinical trials in patients with functional dyspepsia and other functional gastrointestinal disorders, such as the irritable bowel syndrome.[23] In the systematic review of functional dyspepsia trials it varied from 13 to 73%.[16] An explanation for the high placebo response rate may be the reassurance effect of a "normal" endoscopy. Fear of cancer is a frequent reason for concern among functional dyspepsia patients undergoing gastroscopy.[9,11,24] In a recent study, Wiklund *et al* measured quality of life and GI symptoms just prior to endoscopy and 7 days later.[25] In patients in whom no significant endoscopic abnormalities were found overall quality of life improved, although there was little change in the severity of individual gastrointestinal symptoms. This observation supports the concept that endoscopy has a powerful placebo effect through reassurance of patients. The higher satisfaction with care in the study by Bytzer *et al*[12] may also be explained by a reassurance effect.

FUNCTIONAL VERSUS UNINVESTIGATED DYSPEPSIA

It is important to distinguish between uninvestigated dyspepsia and functional dyspepsia. The diagnosis of functional dyspepsia is generally considered to require an endoscopy. Most studies to date have dealt with investigated dyspepsia. Studies of uninvestigated dyspepsia will include a proportion of patients with duodenal or gastric ulcer, esophagitis and, rarely, gastric cancer. The frequency with which structural abnormalities are found is up to 25% for duodenal ulcer, 14% for gastric ulcer, 29% for esophagitis, and 3% for gastric cancer.[9,11] However, these rates clearly depend on the prevalence of these disorders in the population being studied. Gastric cancer is rare below the age of 50 years. In most endoscopic dyspepsia studies the rate of functional dyspepsia is high and varies between 30 and 60%.[9,11] Several studies of patients with uninvestigated dyspepsia are currently being carried out in general practice. Such studies are contaminated with patients with undiagnosed duodenal or gastric ulcer and GERD. However, this situation will better mimic the real life situation in general practice, where treatment in most patients is instituted without endoscopic investigations. In this chapter we will focus on patients with investigated dyspepsia, ie functional dyspepsia.

Given the problems in study design, especially the large variation in the way outcome measures have been used, it is difficult to perform quantitative meta-analysis. Therefore, the results are presented in a qualitative fashion.

DRUG TREATMENT

Antacids

R Grade A

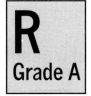

Over-the-counter medications, especially antacids, are commonly prescribed as first line treatment. Many patients will probably have tried these medications before consulting a physician. As several reviews have been written on the use of antacids, the details of individual studies will not be discussed here. Clinical trials have generally not shown significant benefit from antacids.[16,26–28] The frequently cited and methodologically strong randomized controlled trial reported by Nyren *et al* did not show benefit of antacids over placebo over a 3-week treatment period.[27]

H_2-receptor antagonists

Antisecretory therapy with H_2-receptor antagonists (H_2RA) is probably the most commonly prescribed therapy for functional dyspepsia.[2,29] These agents are effective in the treatment of GERD and duodenal and gastric ulcers. Results in functional dyspepsia trials have varied, but in several randomized controlled trials which showed a benefit from H_2RA, the benefit possibly was due to inclusion of GERD patients.[16,26,30–38] This factor may explain why the meta-analysis by Dobrilla *et al* showed a therapeutic gain of 20% of active treatment over placebo.[30] Two methodologically strong studies did not show a benefit of either cimetidine or nizatidine over placebo.[29,39] Most studies have used low doses of H_2RA, eg ranitidine 150 mg twice a day. It is possible that higher doses of H_2RA might yield larger and more consistent treatment effects, but this possibility can only be proven by appropriate randomized controlled trials.

Proton pump inhibitors

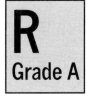

Until recently, the use of proton pump inhibitors (PPIs) was mainly restricted to patients with peptic ulcer disease or GERD. This increased efficacy compared to H_2RA in these patient populations is explained by the more profound acid suppression induced by proton pump inhibition. Recently a large randomized controlled trial evaluated the role of PPI therapy in functional dyspepsia.[40] In this 4-week trial, 1262 functional dyspepsia patients were randomized to either omeprazole (20 or 10 mg) or placebo. Complete relief of symptoms was achieved in 38% of patients on omeprazole 20 mg, 36% on omeprazole 10 mg, and 28% on placebo (P <0.001). The absolute risk reduction (ARR) of 10% and 8% correspond to an NNT (the number of patients needed to treat with omeprazole to yield one additional patient with a complete response) of 10 for 20 mg omeprazole and 12 for 10 mg omeprazole. Subgroup analysis suggested that patients with ulcer-like and

R Grade A

reflux-like dyspepsia benefited from omeprazole therapy, while patients fulfilling the criteria for dysmotility-like dyspepsia did not. Although it is generally not useful to make a diagnosis of specific dyspepsia subgroups, the results of this study suggest that use of the two subgroups – ulcer-like and reflux-like dyspepsia – may be useful to predict a response to PPI therapy. Further randomized trials are needed to confirm the results of this subgroup analysis. The large sample size and strong design aspects of this trial make it likely that the results will be reproducible, and consideration of the participants in the study suggests that the results will be generalizable. It remains to be determined whether the dyspepsia responders in such trials of omeprazole are in fact patients with unrecognized endoscopy negative GERD. Omeprazole was superior to antacids in combination with ranitidine[41,42] or cimetidine alone[43] in three trials in patients with ulcer-like or reflux-like dyspepsia. Two large studies in primary care have shown that omeprazole 20 and 10 mg are efficacious in patients with reflux symptoms.[44,45] Both studies included patients with reflux-like dyspepsia and endoscopy negative GERD.

R
Grade A

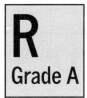

Domperidone and cisapride

Prokinetics have been evaluated in functional dyspepsia because of the hypothesis that disturbed gastrointestinal motility may in part be responsible for the dyspepsia symptoms. Domperidone is a dopamine receptor antagonist, which has shown a benefit in several randomized placebo controlled trials in functional dyspepsia. However, many of these trials enrolled only small numbers of patients and had other weaknesses.[16,26] Cisapride is a prokinetic agent with $5HT_4$-agonist activity. Cisapride is effective for the treatment of mild to moderate GERD and of delayed gastric emptying, especially associated with diabetic gastroparesis. Most randomized trials of cisapride in functional dyspepsia have recruited patients specifically with dysmotility-like dyspepsia.[46–50] A meta-analysis, which thus far is published only in abstract form, combined the results of 18 published trials.[51] Grade A Owing to differences in study design, the results of only 14 trials could be used for a pooled statistical analysis. Using global assessment of improvement as the outcome, patients treated with cisapride were more likely to show an improvement in overall severity of symptoms (OR 2.8). However, caution in the interpretation of these findings is warranted, since several of the included studies had methodological problems. In some studies patients with possible GERD were not excluded, and the sample size of several of the studies was small. Two recent methodologically strong studies with adequate sample size did not show a benefit of cisapride over placebo.[39,52] Grade A In the study of 330 patients by Hansen *et al*[39] there were no statistically significant differences in response to 2 weeks' treatment with cisapride 10 mg tid (62%), nizatidine 300 mg od (54%), or placebo (62%). In the study of 123 patients by Champion *et al* there were no statistically significant differences in good or excellent response to treatment among patients treated with cisapride 10 mg tid (47%), cisapride 20 mg tid (38%), and placebo (33%), P = ns. Grade A

Anti-helicobacter therapy

The prevalence of *Helicobacter pylori* in functional dyspepsia varies from 30 to 70%, but this is in large part dependent on known risk factors for *H. pylori* infection: age, socioeconomic status, and race.[53,54]

Due to differences in study design and problems with selection bias, it is still unclear whether the prevalence of *H. pylori* infection is increased in patients with functional dyspepsia compared to normal controls, although a recent meta-analysis suggested that it is.[55] Currently one of the most important unresolved clinical questions about the role of *H. pylori* is whether cure of the infection leads to a sustained improvement in symptoms of functional dyspepsia. Until 1997 all published trials have been small and results have been conflicting, with some studies showing no benefit and others reporting a positive outcome.[56–59] Four large randomized controlled trials have been reported recently.[60–63] In the study published by Gillvary *et al* a symptom score with a range of 0–20 was used as the outcome measure.[60] This score includes an assessment of the frequency and severity of four symptoms. Gillvary reported the results according to the success or failure of anti-helicobacter therapy, rather than according to the intention to treat principle. A statistically significant improvement in symptoms, reported as the average improvement for the group, was found in patients in whom *H. pylori* was cured. The study did not a priori define a patient response. Consequently, the more appropriate outcome measure, the proportion of patients who achieved a defined degree of improvement, was not used.

R Grade A

The UK MRC trial of *H. pylori* eradication therapy for functional dyspepsia was a single-center randomized controlled trial conducted in Scotland.[61] Three hundred and eighteen patients were randomized to 14 days of treatment with anti-helicobacter therapy (omeprazole, metronidazole, and amoxycillin) or omeprazole alone and followed for 12 months. The primary outcome measure was the validated GDSS.[21] This score assesses the frequency of dyspepsia symptoms and the impact they have on daily activities, the number of doctor visits and diagnostic tests for dyspepsia, and the need for either over-the-counter medication or prescription drugs to treat the symptoms. The proportion of patients who became *H. pylori* negative was 87% for patients randomized to anti-helicobacter therapy compared to 4% for the omeprazole group. Improvement, defined as a score of 0 or 1 on the dyspepsia score, was achieved in 21% of anti-helicobacter treated patients and 7% of the control group (P <0.001, ARR 14%, NNT = 7).

R Grade A

Two recently reported randomized controlled trials compared responses in patients randomized to receive OAC (omeprazole, clarithromycin, and amoxycillin) triple therapy or control therapy (omeprazole alone or placebo) for 1 week . Both studies used the relief of dyspepsia symptoms, measured on a 7-point scale, as the primary outcome measure. Patients were classified as responders if they had no or minimal symptoms of dyspepsia during the last week of the 52-week follow-up period. In the OCAY trial,[62] 348 patients were randomized and followed for 12 months. *H. pylori* was eradicated in 79% of OAC treated patients, compared to a rate of 2% in the omeprazole group. There was no statistically significant difference in the response rate (OAC 27%, omeprazole alone 21%, P = 0.17). In the ORCHID trial,[63] 275 patients were randomized and also followed for 12 months. The eradication rates for *H. pylori* (OAC 85%, placebo 4%) and the response rates (OAC 28%, placebo 21%, P >0.05) were comparable to those in the OCAY trial.

R Grade A

R Grade A

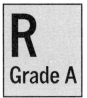

The results of the OCAY and ORCHID studies, which used the same outcome measure and had similar study design, did not show a statistically significant improvement in symptoms associated with eradication of *H. pylori* infection, in contrast to the studies of Gillvary *et al*[60] and McColl *et al.*[61] The UK/MRC trial by McColl *et al* used a previously validated multidimensional outcome measure, the GDSS, to determine treatment success. Treatment success was defined as the presence of no or minimal symptoms as indicated by a GDSS score of either 0 or 1. It is important to point out that the GDSS score asks patients to rate their symptoms over the preceding 6-month period, while the global scale used to assess the severity of dyspepsia symptoms in the OCAY and ORCHID studies required patients to fill in their responses on a diary card during the 7 days preceding the final study visit. Whether the time frame over which symptoms were assessed to define treatment success is the explanation for the benefit of *H. pylori* eradication observed in the UK/MRC trial, and the lack of a statistically significant effect in the ORCHID and OCAY studies, is unclear. There may be other reasons for the discrepant results. The patients in the McColl study were recruited at a single center and may have been more homogeneous than those in the other trials. The disadvantage which accompanies this greater homogeneity is that results may be less generalizable. The population in which such a study is carried out may influence outcome. Endoscopic studies of asymptomatic *H. pylori* positive individuals or *H. pylori* positive blood donors, have revealed marked differences in the prevalence of peptic ulcers. For example, in an Italian study 42% of 1010 predominantly asymptomatic blood donors were *H. pylori* positive. Of the *H. pylori* positive patients, 15% had a duodenal ulcer and 5% a gastric ulcer.[64] By contrast, in a study of asymptomatic *H. pylori* positive volunteers in Texas the point prevalence of duodenal ulcer was only 1%.[65] McColl *et al* found a prevalence of duodenal ulcer of 40% in patients presenting with dyspepsia in Scotland.[66] The incidence and prevalence of duodenal and gastric ulcer have been in decline now for quite some time in Western countries, and individual countries may be at different stages along this slope of change. The consequence for interpretation of *H. pylori* eradication trials is that in countries with a continuing high background of duodenal ulcers there will also be a higher proportion of patients among the functional dyspepsia patients who ultimately will develop duodenal ulcers. It is possible that functional dyspepsia trials carried out in these countries are more likely to demonstrate a beneficial effect on symptoms after eradication of *H. pylori*.

The evidence relating to *H. pylori* eradication in functional dyspepsia is not conclusive to date. If there is an overall benefit of treatment the proportion of patients who benefit is likely to be associated with values of NNT in the range 7–15. Many physicians are currently treating all *H. pylori* positive functional dyspepsia patients with eradication therapy, despite the equivocal evidence that treatment will relieve symptoms. This is done because of the widely accepted belief that the organism is a true pathogen which causes peptic ulcer disease and perhaps gastric cancer.

CONCLUSION

There are methodological shortcomings in many of the functional dyspepsia treatment trials which make it difficult to provide firm guidelines. Trials that have carried out head to head comparisons among the main treatment options have not been performed. These options include H_2-receptor antagonists, proton pump inhibitors, cisapride, and anti-helicobacter therapy for patients who are *H. pylori* positive. Endoscopy may give a patient reassurance that there is no serious underlying disease and this may have a powerful beneficial therapeutic effect. It is reasonable to prescribe a period of acid suppression with either an H_2RA or a PPI in patients with functional dyspepsia. The evidence for effectiveness of PPIs is stronger. For all these treatments it is possible that patients with unrecognized GERD represent the main responders. Whether eradication therapy for *H. pylori* will lead to a sustained improvement of functional dyspepsia symptoms is currently unresolved. However, given that *H. pylori* is a true pathogen, capable of producing peptic ulcers and sometimes gastric cancer, the author recommends that eradication therapy should be prescribed when the presence of the infection is documented.

R Grade **A/C**

ACKNOWLEDGEMENT

Dr Veldhuyzen van Zanten holds a Nova Scotia Clinical Scholar Award from the Nova Scotia Government, Canada.

REFERENCES

1 Nyrén O, Lindberg G, Lindstrom E *et al.* *Economic costs of functional dyspepsia.* PharmacoEconomics, Adis International Ltd,1992, pp 312–24.

2 Chiba N, Bernard L, O'Brien BJ *et al.* A Canadian physician survey of dyspepsia management. *Can J Gastroenterol* 1998; **12**: 183–90.

3 Veldhuyzen van Zanten SJO. Treatment of functional dyspepsia. *Balliere's Clin Gastroenterol* 1998; **12**: 573–86.

4 Drossman DA, Thompson G, Talley NJ *et al.* Identification of subgroups of functional gastrointestinal disorders. *Gastroenterol Int* 1991; **4**: 145–60.

5 Talley NJ, Colin-Jones D, Koch KL *et al.* Functional dyspepsia: a classification with guidelines for diagnosis and management. *Gastroenterol Int* 1991; **4**: 145–60.

6 Talley NJ, Zinsmeister AR, Schleck CD *et al.* Dyspepsia and dyspepsia subgroups: a population-based study. *Gastroenterol* 1992; **102**: 1259–68.

7 Talley NJ, Weaver AL, Tesmer DL *et al.* Lack of discriminant value of dyspepsia subgroups in patients referred for upper endoscopy. *Gastroenterol* 1993; **105**: 1378–86.

8 Klauser A, Voderholzer WA, Knesewitsch PA *et al.* What is behind dyspepsia. *Dig Dis Sci* 1993; **38**: 147–54.

9 Talley NJ, Silverstein MC, Agreus L *et al.* AGA Technical Review: evaluation of dyspepsia. *Gastroenterol* 1998; **114**: 582–95.

10 Veldhuyzen van Zanten SJO. Can the age limit for endoscopy be increased in dyspepsia patients who do not have alarm symptoms? *Am J Gastroenterol* 1999; **94**: 9–11.

11 Axon ATR. Chronic dyspepsia: who needs endoscopy? *Gastroenterol* 1997; **112**: 1376–80.

12 Bytzer P, Hansen JM, Schaffalitzky de Muckadell OB. Empirical H_2-blocker therapy or prompt endoscopy in management of dyspepsia. *Lancet* 1994; **343**: 811–16.

13 Talley NJ, Phillips SF. Non-ulcer dyspepsia: potential causes and pathophysiology. *Ann Intern Med* 1988; **108**: 865–79.

14 Talley NJ, Hunt RH. What role does *H. pylori* play in dyspepsia and non-ulcer dyspepsia: arguments for and against *H. pylori* being associated with dyspeptic symptoms. *Gastroenterol* 1997; **113**: S67–77.

15 Veldhuyzen van Zanten SJO. The role of *H. pylori* in non-ulcer dyspepsia. *Scand J Gastroenterol* 1997; **11(51)**: 63–9.

16 Veldhuyzen van Zanten SJO, Cleary C, Talley NJ *et al.* Drug treatment of functional dyspepsia: a systematic analysis of trial methodology with recommendations for design of future trials. *Am J Gastroenterol* 1996; **91**: 660–71.

17 Guyatt GH, Veldhuyzen van Zanten SJO, Feeney DH *et al.* Measuring quality of life in clinical trials. A taxonomy and review. *Can Med J Assoc* 1989; **140**: 1441–8.

18 Nyrén O, Adami HO, Bates S *et al.* Self-rating of pain in nonulcer dyspepsia. *J Clin Gastroenterol* 1987; **9**: 408–14.

19 Dimenas E, Glise H, Ballerback B *et al.* Well-being and gastrointestinal symptoms among patients referred to endoscopy due to suspected duodenal ulcer. *Scand J Gastroenterol* 1995; **30**: 1046–52.

20 Veldhuyzen van Zanten SJO, Tytgat KMAJ, Pollak PT *et al.* Can severity of symptoms be used as outcome measures in trials of non-ulcer dyspepsia and *Helicobacter pylori. J Clin Epidemiol* 1993; **46**: 273–9.

21 El-Omar EM, Banerjee S, Wirz A *et al.* The Glasgow Dyspepsia Severity Score – a tool for the global measurement of dyspepsia. *Eur J Gastroenterol Hepatol* 1996; **8**: 967–71.

22 Buckley MJ, Seatko C, McGuigan J *et al.* A validated dyspepsia symptom score. *It J Gastroenterol* 1998; **18**: 495–500.

23 Klein KB. Controlled treatment trials in the irritable bowel syndrome: a critique. *Gastroenterol* 1988; **95**: 232–41.

24 Christie J, Shepherd NA, Codling BW *et al.* Gastric cancer below the age of 55: implications for screening patients with uncomplicated dyspepsia. *Gut* 1997; **41**: 513–17.

25 Wiklund I, Glise H, Jerndal P I *et al.* Does endoscopy have a positive impact on quality of life in dyspepsia? *Gastrointest Endosc* 1998; **47**: 449–54.

26 Talley NJ. Drug treatment of functional dyspepsia. *Scand J Gastroenterol* 1991; **26(S182)**: 47–60.

27 Nyren O, Adami HO, Bates S *et al.* Absence of therapeutic benefit from antacids or cimetidine in non-ulcer dyspepsia. *N Engl J Med* 1986; **314**: 339–43.

28 Gotthard R, Bodemar G, Brodin U *et al.* Treatment with cimetidine, antacids, or placebo in patients with dyspepsia of unknown origin. *Scand J Gastroenterol* 1988; **23**: 7–18.

29 Bodger K, Daly MJ, Heatley RV. Prescribing patterns for dyspepsia in primary care: a prospective study of selected general practitioners. *Aliment Pharmacol Ther* 1996; **10**: 889–95.

30 Dobrilla G, Comberlato L, Steele A *et al.* Drug treatment of functional dyspepsia. A meta-analysis of randomized controlled clinical trials. *J Clin Gastroenterol* 1989; **11**: 169–77.

31 Delattre M, Malesky M, Prinzie A. Symptomatic treatment of non-ulcer dyspepsia with cimetidine. *Curr Ther Res* 1985; **37**: 980–91.

32 Nesland A, Berstad A. Effect of cimetidine in patients with non-ulcer dyspepsia and erosive prepyloric changes. *Scand J Gastroenterol* 1985; **20**: 629–35.

33 Talley NJ, McNeil D, Hayden A *et al.* Randomized, double-blind, placebo-controlled crossover trial of cimetidine and pirenzepine in nonulcer dyspepsia. *Gastroenterol* 1986; **91**: 149–56.

34 Gotthard R, Bodemar G, Brodin U *et al.* Treatment with cimetidine, antacids, or placebo in patients with dyspepsia of unknown origin. *Scand J Gastroenterol* 1988; **23**: 7–18.

35 Johannessen T, Fjosne U, Kleveland P *et al.* Cimetidine responders in non-ulcer dyspepsia. *Scand J Gastroenterol* 1988; **23**: 327–36.

36 Johannessen T, Kristensen P, Petersen H *et al.* The symptomatic effect of 1-day treatment periods with cimetidine in dyspepsia. Combined results from randomized, controlled, single-subject trials. *Scand J Gastroenterol* 1991; **26**: 974–80.

37 Saunders J, Oliver R, Higson D. Dyspepsia: incidence of non-ulcer disease in a controlled trial of ranitidine in general practice. *Br Med J* 1986; **292**: 665–8.

38 Farup P, Larsen S, Ulshagen K *et al.* Ranitidine for non-ulcer dyspepsia. A clinical study of the symptomatic effect of ranitidine and a classification and characterization of the responders to treatment. *Scand J Gastroenterol* 1991; **26**: 1209–16.

39 Hansen JM, Bytzer P, Schaffalitzky de Muckadell OB. Placebo-controlled trial of cisapride and nizatidine in unselected patients with functional dyspepsia. *Am J Gastroenterol* 1998; **93**: 368–74.

40 Talley NJ, Meineche-Schmidt V, Pare P *et al.* Efficacy of omeprazole in functional dyspepsia: double-blind, randomized placebo-controlled trials (the Bond and Opera studies). *Aliment Pharmacol Ther* 1998; **12**: 1055–65.

41 Mason I, LJ Millar, RR Sheikh *et al.* The management of acid-related dyspepsia in general practice: a comparison of an omeprazole versus an antacid-alginate/ranitidine management strategy. *Aliment Pharmacol Ther* 1998; **12**: 263–71.

42 Goves H, Oldring JK, Kerr D *et al.* First line treatment with omeprazole provides an effective and superior alternative strategy in the management of dyspepsia compared to antacid/alginate liquid: a multicentre study in general practice. *Aliment Pharmacol Ther* 1998; **2**: 147–57.

43 Meineche-Schmidt V, Krag E. Antisecretory therapy in 1017 patients with ulcerlike or reflux-like dyspepsia in general practice. *Eur J Gen Prac* 1997; **3**: 125–30.

44 Venables TL, Newland RD, Patel AC *et al.* Omeprazole 10 mg once daily, omeprazole 20 mg once daily, or ranitidine 150 mg twice daily, evaluated as initial therapy for the relief of symptoms of gastro-esophageal reflux disease in general practice. *Scand J Gastroenterol* 1997; **32**: 965–73.

45 Carlsson R, Dent J, Watts R *et al*, the International GORD Study Group. Gastroesophageal reflux disease in primary care: an international study of different treatment strategies with omeprazole. *Eur J Gastroenterol Hepatol* 1998; **10**: 119–24.

46 Rösch W. Cisapride in non-ulcer dyspepsia. Results of a placebo-controlled trial. *Scand J Gastroenterol* 1987; **22**: 161–4.

47 Rösch W. Efficacy of cisapride in the treatment of epigastric pain and concomitant symptoms in non-ulcer dyspepsia. *Scand J Gastroenterol* 1989; **24(S165)**: 54–8.

48 Deruyttere M, Lepoutre L, Heylen H *et al.* Cisapride in the management of chronic functional dyspepsia: a multicenter, double-blind, placebo-controlled study. *Clin Ther* 1987: **10**: 44–51.

49 François, De Nutte N. Nonulcer dyspepsia: effect of the gastrointestinal prokinetic drug cisapride. *Curr Ther Res* 1987; **41**: 891–8.

50 Hausken T, Berstad A. Cisapride treatment of patients with nonulcer dyspepsia and erosive prepyloric changes. A double-blind, placebo controlled trial. *Scand J Gastroenterol* 1992; **27**: 213–17.

51 Veldhuyzen van Zanten SJO, Jones M, Talley NJ. Cisapride for treatment of non-ulcer dyspepsia: a meta-analysis of randomized controlled trials. *Gastroenterology* 1998; **114**(4 – Part 2): A323(G1322).

52 Champion MC, Mac Cannell K, Thomson A *et al.* A double-blind randomized study of cisapride in the treatment of non-ulcer dyspepsia. The Canadian Cisapride NUD study group. *Canad J Gastroenterol* 1997; **11**: 127–34.

53 Graham DY, Malaty HM, Evans DG *et al.* Epidemiology of *H. pylori* in an asymptomatic population in the United States: effect of age, race and socioeconomic status. *Gastroenterol* 1991; **100**: 1495–501.

54 Veldhuyzen van Zanten SJO. *H. pylori*, socioeconomic status, marital status and occupation. *Aliment Pharmacol Ther* 1995; **9(S2)**: 41–4.

55 Armstrong D. *H. pylori* and dyspepsia. *Scand J Gastroenterol* 1996; **31(Suppl 215)**: 38–47.

56 Laheij RJF, Jansen JBMJ, van De Lisconk EH *et al.* Review article: symptom improvement through eradication of *H. pylori* in patients with non-ulcer dyspepsia. *Aliment Pharmacol Ther* 1996; **10**: 843–50.

57 Talley NJ. A critique of therapeutic trials in *Helicobacter pylori* positive functional dyspepsia. *Gastroenterol* **106**: 1174–83.

58 Trespi E, Broglia F, Villani L *et al.* Distinct profiles of gastritis in dyspepsia subgroups. Their different clinical responses to gastritis healing after *H. pylori* eradication. *Scand J Gastroenterol* 1994; **29**: 884–8.

59 Sheu B-S, Lin C-Y, Lin X-Z *et al.* Long-term outcome of triple therapy in *H. pylori*-related non-ulcer dyspepsia: a prospective controlled assessment. *Am J Gastroenterol* 1996; **91**: 441–7.

60 Gillvary J, Buckley M, Beattie S *et al.* Eradication of *H. pylori* affects symptoms in non-ulcer dyspepsia. *Scand J Gastroenterol* 1997; **32**: 535–40.

61 McColl KEL, Murray LS, El-Omar E *et al.* Symptomatic benefit from eradicating *H. pylori* in patients with non-ulcer dyspepsia. *N Engl J Med* 1998; **339**: 1869–74.

62 Blum AL, Talley NJ, O'Morain C *et al.* Lack of effect of treating *H. pylori* infection in patients with non-ulcer dyspepsia. *N Engl J Med* 1998; **339**: 1875–81.

63 Talley NJ, Janssens J, Lauritsen K *et al.* Cure of *H. pylori* and symptoms in functional dyspepsia. A randomized double-blind placebo-controlled trial. *Br Med J* 1999.

64 Vaira D, Miglioli M, Mule P *et al.* Prevalence of peptic ulcer in *H. pylori* positive blood donors. *Gut* 1994; **35**: 309–12.

65 Anand BS, Raed AK, Malaty HM *et al.* Low point prevalence of peptic ulcer in normal individuals with *H. pylori* infection. *Am J Gastroenterol* 1996; **91**: 1112–15.

66 McColl KEL, El-Nujumi A, Murray L *et al.* The *H. pylori* breath test: a surrogate marker for peptic ulcer disease in dyspeptic patients. *Gut* 1997; **40**: 302–6.

Celiac disease: diagnosis, treatment, and prognosis

7

James Gregor

Since its first description in children by Gee[1] over a century ago, the term celiac disease has been used interchangeably with such designations as primary malabsorption, gluten-sensitive enteropathy, and non-tropical or celiac sprue. Due to the protean nature of its clinical manifestations and their consistent improvement with appropriate therapy, few medical conditions can rival celiac disease for both the frustration and gratification experienced by clinicians and patients.

The first clinical description of celiac disease in adults was provided by Thaysen[2] in 1932. In the early 1950s the link between the disease and the ingestion of certain grains[3] was suggested, and over the next decade the characteristic intestinal lesion was described in both surgical specimens[4] and those obtained using the newly developed peroral suction biopsy technique.[5]

Though reported worldwide, celiac disease is rare in populations of African and Oriental origin. In populations of European descent *reported* prevalences range from 50 to 500 per 100 000 and tend to vary with geographic location. The *apparent* prevalence also varies with the intensity of screening.[6]

CLINICAL MANIFESTATIONS

The clinical manifestations of celiac disease are largely due to nutrient malabsorption. The most frequently reported gastrointestinal symptoms are diarrhea and flatulence. Other symptoms such as severe abdominal pain, nausea, and vomiting are much less common. Although some patients may even complain of constipation, most describe increased stool volume. The diarrhea of celiac disease is classically described as high volume, pale, loose to semi-formed, and foul smelling. However, in many cases it is watery, probably due to the effects of malabsorbed fat and its bacterial degradation products on the secretory mechanisms of intestinal mucosal cells. A high fat content may produce an oily or frothy appearance, and a high gas content can make the stools difficult to flush from the toilet bowl.

Constitutional symptoms of fatigue, weakness, and weight loss, often despite a history of hyperphagia, are common. Many of these symptoms can be attributed to the presence of nutritional deficiencies. In some patients insufficient calories and protein are absorbed to meet nutritional requirements and weight loss and muscle wasting ensue. Specific deficiencies resulting in anemia, bleeding diathesis, tetany, neuropathy, and dermatitis can also occur.

Given the genetic and immunological factors felt to be important in the pathogenesis of the disease, it is not surprising that investigators have sought and reported an association between celiac disease and over 100 medical conditions[7]. By far the most common of these is dermatitis herpetiformis. This pruritic rash is typically papulovesicular and characterized by IgA deposits at the dermal–epidermal junction. If adequate biopsies are performed, villous atrophy has been identified in up to 95% of these patients. In support of the validity of this association is the observation that the characteristic blistering skin lesions tend to improve in response to a gluten-free diet, although at a slower rate (up to 2 years) than the intestinal lesions.[8]

Lymphocytic infiltration of the epithelium of the colon and even stomach has been widely reported in celiac disease. Recent data suggest, however, that the majority of patients with microscopic or collagenous colitis do not have serological evidence of celiac disease.[9]

Type I diabetes mellitus has been described in up to 5% of patients with celiac disease[7] and a similar proportion of insulin dependent diabetics have been reported to have occult villous atrophy.[10,11] Autoimmune thyroid disease[7] and selective IgA deficiency[12] also appear to be more prevalent in patients with celiac disease. Studies linking celiac disease to other autoimmune diseases such as ulcerative colitis,[13] primary biliary cirrhosis,[14] and sclerosing cholangitis[15] are primarily family studies or small case series. Screening studies suggest an increased prevalence (up to 7%) of celiac disease in patients with Down's syndrome.[16,17] In one study this generated an odds ratio as high as 100, compared to the general population.[18] However, due to the small number of celiac patients diagnosed in the groups with Down's syndrome, a statistically significantly increased prevalence has not been demonstrated uniformly.

PATHOLOGY

Celiac disease primarily affects the mucosal layer of the small intestine. The characteristic lesion includes lymphocytic infiltration of the lamina propria and, in particular, the surface epithelium, resulting in villous atrophy and crypt hyperplasia. The degree of villous damage ranges from mere blunting to total atrophy. The involvement may be restricted to the duodenum and proximal jejunum or may involve the entire length of the small bowel. The degree and extent of disease involvement grossly correlates with severity of symptoms.[19] In some studies the prevalence of asymptomatic celiac disease is fourfold greater than the prevalence of symptomatic disease.[20]

Historically, the gold standard for the diagnosis of celiac disease has required not only the identification of the typical histological lesion, but also clinical and histological improvement with appropriate dietary therapy. It has been clearly demonstrated in human subjects that the instillation into the small bowel of wheat, rye, or barley flour or their alcohol-soluble protein components, "prolamins", produces both clinical symptoms and histological lesions.[21]

Much of the fundamental research relating to celiac disease in recent years has focussed on the immunological and genetic factors associated with sensitivity to gliadin and the other prolamins. In clinical practice the diagnosis and treatment of the disease are well defined. Thus most of the recently published clinical research has focussed on a few specific questions:

1 **Diagnosis**: the role of the antiendomysial antibody for screening populations at risk, diagnosing symptomatic individuals, and following the response to a gluten-free diet.
2 **Treatment**: whether oats (or specifically the oat prolamin avenin) can safely be consumed by patients with celiac disease or dermatitis herpetiformis.
3 **Prognosis**: whether patients are at an increased risk of malignancy and whether adherence to a gluten-free diet reduces that risk.

SEROLOGICAL TESTING

In patients with typical signs, symptoms, and laboratory parameters the diagnosis of celiac disease is usually made by performing a mucosal biopsy of the small bowel. Though the differential diagnosis of villous injury is long (including tropical sprue, lymphoma, cows' milk induced enteritis, Zollinger–Ellison syndrome, Whipple's disease, eosinophilic gastroenteritis, bacterial overgrowth, and even viral gastroenteritis), in most patients the diagnosis is not in doubt. From the 1950s until the introduction of flexible endoscopic equipment, specimens were usually obtained using peroral suction instruments, a cumbersome procedure which was uncomfortable for the patient. With the recognition of the immunological nature of the disease it was predictable that serological testing would be developed and evaluated to simplify diagnosis and to facilitate the institution of screening programs in areas of high prevalence.

A number of serological tests have been developed employing antireticulin antibodies (ARA), antigliadin antibodies (AGA), and more recently antibodies to smooth muscle endomysium (EMA). Given that the pathogenesis of celiac disease appears to involve the interaction between cereal grain gluten, or more specifically the alcohol-soluble gliadins, it is not surprising that many of the early reports have focussed on AGA as the primary serological test. As is often the case following the introduction of a new diagnostic test, the initial promise has to some degree yielded to acknowledgement of the test's limitations. Most studies have examined both the IgG and IgA subsets of AGA.[22,23] The data demonstrate reasonable sensitivity (69–91%) but poor specificity (2–79%) for the IgG antibody, suggesting that it may be a general marker for increased gut permeability of any cause rather than an important factor in disease pathogenesis. The IgA AGA has improved specificity (9–94%) at the expense of sensitivity (66–87%).

The development of the antiendomysial antibody test has produced a renewed interest in serological diagnosis. Initial reports suggested almost perfect test accuracy in subjects not restricted to a gluten-free diet. Because it employs an IgA antibody, it is acknowledged that the test may be falsely negative in a celiac patient with associated IgA deficiency. The test is generally performed on serum diluted at 1:10 and 1:20 concentrations, using an immunofluorescence technique. The substrate used is derived from monkey esophagus which has the disadvantages of being expensive (US$20–40) and morally controversial. Recently studies have shown that using human umbilical cord as a substrate (UCA) produces similar test results.[24–27] In addition, an enzyme-linked immunosorbent assay (ELISA) for endomysial antibodies to tissue transglutaminase has been developed.[27] Preliminary results suggest similar diagnostic accuracy without the subjectivity inherent in immunofluorescence.

One of the largest studies evaluating the EMA assay involved 22 pediatric gastroenterology centers throughout Italy.[28] Almost 4000 children underwent testing with both AGA (IgA and IgG) and IgA EMA. "Gold standard" biopsies had been obtained from all patients with a diagnosis of celiac disease who had not yet been placed on dietary therapy ($n = 688$) and from those with compatible gastrointestinal symptoms who subsequently were given a different diagnosis ($n = 797$). Limiting the analysis to these two groups, the EMA assay was more sensitive than the IgG AGA assay (94% vs 90%) and more specific than the IgA AGA assay (97 vs 90%), both differences being statistically significant. Healthy first degree relatives ($n = 599$) were also studied. Of the 46 positive EMA results (7.6%), 32 underwent biopsy. Ninety per cent of these patients were found to have pathological changes consistent with a diagnosis of celiac

Table 7.1 Recent studies examining the operating properties of the antiendomysial antibody in patients who have undergone small bowel biopsy

Study	Subjects	Proportion celiac	Sensitivity	Specificity	Positive LR[a]	Negative LR[b]
Cataldo 1995[28]	1485 children with GI disease	46%	94%	97%	**31**	**0.06**
Grodzinsky 1995[29]	97 children with GI symptoms	28%	78%	99%	**78**	0.22
Vogelsang 1995[30]	102 patients with suspected celiac	48%	100%	100%	**100**	**0.01**
Volta 1995[24]	160 patients with GI disease	38%	95%	100%	**95**	**0.05**
Pacht 1995[31]	35 children with GI symptoms	63%	100%	100%	**100**	**0.01**
Stern 1996[32]	66 patients with GI disease	71%	98%	89%	8.9	**0.02**
Grodzinsky 1996[20]	49 AGA-positive blood donors	14%	71%	100%	**71**	0.29
Valdimarsson 1996[33]	144 patients with suspected celiac	17%	74%	100%	**74**	0.26
Ascher 1996[34]	120 patients with GI symptoms	46%	98%	100%	**98**	**0.02**
Sacchetti 1996[35]	74 children with GI symptoms	43%	97%	100%	**97**	**0.03**
de Lecea 1996[36]	65 children of short stature	34%	88%	91%	9.7	0.13
Yiannakou 1996[27]	154 patients – celiac, IBD or normal	30%	89%	100%	**89**	0.11
Carroccio 1996[26]	108 children – celiac or milk allergy	33%	97%	100%	**97**	**0.03**
Bottaro 1996[37]	50 children – celiac or normal	67%	96%	96%	**24**	**0.04**
Atkinson 1997[38]	66 patients with GI symptoms	33%	95%	64%	2.6	**0.08**
Corazza 1997[39]	78 patients with GI symptoms	45%	91%	80%	4.6	0.11
Kolho 1997[25]	167 children with GI symptoms	32%	94%	100%	**94**	**0.06**

Positive LR greater than 10 and negative LR less than 0.1 are shown in bold type because they are generally considered to be quite useful.
[a] Calculated using sensitivity/1 − specificity and assuming specificity = 99% when reported as 100%.
[b] Calculated using 1 − sensitivity/specificity and assuming sensitivity = 99% when reported as 100%.

disease. In patients on a strict gluten-free diet ($n = 96$) it was found that 81% were negative for EMA, suggesting that the test may have a role in monitoring intestinal response after diagnosis.

There have been many studies from several countries[20,24–39] which have evaluated the diagnostic accuracy of EMA (Table 7.1). One useful way of summarizing the utility of a test is to consider both its positive and negative likelihood ratios (LR). In Bayesian analysis the appropriate LR (depending on the positivity or negativity of the test) is multiplied by the estimated pretest odds to determine the likelihood that a particular condition is present or absent. Positive LRs greater than 10 and negative LRs less than 0.1 are generally agreed to be quite useful. Consider an example of a patient with non-specific symptoms and a family history of celiac disease in whom the pretest likelihood of celiac disease was estimated to be 8% (odds of 2:23). Using the LRs from the large Italian study[28] of 31 and 0.06 respectively, the post-test likelihood of celiac disease after a positive test would be 65% and after a negative test 0.5%. In a patient with more specific symptoms and therefore a higher pretest probability estimated at 50%, a positive test would produce a post-test likelihood of 97% while a negative test would reduce this likelihood to 6%. Similarly if one screened the general population (with a prevalence of 0.25%) the post-test probabilities would be much different at 8% and 0.02% respectively, significantly lower than a high risk or symptomatic population.

Though obviously highly dependent on pretest probabilities, the utility of a particular LR also has to be interpreted in light of the implications of misdiagnosis, which in the case of celiac disease would include weighing the tribulations of a gluten-free diet against the potential for future symptoms and complications in an untreated patient. In one recent economic model,[38] it was estimated that using EMA alone for the diagnosis of celiac disease was potentially more costly than small bowel biopsy if the test specificity was under 95%. The authors concluded that the most cost-effective strategy for most patients presenting to a gastroenterologist was to use EMA as the initial diagnostic test and to confirm all positive results with a small bowel biopsy.

Although most studies suggest good diagnostic accuracy, due to differences in test interpretation and the populations studied there are considerable differences of opinion as to whether EMA is more useful in ruling out celiac disease (high sensitivity/negative LR) or confirming the diagnosis (high specificity/positive LR). Of the 17 studies listed in Table 7.1, 13 produced positive LRs above 10, and 11 produced negative LRs below 0.1. At this point in time EMA appears to be a useful diagnostic test that should replace other serological tests, but it probably should not replace small bowel biopsy for the diagnosis of celiac disease. Future effectiveness (as opposed to efficacy) studies are desirable to determine whether the test characteristics are robust as the test is used in general medical practice.

THERAPY

R
Grade B

The mainstay of therapy for celiac disease is a lifelong gluten-free diet. Because biopsy findings suggesting celiac disease may also be compatible with other conditions, some clinicians advocate a follow-up biopsy to confirm remission after implementation of a gluten-free diet . However, most are satisfied with a symptomatic response.[6] In addition to a gluten-free diet, supplemental vitamins such as iron, folic acid, or vitamin K should be given where deficiencies are documented. Calcium and vitamin D may be deficient, and consideration may be given to measuring bone mineral density, particularly in women. Although it is suggested that the institution of a gluten-free diet protects against increasing bone loss,[40] some patients may be candidates for hormone replacement or biphosphonate therapy.

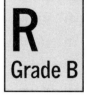

Poor dietary compliance is the most common reason for failure of a gluten-free diet. However, the complications of intestinal lymphoma and adenocarcinoma must be

R
Grade C

considered. Patients with persistent symptoms in whom other diagnoses are excluded are described as having refractory sprue. There are considerable uncontrolled data to support the use of corticosteroids for this indication.[41] Anecdotal evidence suggests that azathioprine[42] and cyclosporin[43] may also be effective in patients who do not respond to corticosteroids.

Currently the greatest controversy pertaining to therapy is the safety of including modest amounts of oats in the diet. Historically, wheat and rye were the first grains demonstrated to be toxic to celiac patients, followed subsequently by reports of toxicity with oats and barley. Similar injurious effects were not found with corn, rice, and potatoes.[44] Although it appears that grain prolamins contain the antigen responsible for the toxic immune response, the exact amino acid sequence of the responsible peptide has yet to be fully elucidated.[8] A proline containing sequence may be particularly important. Wheat, rye, and barley are grasses of the tribe Triticeae while oats belong to the tribe Aveneae. The oat protein avenin has been found to have a lower proline content, giving biological plausibility to the hypothesis that oats may be less toxic. Contrary immunological evidence suggests that antigliadin antibodies from patients with celiac disease and dermatitis herpetiformis and those produced using monoclonal techniques react not only against Triticae proteins but also against avenin.[45] The relevance of this finding is questionable, since immune reactivity was also observed with corn extract.

Few clinical trials have been performed to answer the question of whether oats are toxic. A small cohort study followed 10 patients with celiac disease for 3 months during which time they consumed porridge containing 50 g of oats daily.[46] The patients remained symptom-free without showing an elevation in antiendomysial or antigliadin antibodies or any histological deterioration. Based only on this result, and the estimation that the upper limit of the 95% confidence interval for a harmful effect in a study failing to show harm is approximately $3/n$, where n is the number of subjects,[47] the true incidence of toxic effects could be as high as 30%.

R
Grade C

A study using a similar design was undertaken to determine the effects of oats on patients with dermatitis herpetiformis. This manifestation often requires even longer periods of gluten withdrawal (2 years on average) to achieve clinical remission, while recurrence usually occurs within 12 weeks of gluten reintroduction.[8] All 10 patients in the study continued with the diet, consuming on average 62.5 g of oats daily. No symptomatic, antibody, or histological relapses were noted.

A larger, Finnish study randomized 92 patients with newly diagnosed celiac disease to a strict gluten-free diet or one containing 50 g of oats daily[48] for 6 months. The authors excluded patients who had severe disease or were not well controlled on their present diet and those with co-morbid illnesses. The patients were well matched with regards to clinical, histological and nutritional parameters. The investigators but not the patients were blinded to treatment. Seventy-six per cent of the oat group consumed more than 30 g daily. Six patients in the oat consuming group withdrew because of cutaneous or abdominal symptoms or for unspecified reasons, but a similar withdrawal rate was observed in the control group. No significant change was found in nutritional laboratory parameters or in small bowel histology. The authors concluded that moderate amounts of oats are safe in most patients. Skeptics could point out that even under these controlled circumstances, 24% of patients may have been intolerant, with a 95% confidence interval of 12–36%. The questions concerning possible oat contamination with other grains secondary to crop rotation and processing and possible long term effects of oat use have not been addressed.

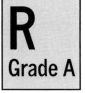

R
Grade A

Table 7.2 A subjective assessment of current evidence attempting to establish a causal or non-causal relationship (see text)

	Hypothesis	
Criteria	Untreated celiac causes gastro-intestinal malignancy/lymphoma	Oats may be consumed as part of a gluten-free diet
Biological plausibility	Yes	Yes
Study designs	Case–control/Cohort	Randomized controlled
Study consistency	**Moderate**	Good
Control groups used	Yes	Yes
Group similarity	**Questionable**	Yes
Adequate follow-up	Yes	**Questionable**
Temporal relationship	Probable	Yes
Exposure gradient	**Not shown**	**Not shown**
Strength of association	Strong	Strong
Precision of estimate	**Poor**	Good

The right-hand column of Table 7.2 summarizes some of the important questions that need to be addressed in order to establish causation. For the most part recent studies establish that moderate amounts of oats are not harmful for the majority of patients with gluten-sensitive disease. A good case can be made, however, for a long term effectiveness (as opposed to efficacy) study looking at the effects of the consumption of oat-containing products in patients with celiac disease.

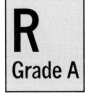

R
Grade A

PROGNOSIS

Celiac disease, if left unrecognized and untreated, has the potential to result in severe complications which are for the most part secondary to malnutrition. When appropriate dietary therapy is instituted the prognosis is usually good. Past studies have suggested an increase in age-adjusted mortality attributable to the disease.[19] However, these studies may have been biassed because of the inclusion of substantial numbers of untreated patients. More recent studies have suggested that at least short term survival is not different from that of the general population[7]. Despite this finding there is evidence, both from retrospective and cohort studies, which suggests an increased risk of certain malignancies.[49]

Immunological stimulation and increased permeability are among the characteristics of the gut in celiac disease which lend biological credence to the possibility that celiac patients are at increased risk for malignancies such as lymphoma and adenocarcinoma of the small bowel. Although the epidemiological studies are heterogeneous in their design and findings, most of the epidemiological evidence to date confirms a general increase in morbidity. The left-hand column of Table 7.2 summarizes some of the data from these studies.

Most of the reports are based on case–control studies. This design is particularly subject to problems with *bias* and *confounding*. A *selection bias* toward the inclusion of particularly ill or refractory patients is one of the most frequently cited criticisms of the studies, which show a mortality rate which is increased as much as 3.4-fold over that of the general population[50–52] and complicating malignancy rates as high as 14%.[53]

Measurement bias is another potential problem. Patients presenting with abdominal symptoms secondary to a malignancy may be more likely to undergo investigations like small bowel biopsy which could lead to a diagnosis of celiac disease. Moreover, it is not always entirely clear that the changes identified on biopsy are diagnostic of celiac disease or whether they could have been induced by the malignancy. Finally, some of the risk factors for celiac disease such as ethnic/geographic origin or immune markers (for example the class II HLA antigens HLA-DR3 and HLA-DQw2) could potentially be independent risks for certain diseases.

Despite these concerns, it is unlikely that the excess risk of small bowel lymphoma and adenocarcinoma seen in most studies can be explained by methodological flaws. In the early 1980s, a British registry collected data on approximately 400 cases of celiac disease and various cancers. The data were analyzed and compared to individual cancer rates in the local population.[54] Two hundred and fifty-nine tumors were histologically confirmed. Slightly more than half of these were lymphomas, the majority of which had arisen in the small bowel. Two-thirds were discovered after the diagnosis of celiac disease was established at a mean interval of 7.3 years. A number of other studies have shown similarly high rates of lymphoma with death rates due to this complication varying from 2.6% to 8.9% translating into relative risks of 25–122.[55]

Of non-lymphomatous malignancies only those of the gastrointestinal tract were seen in excess, compared to the rates expected in the general population. A statistically significant increased risk of adenocarcinomas of the pharynx, esophagus, and small bowel was observed. The relative risk of pharyngeal or esophageal cancer was relatively small (five to six) and could possibly be explained by confounding risk factors. However, the relative risk of small bowel carcinoma, a rare malignancy in the general population, was markedly increased at 83 (95% confidence limits 46–117).

Another British series of 210 patients reported in 1976[56] produced similar results. It was followed by a prospective cohort study published in 1989[57] which also demonstrated increased cancer risk. In the initial report an effect of a gluten-free diet on cancer risk was not demonstrated. Short of a randomized controlled trial, which is not a feasible approach to this problem, reduction in cancer risk corresponding to reduced gluten intake and intestinal damage would provide the strongest evidence of causation. The patients were a priori divided into three groups – patients following a strict gluten-free diet ($n = 108$), patients intermittently adherent or adherent less than 5 years ($n = 56$), and patients not adhering to any dietary restrictions ($n = 46$). Increased risk was seen overall for cancers of the mouth, pharynx, and oesophagus (ratio of observed to expected (O/E) approximately 10). The increase in risk was particularly strong for non-Hodgkin's lymphoma ($n = 9$; O/E = 42.7). For these cancers there was a statistically significant reduced risk for the strict gluten-free diet group (O/E approximately 40 vs 6.5) but an effect of degree of gluten exposure in terms of a gradient of risk was not shown.

The risk of malignancy in patients with dermatitis herpetiformis has also been studied. One study used a retrospective cohort design[58] to evaluate 109 patients who were followed for 13 years at one clinic, with almost complete follow-up. Seven patients (6.4%) developed a malignancy, three of which were lymphomas, one without small intestinal involvement. This translated into a relative risk of lymphoma of 100. The overall relative risk of malignancy was 2.38 (95% confidence intervals, 1.22–3.56). However, in those patients adhering to a gluten-free diet, no increased risk was seen. A subsequent Finnish study[59] of 305 patients in whom 81% were compliant with a gluten-free diet also showed no excess risk of malignancy with the exception of non-Hodgkin's lymphoma ($n = 4$) (RR = 10, 95% confidence intervals, 2.8–26.3).

In contrast to these results, another retrospective cohort study originating in Finland[7] compared 335 celiac patients to age- and sex-matched controls with other gastrointestinal disease and normal villous architecture. A statistically significant increased incidence of endocrine disease (12%) and connective tissue disease (7%) was observed, but no increased incidence of malignancy was detected. Notably, no cases of small bowel adenocarcinoma or non-Hodgkin's lymphoma were identified. This negative finding may be accounted for by either the relatively short mean follow-up (3.1 years) or the high rate of dietary compliance with a strict gluten-free diet (83%).

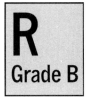

Though debate persists on the magnitude and type of cancer for which untreated celiac patients are at risk, there is a general acceptance among clinicians that the risk is significant enough to warrant lifelong strict dietary compliance even in asymptomatic patients. This concern is foremost among those advocating that oats should not be included in a gluten-free diet[60]. Table 7.2 suggests that the evidence supporting the view that the inclusion of modest amounts of oats in a celiac diet is safe may actually be stronger than the data demonstrating an increased cancer risk in celiac patients.

R
Grade B

Other complications of celiac disease are much more rare. These include refractory sprue which often requires immunosuppressive therapy. Ulcerative jejunoileitis manifesting as chronic ulcers of the small and occasionally large bowel can rarely occur and may lead to the diagnosis of celiac disease.[49] This condition can be difficult to distinguish from intestinal lymphoma and may actually progress to this disease. Collagenous sprue, an even more rare complication of celiac disease, is histologically distinguished by a thick subepithelial band of collagen. No effective therapy has been described and patients generally go on to parenteral alimentation.[6,61]

CONCLUSION

The gold standard for the diagnosis of celiac disease remains the small bowel biopsy. Serological testing, particularly the antiendomysial antibody, can be very useful in the appropriate clinical situation to both diagnose and to monitor the response to a gluten-free diet. The threshold for initial and follow-up biopsy if necessary should be low given the limitations of the test and the general ease of upper gastrointestinal endoscopy and biopsy. A gluten-free diet remains the cornerstone of management. The available evidence suggests that a substantial proportion of patients will tolerate a moderate amount of oats in their diet with the appropriate clinical follow-up. To prevent symptomatic recurrences, nutritional deficiencies (particularly bone disease), and malignant complications, a strict gluten-free diet should be encouraged in all patients.

REFERENCES

1 Gee S. On the coeliac affection. *St Barth Hosp Rep* 1888; **24**: 17–20.
2 Thaysen TEH. *Non-tropical sprue*. Copenhagen: Levin & Munksgaard, 1932.
3 Dicke WK, Weijers HA, van de Kamer JH. Coeliac disease. II: The presence in wheat of a factor having a deleterious effect in cases of coeliac disease. *Acta Paediatr Scand* 1953; **42**: 34–42.
4 Paulley LW. Observations on the aetiology of idiopathic steatorrhea. *Br Med J* 1954; **2**: 1318–21.
5 Rubin CE, Brandborg LL, Phelps PC *et al*. Studies of coeliac disease I. The apparent identical and specific nature of the duodenal and proximal jejunal lesion in coeliac disease and idiopathic sprue. *Gastroenterology* 1960; **38**: 28–49.
6 Trier JS. Coeliac sprue. *N Engl J Med* 1991; **325**: 1709–19.

7 Collin R, Reunala T, Pukkala E *et al.* Coeliac disease – associated disorders and survival. *Gut* 1994; **35**: 1215–18.

8 Hardman C, Garioch, JJ, Leonard JN *et al.* Absence of toxicity of oats in patients with dermatitis herpetiformis. *N Engl J Med* 1997; **337**: 1884–7.

9 Bohr J, Tysk C, Yang P *et al.* Autoantibodies and immunoglobulins in collagenous colitis. *Gut* 1996; **39**: 73–6.

10 Mäki M, Huupponen T, Holm K *et al.* Seroconversion of reticulin autoantibodies predicts coeliac disease in insulin dependent diabetes mellitus. *Gut* 1995; **36**: 239–42.

11 Rensch MJ, Merenich JA, Lieberman M *et al.* Gluten-sensitive enteropathy in patients with insulin-dependent diabetes mellitus. *Ann Intern Med* 1996; **124**: 564–7.

12 Rittmeyer C, Rhoads JM. IgA deficiency causes false-negative endomysial antibody results in coeliac disease. *J Pediatr Gastroenterol Nutr* 1996; **23**: 504–6.

13 Shah A, Mayberry JF, Williams G *et al.* Epidemiological survey of coeliac disease and inflammatory bowel disease in first-degree relatives of coeliac patients. *Q J Med* 1990; **74**: 283–8.

14 Logan RF, Finlayson NDC, Weir DG. Primary biliary cirrhosis and coeliac disease: an association? *Lancet* 1978; **i**: 230–3.

15 Hay JE, Wiesner RH, Shorter R *et al.* Primary sclerosing cholangitis and coeliac disease. *Ann Intern Med* 1988; **109**: 713–17.

16 George EK, Mearin ML, Bouquet J *et al.* High frequency of coeliac disease in Down's syndrome. *J Pediatr* 1996; **128**: 555–7.

17 Bonamico M, Rasore-Quartino A, Mariani P *et al.* Down syndrome and coeliac disease: usefulness of antigliadin and antiendomysium antibodies. *Acta Paediatr* 1996; **85**: 1503–5.

18 Gale L, Wimalaratna H, Brotodihargo A *et al.* Down's syndrome is strongly associated with coeliac disease. *Gut* 1997; **40**: 492–6.

19 Trier JS. *Coeliac sprue and refractory sprue.* Toronto: WB Saunders, 1998.

20 Grodzinsky E. Screening for coeliac disease in apparently healthy blood donors. *Acta Paediatr* 1996; **412**(Suppl): 36–8.

21 van de Kamer JH, Weijers HA, Dicke WK. Coeliac disease. IV. An investigation into the injurious constituents of wheat in connection with their action on patients with coeliac disease. *Acta Paediatr Scand* 1953; **42**: 223–31.

22 Berger R, Schmidt G. Evaluation of six antigliadin antibody assays. *J Immunol Methods* 1996; **91**: 77–86.

23 Chartrand LJ, Agulnik J, Vanounou T *et al.* Effectiveness of antigliadin antibodies as a screening test for coeliac disease in children. *Can Med Assoc J* 1997; **157**: 527–33.

24 Volta U, Molinaro N, De Franceshi L *et al.* IgA anti-endomysial antibodies on human umbilical cord tissue for coeliac disease screening save both money and monkeys. *Dig Dis Sci* 1995; **40**: 1902–5.

25 Kolho KL, Savilahti E. IgA endomysium antibodies on human umbilical cord: an excellent diagnostic tool for coeliac disease in childhood. *J Pediatr Gastroenterol Nutr* 1997; **24**: 563–7.

26 Carroccio A, Cavataio F, Iacono G *et al.* IgA antiendomysial antibodies on the umbilical cord in diagnosing coeliac disease. Sensitivity, specificity, and comparative evaluation with the traditional kit. *Scand J Gastroenterol* 1996; **31**: 759–63.

27 Sulkanen S, Halttunen T, Laurila K *et al.* Tissue transglutaminase autoantibody enzyme-linked immunosorbent assay in detecting celiac disease. *Gastroenterology* 1998; **115**: 1322–8.

28 Cataldo F, Ventura A, Lazzari R *et al.* Antiendomysium antibodies and coeliac disease: solved and unsolved questions. An Italian multicentre study. *Acta Paediatr* 1995; **84**: 1125–31.

29 Grodzinsky E, Jansson G, Skogh T *et al.* Anti-endomysium and anti-gliadin antibodies as serological markers for coeliac disease in childhood: a clinical study to develop a practical routine. *Acta Paediatr* 1995; **84**: 294–8.

30 Vogelsang H, Genser D, Wyatt J *et al.* Screening for coeliac disease: a prospective study on the value of noninvasive tests. *Am J Gastroenterol* 1995; **90**: 394–8.

31 Pacht A, Sinai N, Hornstein L. The diagnostic reliability of anti-endomysial antibody in coeliac disease: the north Israel experience. *Isr J Med Sci* 1995; **31**: 218–20.

32 Stern M, Teuscher M, Wechmann T. Serological screening for coeliac disease: methodological standards and quality control. *Acta Paediatr Suppl* 1996; **412**: 49–51.

33 Valdimarsson T, Franzen L, Grodzinsky E. Is small bowel biopsy necessary in adults with suspected coeliac disease and IgA anti-endomysium antibodies? 100% positive predictive value for coeliac disease in adults. *Dig Dis Sci* 1996; **41**: 83–7.

34 Ascher H, Hahn-Zoric M, Hanson LÅ *et al.* Value of serologic markers for clinical diagnosis and population studies of coeliac disease. *Scand J Gastroenterol* 1996; **31**: 61–7.

35 Sacchetti L, Ferrajolo A, Salerno G *et al.* Diagnostic value of various serum antibodies detected by diverse methods in childhood coeliac disease. *Clin Chem* 1996; **42**: 1838–42.

36 de Lecea A, Ribes-Koninckx C, Polanco I, Calvete JF. Serological screening (antigliadin and antiendomysium antibodies) for non-overt coeliac disease in children of short stature. *Acta Paediatr* 1996; **412**(Suppl): 54–5.

37 Bottaro G, Volta U, Spina M *et al.* Antibody pattern in childhood coeliac disease. *J Pediatr Gastroenterol Nutr* 1997; **24**: 559–62.

38 Atkinson K, Tokmakajian S, Watson W. Evaluation of the endomysial antibody for coeliac disease: operating properties and associated cost implications in clinical practice. *Can J Gastroenterol* 1997; **11**: 673–7.

39 Corazza GR, Biagi F, Andreani ML *et al.* Screening test for coeliac disease. *Lancet* 1997; **349**: 325–6.

40 Valdimarsson T, Löfman O, Toss G *et al.* Reversal of osteopenia with diet in adult coeliac disease. *Gut* 1996; **38**: 322–7.

41 Trier JS. Coeliac sprue and refractory sprue. *Gastroenterology* 1978; **75**: 307–8.

42 Sinclair TS, Kumar PJ, Dawson AM. Azathioprine responsive villous atrophy. *Gut* 1983; **24**: A494 (abstract).

43 Longstreth GF. Successful treatment of refractory sprue with cyclosporine. *Ann Intern Med* 1993; **119**: 1014–16.

44 Schmitz J. Lack of oats toxicity in coeliac disease (editorial). *Br Med J* 1997; **314**: 159–60.

45 Vainio E, Varjonen E. Antibody response against wheat, rye, barley, oats and corn: comparison between gluten-sensitive patients and monoclonal antigliadin antibodies. *Int Arch Allerg Immunol* 1995; **106**: 134–8.

46 Srinivasan U, Leonard N, Jones E *et al.* Absence of oats toxicity in adult coeliac disease. *Br Med J* 1996; **313**: 1300–1.

47 Hanley J, Lippman-Hand A. If nothing goes wrong is everything all right? Interpreting zero numerators. *JAMA* 1983; **249**: 1743–5.

48 Janatuinen EK, Pikkarainen PH, Kemppainen TA *et al.* A comparison of diets with and without oats in adults with coeliac disease. *N Engl J Med* 1995; **333**: 1033–7.

49 Holmes GKT. Coeliac disease and malignancy. *J Pediatr Gastroenterol Nutr* 1997; **24**: S20–4.

50 Nielsen OH, Jacobsen O, Pedersen EF *et al.* Non-tropical sprue: malignant diseases and mortality rate. *Scand J Gastroenterol* 1985; **20**: 13–18.

51 Logan RF, Rifkind EA, Turner ID *et al.* Mortality in coeliac disease. *Gastroenterology* 1989; **97**: 265–71.

52 Ferguson A, Kingstone K. Coeliac disease and malignancies. *Acta Paediatr* 1996; **412**(Suppl): 78–81.

53 Harris OD, Cooke WT, Thompson H *et al.* Malignancy in adult coeliac disease and idiopathic steatorrhoea. *Am J Med* 1967; **42**: 899–912.

54 Swinson CM, Coles EC, Slavin G *et al.* Coeliac disease and malignancy. Lancet1983; **i**: 111–15.

55 Mathus-Vliegen EMH. Coeliac disease and lymphoma: current status. *Neth J Med* 1996; **49**: 212–20.

56 Holmes GKT, Stokes PL, Sorahan TM *et al.* Coeliac disease, gluten-free diet, and malignancy. *Gut* 1976; **17**: 612–19.

57 Holmes GKT, Prior P, Lane MR *et al.* Malignancy in coeliac disease – effect of a gluten free diet. *Gut* 1989; **30**: 333–8.

58 Leonard JN, Tucker WFG, Fry JS *et al.* Increased incidence of malignancy in dermatitis herpetiformis. *Br Med J* 1983; **286**: 16–18.

59 Collin P, Pukkala E, Reunala T. Malignancy and survival in dermatitis herpetiformis: a comparison with coeliac disease. *Gut* 1996; **38**: 528–30.

60 Branski D, Shine M. Oats in coeliac disease (Letter). *N Engl J Med* 1996; **334**: 865–6.

61 Trier JS. Complications of coeliac sprue and potentially related diseases with similar intestinal histopathology. *Gastroenterology* 1978; **75**: 314–15.

8 Crohn's disease: treatment

Brian G Feagan, John WD McDonald

The use of non-specific anti-inflammatory drugs such as the 5-aminosalicylates, glucocorticoids, and antimetabolites is the foundation of the current treatment for Crohn's disease (CD). However, recent advances in molecular biology have yielded novel approaches for therapy which may be more relevant to the pathophysiology of the disease. This review offers an evidence based approach to the management of active CD. A brief overview of maintenance therapy is also given.

INDUCTION OF REMISSION

An ideal treatment for active CD should rapidly and reliably induce a remission of symptoms. In clinical trials the most frequently utilized metric is a decrease in the Crohn's Disease Activity Index (CDAI) of from 50 to 100 points with a final score below 150.[1] A substantial placebo response (20–30%) is observed in short term (8–16 week) studies. Three classes of drugs have been most frequently evaluated for treatment of active disease: 5-aminosalicylates (5-ASA), glucocorticoids, and antibiotics.

5-Aminosalicylates

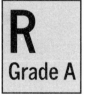

R
Grade A

The prototypic 5-ASA compound sulphasalazine (SPS) has been used to treat CD for more than 40 years.[2] Although highly effective for ulcerative colitis, randomized trials showed that SPS was only marginally superior to a placebo for the induction of remission in active CD[3,4] (Figure 8.1). Since the sulfa related adverse effects of SPS often limit the maximum drug dose that can be administered, the development of 5-ASA formulations which lack a sulfa moiety and which target specific regions of the gastrointestinal tract raised the possibility that greater efficacy was possible. Multiple RCTs have compared the newer 5-ASA compounds with either a placebo (Table 8.1) or an active treatment (SPS, glucocorticoids). Although many of these trials were at a high risk of a type II statistical error due to a small sample size, some definite conclusions can be derived.

Initial experience with 5-ASA doses of 1.5 g/day showed no clear benefit over a placebo.[5,6] These negative studies led to the evaluation of higher dose regimens. Singleton and colleagues[7] allocated over 300 patients with moderate disease activity to receive either 1 g, 2 g or 4 g of Pentasa daily or a placebo for a period of 16 weeks. Although 5-ASA was well tolerated, only a modest benefit of treatment was observed; 43% of the patients who received 4 g/day of Pentasa entered remission as compared with 18% of those who were

Table 8.1 Response rates of remission in studies comparing 5-ASA to placebo or glucocorticoid therapy

Study	Drug dose	No. of patients	Duration (wk)	PL	% remission 5-ASA	GL
NCCDS, 1979[3]	SPS 4–6 g/day	236	17	30	43	—
ECCDS, 1984[4]	SPS 3 g/day	159	18	38	50	82
Rasmussen, 1987[5]	Pentasa 1.5 g/day	67	16	30	40	—
Mahida, 1990[6]	Pentasa 1.5 g/day	40	6	—	—	—
Singleton, 1993[7]	Pentasa 1,2,4 g	310	16	18 placebo vs 4 g 18	43	—
Schölmerich, 1990[9]	Pentasa 2 g	62	24	—	27	66
Martin, 1990[10]	Salofalk 3 g/day	55	12	—	47	46
Maier, 1990[11]	Salofalk 3 g/day	52	12	—	83	88
Thomsen, 1996[12]	Pentasa 4 g	182	16	—	36	62
Prantera, 1993[13]	Asacol 4 g, 5-ASA microgranules	94	12	—	60	61
Gross, 1995[14]	Salofalk 4.5 g	34	8	—	40	56.3

PL, placebo; GL, glucocorticoids.
Source: Feagan B. Aminosalicylates for active disease and in the maintenance of remission in Crohn's disease. *Eur J Surg* 1998;**164**(12):903–9

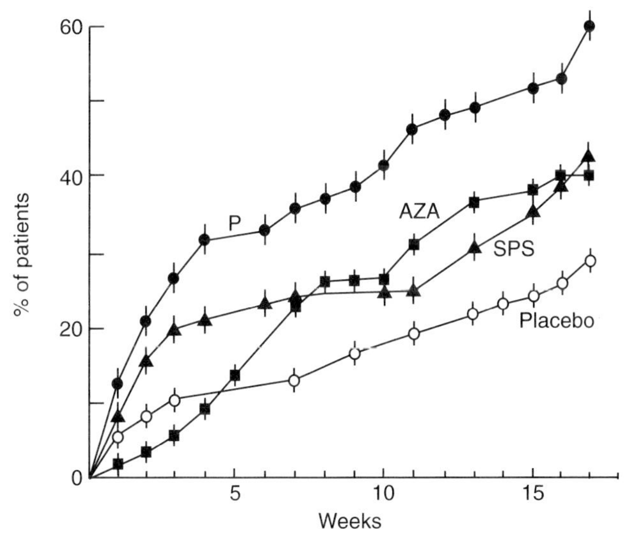

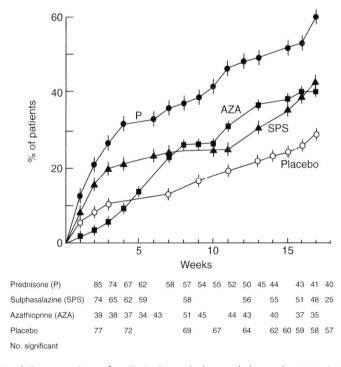

Prednisone (P) 85 74 67 62 58 57 54 55 52 50 45 44 43 41 40
Sulphasalazine (SPS) 74 65 62 59 58 56 55 51 48 25
Azathioprine (AZA) 39 38 37 34 43 51 45 44 43 40 37 35
Placebo 77 72 69 67 64 62 60 59 58 57
No. significant

Figure 8.1 Cumulative percentage of patients in remission week by week: comparison of prednisone, sulphasalazine, azathioprine, and placebo. Remission is defined as CDAI less than 150 and continuing below 150 through week 17 (life table using Kaplan–Meier method). (Adapted with permission from Summers RW, Switz DM, Sessions JT Jr *et al.* National Cooperative Crohn's Disease Study: results of drug treatment. *Gastroenterology* 1979;**77**:847–69)

assigned to the placebo (ARR 25%, NNT = 4, $P = 0.017$). No improvement over placebo was observed for those individuals who received the lower doses of 5-ASA. Subgroup analyses failed to identify any specific predictors of response. Pentasa was well tolerated; more patients who received the placebo were withdrawn from treatment due to adverse events than those who received the highest dose of the active drug.

Although this trial suggested a benefit of high dose 5-ASA therapy, a cautionary note was raised subsequently by the principal investigator,[8] who described a second evaluation of Pentasa in 232 patients. This study, which was similar in design to the previous trial and showed no benefit of 5-ASA therapy, has not been published.

No trials of adequate power have compared the efficacy of the newer 5-ASA drugs and SPS. However, several studies have compared 5-ASA to glucocorticoid therapy for induction of remission (Table 8.1). Schölmerich[9] randomized 62 patients to receive either 5-ASA at a dose of 2 g/day or a standard tapering regimen of methyl prednisolone. In this 24 week trial 73% of the 5-ASA treated patients failed therapy compared with 34% of those who received methyl prednisolone (ARR 39%, NNT = 3, $P = 0.0019$). The authors concluded that treatment with 5-ASA, although well tolerated, was inferior to steroid therapy. Martin *et al*[10] compared a 3 g/day dose of Salofalk to a standard oral prednisone regimen. Although a similar proportion of individuals in the two treatment groups entered remission (47% 5-ASA vs 46% prednisone $P = 0.59$), an analysis of the change in mean CDAI and quality of life scores demonstrated a more rapid improvement in patients treated with prednisone. A study by Thomsen and colleagues provides important information on the relative efficacy of glucocorticoids and 5-ASA.[12] In this methodologically rigorous trial 182 patients with active disease were assigned to receive either 9 mg/day of a controlled ileal release preparation of budesonide (a locally active steroid) or 4 g/day of Pentasa. Following 16 weeks of treatment, 62% of budesonide treated patients were in remission compared with only 36% of the patients who received 5-ASA (ARR 26%, NNT = 4, $P < 0.01$).

R
Grade A

What conclusions can be drawn from these trials? The existing data show that the newer 5-ASA compounds are not more effective than SPS and are, at best, only marginally superior to a placebo for the induction of remission. A single clinical trial has demonstrated the superiority of budesonide over high dose 5-ASA with no increased frequency of adverse events. Although many clinicians prescribe 5-ASA compounds as first line therapy for mild disease activity and treat those patients who fail to achieve a remission with glucocorticoids, the wisdom of this approach is questionable. Although the reluctance of physicians to expose individuals to glucocorticoid therapy is understandable, the likelihood of a response to 5-ASA is so low that the strategy is inefficient. Most patients will ultimately require glucocorticoid treatment to induce remission.

The glucocorticoids

CONVENTIONAL STEROIDS

R
Grade A

The conventional glucocorticoid compounds, prednisone and 6-methyl prednisolone, are highly effective drugs for the treatment of active CD. The National Cooperative Crohn's Disease Study (NCCDS) and the European Cooperative Crohn's Disease Study (ECCDS) both showed that approximately 70% of patients who are treated with 40–60 mg/day of prednisone for 3–4 months enter remission,[3,4] compared to 30% of patients treated with placebo (Figure 8.1).

BUDESONIDE

Glucocorticoids have pluripotent actions on the immune system, including effects on the synthesis of inflammatory mediators, cellular immunity, and neutrophil function.[15] Since the glucocorticoid receptor is widely expressed in tissues, the biological actions of these drugs are not restricted to the immune system. Unpleasant cosmetic effects (acne, moon faces, bruising) and more serious metabolic disturbances (hypertension, metabolic bone disease, and diabetes) are common[16] and limit the usefulness of these agents. An ideal glucocorticoid should retain the efficacy of conventional glucocorticoid drugs while minimizing systemic effects. One possible means of achieving this objective is to specifically target the bowel wall as the therapeutic compartment of interest.[17] The development of budesonide as a treatment for active CD is an example of this approach.

Budesonide is a novel glucocorticoid with a potency approximately five times that of prednisone. The systemic effects of budesonide are reduced in comparison to conventional steroid drugs as a result of extensive first pass metabolism to inactive compounds. Thus a high local anti-inflammatory effect on mucosal surfaces is possible with low systemic activity.[18] Proof of this concept was first demonstrated in asthma therapy, where topical budesonide was shown to be highly effective with few or no systemic adverse effects.[19] An oral controlled ileal release formulation of budesonide was developed for the treatment of active CD of the ileum and right colon. A Canadian multicenter dose finding study [20] found that, first, 9 mg/day of budesonide was more effective than a placebo for the induction of remission in patients with moderately active CD (51% vs 20%, $P<0.001$) and, second, the proportion of patients experiencing glucocorticoid related adverse effects with this drug was not greater than with placebo treatment (26% 9 mg budesonide vs 26% placebo, $P>0.05$). In a second study, Rutgeerts and colleagues[21] compared 9 mg/day of budesonide to a standard prednisolone regimen. Although a favorable trend in response rate was observed in favor of prednisolone therapy, the difference in efficacy between the treatment groups was not large (65% vs 52%, $P=0.12$). There were fewer glucocorticoid related adverse events in patients who received budesonide (budesonide 29%, prednisolone 55%, ARR 26%, NNT = 4, $P=0.003$). Finally, as described earlier, Thomsen and colleagues[12] have shown that 9 mg/day of budesonide is more effective than 4 g/day of 5-ASA and is equally well tolerated. Thus, budesonide is an attractive alternative to 5-ASA or prednisone in patients whose disease is restricted to the appropriate anatomical sites. Whether the chronic administration of such a high dose of budesonide is safe and effective as a chronic treatment remains to be determined.

R Grade A

Antibiotics

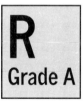

A substantial body of experimental evidence supports the notion that bacteria play an important role in initiating and/or sustaining the pathological inflammatory reaction in the bowel wall.[22,23] Antibiotics have been used empirically for the treatment of active CD for many years, and review articles and textbooks of medicine commonly advocate their use. However, few good data exist to support this endorsement. The Cooperative Crohn's Disease Study in Sweden[24] compared 800 mg/day of metronidazole to 1.5 g/day of SPS in 78 patients with active disease. A 25% response rate for both treatments was shown. Accordingly, it is debatable whether these results are more consistent with an equivalent benefit of metronidazole or the lack of any therapeutic effect for either treatment. The largest trial of metronidazole, performed by Sutherland and colleagues,[25] randomized patients to receive metronidazole (10 or 20 mg/kg/day) or a placebo for 16 weeks (n = 105). Metronidazole therapy produced a dose dependent decrease of disease activity (decrease in CDAI: metronidazole 20 mg/kg 97, 10 mg/kg 60, placebo 1; $P = 0.001$). However, no difference in remission rate was observed (proportion in remission: placebo 25%, metronidazole 10 mg/kg 36%, 20 mg/kg 27%). Thus, the controlled data that support the efficacy of metronidazole are not impressive.

More recently the quinolone antibiotic ciprofloxacin has been utilized in combination with metronidazole. Prantera and colleagues randomized 41 patients to receive combined antibiotics (ciprofloxacin 500 mg bid *and* 250 mg of metronidazole qid) or methyl prednisolone 0.7–1.0 mg/kg for 12 weeks.[26] A statistically significant difference in patients entering remission was not demonstrated (combined antibiotic therapy 10/22 (46%), steroid therapy 12/19 (63%), $P > 0.05$). The small number of patients in this trial does not permit any definitive conclusion regarding the value of combined antibiotic therapy; however, the 17% difference in remission rates in favor of methyl prednisolone is most consistent with a clinically meaningful treatment advantage in favor of glucocorticoid therapy.

R
Grade A

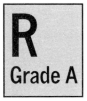

In summary, glucocorticoids are the most effective treatment for active CD. For those patients whose disease is confined to the terminal ileum and/or right colon, budesonide is an attractive alternative to the conventional glucocorticoids because of the lower incidence of adverse events. Although the newer 5-ASA compounds and antibiotics are used by many clinicians to treat patients with milder forms of the disease, limited data exist to support the efficacy of these drugs.

TREATMENT OF THERAPY RESISTANT OR STEROID DEPENDENT PATIENTS

Munkholm and colleagues[27] have documented the natural history of an acute exacerbation of CD in a cohort of patients from Copenhagen County. One year after an initial course of treatment a high proportion (56%) of their patients were either therapy resistant (20%) or steroid dependent (36%). This observation has led many clinicians to conclude that earlier and more aggressive treatment with immunosuppressives may be warranted in selected patients.

Conventional immunosuppressive drugs

Three classes of drugs have been most frequently utilized: the purine antimetabolites (azathioprine/6-MP), cyclosporin, and methotrexate.

THE PURINE ANTIMETABOLITES

Until recently the use of the purine antimetabolites for the treatment of refractory patients was not widely accepted, perhaps because of the inconsistent results obtained from the early randomized trials of these drugs. However, recent studies have for the most part confirmed their efficacy. One of the more important trials was conducted by Candy *et al*,[28]

Review: Azathioprine or 6-mercaptopurine for inducing remission in Crohn's disease
Comparison: Antimetabolite Therapy: Active Disease
Outcome: Antimetabolite studies: azathoprine, 6-mercaptopurine, combined azathioprine and 6-mercaptopurine

Study	Expt n/N	Ctrl n/N	Peto OR (95%CI Fixed)	Weight %	Peto OR (95%CI Fixed)
Azathioprine vs. placebo trials					
Candy 1995	25 / 33	20 / 30		13.9	1.55 [0.52,4.59]
Ewe 1993	16 / 21	8 / 21		11.2	4.57 [1.35,15.27]
Klein 1974	6 / 13	6 / 13		7.1	1.00 [0.22,4.54]
Rhodes 1971	0 / 9	0 / 7		0.0	Not estimable
Summers 1979	21 / 59	20 / 77		30.1	1.57 [0.75,3.29]
Wiloughby 1971	6 / 6	1 / 6		3.4	23.17 [2.57,206.81]
Subtotal (95%CI)	74 / 141	55 / 154		65.7	2.06 [1.25,3.39]
Chi-square 7.98 (df=4) Z=2.83					
6-Mercaptopurine vs. placebo trials					
Oren 1997	13 / 32	12 / 28		15.2	0.80 [0.26,2.26]
Present 1980	25 / 36	5 / 36		19.0	10.45 [4.14,26.38]
Subtotal (95%CI)	39 / 68	17 / 62		34.3	3.34 [1.67,6.66]
Chi-square 13.11 (df=1) Z=3.42					
Total (95%CI)	113 / 209	72 / 216		100.0	2.43 [1.62,3.64]
Chi-square 22.34 (df=6) Z=4.30					

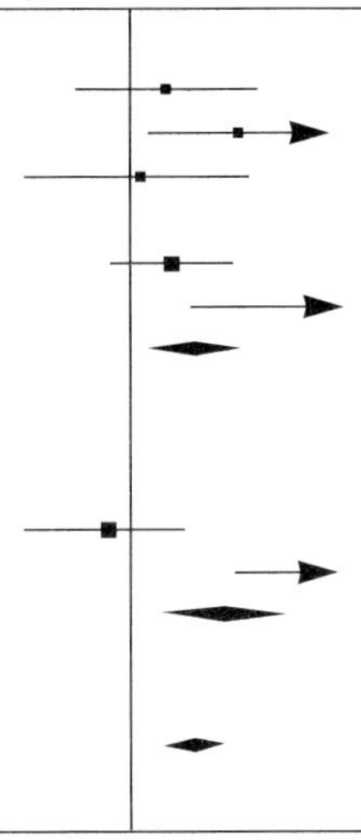

Figure 8.2 Azathioprine or 6-mercaptopurine for inducing remission in Crohn's disease. (*Source*: Sandborn WJ, Sutherland L, Pearson D *et al.* Azathioprine or 6-mercaptopurine for inducing remission of Crohn's disease (Cochrane Review). In: *The Cochrane Library*, issue 2, 1999. Oxford: Update Software)

who randomized 63 patients with active CD to receive a standard tapering induction regimen of prednisone over 3 months and either azathioprine (AZA) 2.5 mg/kg daily or a placebo for 15 months. Although no early (3 months) benefit of AZA was identified with respect to remission rates (CDAI <150 and no prednisone), the proportion of patients who remained in remission over the entire follow-up time was greater in the AZA group (42% vs 7%, ARR 35%, NNT = 3, $P = 0.001$). This result is consistent with observational data that suggest that the purine antimetabolites require a minimum of 3 months to show a treatment effect. In an attempt to overcome this theoretical limitation Sandborn *et al*[29] performed a small, uncontrolled study in which patients with active CD received an intravenous 1800 mg loading dose of AZA. This strategy rapidly achieved stable erythrocyte concentrations of the thiol metabolites, which are believed responsible for the immunosuppressive effects of AZA. Despite this promising finding, a subsequent randomized controlled trial which evaluated 96 patients showed equally low (8 week) remission rates in patients who received either loading or conventional AZA regimens (25% vs 24%)[30] in spite of achieving steady state nucleotide levels by week 2. Furthermore, the proportion of patients entering remission did not increase after 8 weeks of treatment.

The data from the RCTs which have evaluated the purine antimetabolites for the treatment of active CD have been summarized in a meta-analysis[31] in which the pooled ARR for azathioprine treatment for induction of remission is approximately 20% (NNT = 5) (Figure 8.2). A steroid sparing effect was also demonstrated. The NNT for steroid sparing (the number of patients needed to treat with azathioprine for one additional

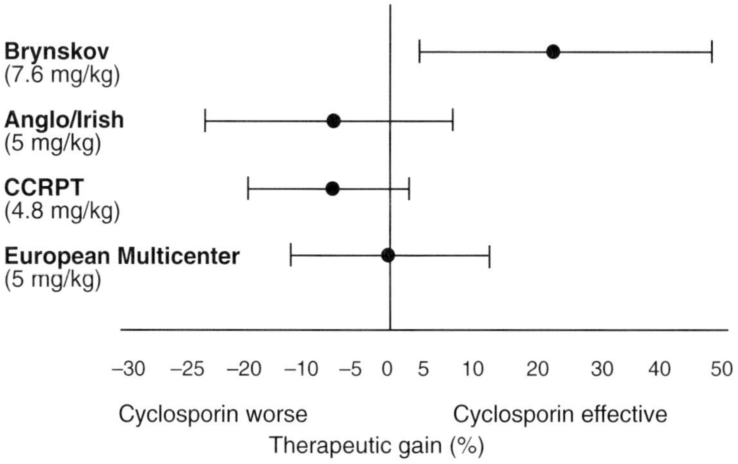

Figure 8.3 Point estimates (•) and 95% confidence limits (⊢—⊣) of the therapeutic gain (% response cyclosporin–% response placebo) for four RCTs of cyclosporin for Crohn's disease. (Reproduced with permission from Feagan B. Cyclosporin has no proven role as a therapy for Crohn's disease. *Inflammatory Bowel Diseases* 1995; 1:335–9)

R Grade A

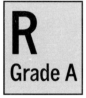

patient to reduce steroids to <10 mg/day) was estimated to be 3. These results should be interpreted with a degree of caution, since important clinical heterogeneity exists among the studies in their definitions of treatment response, duration, and the use of co-interventions. Nevertheless, an overall beneficial effect is apparent, and the use of these drugs can be recommended for treatment of patients who fail to respond to steroid therapy or develop steroid dependence.

CYCLOSPORIN

The emergence of this drug as a standard therapy for organ transplantation led to large scale evaluations for the treatment of chronically active CD. The results of four RCTs (Figure 8.3) have shown that the therapeutic index of cyclosporin is low,[32–35] if there is any efficacy. The study of Brynskov,[32] which demonstrated only a modest benefit, used a high cyclosporin dose (7.6 mg/kg per day), which cannot be recommended for chronic treatment, since the risk of nephrotoxicity is unacceptably high.[36] The three trials[33–35] which assessed a dose of cyclosporin that is tolerable for long term treatment (5 mg/kg per day) showed no benefit with this drug. Thus cyclosporin is not a practical therapy for long term management. Although uncontrolled studies[37,38] have suggested that short duration, high dose intravenous therapy may be beneficial in patients with refractory CD, data from controlled trials are required before this intervention can be advocated for widespread use.

METHOTREXATE

The success of low dose (5–25 mg/weekly) methotrexate (MTX) as a treatment for rheumatoid arthritis led to its evaluation in patients with chronically active CD. In 1989 Kozarek[39] reported the results of an open study in which two-thirds of patients with steroid refractory disease showed an improvement in symptoms and a concomitant reduction in prednisone requirements. Some patients demonstrated an endoscopic

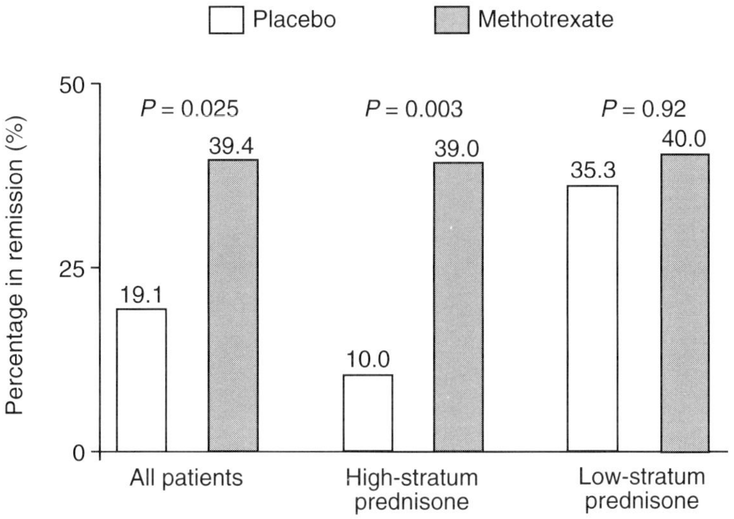

Figure 8.4 Percentages of patients in remission at week 16 according to study group and stratum of daily prednisone dose before entry into the study. The high prednisone stratum was receiving a daily dose of more than 20 mg prednisone, and the low prednisone stratum a daily dose of 20 mg or less more than 2 weeks before randomization. The actual percentages are shown above the bars. *P* values were derived by the Mantel–Haenzel chi-square test, with adjustment for study center. (Reproduced with permission from Feagan BG, Rochon J, Fedorak RN *et al.* Methotrexate for the treatment of Crohn's disease. *N Engl J Med* 1995;**332**:292–7)

remission. A controlled trial[40] was subsequently conducted in which 141 patients who had failed previous attempts to discontinue prednisone were randomized to receive either MTX 25 mg/weekly IM or a placebo for 16 weeks. All of the patients received 20 mg of prednisone per day at the initiation of the trial; a standardized prednisone withdrawal regimen was then used. Patients who responded to therapy discontinued prednisone entirely 12 weeks following randomization. A significant benefit of MTX therapy was observed for the primary outcome measure, the proportion of patients who were completely withdrawn from prednisone *and* in clinical remission as defined by a CDAI score of <150 points (MTX 39%, placebo 19%, ARR 20%, NNT = 5, $P = 0.025$) (Figure 8.4). Improvements in the median prednisone dose, Health Related Quality of Life and mean CDAI scores, and concentration of serum acute phase reactants were also associated with methotrexate therapy. In this short term trial, no serious toxicity was observed, although withdrawals from treatment due to nausea were more common with MTX.

R Grade A

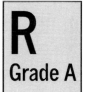

NOVEL IMMUNOSUPPRESSIVE DRUGS

New knowledge of the human immune system and the growth of the biotechnology industry have combined to yield an abundance of new treatments for chronic inflammatory diseases. The development of infliximab as a therapy for CD is a most dramatic example of the promise of this new technology.

Tumor necrosis factor alpha (TNF-α) is a proinflammatory cytokine which plays an important part in the pathophysiology of Crohn's disease.[41] Following the successful treatment of a young woman with a chimeric anti-TNF-α antibody by investigators in

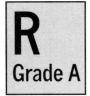

Amsterdam,[42] a series of controlled studies were initiated. Targan and colleagues[43] performed a multicenter dose finding study that evaluated 108 patients whose disease was refractory to other forms of treatment. Patients with moderately severe disease received one of three doses of infliximab (5, 10, 20 mg/kg) or a placebo administered as a single intravenous infusion. Patients continued to receive other treatments at a fixed dose. The primary endpoint of the study was the occurrence of a clinical response as defined by a decrement of 70 points in the CDAI score from the baseline value. No dose–response relationship was identified; 81.5% of infliximab treated patients responded as compared to 16.7% of those who received the placebo (ARR 65%, NNT = 2, P <0.001). Minor allergic reactions to the antibody occurred infrequently but clinically significant adverse effects were not encountered in this short term study.

R
Grade A

In a second pivotal trial colleagues evaluated the efficacy of infliximab for the treatment of patients with fistulizing Crohn's disease[44] (no previous controlled trials had evaluated this population of patients). The patients studied had active, fistulizing disease for a minimum of 3 months prior to randomization. Concomitant treatment with steroids, 6-MP or azathioprine, and antibiotics was permitted although the dose of these co-interventions was maintained at a stable level throughout the trial. The primary measure of response was a 50% reduction in the number of open fistulae. Ninety-four patients received three intravenous infusions of either a placebo or one of two dose regimens of antibody (5 or 10 mg/kg) during a total of 18 weeks of follow-up. Patients treated with infliximab were significantly more likely to respond (61.9% vs 25.8%, ARR 36.1%, NNT = 3, P = 0.002). The response to treatment was rapid and in many cases dramatic. Again, no dose–response relationship was identifiable.

The data from these two landmark studies were sufficient for the FDA to approve infliximab for the treatment of active CD based on the demonstration of efficacy in a patient population refractory to other treatments and the absence of serious short term toxicity. However, additional data are desirable regarding the safety and long term efficacy of this drug. Potential safety concerns include the formation of autoantibodies, the risk of infusion reactions with retreatment, and a possible increased risk of lymphoproliferative disease. At present it is unknown whether in patients who respond to therapy repeated infusions of infliximab at regular intervals is a preferable strategy to retreatment when the disease becomes active. A multicenter study which will evaluate the use of maintenance therapy over 1 year is under way. Until data from this trial are available, it is most appropriate to reserve infliximab as an induction treatment for individuals who have failed to respond to or are intolerant of conventional drug treatments. Patients who receive treatment should be carefully followed for the possible development of autoimmune or lymphoproliferative disorders.

MAINTENANCE OF REMISSION

The objectives of maintenance therapy are to prevent the recurrence of symptoms, to reduce the risk of complications, and to avoid the need for surgery and hospitalization. One year after a medically induced remission of CD approximately 30–40% of patients will experience a relapse of disease;[45] and following surgery symptoms recur at a rate of approximately 15% per year.[46] The failure of the maintenance therapy components of the NCCD[3] and ECCDS[4] trials to demonstrate a long term benefit of SPS or conventional, low dose glucocorticoid therapy led to the extensive evaluation of the newer 5-aminosalicylates and budesonide for this indication.

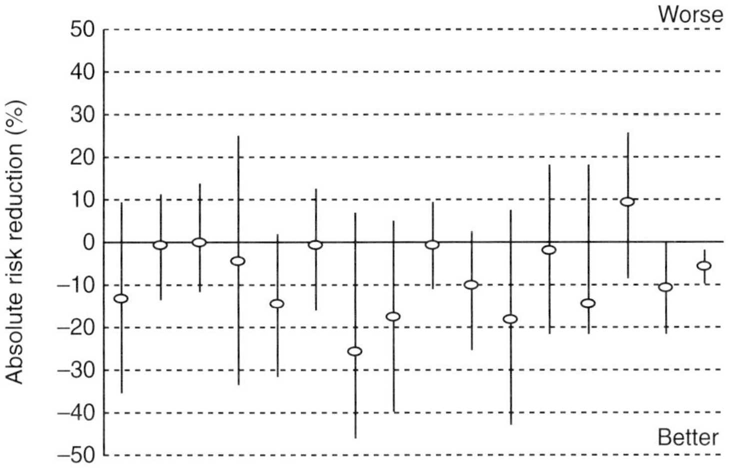

Figure 8.5 Meta-analysis of 5-ASA drugs for maintenance therapy in Crohn's disease. (Adapted with permission from Camma C, Giunta M, Roselli M *et al.* Mesalamine in the maintenance treatment of Crohn's disease: a meta-analysis adjusted for confounding variables. *Gastroenterology* 1997;**13**:1465–73)

The aminosalicylates

Over 20 clinical trials have compared a 5-ASA drug to a placebo for the prevention of a symptomatic recurrence following either surgery or a medically induced remission. The majority of the studies that have evaluated 5-ASA for the latter indication show a 1-year reduction in the rate of relapse of about 10–20%. In the "typical" trial the size of the treatment effect observed is less than that which the investigators considered to be clinically important when the sample size for the trial was determined. Thus statistical significance has not often been demonstrated. To illustrate this point, consider the results of the trial performed by Sutherland *et al*,[47] who randomized 293 patients with quiescent disease to receive either 3 g/day of 5-ASA or placebo for 1 year. A total of 25% of the patients who received the active treatment experienced a relapse compared with 36% of those who received the placebo (ARR 11%, $P = 0.056$).

In an attempt to provide a more precise estimate of the magnitude of the treatment effect of 5-ASA several meta-analyses[48–50] have been performed. Some caution is warranted when considering the data from these overview analyses. First, meta-analysis is an observational procedure (unlike the RCT) which is susceptible to bias.[51] As noted previously, Singleton has documented the occurrence of publication bias with respect to the trials which evaluated 5-ASA for the therapy of active disease. Another issue is the considerable heterogeneity which exists in the published literature. The variability of study design, patient populations, and the drug formulations/doses which have been evaluated is a concern. Notwithstanding these considerations, meta-analysis does provide important information. In the most recent overview Camma[50] evaluated 15 maintenance trials, which included a total of 2097 patients (Figure 8.5). An overall ARR of 6.3% per year was identified for 5-ASA therapy in comparison to a placebo (95% CI −2.1% to −10.4 %). The results of a subgroup analysis demonstrated that the benefit of 5-ASA was most apparent in the post-surgical trials where an ARR of 13.1% was calculated (95% CI −4.5% to −21.8%). No statistically significant result was observed for those trials that evaluated 5-ASA after a medically induced remission (ARR 4.7%; 95%

CI −9.6% to 2.8%). Patients with ileal disease and prolonged disease duration were most likely to benefit from therapy.

R
Grade A

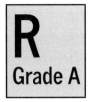

Thus a relatively clear picture of the efficacy of 5-ASA maintenance therapy has emerged. The majority of RCTs show a modest effect of treatment. If the ARR of 13% identified by the Camma meta-analysis is accepted as the best estimate of the true value of 5-ASA therapy, the NNT, the number of patients it is necessary to treat for 1 year to prevent one symptomatic recurrence of the disease, is 8. Whether a benefit of this magnitude is meaningful given the cost[51] and inconvenience of the drug depends on the patients' wishes, previous disease severity, the anatomical location of disease and whether or not maintenance treatment follows surgery.

Budesonide

The efficacy of budesonide for induction of remission in CD suggested that chronic therapy might be an effective and safe maintenance strategy. Three randomized placebo controlled trials[52–54] have evaluated the use of either 6 mg/day or 3 mg/day of budesonide for 1 year of treatment. The studies were of similar design, following treatment of active CD with either budesonide, prednisolone or a placebo. Patients who responded to treatment were randomized to receive either one of the two doses of budesonide or a placebo. No other treatments for CD were permitted. The primary outcome measure of these studies was the proportion of symptomatic relapses of CD as defined by a 60 point increase in the CDAI and a minimum CDAI score of 200 at the time of the disease exacerbation.

Greenberg *et al*[52] ($n = 105$) found that the median time to relapse or withdrawal from treatment differed significantly between the three treatment groups: budesonide treated patients remained in remission longer than those who received the placebo (178 days 6 mg vs 124 days 3 mg vs 39 days placebo; $P = 0.027$); however, the treatment effect was not durable. The greatest difference in remission rates was observed 3 months after randomization whereas at 1 year no significant differences were present (39% 6 mg vs 30% 3 mg vs 33% placebo). Budesonide therapy was well tolerated. No differences were observed among the treatment groups in the proportion of patients who experienced adverse events (78% 6 mg vs 70% 3 mg vs 89% placebo). Although glucocorticoid related adverse events occurred more frequently in patients who were treated with budesonide, the proportion of patients who reported these events decreased throughout the follow-up period and the most common steroid-related adverse event identified was easy bruising. A dose dependent depression of the plasma cortisol concentration was noted in the budesonide treated groups.

Similar results were obtained by Löfberg and colleagues[53] (n = 90) who observed that the median time to relapse or discontinuation of therapy was 258 days for the 6 mg/day group, 139 days for the 3 mg/day group, and 92 days for the patients who received a placebo ($P = 0.021$). Again, the time in remission was significantly prolonged for those patients who received budesonide, but the therapeutic effect was not sustained. At 12 months following randomization, 41%, 26%, and 37% of the 6 mg/day, 3 mg/day, and placebo group respectively remained in remission ($P = 0.44$). Thirty-eight percent of those patients who had received 6 mg/day reported glucocorticoid related adverse events compared to 20% of those who received 3 mg/day and 12% of those who received the placebo.

The third trial, by Ferguson *et al*,[54] which evaluated the smallest number of patients ($n = 75$), failed to demonstrate any benefit of budesonide treatment. The median time to

Review: Azathioprine for maintaining remission of Crohn's disease
Comparison: Antimetabolite vs. placebo: quiescent disease
Outcome: Maintenance of remission

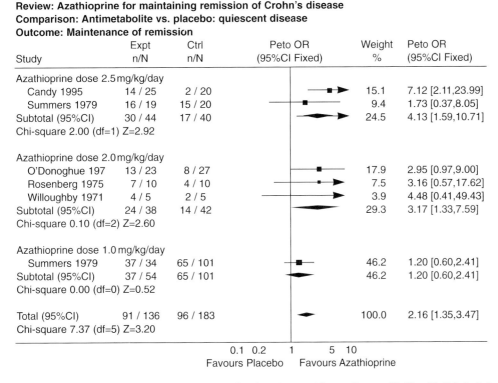

Study	Expt n/N	Ctrl n/N	Weight %	Peto OR (95%CI Fixed)
Azathioprine dose 2.5 mg/kg/day				
Candy 1995	14 / 25	2 / 20	15.1	7.12 [2.11,23.99]
Summers 1979	16 / 19	15 / 20	9.4	1.73 [0.37,8.05]
Subtotal (95%CI)	30 / 44	17 / 40	24.5	4.13 [1.59,10.71]
Chi-square 2.00 (df=1) Z=2.92				
Azathioprine dose 2.0 mg/kg/day				
O'Donoghue 197	13 / 23	8 / 27	17.9	2.95 [0.97,9.00]
Rosenberg 1975	7 / 10	4 / 10	7.5	3.16 [0.57,17.62]
Willoughby 1971	4 / 5	2 / 5	3.9	4.48 [0.41,49.43]
Subtotal (95%CI)	24 / 38	14 / 42	29.3	3.17 [1.33,7.59]
Chi-square 0.10 (df=2) Z=2.60				
Azathioprine dose 1.0 mg/kg/day				
Summers 1979	37 / 34	65 / 101	46.2	1.20 [0.60,2.41]
Subtotal (95%CI)	37 / 54	65 / 101	46.2	1.20 [0.60,2.41]
Chi-square 0.00 (df=0) Z=0.52				
Total (95%CI)	91 / 136	96 / 183	100.0	2.16 [1.35,3.47]
Chi-square 7.37 (df=5) Z=3.20				

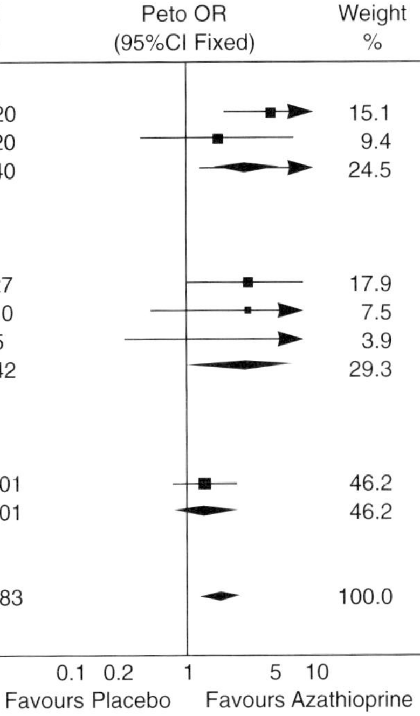

Figure 8.6 Azathioprine for maintaining remission of Crohn's disease. (*Source:* Pearson DC, May GR, Fick G *et al.* Azathioprine for maintaining remission of Crohn's disease (Cochrane Review). In: *The Cochrane Library*, issue 2, 1999. Oxford: Update Software)

relapse or discontinuation of therapy was 272 days in the 6 mg/day group, 321 days in the 3 mg/day group, and 290 days in the placebo group ($P = 0.80$). A similar proportion of patients in the three treatment groups experienced glucocorticoid related adverse events (18% 6 mg/day vs 36% 3 mg/day and 15% placebo; $P = 0.79$).

Taken collectively, these three studies suggest that budesonide treatment prolongs remission following an exacerbation of CD. An analysis of the pooled data from these trials[55] shows that on average an additional 110 days of remission is associated with the use of 6 mg/day of budesonide. Unlike the previous trials of low dose systemically active glucocorticoids, which showed no evidence for efficacy, chronic budesonide therapy was not associated with serious toxicity. The reason for the lack of a sustained benefit is currently unknown. Possible explanations such as up-regulation of the glucocorticoid receptor or enhanced drug metabolism require further evaluation. Additional trials are evaluating the use of budesonide at higher doses and with flexible dose schedules. In the meantime, the routine use of budesonide as a maintenance therapy is not recommended.

Antituberculous therapy

A recent systematic review[56] of antituberculous therapy for maintenance of remission in Crohn's disease demonstrated a possible small benefit in patients in whom remission was

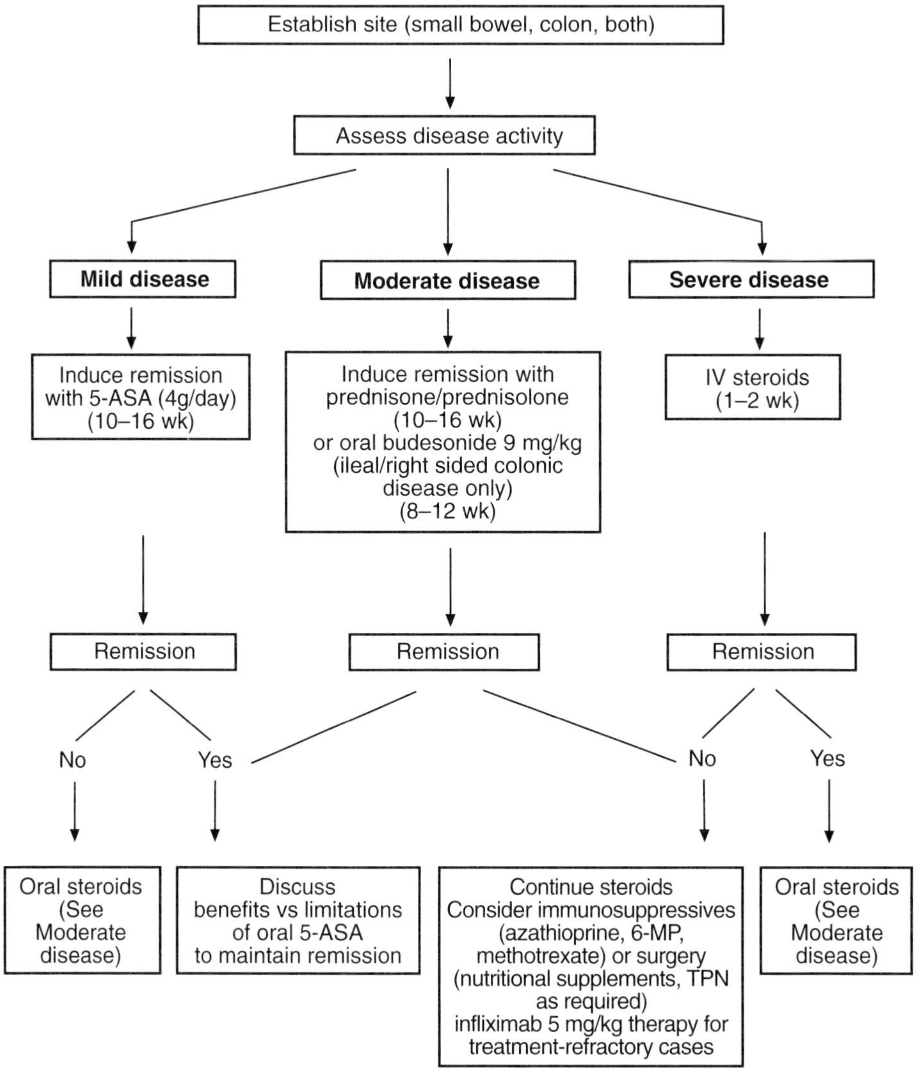

Figure 8.7 Management of Crohn's disease. Several concepts are inherent to this treatment plan. First, only a minority of patients with active disease are considered to be suitable candidates for treatment with 5-ASA. Patients with moderately severe disease and involvement of the terminal ileum and or right colon may be treated with budesonide at a dose of 9 mg/day. Patients with more extensive colonic involvement, those who fail to respond to budesonide or 5-ASA or those with severe disease activity should receive either prednisone or parenteral steroids. Failure to achieve remission with these drugs (therapy resistant disease) is an indication for treatment with either methotrexate, infliximab or surgery. Azathioprine or 6-mercaptopurine are not as attractive for the acutely ill, therapy resistant patient because of the relatively slow onset of action of these drugs. Individuals who respond to glucocorticoid therapy should be withdrawn from steroid therapy over a 12–16 week period. For individuals who attain a remission the advantages and disadvantages of 5-ASA maintenance therapy should be discussed and a decision to initiate chronic maintenance treatment with 5-ASA should be made on a case-by-case basis. In those patients who fail to successfully discontinue prednisone without a reactivation of disease activity (steroid dependent disease), the introduction of either azathioprine or methotrexate treatment is warranted. Furthermore, individuals who experience frequent relapses of the disease are candidates for long term therapy with one of the purine antimetabolites or methotrexate. Surgery remains a highly effective therapy for patients with limited disease who are experiencing adverse effects of medical therapy

induced by steroid. However, this observation was derived from a meta-analysis of subgroups from only two trials involving 90 patients, and the authors of the review do not recommend this form of therapy in the absence of further trials.

Azathioprine

A recent systematic review published by Pearson *et al*[57] analyzed the results of five randomized trials of azathioprine, of which two[58,59] studied only patients with quiescent disease and three[3,7,25] enrolled patients in a separate phase of a trial which also included patients with active disease. These trials were all relatively small, with a total of 319 patients included. The overall rate of maintenance of remission was 91/136 (67%; CI 59–75%) for treatment compared to 96/183 (52%; CI 45–60%) for placebo (Figure 8.6). The analysis suggested that higher doses of azathioprine were more effective than a dose of 1 mg/kg. The Peto odds ratio for response to azathioprine was 2.16 (CI 1.35–3.47). The number needed to treat to prevent one recurrence was 7. There was some evidence of a steroid sparing effect, although this was based on the analysis of only 30 patients in two trials. Patients who received azathioprine were at greater risk of withdrawal from studies due to adverse events compared to those on placebo (Peto odds ratio 4.36 , CI 1.63–11.67). The number needed to harm (NNH) was estimated to be 19. Withdrawals due to adverse effects were noted in 5.8% of those patients receiving therapy, and 1.3% of the patients who were not. Common events for withdrawal included pancreatitis, leukopenia, nausea, "allergy", and infection. Azathioprine appears to have a modest benefit for maintenance of remission, but there is strong evidence that a dose of 1 mg/kg is not effective.

R
Grade A

Methotrexate

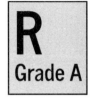

A recent multicenter trial, as yet unpublished, has evaluated the efficacy of methotrexate in a dose of 15 mg per week for maintaining remission in 76 patients with quiescent Crohn's disease. Patients were randomized if they entered remission on steroid and methotrexate as part of the induction phase of the study referred to above[40] or in an "open label" treatment period. Methotrexate was well tolerated and significantly superior to placebo in maintaining clinical remission and reducing the requirement for steroid therapy.[60]

SUMMARY

An algorithm for the treatment of Crohn's disease is given in Figure 8.7.

Although our existing medical management is relatively effective for induction of remission of CD, and improves the quality of life of the majority of patients, current therapy for maintenance of remission is less effective. A substantial proportion of patients still experience morbidity from chronically active disease, complications, or adverse effects of drug therapy. Many patients require surgery and a majority undergo more than one resection. In the future it is highly likely that drugs will become available which are able to favorably modify the natural history of the disease.

REFERENCES

1 Feagan BG, McDonald JWD, Koval JJ. Therapeutics and inflammatory bowel disease: a guide to the interpretation of randomized controlled trials. *Gastroenterology* 1996; **110**(1): 275–83.

2 Azad Khan AK, Piris J, Truelove SC. An experiment to determine the active therapeutic mocity of sulphasalazine. *Lancet* 1977; **ii**: 892–5.

3 Summers RW, Switz DM, Sessions JT Jr *et al.* National Cooperative Crohn's Disease Study: results of drug treatment. *Gastroenterology* 1979; **77**: 847–69.

4 Malchow H, Ewe K, Brandes JW *et al.* European Cooperative Crohn's Disease Study (ECCDS): results of drug treatment. *Gastroenterology* 1984; **86**: 249–66.

5 Rasmussen SN, Lauritsen K, Tage-Jensen U *et al.* 5-aminosalicylic acid in the treatment of Crohn's disease. A 16-week double blind, placebo-controlled, multicentre study with Pentasa®. *Scand J Gastroenterol* 1987; **22**: 877–83.

6 Mahida YR, Jewell DP. Slow-release 5-amino-salicylic acid (Pentasa) for the treatment of active Crohn's disease. *Digestion* 1990; **45**(2): 88–92.

7 Singleton JW, Hanauer SB, Gitnick GL *et al.* Mesalamine capsules for the treatment of active Crohn's disease: results of a 16-week trial. *Gastroenterology* 1993; **104**: 1293–301.

8 Singleton J. Second trial of mesalamine therapy in the treatment of active Crohn's disease. *Gastroenterology* 1994; **107**(2): 632–3.

9 Schölmerich J, Jenss H, Hartmann F *et al.* The German 5-ASA Study Group. Oral 5-aminosalicylic acid versus 6-methylprednisolone in active Crohn's disease. *Can J Gastroenterol* 1990; **4**(7): 446–51.

10 Martin F, Sutherland L, Beck IT *et al.* Oral 5-ASA versus prednisone in short term treatment of Crohn's disease: a multicentre controlled trial. *Can J Gastroenterol* 1990; **4**(7): 452–7.

11 Maier K, Frick H-J, von Gaisberg U, Teufel T, Klotz U. Clinical efficacy of oral mesalazine in Crohn's disease. *Can J Gastroenterol* 1990; **4**(1): 13–18.

12 Thomsen OO, Cortot A, Jewell D *et al.* Budesonide CIR is more effective than mesalazine in active Crohn's disease. A 16 week, international randomized, double-blind multicenter trial. *AGA Abstracts* 1996; **112**(4): A1104.

13 Prantera C, Pallone F, Brunetti G, Cottone M, Miglioli M, The Italian IBD Study Group. Oral 5-aminosalicylic acid (Asacol) in the maintenance treatment of Crohn's disease. *Gastroenterology* 1992; **103**: 363–8.

14 Gross V, Andus T, Fischbach W *et al.* Comparison between high dose 5-aminosalicylic acid and 6-methylprednisolone in active Crohn's ileocolitis. A multicenter randomized double-blind study. *Z Gastroenterol* 1995; **33**(10): 581–4.

15 Fahey JV, Guyer PM, Munck A. Mechanisms of anti-inflammatory actions of glucocorticoids. In: Weissman G (ed), *Advances in inflammation research, 2.* New York: Raven Press, 1981: pp 21–51.

16 Singleton JW, Law DH, Kelley ML *et al.* National Cooperative Crohn's Disease Study: adverse reactions to study drugs. *Gastroenterology* 1979; **77**: 870–82.

17 Hamedani R, Feldman RD, Feagan BG. Review article: drug development in inflammatory bowel disease: budesonide – a model of targeted therapy. *Aliment Pharmacol Ther* 1997; **3** (Suppl): 98–108.

18 Brattsand R. Overview of newer gluco-corticosteroid preparations for inflammatory bowel disease. *Can J Gastroenterol* 1990; **4**: 407–14.

19 Pauwels RA, Lofdahl CG, Postma DS *et al.* Effect of inhaled formoterol and budesonide on exacerbations of asthma. Formoterol and Corticosteroids Establishing Therapy (FACET) International Study Group. *N Engl J Med* 1997; **337**(20): 1405–11.

20 Greenberg GR, Feagan BG, Martin F *et al.* Oral budesonide for active Crohn's disease. Canadian Inflammatory Bowel Disease Study Group. *N Engl J Med* 1994; **331**: 836–41.

21 Rutgeerts P, Lofberg R, Malchow H *et al.* A comparison of budesonide with prednisolone for active Crohn's disease. *N Engl J Med* 1994; **331**(13): 842–5.

22 Herfarth HH, Mohanty SP, Rath HC, Tonkonogy S, Sartor RB. Interleukin 10 suppresses experimental chronic, granulomatous inflammation induced by bacterial cell wall polymers. *Gut* 1996; **39**(96): 836–45.

23 Duchmann R, Schmitt E, Knolle P *et al.* Tolerance towards resident intestinal flora in mice is abrogated in experimental colitis and restored by treatment with interleukin-10 or antibodies to interleukin-12. *Eur J Immunol* 1996; **26**: 934–8.

24 Ursing B, Alm T, Barany F *et al.* A comparative study of metronidazole and sulfasalazine for active Crohn's disease: the Cooperative Crohn's Disease Study in Sweden II. Result. *Gastroenterology* 1982; **83**: 550–62.

25 Sutherland L, Singleton J, Sessions J *et al.* Double blind, placebo controlled trial of metronidazole in Crohn' s disease. *Gut* 1991; **32**: 1071–5.

26 Prantera C, Zannoni F, Scribano ML *et al.* An antibiotic regimen for the treatment of active Crohn's disease: a randomized, controlled clinical trial of metronidazole plus ciprofloxacin. *Am J Gastroenterol* 1996; **2**: 328–32.

27 Munkholm P, Langholz E, Davidsen *et al.* Disease activity courses in a regional cohort of Crohn's disease patients. *Scand J Gastroenterol* 1995; **30**(7): 699–706.
28 Candy S, Wright J, Gerber M *et al.* A controlled double blind study of azathioprine in the management of Crohn's disease. *Gut* 1995; **37**: 674–8.
29 Sandborn WJ, Van O EC, Zins BJ *et al.* An intravenous loading dose of azathioprine decreases the time to response in patients with Crohn's disease. *Gastroenterology* 1995; **109**(6): 1808–17.
30 Sandborn WJ, Tremaine WJ, Wolf DC *et al.* Lack of effect of intravenous administration on time response to azathioprine for steroid treated Crohn's disease. *Gastroenterology* 1999; **117**: 527–35.
31 Sandborn WJ, Sutherland L, Pearson D *et al.* Azathioprine or 6-mercaptopurine for inducing remission of Crohn's disease. In: *The Cochrane Library* (database on disk and CD-ROM). Oxford: The Cochrane Collaboration. Update Software; 1999, issue 2.
32 Brynskov J, Freund L, Rasmussen SN *et al.* A placebo-controlled, double-blind, randomized trial of cyclosporine therapy in active chronic Crohn's disease. *N Engl J Med* 1989; **321**(13): 845–50.
33 Feagan BG. Cyclosporine has no proven role as a therapy for Crohn's disease. *Inflamm Bowel Dis* 1995; **1**: 335–9.
34 Jewell DP, Lennard-Jones JE, the Cyclosporin Study Group of Great Britain and Ireland. Oral cyclosporin for chronic active Crohn's disease: a multicentre controlled trial. *Eur J Gastroenterol Hepatol* 1994; **6**: 499–505.
35 Stange EF, Modigliani R, Peña AS *et al.* European trial of cyclosporin in chronic active Crohn's disease: a 12-month study. *Gastroenterology* 1995; **109**: 774–82.
36 Feutren G, Mihatsch MJ. Risk factors for cyclosporine-induced nephrotoxicity in patients with autoimmune diseases. International Kidney Biopsy Registry of Cyclosporine in Autoimmune Diseases. *N Engl J Med* 1992; **326**(25): 1654–60.
37 Hanauer SB, Smith MB. Rapid closure of Crohn's disease fistulas with continuous intravenous cyclosporin A. *Am J Gastroenterol* 1993; **88**: 646–9.
38 Present DH, Lichtiger S. Efficacy of cyclosporine in treatment of fistula of Crohn's disease. *Dig Dis Sci* 1994; **39**(2): 374–80.
39 Kozarek RA, Patterson DJ, Geland MD *et al.* Methotrexate induces clinical and histologic remission in patients with refractory inflammatory bowel disease. *Ann Intern Med* 1989; **110**: 353–6.
40 Feagan BG, Rochon J, Fedorak RN *et al.* Methotrexate for the treatment of Crohn's disease. *N Engl J Med* 1995; **332**: 292–7.
41 Van Deventer SJH. Tumour necrosis factor and Crohn's disease. *Gut* 1997; **40**: 443–8.
42 Derkx HHF, Taminiau J, Radema SA *et al.* Tumour necrosis factor antibody treatment in Crohn's disease. *Lancet* 1993; **342**: 173–4.
43 Targan SR, Hanauer SB, van Deventer SJH *et al.* A short-term study of chimeric monoclonal antibody cA2 to tumor necrosis factor α for Crohn's disease. *N Engl J Med* 1997; **337**: 1029–35.
44 Present DH, Rutgeerts P, Targan S *et al.* Infliximab for the treatment of fistulas in patients with Crohn's disease. *New Engl J Med* 1999; **340**(6): 1398–405.
45 Feagan BG. Aminosalicylates for active disease and in the maintenance of remission in Crohn's disease. *Eur J Surg* 1998; **164**(12): 903–9.
46 Lapidus A, Bernell O, Hellers G, Lofberg R. Clinical course of colorectal Crohn's disease: a 35-year follow-up study of 507 patients. *Gastroenterology* 1998; **114**(6): 1151–60.
47 Sutherland LR, Martin F, Bailey RJ *et al.* A randomized, placebo-controlled, double-blind trial of mesalamine in the maintenance of remission of Crohn's disease. *Gastroenterology* 1997; **112**(4): 1069–77.
48 Messori A, Brignola C, Trallori G *et al.* Effectiveness of 5-aminosalicylic acid for maintaining remission in patients with Crohn's disease: a meta-analysis. *Am J Gastroenterol* 1994; **89**(5): 692–8.
49 Steinhart AH, Hemphill D, Greenberg GR. Sulfasalazine and mesalamine for the maintenance therapy of Crohn's disease: a meta-analysis. *Am J Gastroenterol* 1994; **89**(12): 2116–24.
50 Camma C, Giunta M, Roselli M *et al.* Mesalamine in the maintenance treatment of Crohn's disease: a meta-analysis adjusted for confounding variables. *Gastroenterology* 1997; **13**: 1465–73.
51 Trallori G, Messori A. Drug treatments for maintaining remission in Crohn's disease: a lifetime cost–utility analysis. *Pharmaco Economics* 1997; **11**(5): 444–53.
52 Greenberg G, Feagan B, Martin F *et al.* Oral budesonide as maintenance treatment for Crohn's disease: a placebo-controlled, dose-ranging study. Canadian Inflammatory Bowel Disease Study Group. *Gastroenterology* 1996; **110**(1): 45–51.
53 Löfberg R, Rutgeerts P, Malchow H *et al.* Budesonide prolongs time to relapse in ileal and ileocaecal Crohn's disease. A placebo controlled one year study. *Gut* 1996; **39**(1): 82–6.

54 Ferguson A, Campieri M, Doe W *et al.* Oral budesonide as maintenance therapy in Crohn's disease – results of a 12 month study. *Aliment Pharmacol Ther* 1998; **12**: 175–83.
55 Feagan BG, Greenburg GR, Lofberg R *et al.* Budesonide controlled Ileal release prolongs remission in Crohn's disease: a pooled analysis. *Gastroenterology* 1997; **112**(Suppl): A970.
56 Borgaonkar M, MacIntosh D, Fardy J *et al.* Antituberculous therapy for maintaining remission of Crohn's disease. In: *The Cochrane Library* (database on disk and CD-ROM). Oxford: The Cochrane Collaboration. Update Software; 1999, issue 2.
57 Pearson DC, May GR, Fick G *et al.* Azathioprine for maintaining remission of Crohn's disease. In: *The Cochrane Library* (database on disk and CD-ROM). Oxford: The Cochrane Collaboration. Update Software; 1999, issue 2.
58 Rosenberg JL, Levin B, Wall AJ *et al.* A controlled trial of azathioprine in Crohn's disease. *Am J Dig Dis* 1975; **20**: 721–6.
59 O'Donoghue DP, Dawson AM, Powell-Tuck J *et al.* Double-blind withdrawal trial of azathioprine as maintenance treatment for Crohn's disease. *Lancet* 1978; **ii**: 955–7.
60 Feagan BG, McDonald J, Hopkins M et al. A randomized controlled trial of methotrexate (MTX) as a maintenance therapy for chronically active Crohn's disease (CD). *Gut* 1999; in press (abstract).

Ulcerative colitis: diagnosis, prognosis, and treatment

9

DEREK P JEWELL, LLOYD R SUTHERLAND

INTRODUCTION

Patients with ulcerative colitis have a variety of questions for those practitioners who treat their disease. This chapter focusses on the evidence on which decisions relating to patient advice (prognosis for the first attack, extension of disease, risk of cancer) and treatment options should be made. Our recommendations have been based wherever possible on evidence from published population based studies and from randomized controlled clinical trials. Where several clinical trials have addressed the same question we have frequently used meta-analyses to summarize results.

HISTOLOGICAL DIAGNOSIS

The diagnosis of ulcerative colitis and Crohn's disease together with accurate differentiation between them and other inflammatory diseases of the colon relies on a combination of clinical, radiological, endoscopic, and histological features. Accurate histological interpretation is crucial but is confounded by at least four major problems:

1 Variability in assessing normal colorectal histology and assessing minimal degrees of information.
2 Considerable overlap in the histological changes of most colonic inflammatory conditions.
3 The accuracy and reproducibility of many histological features commonly used for diagnosis have not been determined.
4 An absence of standard nomenclature.

Recently a working party of the British Society of Gastroenterology has published guidelines for the biopsy diagnosis of suspected chronic inflammatory bowel disease.[1] Databases were searched for papers relating to reproducibility, sensitivity, and specificity of histological features used for the differential diagnosis of inflammatory bowel disease. Only those achieving moderate reproducibility (a minimum kappa statistic of 0.4 or a percentage agreement of 80% or more) were included. Precise definitions of mucosal architectural changes, lamina propria cellularity, neutrophil infiltration, and epithelial cell abnormalities were derived from the systematic review of the literature. Then the quality of the evidence for these features with respect to differential diagnosis was rated according to the criteria recommended by the Evidence Based Working Party. Figure 9.1 lists those features for which the literature review provided high quality evidence for their use in differential diagnosis. Such guidelines should prove very valuable in clinical practice and should provide for much improved consistency in reporting biopsy specimens.

Normal or inflamed?
Normal crypt density
Crypt architecture not disturbed
Normal density, distribution of cells within lamina propria
No neutrophil infiltration
Surface epithelium – columnar not intact
Goblet cells – normal mucin content**

Chronic IBD (UC, CD, indeterminate)
Crypt architectural distortion
Crypt density decreased
Surface irregular
Increased cellularity of lamina propria – transmucosal or discontinuous
Epithelial granulomas
Surface epithelial flattening
Neutrophil infiltration**

Acute infective colitis
Crypt architecture normal
Lamina propria – superficial increase of cellularity
Neutrophil infiltration**
Mucin depletion**
Discontinuous inflammation**
Focal cryptitis**

Ulcerative colitis
Crypt distortion severe
Crypt density – severity reduced and widespread
Villous surface
Lamina propria cellularity
– diffuse and transmural
– dense
Mucin depletion severe**

Crohn's disease
Epithelial granulomas
Crypt distortion focal
Inflammation discontinuous**
Cryptitis focal*

Note: All features have the highest quality of evidence except for:
**evidence of diagnostic value from single studies only
*no published evidence of accuracy or reproducibility

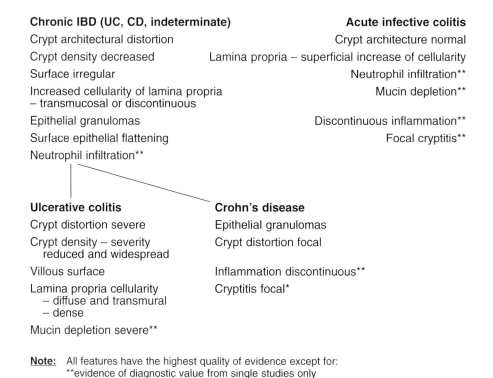

Figure 9.1 Evidence based features for histological diagnosis of colonic biopsy specimens. (IBD, inflammatory bowel disease; UC, ulcerative colitis; CD, Crohn's disease)

PROGNOSIS

Population based studies

The importance of recognizing that the prognosis for referred patients differs from that of a regional population was recognized by Truelove and Pena nearly two decades ago.[2] They found that the survival of patients who were referred to Oxford (UK) from other regions was significantly reduced compared to that of patients who actually resided in the Oxford catchment area.

There are several population based studies regarding the prognosis for patients with ulcerative colitis. Sinclair and associates described the prognosis of 537 patients with ulcerative colitis, seen between 1967 and 1976 in northeastern Scotland.[3] They found a high proportion of cases with distal disease (70%). The overall mortality and surgical resection rates in the first attack were both 3%. During this period of time, the mortality rate for severe, first time attacks was 23%. However, there were only modest differences in the observed/expected mortality rates for the ulcerative colitis population. The colectomy rate after 5 years was 8%.

The prognosis and mortality associated with ulcerative colitis in Stockholm county was reported by Persson *et al.*[4] In their review of 1547 patients followed from 1955 to 1984, they found that the mortality rate in the patient population was higher than the rate expected in the general population. After 15 years of follow-up, the survival rate was 94% of that expected based on the study population's age and gender. The relative survival rates differed more for patients with pancolitis than for patients with proctitis, but the confidence intervals overlapped. While ulcerative colitis was the most important influence on the increased mortality rate, deaths from colorectal cancer, asthma, and non-alcoholic liver disease were also increased.

Danish investigators have also reported the results of their population based assessment of the prognosis of ulcerative colitis. Their population included 1161 patients with ulcerative colitis followed for up to 25 years (median 11 years).[5] Of the 1161 patients, 235 underwent colectomy. Interestingly, 60 of these patients presented with proctosigmoiditis initially. The cumulative colectomy rate was 9%, 24%, 30%, and 32% at 1, 10, 15, and 25 years after diagnosis. At any one time, nearly half of the clinic population was in remission. Prognostic factors associated with frequent relapses included: the number of relapses in the first 3 years after diagnosis and the year of diagnosis (1960s vs 1970s, vs 1980s). Surprisingly, signs and symptoms of weight loss or fever were associated with fewer relapses on follow-up.

A more recent report by the same investigators focussed on the prognosis in children with ulcerative colitis.[6] Eighty of the 1161 patients in the cohort were children who presented with more extensive disease compared to adults. The cumulative colectomy rate did not differ from that of adults (29% at 20 years). At any interval from diagnosis, the majority of children were thought to be in remission.

Extension of disease

Ayres and associates reported their experience with extension of disease in 145 patients presenting with proctitis or proctosigmoiditis, followed prospectively for a median of 11 years. By life table analysis, extension occurred in 16% and 31% of patients at 5 and 10 years of follow-up, respectively. Extension was associated with a clinical exacerbation of disease in most cases but no specific clinical factors were associated with disease extension.[7]

While research for the most part has focussed on extension of disease, Langholz and colleagues report a much more dynamic pattern. After 25 years of follow-up, 53% of patients with limited disease had extension of disease, but in 75% of patients with extensive disease, the disease boundary had regressed.[8] This dynamic process, if confirmed by others, could have implications in terms of cancer surveillance programs. A potential explanation for these findings could be that in the early years of the study, disease extent was assessed by radiological techniques.

CANCER SURVEILLANCE (see also Chapter 12)

Although ulcerative colitis is a premalignant condition, the proportion of patients who develop cancer is small. In a population study using a retrospectively assembled cohort of patients the cumulative risk at 20 years of disease was about 7% and rose to 12% at 30 years.[9] This study is likely to have included all or nearly all patients with ulcerative colitis in two regions of England and one of Sweden and referral bias is probably minimal. Follow-up was both of long duration (17–38 years) and thorough (97%). On the other hand, in centres with an aggressive policy of colectomy, no increased cancer risk has been seen.[10] In all studies, length of history and extent of disease are important factors. Thus, left-sided colitis carries only a slightly increased risk while extensive colitis increases the risk about 20 times over that of an age- and sex-matched population. Whether early age of onset of ulcerative colitis is an independent risk factor is controversial. Children tend to have extensive disease and have a greater life expectancy than adults; they are, therefore, more likely to be at risk.

The major controversy concerns the role of colonoscopic surveillance in order to detect cancer. Most centers perform colonoscopy in patients with extensive disease after 8–10 years from diagnosis. Even at that stage, a few patients with dysplasia or a frank carcinoma will be identified. However, the subsequent pickup rate during the surveillance program is small – about 11% – and in one center only two cancers were detected in 200 patients over a 20-year period.[11] Furthermore, cancers can develop outside the screening program. Thus, the need for colonoscopic surveillance has been questioned and no controlled study has shown that surveillance reduces mortality. However, in the published studies, the 5-year survival rates for cancers detected in asymptomatic patients have been considerably higher than those presenting with symptoms.

R
Grade C

Reviewing the evidence for dysplasia surveillance, Riddell recommends obtaining three to four biopsies every 10 cm.[12] Annual colonoscopy is probably ideal, but 2-yearly colonoscopy with intervening flexible sigmoidoscopy on alternate years is a compromise. Dysplasia detected at the initial screening colonoscopy should lead to colectomy as there is a high chance of concomitant cancer. Indeed, most clinicians advocate colectomy whenever dysplasia is found, even when it is low grade. There is no doubt that such a policy abolishes the cancer risk but justification for it for patients with low grade dysplasia is based more on anecdote than on evidence.

TREATMENT

Discussion of treatment options for ulcerative colitis may be conveniently divided by categories or classes of medication and further grouped into the induction or the maintenance of remission.

Aminosalicylates

With the discovery of sulfasalazine by Svartz,[13] the first effective agent for the treatment of ulcerative colitis became available. The first trial to establish the efficacy of sulfasalazine for the *induction of remission* was reported in 1962.[14] Misiewicz and colleagues were the first to report the efficacy of sulfasalazine as *maintenance therapy*.[15] An early randomized trial performed in the United Kingdom established the importance of continuous

Review: Ulc. colitis: induction of remission, 5-ASA
Comparison: 5-ASA vs. placebo
Outcome: Failure to induce global/clinical remission

Study	Expt n/N	Ctrl n/N	Weight %	Peto OR (95%CI Fixed)
Dose of 5-ASA: <2 g				
Hanauer 1993	73 / 92	26 / 30	13.8	0.62 [0.22,1.78]
Schroeder 1986	10 / 11	36 / 38	2.0	0.52 [0.03,8.31]
Sninsky 1991	47 / 53	25 / 28	5.6	0.40 [0.08,2.07]
Subtotal (95%CI)	130 / 156	87 / 94	21.4	0.55 [0.23,1.27]
Chi-square 0.20 (df=2) Z=1.41				
Dose of 5-ASA: 2–2.9 g				
Hanauer 1993	69 / 97	26 / 30	17.2	0.44 [0.17,1.13]
Hanauer 1996	81 / 92	39 / 45	13.1	1.13 [0.39,3.33]
Sninsky 1991	47 / 53	25 / 26	5.6	0.40 [0.08,2.07]
Subtotal (95%CI)	197 / 242	90 / 101	35.9	0.61 [0.32,1.17]
Chi-square 1.98 (df=2) Z=1.48				
Dose of 5-ASA: ≥3 g				
Hanauer 1993	67 / 95	27 / 30	17.0	0.35 [0.14,0.91]
Hanauer 1996	75 / 91	39 / 45	16.3	0.73 [0.28,1.93]
Schroeder 1986	29 / 38	36 / 38	9.4	0.23 [0.06,0.82]
Subtotal (95%CI)	171 / 224	102 / 113	42.6	0.43 [0.23,0.77]
Chi-square 2.25 (df=2) Z=2.81				
Total (95%CI)	498 / 622	279 / 306	100.0	0.51 [0.35,0.76]
Chi-square 5.12 (df=8) Z=3.37				

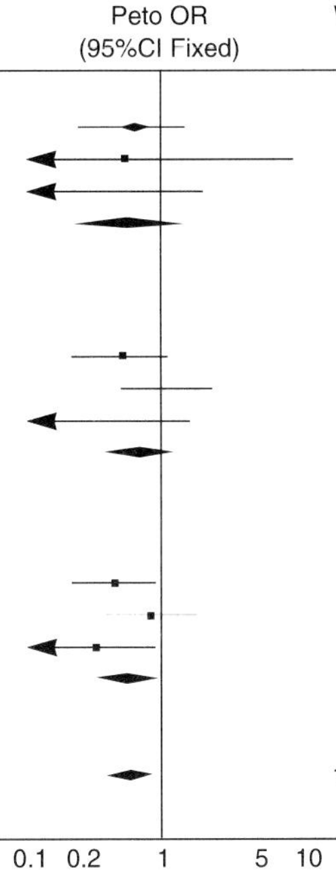

(a)

Review: Ulc. colitis: induction of remission, 5-ASA
Comparison: 5-ASA vs. sulfasalazine
Outcome: Failure to induce global/clinical remission

Study	Expt n/N	Ctrl n/N	Weight %	Peto OR (95%CI Fixed)
5-ASA / SASP < 1/2				
Riley 1988	14 / 20	7 / 9	5.7	0.69 [0.12,3.87]
Subtotal (95%CI)	14 / 20	7 / 9	5.7	0.69 [0.12,3.87]
Chi-square 0.00 (df=0) Z=0.43				
1/1 > 5-ASA / SASP ≥ 1/2				
Andreoli 1987	2 / 6	3 / 6	3.5	0.53 [0.06,4.80]
Rachmilewitz 1989	78 / 115	70 / 105	54.1	1.05 [0.60,1.85]
Rijk 1991	13 / 27	17 / 28	15.5	0.61 [0.21,1.74]
Subtotal (95%CI)	93 / 148	90 / 139	73.2	0.91 [0.56,1.47]
Chi-square 1.05 (df=2) Z=0.39				
5-ASA / SASP ≥ 1/1				
Green 1993	6 / 28	12 / 29	14.0	0.40 [0.13,1.22]
Riley 1988	12 / 21	8 / 10	7.1	0.38 [0.08,1.79]
Subtotal (95%CI)	18 / 49	20 / 39	21.1	0.40 [0.16,0.97]
Chi-square 0.00 (df=1) Z=2.02				
Total (95%CI)	125 / 217	117 / 187	100.0	0.75 [0.50,1.13]
Chi-square 3.60 (df=5) Z=1.37				

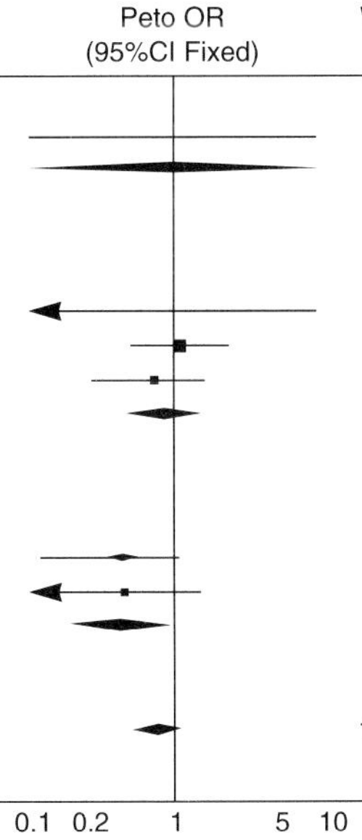

(b)

Figure 9.2 Failure to induce clinical or endoscopic remission in ulcerative colitis. Randomized controlled clinical trials of mesalamine (5-ASA) and sulfasalazine (SASP): (a) mesalamine (Expt) vs placebo (Ctrl); (b) mesalamine (Expt) vs sulfasalazine (Ctrl). (Source: Ulcerative Colitis: induction of remission (Cochrane Review). In : *The Cochrane Library*, Issue 2, 1999. Oxford: Update Software)

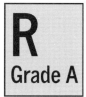

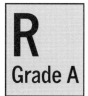

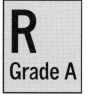

R Grade A

sulfasalazine therapy.[16] Azad Khan and the Oxford group established that 2 g of sulfasalazine offered the optimal tradeoff between efficacy and the adverse events associated with sulfasalazine therapy.[17]

The subsequent finding that mesalamine (5-ASA) was the active moiety of sulfasalazine[18,19] stimulated a decade of trials for induction and maintenance of remission. Numerous aminosalicylate delivery systems have been developed. They include those that require bacterial splitting of the azo bond (sulfasalazine, olsalazine, balsalazide), pH dependent release formulations, such as Asacol (pH = 7) and Claversal/Mesasal/Salofalk (pH = 6), and microspheres (Pentasa).[20]

R Grade A

The efficacy of oral mesalamine has been evaluated by meta-analyses of randomized controlled trials.[21–23] Figure 9.2a shows that mesalamine is more effective than placebo for the *induction of remission*[22] (pooled odds ratio 0.52; CI 0.35–0.77). When compared to the older medication sulfasalazine, no statistically significant difference in effectiveness was demonstrated for the newer 5-ASA preparations. (pooled odds ratio 0.75; CI 0.50–1.13) (Figure 9.2b). However, adverse effects were observed less frequently with the newer preparations (NNT, the number of patients needed to treat with a newer 5-ASA compound rather than sulfasalazine to avoid an adverse effect in one patient is approximately 7).

R Grade A

Figure 9.3a shows the result of the meta-analysis[23] which demonstrates that the aminosalicylates are more effective than placebo for maintenance of remission (pooled odds ratio 0.48; CI 0.35–0.65). When sulfasalazine and mesalamine were compared for their effectiveness for maintenance therapy, the results were conflicting. Figure 9.3b shows that, overall, sulfasalazine appeared to be more effective than mesalamine (pooled odds ratio 1.29; CI 1.06–1.57)). When the analysis was restricted to studies that had a minimum of 12 months' follow-up, there was no statistically significant advantage for sulfasalazine (pooled odds ratio 1.15; CI 0.89–1.50). There are a variety of explanations for the difference in results. First the observation in the overall analysis may be correct, and sulfasalazine is a more effective delivery system. Second, the analysis restricted to a 12 month follow-up may lack the statistical power to detect a subtle difference. Third, the high dropout rate associated with olsalazine therapy may have biassed the overall results against mesalamine. Finally, it should be noted that studies that compare sulphasalazine with newer 5-ASA compounds for either induction or maintenance of remission, may suffer from a selection bias. With the exception of one trial,[24] the inclusion criteria included tolerance of sulfasalazine. This factor would tend to minimize the occurrence of adverse events associated with sulfasalazine therapy.

Topical therapy is an attractive option for patients with disease limited to the distal colon. In theory, it presents a high concentration of mesalamine to the affected area, while minimizing systemic absorption. Marshall and associates have published two meta-analyses of topical therapy. In the first, they established that topical therapy with mesalamine was effective for both induction and maintenance of remission in patients with distal disease.[25] A recent follow-up study reported that mesalamine was more effective than topical corticosteroids for the induction of remission.[26]

Corticosteroids

CONVENTIONAL STEROIDS

Corticosteroids remain the standard of therapy for the treatment of moderate to severe ulcerative colitis. Truelove and Witts were the first to perform a randomized controlled

Review: Ulc. colitis: maintenance of remission, 5-ASA
Comparison: 5-ASA vs. placebo
Outcome: Failure to maintain clinical or endoscopic remission

Study	Expt n/N	Ctrl n/N	Weight %	Peto OR (95%CI Fixed)
Dose of 5-ASA: <1 g				
Hanauer 1996	50 / 90	31 / 43	13.6	0.50 [0.24,1.05]
Subtotal (95%CI)	50 / 90	31 / 43	13.6	0.50 [0.24,1.05]
Chi-square 0.00 (df=0) Z=0.1.82				
Dose of 5-ASA: 1–1.9 g				
Hanauer 1996	49 / 87	31 / 44	13.7	0.56 [0.28,1.16]
Hawkey 1997	40 / 99	66 / 111	25.6	0.47 [0.27,0.80]
Sandberg 1986	12 / 52	22 / 49	11.1	0.38 [0.17,0.86]
Subtotal (95%CI)	101 / 238	119 / 204	50.4	0.47 [0.32,0.69]
Chi-square 0.45 (df=2) Z=3.86				
Dose of 5-ASA: ≥2 g				
Miner 1995	44 / 103	68 / 102	24.9	0.38 [0.22,0.66]
Wright 1993	31 / 49	36 / 52	11.1	0.77 [0.34,1.75]
Subtotal (95%CI)	75 / 152	104 / 154	36.0	0.47 [0.30,0.75]
Chi-square 1.91 (df=1) Z=3.21				
Total (95%CI)	226 / 480	254 / 401	100.0	0.47 [0.36,0.62]
Chi-square 2.39 (df=5) Z=5.33				

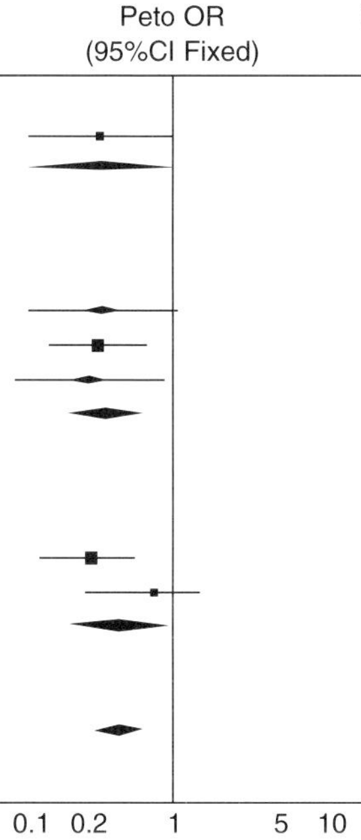

(a)

Review: Ulc. colitis: maintenance remission, 5-ASA
Comparison: 5-ASA vs. sulfasalazine
Outcome: Failure to maintain clinical or endoscopic remission

Study	Expt n/N	Ctrl n/N	Weight %	Peto OR (95%CI Fixed)
Andreoli 1987	3 / 7	1 / 6	0.8	3.11 [0.32,30.11]
Ardizzone 1989	20 / 44	27 / 44	5.7	0.53 [0.23,1.22]
Ireland 1988	35 / 82	21 / 82	9.6	2.13 [1.12,4.05]
Killerich 1992	61 / 114	55 / 112	14.7	1.19 [0.71,2.01]
Kruis 1995	39 / 108	13 / 40	6.9	1.17 [0.55,2.50]
McIntyre 1988	20 / 41	14 / 38	5.1	1.62 [0.67,3.92]
Mulder 1988	19 / 42	20 / 36	5.1	0.67 [0.27,1.61]
Nilsson 1995	88 / 161	76 / 161	20.9	1.35 [0.87,2.08]
Rijk 1992	14 / 23	11 / 23	3.0	1.67 [0.53,5.27]
Riley 1988	20 / 50	23 / 60	6.4	0.78 [0.36,1.73]
Rutgeerts 1989	90 / 167	70 / 167	21.7	1.61 [1.05,2.48]
Total (95%CI)	409 / 839	331 / 759	100.0	1.29 [1.05,1.57]
Chi-square 12.61 (df=10) Z=2.47				

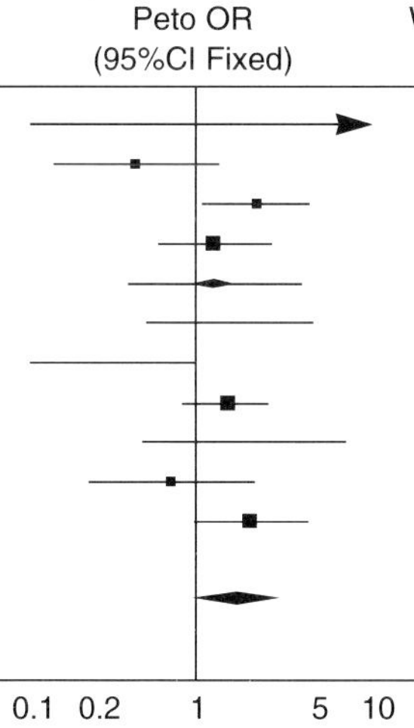

(b)

Figure 9.3 Failure to maintain clinical or endoscopic remission in ulcerative colitis. Randomized controlled clinical trials of mesalamine (5-ASA) and sulfasalazine: (a) mesalamine (Expt) vs placebo (Ctrl); (b) mesalamine (Expt) vs sulfasalazine (Ctrl). (Source: Ulcerative Colitis: maintenance of remission (Cochrane Review). In: *The Cochrane Library*, Issue 2, 1999. Oxford: Update Software)

trial of cortisone (100 mg/day tapering over 6 weeks) in patients with active ulcerative colitis.[27] Grade A

Lennard-Jones and associates reported similar efficacy for prednisone.[28] The assumption that there is no additional benefit from the use of doses of prednisone greater than 40 mg/day is based on a small comparative trial by Baron and associates.[29] Grade A This trial compared the outcomes of 58 outpatients randomized to 20, 40 or 60 mg of prednisone per day. Although it was possible to show that both the 40 and 60 mg doses produced better results than the 20 mg/day regimen, no difference between the groups receiving 40 and 60 mg was demonstrated. However, the trial had insufficient power to rule out a beneficial effect of the higher dose. The frequency of taking steroids (once a day or in divided doses) does not appear to influence efficacy.[30]

Budesonide is a potent second generation corticosteroid with 90% first pass metabolism.[31] The results of the first randomized controlled trial (RCT) using a targeted colonic release formulation have been reported.[32] Budesonide appeared to be as effective as prednisolone and also exhibited a better adverse event profile.

Budesonide enemas have also been used in active distal disease. The meta-analysis by Marshall and Irvine reported that budesonide enemas were as effective as conventional steroid preparations.[25] Grade A To date, only one published trial has compared budesonide enemas with 5-ASA enemas.[33] This study revealed no differences in endoscopic or histopathological scores between the treatment groups, but the clinical remission rate was superior for the 5-ASA group (budesonide 38%, 5-ASA 60 %, $P = 0.03$).

There is no evidence to recommend the use of corticosteroids for maintenance of remission. Most reported trials have identified no benefit.[34–36] Grade A

Immunosuppressive therapy

AZATHIOPRINE

Few trials of azathioprine therapy have been performed in ulcerative colitis and, in general, they have been small. There is no evidence that azathioprine (2.5 mg/kg) combined with prednisolone induces remission more effectively than steroids alone.[37] Nevertheless, for chronic active disease requiring continuing steroid therapy, azathioprine has been shown to have a steroid-sparing effect at doses between 1.5 and 2.5 mg/kg, and this has now become the main indication for using the drug in this disease.[38,39] In the double-blind RCT of Jewell and Truelove, patients who had gone into remission during the acute stage were weaned off steroids, but continued on maintenance therapy with azathioprine or placebo for a year. Overall there was no statistically significant benefit for azathioprine in terms of reducing the relapse rate. However, subgroup analysis of the stratum which was randomized during a relapse of established disease, as opposed to the stratum which was randomized during the initial attack, suggested that there was some benefit in the former group (Table 9.1). Thus, 9 of 24 azathioprine-treated patients in this stratum had no relapses during follow-up compared with only 3 of 25 patients in the placebo group. More detailed *post hoc* analysis revealed that only 7 of the azathioprine group had three relapses or failed compared with 15 of those in the placebo group ($P = 0.055$). This subgroup analysis involving rather small numbers of patients must be interpreted with caution.

R Grade C

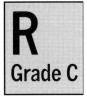

A possible benefit of azathioprine for maintenance of remission was also supported by the withdrawal trial of Hawthorne *et al.*[40] In this study, patients in remission on long term

Table 9.1 Clinical course during **trial** in two treatment groups of patients according to whether patients entered trial in first attack of ulcerative colitis or in relapse. Reproduced from *Br Med J* 1947; 14 December: 629

	Admitted in first attack		Admitted in relapses	
No. of relapses	Azathioprine group	Control group	Azathioprine group	Control group
0	7	6	9	3
1-2	5	6	8	7
3 or failed	4	3	7	15
Total	16	15	24	25
Significance of differences*	NS		$P = 0.055$	

*Fisher's exact test.

azathioprine therapy were randomized to continue azathioprine or to receive a placebo. During the subsequent year of follow-up, patients receiving placebo relapsed significantly more often than those who remained on azathioprine. It should be pointed out, however, that this type of trial design cannot be used to estimate the size of the treatment effect resulting from an intervention. It is possible that only a small proportion of patients can be maintained in remission with azathioprine, yet most of these would relapse if the drug were withdrawn. The use of azathioprine to prevent relapse in ulcerative colitis is based on comparatively weak evidence.

R Grade A

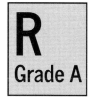

There have been no formal randomized controlled trials of 6-mercaptopurine, as distinct from azathioprine, in ulcerative colitis.

METHOTREXATE

Anecdotal reports of the steroid sparing effects of methotrexate in chronic active ulcerative colitis prompted a double-blind RCT of oral methotrexate in patients with steroid dependent disease. Sixty-seven patients were randomized to methotrexate 12.5 mg (30 patients) or placebo (37 patients), given weekly over a 9-month period. No benefit was seen in terms of improvement in disease activity, remission rate, or steroid dose.[41] However, the 12.5 mg weekly dose chosen in this trial was low compared with that employed in reported anecdotal experiences, which have used 25 mg IM weekly. Larger trials using higher doses of methotrexate would be of interest.

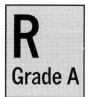

R Grade A

CYCLOSPORIN

There have been no RCTs of oral cyclosporin in ulcerative colitis. Anecdotal experience, as judged by a handful of case reports, has not suggested impressive efficacy. However, the use of intravenous cyclosporin for treating severe attacks has been formally tested in a single small randomized trial following favorable anecdotal experience. Lichtiger *et al* enrolled 20 patients with a severe attack of ulcerative colitis who had failed to respond to 7–10 days of treatment with intravenous hydrocortisone.[42] Patients were randomized to receive cyclosporin (4 mg/kg) or a placebo, by continuous intravenous infusion.

R Grade A

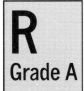

Nine of the 11 cyclosporin-treated patients avoided surgery and went into remission, compared with none of the placebo group. However, five of the placebo-treated patients were offered intravenous cyclosporin subsequently and all entered remission. Since this trial was published, cyclosporin has been used extensively for severe disease. The response rate outside of trials is reported to be between 60 and 65%, and many patients treated in this way subsequently relapse and undergo colectomy.[9,43] Nevertheless, intravenous cyclosporin may be a useful medication especially for patients in their first attack of severe colitis and for those who want time to make up their minds regarding surgery. Confirmation of the effectiveness of this approach by a larger trial would be useful. Other questions that need answers concern dose (2 mg/kg may be as effective as 4 mg/kg), when to begin cyclosporin treatment (7–10 days or earlier), and whether to continue oral cyclosporin once the severe attack settles or add azathioprine, either alone or in combination with cyclosporin.[44] Current practice differs considerably and there is no hard evidence on which to base guidelines.

R Grade B

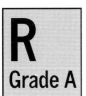

Cyclosporin has also been used as topical therapy for patients with resistant proctitis or distal colitis. Using 250 mg in each enema, plasma concentrations have been minimal and no systemic side effects have been observed. Small series of patients have been reported from Copenhagen, the Mayo Clinic, and Oxford. All patients had failed to respond to oral and topical mesalamine, steroids, and immunosuppression. About 70% appeared to do well on topical cyclosporin, although many relapsed when treatment was stopped. Unfortunately, no formal trial has been conducted in patients with resistant proctitis, largely because of the negative result of the small randomized trial published by Sandborn

R Grade A

et al.[45] This trial, involving only 40 patients, may have lacked power and also enrolled any patient with active distal disease, a different population from the patients with resistant disease studied in the open series. Nevertheless, there is no good evidence to support the use of cyclosporin enemas for proctitis.

NICOTINE

While current smokers have a decreased risk of developing ulcerative colitis, ex-smokers and non-smokers are at increased risk.[46] Three randomized placebo controlled trials have examined the efficacy of the nicotine patch given concurrently with mesalamine and/or corticosteroids in the therapy of ulcerative colitis.[47-49]

R Grade A

The study reported by Pullan *et al* demonstrated that the nicotine patch was effective for the induction of remission (nicotine 49%, placebo 24%) and the trial of Sandborn *et al* showed that the patch produced clinical improvement (nicotine 39%, placebo 9%). The number needed to treat (NNT) for induction of remission or production of clinical improvement with the nicotine patch compared to placebo can be calculated to be 4 and 3 in these studies. Approximately 10% of patients in these trials had to withdraw because of adverse events. A 6-week randomized trial comparing the nicotine patch with 15 mg prednisolone failed to demonstrate any benefit for nicotine compared to steroid.[49]

R Grade A

Two pilot studies assessing the efficacy of enemas containing nicotine have been reported.[50,51] Both trials presented sufficient evidence of efficacy to call for RCTs.

To date, only one trial of the nicotine patch given as *maintenance therapy* has been reported. Thomas and associates found no benefit with nicotine treatment (15 mg daily for 6 months) compared to placebo. Poor compliance by nicotine patch users was suspected.[52]

Pouch surgery

Colectomy with the construction of an ileal pouch–anal anastomosis has largely superseded colectomy with the ileorectal anastomosis or proctocolectomy with an end ileostomy in the major centers as the operation of choice for ulcerative colitis. Precise details of pouch construction may influence subsequent outcome in terms of function although, for most patients, a "J" pouch with 20 cm limbs with a stapled anastomosis 1.0–1.5 cm above the dentate line provides the best design to achieve good quality of life.[53–55] Nevertheless, problems of pouch dysfunction are common. There are many causes of this but "pouchitis" is one of the more frequent. The management of pouchitis is dealt with in Chapter 10.

R
Grade B

REFERENCES

1 Jenkins D, Balsitis M, Gallivan S *et al.* Guidelines for the initial biospy diagnosis of suspected chronic inflammatory bowel disease. The British Society of Gastroenterology Initiative. *J Clin Pathol* 1997; **50**: 93–105.
2 Truelove SC, Pena AS. Course and prognosis of Crohn's disease. *Gut* 1976; **17**: 192–201.
3 Sinclair TS, Brunt PW, Mowat NAG. Nonspecific protocolitis in northeastern Scotland: a community study. *Gastroenterology* 1983; **85**: 1–11.
4 Persson PG, Bernell O, Leijonmarck CE *et al.* Survival and cause-specific mortality in inflammatory bowel disease: a population-based cohort study. *Gastroenterology* 1996; **110**: 1339–45.
5 Langholz E, Munkholm P, Davidsen M *et al.* Course of ulcerative colitis: analysis of changes in disease activity over years. *Gastroenterology* 1994; **107**: 3–11.
6 Langholz E, Munkholm P, Krasilnikoff PA *et al.* Inflammatory bowel diseases with onset in childhood-clinical features, morbidity, and mortality in a regional cohort. *Scand J Gastroenterol* 1997; **32**: 139–47.
7 Ayres RC, Gillen CD, Walmsley RS, Allan RN. Progression of ulcerative proctosigmoiditis: incidence and factors influencing progression. *Eur J Gastroent Hepatol* 1996; **8**: 555–8.
8 Langholz E, Munkholm P, Davidsen M *et al.* Changes in extent of ulcerative colitis – a study on the course and prognostic factors. *Scand J Gastroenterol* 1996; **31**:260–6.
9 Gyde SN, Prior P, Allan RN *et al.* Colorectal cancer in ulcerative colitis: a cohort study of primary referrals from three centres. *Gut* 1988; **29**: 206–17.
10 Langholz E, Munkholm P, Davidsen M *et al.* Colorectal cancer risk and mortality in patients with ulcerative colitis. *Gastroenterology* 1992; **103**: 1444–51.
11 Lynch DAF, Lobo AJ, Sobala GM *et al.* Failure of colonoscopic surveillance in ulcerative colitis. *Gut* 1993; **34**: 1075–80.
12 Riddell RH. Cancer surveillance in IBD does not work: the argument against. In: Tytgat GNJ, Bartelsman JFWM, Deventer SJH (eds), *Inflammatory bowel diseases.* New York: Kluwer Academic, 1995, pp 690–700.
13 Svartz N. Salazopyrin, a new sulfanilamide preparation. A: Therapeutic results in rheumatic polyarthritis. B: Therapeutic results in ulcerative colitis. C: Toxic manifestations in treatment with sulfanilamide preparation. *Acta Med Scand* 1942; **110**: 557–90.
14 Baron JH, Connell AM, Lennard-Jones JE *et al.* Sulphasalazine and salicylazosulphadimidine in ulcerative colitis. *Lancet* 1962; **i**: 1094–6.
15 Misiewicz JJ, Lennard-Jones JE, Connell AM *et al.* Controlled trial of sulphasalazine in maintenance therapy for ulcerative colitis. *Lancet* 1965; **i**: 185–8.
16 Dissanayake AS, Truelove SC. A controlled therapeutic trial of long-term maintenance treatment of ulcerative colitis with sulphasalazine (Salazopyrin). *Gut* 1973; **14**: 923–6.
17 Azad Khan AK, Piris J, Truelove SC *et al.* An optimum dose of sulfasalazine for maintenance treatment in ulcerative colitis. *Gut* 1980; **21**: 232–40.
18 Azad Khan AK, Piris J, Truelove SC. An experiment to determine the active therapeutic moiety of sulphasalazine. *Lancet* 1977; **ii**: 892–5.
19 Van Hees PAM, Bakker JH, Van Tongeren JHM. Effect of sulphapyridine, 5-aminosalicylic acid, and placebo in patients with idiopathic proctitis: a study to determine the active therapeutic moiety of sulphasalazine. *Gut* 1980; **21**: 632–5.
20 Williams CN. Overview of 5-ASA in the therapy of IBD In: Sutherland LR, Collins SM, Martin F *et al* (eds), *Bowel disease: basic research, clinical implications and trends in therapy.* Dordrecht: Kluwer Academic, 1994, pp. 361–6.

21 Sutherland LR, Roth DE, Beck PL. Alternatives to sulfasalazine: a meta-analysis of 5-ASA in the treatment of ulcerative colitis. *Inflammatory Bowel Dis* 1997; **3**: 65–78.
22 Sutherland L, Roth D, Beck P *et al.* The use of oral 5-aminosalicylic acid in the induction of remission in ulcerative colitis. In: The Cochrane Library (database on disk and CD-ROM). Oxford: The Cochrane Collaboration. Update Software; 1998, issue 4.
23 Sutherland L, Roth D, Beck P *et al.* The use of oral 5-aminosalicylic acid for maintenance of remission in ulcerative colitis. In: The Cochrane Library (database on disk and CD-ROM). Oxford: The Cochrane Collaboration. Update Software; 1998, issue 4.
24 Rao SSC, Dundas SAC, Holdsworth CD *et al.* Olsalazine or sulphasalazine in first attacks of ulcerative colitis? A double blind study. *Gut* 1989; **30**: 675–9.
25 Marshall JK, Irvine EJ. Rectal aminosalicylate therapy for distal ulcerative colitis: a meta-analysis. *Aliment Pharmacol Ther* 1995; **9**: 293–300.
26 Marshall JK, Irvine EJ. Rectal corticosteroids versus alternative treatments in ulcerative colitis: a meta-analysis. *Gut* 1997; **40**: 775–81.
27 Truelove SC, Witts LJ. Cortisone in ulcerative colitis. Final report on a therapeutic trial. *Br Med J* 1955; no 4947: 1041–8.
28 Lennard-Jones JE, Longmore AJ, Newell AC *et al.* An assessment of prednisone, salazopyrin, and topical hydrocortisone hemisuccinate used as out-patient treatment for ulcerative colitis. *Gut* 1960;**1**:217–22.
29 Baron JH, Connell AM, Kanaghinis TG *et al.* Out-patient treatment of ulcerative colitis. Comparison between three doses of oral prednisone. *Br Med J* 1962; **2**: 441–3.
30 Powell-Tuck J, Bown RL, Lennard-Jones JE. A comparison of oral prednisolone given as single or multiple daily doses for active proctocolitis. *Scand J Gastroenterol* 1978; **13**: 833–7.
31 Brattsand R. Overview of newer glucocorticosteroid preparations for inflammatory bowel disease. *Can J Gastroenterol* 1990; **4**: 407–14.
32 Lofberg R, Danielsson A, Suhr O *et al.* Oral budesonide versus prednisolone in patients with active extensive and left sided colitis. *Gastroenterology* 1996; **110**: 1713–18.
33 Lemann M, Galian A, Rutgeerts P. Comparison of budesonide and 5-aminosalicylic acid enemas in active distal ulcerative colitis. *Aliment Pharmacol Ther* 1995; **9**: 557–62.
34 Truelove SC, Witts LJ. Cortisone and corticotrophin in ulcerative colitis. *Br Med J* 1959; **1**: 387–94.
35 Truelove SC. Treatment of ulcerative colitis with local hydrocortisone hemisuccinate sodium: a report on a controlled therapeutic trial. *Br Med J* 1958; **2**: 1072–7.
36 Lennard-Jones JE, Misiewicz JJ, Connell AM. Prednisone as maintenance treatment for ulcerative colitis in remission. *Lancet* 1965; **i**: 188–9.
37 Jewell DP, Truelove SC. Azathioprine in ulcerative colitis: final report on controlled therapeutic trial. *Br Med J* 1974; **iv**: 627–30.
38 Rosenberg JL. A controlled trial of azathioprine in the management of chronic ulcerative colitis. *Gastroenterology* 1975; **69**: 96–9.
39 Kirk AP, Lennard-Jones JE. Controlled trial of azathioprine in chronic ulcerative colitis. *Br Med J* 1982; **284**: 1291–2.
40 Hawthorne AB, Logan RFA, Hawkey CJ *et al.* Randomised controlled trial of azathioprine withdrawal in ulcerative colitis. *Br Med J* 1992; **305**: 20–2.
41 Oren R, Arber N, Odes S *et al.* Methotrexate in chronic active ulcerative colitis: a double-blind, randomized, Israeli multicentre trial. *Gastroenterology* 1996; **110**: 1416–21.
42 Lichtiger S, Present DH, Kornbluth A. Cyclosporin in severe ulcerative colitis refractory to steroid therapy. *N Engl J Med* 1994; **330**: 1841–5.
43 Hyde GM, Thillainayagam AV, Jewell DP. Intravenous cyclosporin as rescue therapy in severe ulcerative colitis: time for reappraisal? *Eur J Gastroenterol Hepatol* 1998; **10**: 411–13.
44 Severe ulcerative colitis: cyclosporin or colectomy? A European view. In: Jewell DP, Hyde GM. Modigliani R (eds), *IBD and salicylates, 3.* Wells Medical, 1998, pp 104–10.
45 Sandborn WJ, Tremaine WJ, Schroeder KW *et al.* A placebo-controlled trial of cyclosporin enemas for mildly to moderately active left-sided ulcerative colitis. *Gastroenterology* 1994; **106**: 1429–35.
46 Calkins BM. A meta-analysis of the role of smoking in inflammatory bowel disease. *Dig Dis Sci* 1989; **34**: 1841–54.
47 Pullan RD, Rhodes J, Ganesh S *et al.* Transdermal nicotine for active ulcerative colitis [see comments]. *N Engl J Med* 1994; **330**: 811–15.
48 Sandborn WJ, Tremaine WJ, Offord KP *et al.* Transdermal nicotine for mildly to moderately active ulcerative colitis – a randomized, double-blind, placebo-controlled trial. *Ann Intern Med* 1997; **126**: 364–71.
49 Thomas GA, Rhodes J, Ragunath K *et al.* Transdermal nicotine compared with oral prednisolone therapy for active ulcerative colitis. *Eur J Gastroenterol Hepatol* 1996; **8**: 769–76.
50 Sandborn WJ, Tremaine WJ, Leighton JA *et al.* Nicotine tartrate liquid enemas for mildly to moderately active left-sided ulcerative colitis unresponsive to first-line therapy: a pilot study. *Aliment Pharmacol Ther* 1997; **11**: 661–71.

51 Green JT, Thomas AG, Rhodes J *et al.* Nicotine enemas for active ulcerative colitis – a pilot study. *Ann Intern Med* 1997; **123**: 132–42.
52 Thomas AOT, Rhodes J, Mani V *et al.* Transdermal nicotine as maintenance therapy for ulcerative colitis. *N Engl J Med* 1995; **332**: 988–92.
53 Romanos J, Samarasekera DN, Stebbing J *et al.* Outcome of 200 restorative proctocolectomy operations: the John Radcliffe Hospital experience. *Br J Surg* 1997; **84**: 814–18.
54 Setti-Carraro P, Ritchie JK, Wilkinson KH *et al.* The first 10 years' experience of restorative proctocolectomy for ulcerative colitis. *Gut* 1994; **35**: 1070–5.
55 McIntyre PB, Pemberton JH, Wolff BG *et al.* Comparing functional results one year and ten years after ileal pouch–anal anastomosis for chronic ulcerative colitis. *Dis Colon Rectum* 1994; **37**: 303–7.

10 Pouchitis after restorative proctocolectomy: diagnosis and treatment

William J Sandborn

INTRODUCTION

Pouchitis is an idiopathic chronic inflammatory disease which may occur in the ileal pouch after restorative proctocolectomy with ileal pouch–anal anastomosis (IPAA) for ulcerative colitis (UC).[1] It is expected that the total number of patients with pouchitis in the United States will eventually stabilize at 30 000–45 000 persons (prevalence of $12–18/10^5$).[2] Thus, pouchitis is emerging as an important third form of inflammatory bowel disease (IBD).

Because pouchitis is a relatively new disease, criteria for diagnosis, classification, and measurement of disease activity were only recently proposed. The previous lack of consensus on these issues has hampered the design and conduct of randomized, double-blind, placebo controlled treatment trials, and medical therapy for pouchitis has been largely empirical. The medical therapies reported to be of benefit for pouchitis are shown in Table 10.1. Only four small placebo controlled trials have been performed, evaluating treatment with metronidazole, probiotic bacteria, and bismuth carbomer foam enemas .[3–6] This chapter will assist physicians and surgeons in becoming familiar with the diagnosis and classification of pouchitis, and will review the clinical results from empirical medical therapies and the rationale for using them.

DIAGNOSIS AND DISEASE ACTIVITY MEASUREMENT

The diagnosis of pouchitis is suggested by variable clinical symptoms of increased stool frequency, rectal bleeding, abdominal cramping, rectal urgency and tenesmus, incontinence, and fever. A clinical diagnosis of pouchitis should be confirmed by endoscopy and mucosal biopsy of the pouch.[1] Endoscopic examination shows inflammatory changes, which may include mucosal edema, granularity, contact bleeding, loss of vascular pattern, hemorrhage, and ulceration.[7,8] Histological examination shows acute inflammation including neutrophil infiltration and mucosal ulceration, superimposed on a background of chronic inflammation including villous atrophy, crypt hyperplasia, and chronic inflammatory cell infiltration.[8,9] Endoscopic examination of the neo-terminal ileum above the ileal pouch should be normal. The Pouchitis Disease Activity Index (PDAI) is a quantitative 19 point index of pouchitis activity based on both clinical symptoms and endoscopic and histological findings (Table 10.2).[10] Active pouchitis is defined as a PDAI score ≥ 7 points and remission is defined as a PDAI score <7 points in a patient with a history of pouchitis.

Table 10.1 Treatments reported to be beneficial for pouchitis

Class example
1 **Antibiotics**
A Metronidazole
B Ciprofloxacin
C Amoxicillin/clavulanic acid
D Erythromycin
E Tetracycline
2 **Probiotic bacteria**
A Lactobacilli, Bifidobacteria, *S. thermophilus*
3 **5-Aminosalicylates**
A Mesalamine enemas
B Sulfasalazine
C Oral mesalamine
4 **Corticosteroids**
A Conventional corticosteroid enemas
B Budesonide enemas
C Oral corticosteroids
5 **Immune modifier agents**
A Cyclosporin enemas
B Azathioprine
6 **Nutritional agents**
A SCFA enemas or suppositories
B Glutamine suppositories
7 **Oxygen radical inhibitors**
A Allopurinol
8 **Antidiarrheal/antimicrobial**
A Bismuth carbomer enemas
B Bismuth subsalicylate

Modified with permission from Sandborn WJ. Pouchitis following ileal pouch–anal anastomosis: definition, pathogenesis, and treatment. *Gastroenterology* 1994; **107**: 1856–60

CLASSIFICATION

Patients with pouchitis can be classified according to disease activity, symptom duration, and disease pattern.[2] Disease activity can be classified as: remission (no active pouchitis), mildly to moderately active (increased stool frequency, urgency, infrequent incontinence), or severely active (hospitalization for dehydration, frequent incontinence). Symptom duration can be classified as: acute (<4 weeks) or chronic (≥4 weeks). Finally, the disease pattern can be classified as: infrequent (1–2 acute episodes), relapsing (≥3 acute episodes), or continuous.

These classifications allow the physician to predict, based on the natural history of pouchitis, the need for suppressive medical therapy.

Table 10.2 Pouchitis disease activity index (PDAI)

Clinical criteria	Score
Stool frequency	
Usual postop stool frequency	0
1–2 stools/day > postop usual	1
3 or more stools/day > postop usual	2
Rectal bleeding	
None or rare	0
Present daily	1
Fecal urgency/Abdominal cramps	
None	0
Occasional	1
Usual	2
Fever (temperature > 100.5)	
Absent	0
Present	1
Endoscopic criteria	
Edema	1
Granularity	1
Friability	1
Loss of vascular pattern	1
Mucus exudate	1
Ulceration	1
Acute histological criteria	
Polymorph infiltration:	
Mild	1
Moderate + crypt abscess	2
Severe + crypt abscess	3
Ulceration per low power field:	
(average) < 25%	1
⩾ 25% ⩾ 50%	2
> 50%	3

Pouchitis is defined as a total PDAI score ⩾7 points

Adapted with permission from Sandborn WJ, Tremaine WJ, Batts KP *et al.* Pouchitis following ileal pouch–anal anastomosis: a pouchitis disease activity index. *Mayo Clin Proc* 1994; **69**: 409–15

TREATMENT WITH ANTIBIOTICS AND PROBIOTIC BACTERIA

Rationale

After IPAA, the primary function of the terminal ileum changes from absorption to storage, and bacterial overgrowth occurs with bacterial concentrations increasing to levels that are intermediate between end ileostomy and colon.[11,12] There is no correlation between fecal bacterial concentrations and histological changes of acute inflammation,[11,12] demonstrating that pouchitis and bacterial overgrowth are not directly related. However, anerobic bacterial overgrowth of the pouch is associated with transformation of the ileal mucosa to a "colon-like" morphology (villous atrophy, chronic inflammatory cell infiltration).[11,13] Thus, pouch bacterial overgrowth may indirectly set the stage for pouchitis to the extent that "colon-like" ileal mucosa may be more susceptible to a recurrence of UC. Strategies directed towards reducing fecal concentrations of anerobic bacteria through the use of antibiotics, or altering the relative balance of anerobes and other bacteria using probiotic bacteria therapy, may be useful in treating pouchitis.

Clinical results

ANTIBIOTIC THERAPY

Clinicians have observed that most patients with pouchitis who are empirically treated with antibiotics experience clinical improvement. In the absence of controlled trials, antibiotics have become the *de facto* "standard medical therapy" for pouchitis. The most commonly used antibiotic for pouchitis is metronidazole.[1,3,4,8,12,14–26] The primary alternative to metronidazole is ciprofloxacin.[21] Amoxicillin/clavulanic acid, erythromycin, and tetracycline have also been reported to be of benefit.[23] Most patients with pouchitis initially appear to respond to metronidazole at doses of 750–1500 mg/day. Symptomatic improvement usually occurs within 1–2 days. Patients with relapsing or continuous pouchitis may require chronic maintenance metronidazole therapy, with doses ranging from 250 mg every third day up to 750 mg/day. In the only controlled trial of this form of therapy reported Madden treated 13 patients with active

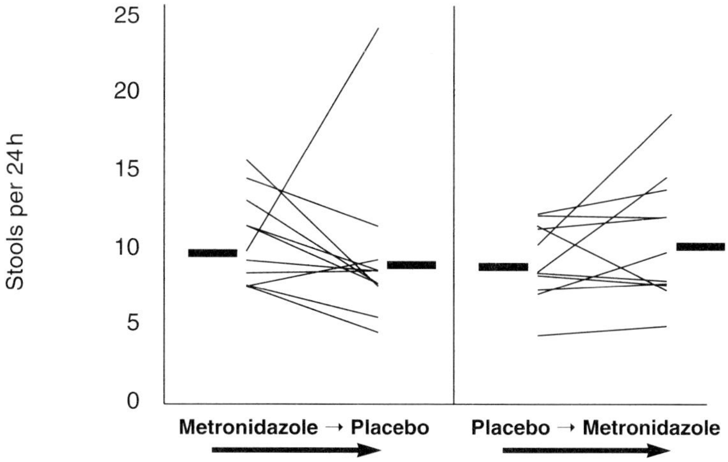

Figure 10.1 Stool frequency before and after metronidazole and placebo. Bars represent mean values. (Reproduced with permission from Madden MV, McIntyre AS, Nicholls RJ. Double-blind trial of metronidazole versus placebo in chronic unremitting pouchitis. *Dig Dis Sci* 1994;**39**:1193–6)

R
Grade A

chronic pouchitis in a crossover trial of oral metronidazole 400 mg t.i.d. or placebo for 14 days.[4] Each patient had a 7 day washout period before crossing over from the first to the second therapy. Eleven of 13 patients completed the study. Metronidazole reduced the daily stool frequency from 10.0 ± 2.8 to 9.0 ± 5.2 (mean ± SD) in 12 patients whereas the 11 placebo treated patients had an increase in daily stool frequency from 8.9 ± 2.5 up to 10.7 ± 4.1 (mean ± SD, $P<0.05$) (Figure 10.1). The clinical significance of such a small change in mean stool frequency may be questioned, and the confidence limits around the difference in means would be very wide in this small study. Adverse effects occurred in 55% of patients during metronidazole treatment, including nausea, vomiting, abdominal discomfort, headache, and skin rash.

In an attempt to reduce adverse effects from metronidazole, Nygaard used a topical metronidazole suspension to treat pouchitis in patients with an IPAA ($n = 4$) or a Kock continent ileostomy ($n = 7$).[27] Seven of the 11 patients had active chronic pouchitis, and three metronidazole-intolerant patients had active acute pouchitis. Treatment consisted of open therapy with a liquid metronidazole suspension (40 mg) instilled into the IPAA or continent ileostomy 1–4 times per day. All 11 patients improved within 2–3 days of beginning treatment with topical metronidazole. Nine of the 11 patients had continued improvement on either maintenance ($n = 3$) or intermittent ($n = 8$) treatment. Four of 8 patients had undetectable serum metronidazole concentrations and 4 had low serum concentrations following instillation of metronidazole into the pouch. In another uncontrolled study a vaginal formulation of metronidazole (37.5 mg) was administered transanally 2–4 times per day with an applicator into the ileal pouch of 6 patients with active pouchitis (4 of whom were metronidazole-intolerant).[28] Six of 6 patients improved, and only one of 6 patients experienced metronidazole-induced adverse effects. Gionchetti also used this "topical" antibiotic approach, reporting that oral ciprofloxacin 1 g/day in combination with an orally administered non-absorbable antibiotic, rifaximin, was beneficial in patients with active chronic pouchitis resistant to standard antibiotic therapy.[29]

PROBIOTIC BACTERIA

R
Grade A

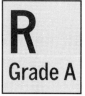

Another therapeutic approach to altering pouch bacterial contents is to administer probiotic bacteria. In what appears to be the largest clinical trial performed in this disease Gionchetti randomized 40 patients with chronic pouchitis in remission (PDAI score = 0 after induction therapy with antibiotics) to treatment with either a new oral probiotic preparation (VSL-3) 6 g/day or placebo for 9 months.[5] The VSL-3 preparation contained 10^{11}/g of viable lyophilized bacteria: four strains of lactobacilli (*L. acidophilus, L. delbrueckii* subsp. *bulgaricus, L. plantarum, L. casei*), three strains of bifidobacteria (*B. infantis, B. longum, B. breve*), and one strain of *Streptococcus salivarius* subsp. *thermophilus*. Relapse was defined as an increase in the clinical component of the PDAI of >2 points (6 points is the maximum possible). At 9 months, the relapse rate in the VSL-3 group was 15% as compared to 100% in the placebo group ($P<0.01$). The NNT, the number needed to treat with this therapy to prevent relapse, is 2, indicating that this is a very effective form of therapy. Fecal concentrations of lactobacilli, bifidobacteria, and *S. thermophilus* increased significantly from baseline in the VSL-3 group but not in the placebo group. There was no change from baseline in the fecal concentrations of anaerobic bacteria in either group.

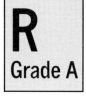

TREATMENT WITH ANTI-INFLAMMATORY AND IMMUNE MODIFIER AGENTS

Rationale

Pouchitis may be a recurrence of inflammatory bowel disease in the ileoanal pouch.[1] Data to support this view include: an increased frequency of pouchitis in patients with UC as compared to familial polyposis; an increased frequency of pouchitis in patients with extra-intestinal manifestations of UC; an increased frequency of pouchitis in patients with primary sclerosing cholangitis; an increased frequency of pouchitis in patients with antineutrophil cytoplasmic antibodies with a perinuclear staining pattern (pANCA); and a protective effect against developing pouchitis in current smokers. Strategies directed towards empirical medical therapy with agents known to be efficacious in UC may be useful in treating pouchitis. Unfortunately no controlled trials have been reported to provide evidence for the efficacy of these approaches.

Clinical results

R Grade B

Uncontrolled studies suggest that topical mesalamine (enemas or suppositories) may be beneficial for active pouchitis.[7,12,22,30–31] Grade B Anecdotal experience suggests that sulfasalazine and oral mesalamine may also be of benefit. An *in vitro* study measuring the azoreductase enzyme activity of fecal bacteria from patients with ileoanal pouches demonstrated adequate enzyme activity to cleave the azo bond necessary to activate sulfasalazine.[32] An *in vivo* study demonstrated that the azo bond of sulfasalazine was cleaved in patients with ileal pouches.[33] It is reasonable to assume that at least a portion of the Pentasa formulation of mesalamine will release into the ileoanal pouch. Whether the Asacol formulation of mesalamine will release into the pouch is unknown.

Uncontrolled reports have suggested that oral and topical corticosteroids may be of benefit in patients with active pouchitis.[12,22–23,25] Grade B Budesonide suppositories 0.5 mg t.i.d. resulted in clinical and endoscopic improvement or remission in 10/10 patients with active acute pouchitis,[34] and decreased pouch luminal concentrations of inflammatory mediators.[31,34]

R Grade A

Cyclosporin enemas (250 mg/day) were reported to be beneficial in one patient with active chronic pouchitis,[35] although a small placebo controlled trial of cyclosporin enemas in patients with left-sided UC was negative. Two studies involving 11 patients with both IPAA for UC and liver transplantation for primary sclerosing cholangitis have reported on the clinical disease course of pouchitis following liver transplantation.[36,37] Five of 11 patients had chronic pouchitis following liver transplantation, despite immunosuppression with cyclosporin or FK506, prednisone, and azathioprine, suggesting that immunosuppression may not be efficacious for pouchitis. One case report suggested a beneficial effect of azathioprine in patients with Crohn's disease and an IPAA.[38]

TREATMENT WITH NUTRITIONAL AGENTS

Rationale

In the well-functioning ileal pouch, the bacterial flora produce short chain fatty acids (SCFA) including acetate, propionate, and butyrate at concentrations similar to those in the colon of healthy controls, and increased compared to stomal SCFA concentrations in ileostomy patients.[11,39] Some[40,41] but not all[11] studies have reported that patients with pouchitis have significantly lower fecal concentrations of SCFAs than patients with well-functioning IPAAs, perhaps from dilution.[40] Strategies directed at replacing fecal SCFA deficiencies by administering SCFA enemas may theoretically be useful in treating pouchitis. Unfortunately no controlled clinical trials have been performed.

Clinical results

Short chain fatty acid 60 ml enemas containing 60 mmol sodium acetate, 30 mmol sodium propionate, 40 mmol sodium n-butyrate, and sodium chloride titrated to a concentration of 280–290 mosmol, were not of benefit in two patients with active pouchitis.[42] Similarly, another study using an identical SCFA enema formulation reported improvement in only 3/8 patients with active pouchitis.[43] In contrast, a third study in patients with active chronic pouchitis reported improvement in 3/9 patients treated with 40 mmol sodium butyrate suppositories compared to 6/10 patients treated with 1 g L-glutamine suppositories.[41] Finally, a case report using the SCFA enema formulation described above reported success in a single patient with active chronic pouchitis.[44] While only small numbers of patients were treated in these open studies, the low overall clinical response rates suggest that SCFA enemas or suppositories are not highly beneficial for active pouchitis.

TREATMENT WITH ALLOPURINOL

Rationale

During surgical construction of the IPAA, the mesenteric vessels may be divided to avoid tension on the pouch–anal anastomosis.[45] This ligation of the arterial blood supply has the potential to cause ischemic injury to the ileal pouch, and oxygen free radical formation is known to be one the mechanisms by which ischemic injury occurs. However, there have been no studies which measured either ileal blood flow or oxygen free radical formation in patients with and without pouchitis. Thus, there is no objective data demonstrating that pouch ischemia occurs, much less data demonstrating a relationship between pouch ischemia and pouchitis. If intestinal ischemia contributed to the pathogenesis of pouchitis, then medical therapy directed towards reducing oxygen free radical formation might be a useful strategy. For this reason, the xanthine oxidase inhibitor allopurinol has been proposed as a treatment for pouchitis.

Clinical results

An uncontrolled study reported that allopurinol 300 b.i.d. induced clinical improvement in 4/8 patients with active acute pouchitis and maintained remission despite the withdrawal of suppressive antibiotic therapy in 7/14 patients with chronic pouchitis.[46] A controlled trial of allopurinol for pouchitis is under way in Scandinavia to verify these preliminary observations.

TREATMENT WITH BISMUTH

Rationale

Bismuth has both antimicrobial and antidiarrheal properties, and has been useful in the treatment of traveler's diarrhea. A randomized, double-blind controlled trial suggested that bismuth citrate may have efficacy comparable to mesalamine for the treatment of active left-sided UC.[47] Given the proven benefit of bismuth for traveler's diarrhea, and its potential benefit in UC, therapeutic trials of bismuth in patients with pouchitis seemed reasonable.

Clinical results

R
Grade A

An uncontrolled study of bismuth complexed to carbomer (an acrylic acid polymer) suggested beneficial effects for both inducing improvement and maintaining remission in patients with chronic pouchitis.[48] A randomized, double-blind placebo controlled trial of bismuth carbomer foam enemas in 40 patients with active chronic pouchitis showed no benefit of bismuth carbomer compared to a placebo containing xanthan gum (45% response in both groups).[6] However, the fact that the placebo response rate is rather high and that a recent uncontrolled study suggests that *Boswella serrata* gum resin may be beneficial in patients with active UC,[49] there is the possibility that both the bismuth carbomer and the xanthan gum were effective therapies, and that the controlled trial simply demonstrated therapeutic equivalence of the two agents. A long term uncontrolled maintenance/toxicity study of bismuth carbomer foam enemas in patients with pouchitis demonstrated minimal systemic absorption of bismuth, no toxicity, and possible continued clinical benefit in patients with chronic pouchitis after treatment for 9–128 weeks.[50] Further support for a potential therapeutic effect of bismuth in pouchitis comes from an uncontrolled study of oral bismuth subsalicylate, administered as two 262 mg tablets 4 times per day for 4 weeks, which suggested a beneficial effect in 11/13 patients with active chronic pouchitis.[51] Controlled trials, using an inactive placebo control, are needed to determine whether bismuth has a role in the treatment of pouchitis.

TREATMENT ALGORITHM FOR POUCHITIS

An algorithm of the approach to treatment of pouchitis is shown in Figure 10.2. A presumptive diagnosis of pouchitis in patients with compatible symptoms should be confirmed by pouch endoscopy and biopsy. After the diagnosis is confirmed, treatment with metronidazole is initiated. For patients who are metronidazole-intolerant or who fail to respond, treatment with other types of antibiotics with anerobic activity is often the next step. When patients who require suppressive antibiotic therapy develop bacterial resistance after prolonged treatment, cycling of three or four antibiotics in 1-week intervals may be beneficial. Those patients who do not respond to metronidazole or other antibiotics should receive topical pouch therapy with mesalamine enemas or suppositories, or with steroid enemas. In more refractory cases, sulfasalazine, oral mesalamine in the form of Pentasa, and oral steroids may be useful. Some patients may require combination therapy with multiple agents similar to the situation in patients with IBD. There is little data or rationale to support empirical therapy with SCFA enemas, glutamine suppositories, or allopurinol. A small number of patients will be refractory to all forms of medical therapy and these patients should be referred to a surgeon for consideration of permanent ileostomy with pouch exclusion or excision.

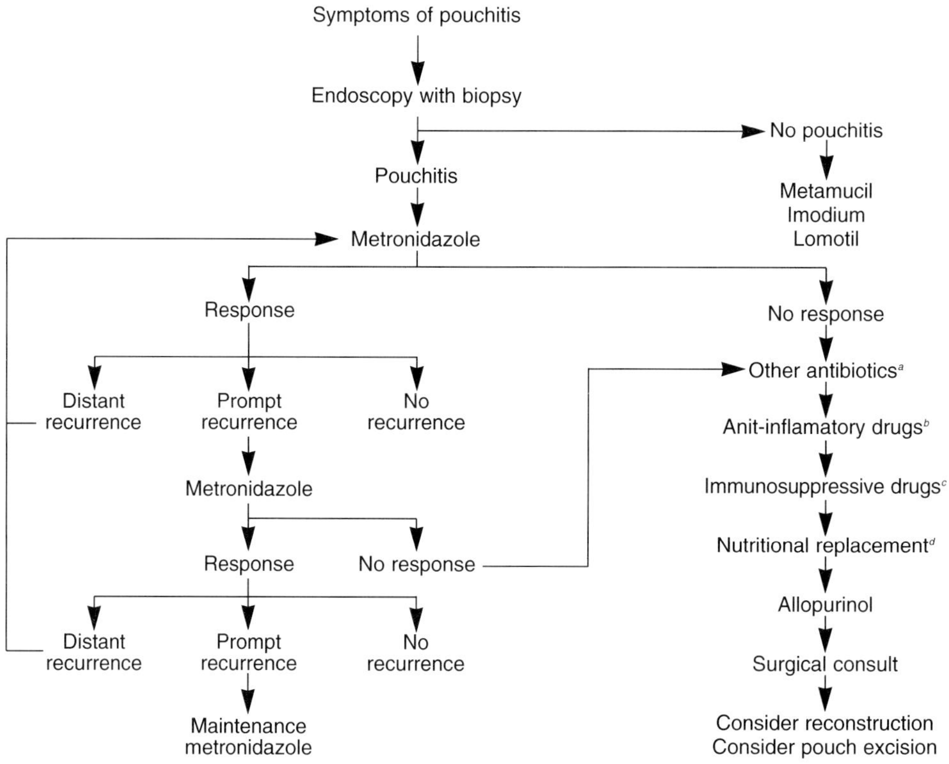

Figure 10.2 Treatment algorithm for pouchitis. Other antibiotics[a] indicates: ciprofloxacin; amoxicillin/clavulanate; erythromycin; tetracycline; and cycling of multiple antibiotics. Anti-inflammatory drugs[b] indicates: mesalamine enemas; sulfasalazine; and oral mesalamine. Immunosuppressive drugs[c] indicates: steroid enemas; oral steroids; azathioprine; and cyclosporine enemas. Nutritional replacement[d] indicates: SCFA enemas and glutamine suppositories. (Reproduced with permission from Sandborn WJ. Pouchitis following ileal pouch–anal anastomosis: definition, pathogenesis, and treatment. *Gastroenterology* 1994; **107**: 1856– 60)

RESPONSE TO TREATMENT OF POUCHITIS (NATURAL HISTORY)

In patients with IPAA for UC, the cumulative risk of developing at least one episode of pouchitis is 32%.[5] Of those patients who develop pouchitis, 36% have one or two acute pouchitis episodes which respond to treatment with antibiotics, 49% relapse more frequently (at least three acute episodes) but respond to antibiotics, and 15% require maintenance suppressive therapy and have been classified as having chronic pouchitis.[52] Of patients with chronic pouchitis, almost 50% require surgical exclusion or excision of the pouch. An algorithm showing the clinical course of pouchitis in IPAA patients is shown in Figure 10.3.

CONCLUSION

Medical treatment of acute and chronic pouchitis is often required. A single small placebo controlled trials has suggested efficacy of metronidazole for active chronic pouchitis. Another somewhat larger placebo controlled trial suggested that treatment with probiotic bacteria may be useful in maintaining remission of pouchitis. A small placebo controlled trial of bismuth carbomer foam enemas did not demonstrate efficacy in active chronic pouchitis. Uncontrolled studies suggest possible benefit from empirical therapy with

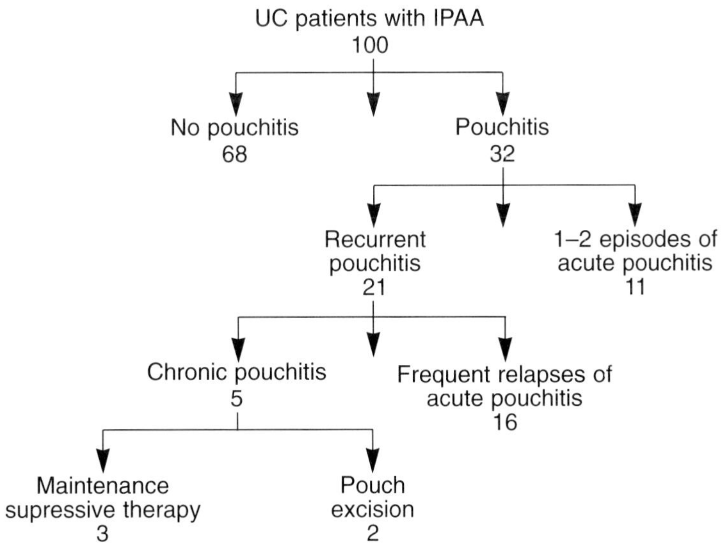

Figure 10.3 Clinical outcome with regard to pouchitis in 100 UC patients undergoing abdominal colectomy with ileal pouch–anal anastomosis. (Reproduced with permission from Sandborn WJ. Pouchitis: definition, risk factors, frequency, natural history, classification, and public health perspective. In: McLeod RS, Martin F, Sutherland LR *et al* (eds), *Trends in inflammatory bowel disease.* Lancaster, UK: Kluwer Academic, 1997, pp 51–63)

antibiotics, sulfasalazine, mesalamine, corticosteroids, and bismuth. There are few data that immune modifiers, SCFA enemas, or allopurinol are of benefit. Natural history studies suggest that most patients with pouchitis respond to a short course of antibiotic therapy. Some patients with chronic pouchitis require suppressive medical therapy, and some will require permanent ileostomy with pouch exclusion or excision. Additional randomized, double-blind placebo controlled trials are needed to determine the efficacy of empirical medical therapies currently being used in patients with pouchitis.

REFERENCES

1 Sandborn WJ. Pouchitis following ileal pouch–anal anastomosis: definition, pathogenesis, and treatment. *Gastroenterology* 1994; **107**: 1856–60.

2 Sandborn WJ. Pouchitis: definition, risk factors, frequency, natural history, classification, and public health perspective. In: McLeod RS, Martin F, Sutherland Lr *et al* (eds), *Trends in inflammatory bowel disease*. Lancaster, UK: Kluwer Academic, 1997, pp 51–63.

3 McLeod RS, Cohen Z, Taylor DW *et al*. Single-patient randomized clinical trial. Use in determining optimum treatment for patient with inflammation of Kock continent ileostomy reservoir. *Lancet* 1986; **i**: 726–8.

4 Madden MV, McIntyre AS, Nicholls RJ. Double-blind trial of metronidazole versus placebo in chronic unremitting pouchitis. *Dig Dis Sci* 1994; **39**: 1193–6.

5 Gionchetti P, Rizzello F, Venturi A *et al*. Maintenance treatment of chronic pouchitis: a randomised placebo controlled, double-blind trial with a new probiotic preparation. *Gastroenterology* 1998; **114**: A985.

6 Tremaine WJ, Sandborn WJ, Wolff BG *et al*. Bismuth carbomer foam enemas for active chronic pouchitis: a randomized, double-blind, placebo controlled trial. *Aliment Pharmacol Ther* 1997; **11**: 1041–6.

7 Di Febo G, Miglioli M, Lauri A *et al*. Endoscopic assessment of acute inflammation of the reservoir after restorative ileo-anal anastomosis. *Gastrointest Endosc* 1990; **36**: 6–9.

8 Moskowitz RL, Shepherd NA, Nicholls RJ. An assessment of inflammation in the reservoir after restorative proctocolectomy with ileoanal ileal reservoir. *Int J Colorectal Dis* 1986; **1**: 167–74.

9 Shepherd NA, Jass JR, Duval I *et al*. Restorative proctocolectomy with ileal reservoir: pathological and histochemical study of mucosal biopsy specimens. *J Clin Pathol* 1987; **40**: 601–7.

10 Sandborn WJ, Tremaine WJ, Batts KP *et al*. Pouchitis following ileal pouch–anal anastomosis: a pouchitis disease activity index. *Mayo Clin Proc* 1994; **69**: 409–15.

11 Sandborn WJ, Tremaine WJ, Batts KP *et al*. Fecal bile acids, short chain fatty acids, and bacteria after ileal pouch anal anastomosis do not differ in patients with pouchitis. *Dig Dis Sci* 1995; **40**: 1474–83.

12 Shepherd NA, Hulten L, Tytgat GNJ *et al*. Workshop: pouchitis. *Int J Colorect Dis* 1989; **4**: 205–29.

13 Natori H, Utsunomiya J, Yamamaura T *et al*. Fecal and stomal bile acid composition after ileostomy or ileoanal anastomosis in patients with chronic ulcerative colitis and adenomatous coli. *Gastroenterology* 1992; **102**: 1278–88.

14 Zuccaro G, Fazio VW, Church JW *et al*. Pouch ileitis. *Dig Dis Sci* 1989; **34**: 1505–10.

15 Lohmuller JL, Pemberton JH, Dozois RR *et al*. Pouchitis and extraintestinal manifestations of inflammatory bowel disease after ileal pouch–anal anastomosis. *Ann Surg* 1990; **211**: 622–9.

16 Svaninger G, Nordgren S, Oresland T *et al*. Incidence and characteristics of pouchitis in the Kock continent ileostomy and the pelvic pouch. *Scand J Gastroenterol* 1993;**28**: 695–700.

17 Kelly DG, Phillips SF, Kelly KA *et al*. Dysfunction of the continent ileostomy: clinical features and bacteriology. *Gut* 1983; **24**: 193–201.

18 Boerr LA, Sambuelli AM, Sugai E *et al*. Faecal alpha1-antitrypsin concentration in the diagnosis and management of patients with pouchitis. *Eur J Gastroenterol Hepatol* 1995; **7**: 129–33.

19 Boerr LAR, Sambuelli AM, Filinger E *et al*. Increased mucosal levels of leukotriene B4 in pouchitis: evidence for a persistent inflammatory state. *Eur J Gastroenterol Hepatol* 1996; **8**: 57–61.

20 Kmiot WA, Hesslewood SR, Smith N *et al*. Evaluation of the inflammatory infiltrate in pouchitis with ^{111}In-labeled granulocytes. *Gastroenterology* 1993; **104**: 981–8.

21 Hurst RD, Molinari M, Chung TP *et al*. Prospective study of the incidence, timing, and treatment of pouchitis in 104 consecutive patients after restorative proctocolectomy. *Arch Surg* 1996; **131**: 497–502.

22 Tytgat GNJ, van Deventer SJH. Pouchitis. *Int J Colorect Dis* 1988; **3**: 226–8

23 Scott AD, Phillips RKS. Ileitis and pouchitis after colectomy for ulcerative colitis. *Br J Surg* 1989; **76**: 668–9.

24 Bonello JC, Thow GB, Manson RR. Mucosal enteritis: a complication of the continent ileostomy. *Dis Colon Rectum* 1981;**24**: 37–41.

25 Klein K, Stenzel P, Katon RM. Pouch ileitis: report of a case with severe systemic manifestations. *J Clin Gastroenterol* 1983; **5**: 149–53.
26 Knobler H, Ligumsky M, Okon E. *et al.* Pouch ileitis – recurrence of the inflammatory bowel disease in the ileal reservoir. *Am J Gastroenterol* 1986; **81**: 199–201.
27 Nygaard K, Bergan T, Bjorneklett A *et al.* Topical metronidazole treatment in pouchitis. *Scand J Gastroenterol* 1994; **29**: 462–7.
28 Isaacs K, Klenzak J, Koruda M. Topical metronidazole for the treatment of pouchitis. *Gastrointest Endosc* 1997; **45**: AB108.
29 Gionchetti P, Rizzello F, Venturi A *et al.* Antibiotic association in patients with chronic treatment-resistant pouchitis. *Gastroenterology* 1997;**112**: A981.
30 Miglioli M, Barbara L, Di Febo G *et al.* Topical administration of 5-aminosalicylic acid: a therapeutic proposal for the treatment of pouchitis. *N Engl J Med* 1989; **320**: 257.
31 Belluzzi A, Campieri M, Gionchetti P *et al.* Acute pouchitis: 5-aminosalicylic acid and budesonide suppositories effectiveness on inflammatory mediator production. *Gastroenterology* 1993; **104**: A665.
32 Rafii F, Ruseler van-Embden JGH, Asad Y. Azoreductase and nitroreductase activity of bacteria in feces from patients with an ileal reservoir. *Dig Dis Sci* 1997; **42**: 133–6.
33 Ciribilli JM, Chaussade S, Perrin S *et al.* Metabolism of sulfasalazine (SLZ) in patients with ileo-anal anastomosis (IAA) and reservoir. *Gastroenterology* 1991; **100**: A203.
34 Belluzzi A, Campieri M, Miglioli M *et al.* Evaluation of flogistic pattern in "pouchitis" before and after the treatment with budesonide suppositories. *Gastroenterology* 1992; **102**: A593.
35 Winter TA, Dalton HR, Merrett MN *et al.* Cyclosporin A retention enemas in refractory distal ulcerative colitis and "pouchitis". *Scand J Gastroenterol* 1993; **28**: 701–4.
36 Zins BJ, Sandborn WJ, Penna CR *et al.* Pouchitis disease course after orthotopic liver transplantation in patients with primary sclerosing cholangitis and an ileal pouch–anal anastomosis. *Am J Gastroenterol* 1995; **90**: 2177–81.
37 Rowley S, Candinas D, Mayer AD *et al.* Restorative proctocolectomy and pouch anal anastomosis for ulcerative colitis following orthotopic liver transplantation. *Gut* 1995; **37**: 845–7.
38 Berrebi W, Chaussade S, Bruhl AL *et al.* Treatment of Crohn's disease recurrence after ileoanal anastomosis by azathioprine. *Dig Dis Sci* 1993; **38**: 1558–60.
39 Nasmyth DG, Godwin PGR, Dixon MF *et al.* Ileal ecology after pouch–anal anastomosis or ileostomy. *Gastroenterology* 1989; **96**: 817–24.
40 Clausen MR, Tvede M, Mortensen PB. Short-chain fatty acids in pouch contents with and without pouchitis after ileal pouch–anal anastomosis. *Gastroenterology* 1992; **103**: 1144–53.
41 Wischmeyer P, Pemberton JH, Phillips SF. Chronic pouchitis after ileal pouch–anal anastomosis: responses to butyrate and glutamine suppositories in a pilot study. *Mayo Clin Proc* 1993; **68**: 978–81.
42 De Silva HJ, Ireland A, Kettlewell M *et al.* Short-chain fatty acid irrigation in severe pouchitis. *N Engl J Med* 1989; **321**: 416–17.
43 Tremaine WJ, Sandborn WJ, Phillips SF *et al.* Short chain fatty acid (SCFA) enema therapy for treatment-resistant pouchitis following ileal pouch–anal anastomosis (IPAA) for ulcerative colitis (UC). *Gastroenterology* 1994; **106**: A784.
44 den Hoed PT, van Goch JJ, Veen HF *et al.* Severe pouchitis successfully treated with short-chain fatty acids. *Canad J Surg* 1996; **39**: 168–9.
45 Smith L, Friend WG, Medwell SJ. The superior mesenteric artery: the critical factor in the pouch pull-through procedure. *Dis Colon Rectum* 1984; **27**: 271.
46 Levin KE, Pemberton JH, Phillips SF *et al.* Role of oxygen free radicals in the etiology of pouchitis. *Dis Colon Rectum* 1992; **35**: 452–6.
47 Pullan RD, Ganesh S, Mani V *et al.* Comparison of bismuth citrate and 5-aminosalicylic acid enemas in distal ulcerative colitis: a controlled trial. *Gut* 1993; **34**: 676–9.
48 Gionchetti P, Rizzello F, Venturi A *et al.* Long-term efficacy of bismuth carbomer enemas in patients with treatment-resistant chronic pouchitis. *Aliment Pharmacol Ther* 1997; **11**: 673–8.
49 Parihar GA, Malhotra P, Singh GB *et al.* Effects of *Boswella serrata* gum resin in patients with ulcerative colitis. *Eur J Med Res* 1997; **2**: 37–43.
50 Tremaine WJ, Sandborn WJ. Safety of long term open treatment with bismuth carbomer foam enemas for chronic pouchitis. *Gastroenterology* 1997; **112**: A1105.
51 Tremaine WJ, Sandborn WJ, Kenan ML. Bismuth subsalicylate tablets for chronic antibiotic-resistant pouchitis. *Gastroenterology* 1998;**114**: A1101.
52 Penna C, Dozois R, Tremaine W *et al.* Pouchitis after ileal pouch–anal anastomosis for ulcerative colitis occurs with increased frequency in patients with associated primary sclerosing cholangitis. *Gut* 1996; **38**: 234–9.

11 Metabolic bone disease in gastrointestinal disorders: prevalence, prevention, and treatment

ANN CRANNEY, CATHERINE DUBE, ALAA ROSTOM, PETER TUGWELL, GEORGE WELLS

INTRODUCTION

Metabolic bone disease is seen in patients suffering from a variety of gastrointestinal (GI) disorders, including chronic liver disease (CLD), inflammatory bowel disease (IBD), and malabsorption syndromes such as celiac disease. In the setting of GI disorders, bone disease can be broadly divided into osteoporosis and osteomalacia. Osteoporosis is a disorder of reduced bone mass per unit volume (ie bone density) and disrupted micro-architecture, resulting in decreased bone strength and an increased risk of fragility fractures mainly of the hip, wrist, and vertebrae.[1] On the other hand, osteomalacia is characterized by defective mineralization of bone matrix, usually due to a disturbance of vitamin D and phosphocalcic homeostasis. It is clinically associated with pain, bone fractures, occasionally muscle weakness, and radiologically with pseudo fractures (radiolucent bands), and loss of trabeculae.[2]

There are two types of bone: cortical, which primarily makes up the long bones, and trabecular bone, which makes up most of the axial skeleton. Bone formation and resorption is a continuous process in which osteoblasts are responsible for the formation of new bone including the mineralization of bone, and osteoclasts are responsible for bone resorption. Metabolic bone disease results from abnormalities in the normal remodeling cycle.

Assessment of bone mass

Age related bone loss begins during the fourth decade, and in women there is an accelerated bone loss at the time of the menopause. Women experience greater rates of bone loss than men and their lifetime risk of an osteoporotic fracture is about 15% in comparison to 5% in men.[3] Osteoporosis can be detected by measurement of bone mineral density. Bone density is the most accurate predictor of fracture risk[4] and it is a useful guide for monitoring therapy. Prospective trials have established the ability of bone density to predict site-specific fractures.[5] For each reduction in bone density of one standard deviation (SD) from the mean for young normals, the risk of hip fracture increases by a factor of 1.5–2.6.[6] In men, low bone mineral density (BMD) has been demonstrated to be predictive of vertebral fractures.[7] In a prospective study which included 1690 men, it was estimated that a one standard deviation decrease in femoral neck bone density was associated with a two-fold increase in risk of atraumatic fracture.[8]

Bone mass can be evaluated at a number of sites, such as the proximal femur, spine, and distal radius. The most commonly used technique to evaluate bone mineral density is dual energy X-ray absorptiometry (DXA). The reproducibility, accuracy, and precision of DXA are excellent, with a coefficient of variation of 2%. Another technique, quantitative computed tomography (QCT), provides a three-dimensional image which makes it possible to separate trabecular and cortical bone. The accuracy of QCT is not as good (5–15%) as DXA, and it is associated with a higher radiation dose.

Bone mineral content (BMC) is the total amount of mineralized tissue (g) in the bone scan, usually normalized to the length of the scan path (grams per mineral per centimeter of bone or g/cm). BMD, on the other hand, is the amount of mineralized tissue in the scanned area (g/cm^2). BMD can be expressed as a T score (comparison of the patient's bone density with the peak bone mass in young normals) or Z score (comparison of patient's BMD to other age-matched controls). Persons with a T score or BMD less than 1 SD below the mean in young adults are considered to be osteopenic, while those with a BMD less than 2.5 SDs below the young normal value are osteoporotic. [1] A study group on densitometry hosted by the World Health Organization (WHO) in 1993 defined these four diagnostic thresholds based on reference populations of healthy young women. Since these thresholds are based on young women, this definition does not account for biological variation and age-related bone loss and many have argued against the use of T scores.[9]

HEPATIC OSTEODYSTROPHY

Hepatic osteodystrophy (HO), or CLD-associated metabolic bone disease, was previously thought to arise mainly in cholestatic liver diseases, as a result of calcium and vitamin D malabsorption. However, HO has now been described in association with most types of chronic liver diseases, whether cholestatic or non-cholestatic. Increased bone loss and/or increased incidence of fractures have been described in primary biliary cirrhosis (PBC),[10,11] primary sclerosing cholangitis (PSC),[12] alcoholic liver disease (ALD),[13,14] autoimmune hepatitis (AIH),[15] hemochromatosis,[16] as well as viral cirrhosis.[17,18] Additionally, HO has important clinical repercussions in the early period after liver transplant, where immobilization, comorbidity, corticosteroids, and immunosuppressive drugs further reduce an already compromised bone mass,[11] resulting in spontaneous vertebral fractures.[19,20]

Prevalence

The prevalence of HO varies from 13 to 56%,[12,16–18] while the incidence of fractures in ambulant and non-alcoholic patients with CLD ranges from 6 to18%,[12,16,17,22] twice that of age- and sex-matched controls.[16,17] The degree of bone loss correlates with the severity of the cirrhosis,[16–18,21] making patients with endstage liver disease the group most at risk of fractures.

The fracture risk in CLD was best studied by Diamond *et al*, in a case–control study of 115 patients with CLD (72 men and 43 women), which were matched for age, sex, and menopausal status with healthy controls.[16] The etiology of the CLD was ALD (40 patients), CAH (27 patients), hemochromatosis (25 patients), PBC (10 patients), and PSC (13 patients). Fifty-two per cent of the patients were cirrhotics, while 30% had clinical and biochemical evidence of hypogonadism. It is important to note that, in men, hypogonadism correlates with the degree of liver dysfunction. All patients were ambulatory and none was on cholestyramine, vitamin D, estrogen, or calcium. From the data in this study, the relative risk (RR) of either spinal or peripheral fractures can be calculated, based on the absolute number of fractures (as opposed to the number of patients with fractures). In men this RR is 3.03 (95% CI 1.35–11.09), while in women the RR is 2.13 (95% CI 1.38–7.46). These authors performed a stepwise regression analysis to define the main predictors of fracture and osteoporosis. Variables used were: age, sex, gonadal status, presence of cirrhosis, type of liver disease, liver function, 25(OH) vitamin D_3 level, and parathyroid hormone (PTH) level. Spinal bone density, liver dysfunction, and hypogonadism were the main predictors of spinal fracture while hypogonadism and the presence of cirrhosis were the main predictors of peripheral fractures.

Because of the potential for impaired absorption of calcium[23] and vitamin D,[24,25] as well as impaired hepatic uptake and metabolism of vitamin D,[26] osteomalacia (OM) was initially thought to be the major cause of hepatic osteodystrophy in cholestatic liver diseases.[26–28] However, it then became evident that bone disease was still prevalent despite treatment with calcium and vitamin D, and that most patients with cholestatic liver disease and osteopenia did not have low 25(OH) vitamin D_3 levels[12] or osteomorphometric characteristics of osteomalacia.[21,29]

The mechanisms responsible for the osteoporosis in this setting are uncertain, and evidence exists for both decreased bone formation[21,22,31,33] and increased bone resorption.[12,32–34] The presence of cirrhosis seems to play an important role, through several mechanisms. Testosterone, 25(OH) vitamin D, and insulin-like growth factor 1 (IGF-1) levels are all reduced in advanced liver disease and correlate inversely with the degree of osteopenia.[16–18] As well, bone mass starts to increase within 6 months to a year after liver transplantation.[11] Other factors may also affect bone metabolism independently of cirrhosis: bone formation is directly suppressed by alcohol,[14,35] and possibly by iron in hemochromatosis. The majority of patients with advanced PBC are also postmenopausal females, which adds to the list of pathogenic factors of HO.[16] Malnutrition, treatment with corticosteroids,[15,36] immunosuppressives, or cholestyramine[37] play a role in some cases.

Treatment

OSTEOMALACIA

R
Grade B

R
Grade B

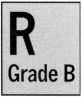

Based on 25(OH) vitamin D level measurement and bone histomorphometry, osteomalacia can be successfully treated and prevented with combined calcium and vitamin D supplementation (oral or parenteral).[25,37,38] Vitamin D does not need to be given as its 25-hydroxy metabolite, since the capacity of the liver to hydroxylate vitamin D is maintained, even in advanced liver disease. However, since its absorption and/or hepatic uptake may be decreased, sufficient doses should be administered.[25] Successful treatment of osteomalacia has been achieved with calcium and either oral vitamin D_2 2000–4000 IU daily,[25] intra muscular vitamin D_2 150 000 IU weekly,[37] or oral 25(OH)D_3 1000–4000 IU daily,[37,38] for a duration of 3–6 months. To prevent osteomalacia in cholestatic liver diseases, clinical trials have used supplementation with calcium 1–1.5 g daily and low doses of vitamin D 100 000 IU im monthly[39] or 266 μg 25(OH)D po weekly.[40]

Table 11.1 Case series of interventions for hepatic osteodystrophy

Study	Disease (no. of patients)	Therapy (duration)	Measurement (site)	Comments
Wagonfeld, 1976[26]	PBC (8)	po or sc D vs 25-OHD_3 100–200 μg/d (3 mth)	X-ray and PBA (hand)	Failure of oral or parenteral vitD to normalize 25-OHD or to prevent accelerated bone loss
Matloff, 1982[41]	PBC (10)	25-OHD_3 40–120 μg/d (1 yr)	PBA (radius)	Normalization of 25-OHD levels but ongoing bone loss and fractures
Herlong, 1982[32]	PBC (15)	25-OHD_3 50–100 μg/d (1 yr)	PBA (radius)	Normalization of 25-OHD levels but ongoing bone loss
Floreani, 1997[42]	PBC (34)	1,25$(OH)_2D_3$ 1 μg/d × 5 d, calcitonin 40 U im 3/wk ×4 wk, $CaCO_3$ 1.5 g/d ×4 wk (3 yr)	DPA (LS)	?Reduced bone loss in treated (uncontrolled)
Neuhaus, 1995[43]	OLT (150)	25-OHD_3 0.25–0.5 μg/d ± Ca 1 g/d ± NaF 25 mg/d (2 yr)	DXA (LS/FN)	Reduced bone loss in any of the treatment groups compared to untreated controls
Riemens, 1996[44]	OLT (53)	1-OHD 1 μg/day; Ca 1 g/day; etidronate 400 mg/day × 2/15 wk (1 yr)	DPA (LS)	No reduction in bone loss compared to historical controls
Crippin, 1992[45]	PBC (107)	Estrogen (low dose oral or patch) (1 yr)	DPA (LS)	Reduction in bone loss in estrogen group

PBC, primary biliary cirrhosis; OLT, orthotopic liver transplantation; CAH, chronic active hepatitis; ALD, alcoholic liver disease; HA, hydroxyapatite; NaF, sodium fluoride; UDCA, ursodeoxycholic acid; DPA, dual photon absorptiometry; DXA, dual X-ray absorptiometry; PBA, photon beam absorptiometry; SPA, single photon absorptiometry; LS, lumbar spine; FN, femoral neck.

OSTEOPOROSIS

The evidence for interventions for the treatment of osteoporosis in CLD is limited (Tables 11.1, 11.2). There are only eight randomized controlled trials (RCTs), most of which included relatively small numbers of patients. The majority of reports are based on case series.

Vitamin D and calcium

Therapy with vitamin D has been studied in osteoporotic patients with either cholestatic[32,41] or non-cholestatic liver disease[13] and low 25(OH)D levels. Uncontrolled studies in PBC (Table 11.1) suggest that normalization of 25(OH)D levels failed to arrest bone loss[32,41] or to prevent spontaneous fractures.[41] In one of these two reports, improvements in bone mass occurred only in patients whose calcium absorption increased as a result of the therapy.[41] However, in an RCT of 18 abstinent patients with alcoholic liver disease, Mobarhan[13]

R Grade C

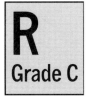

showed that normalization of 25(OH)D levels was associated with a significant increase in BMD after a mean duration of 10 months (Table 11. 2). Unfortunately, bone biopsy to rule out osteomalacia was only performed in 9 out of the 18 patients.

Calcium or hydroxyapatite supplementation appeared to prevent or diminish bone loss compared to untreated controls.[46,49]

Anti-resorptive and bone forming agents

A retrospective study of 107 females with PBC suggested that hormone replacement therapy (HRT) is associated with a significant reduction of annual bone loss[45] (Table 11.1).

Table 11.2 summarizes the results of randomized trials of a variety of other interventions. Guanabens *et al*, in a 2-year randomized controlled trial of 32 women with

Table 11.2 Randomized trials of interventions for hepatic osteodystrophy

Study	Disease (no. of paticnts)	Intervention (duration)	Measurement (sitc)	Commcnts
Epstein, 1982[46]	PBC (64)	HA 8 g/d vs Ca gluconate 2 g/d vs control (14 mth)	X-ray (hand)	Cortical thickness unchanged in Ca; increased in HA; reduced in control
Guanabens, 1997[30]	PBC (32)	Etidronate 400 mg/d × 2/15 wk vs NaF 50 mg/d (2 yr)	DPA (LS)	Significant reduction in bone loss in etidronate group
Guanabens, 1992[40]	PBC (22)	NaF 50 mg/d vs placebo (2 yr)	DPA (LS)	Significant reduction in bone loss in NaF group
[a]Camisasca, 1994[39]	PBC (25)	Carbicalcitonin 40 U sc qod vs porcine calcitonin IU sc 2/wk (15 mth)	DPA (LS)	No difference between groups
Wolfhagen, 1997[47]	PBC (12)	Etidronate 400 mg/d ×2/13 wk + Ca 500 mg/d ×11/13 wk vs Ca 500 mg/d (1 yr)	DXA (LS/FN)	Significant reduction in LS bone loss in etidronate group
Lindor, 1995[48]	PBC (88)	UDCA 13–15 mg/kg/d (3 yr)	DPA (LS)	No difference between groups
Stellon, 1985[49]	CAH (36)	HA 8 g/d (2 yr)	X-ray/SPA	Reduced bone loss in HA group
Mobarhan, 1984[13]	ALD (18)	D_2 50 000 u 2–3×/wk vs 25(OH)D 20–50 μg/d vs control (1 yr)	DPA (LS)	Significant increase in BMD compared to baseline in all groups

[a]Crossover design.
Abbreviations as Table 11.1.

PBC, compared cyclical etidronate at a dose of 400 mg for 2 weeks every 78 days, to NaF 50 mg per day.[30] In the fluoride treated group, the bone density of the lumbar spine decreased by 1.94% and the femoral neck decreased by 1.4%. By contrast, etidronate increased bone mass in the lumbar spine by 0.53% and femoral neck BMD was stable.

Wolfhagen *et al* compared etidronate plus calcium with calcium alone in a randomized trial in 12 women with PBC on corticosteroids.[47] There was a statistically significant difference in the percentage change in mean lumbar BMD between the etidronate and calcium treated groups (etidronate +0.4%, calcium −3.0%, $P = 0.01$).

Camisasca *et al* evaluated the effect of a 6-month course of calcitonin 40 IU every other day, given subcutaneously in a trial with a crossover design.[39] The control group received 1 IU of porcine calcitonin (no metabolic effect). Both groups received calcium and 100 000 IU of parenteral vitamin D_2 ($n = 25$). Treatments were administered for 6 months with a 3-month washout. There was no difference in bone density between the two treatment groups in either of the crossover periods. It is possible that this study was inadequately powered to detect a significant difference.

In another trial of 22 women with PBC followed for 2 years, Guanabens compared sodium fluoride to calcium in a 2-year RCT.[40] In the NaF group, the bone density of the lumbar spine increased by 2.9% compared to the control group that decreased by 6.6%. However, there was a high frequency of adverse effects, mainly in the gastrointestinal system. Since NaF therapy was also less effective than etidronate in another study,[30] this intervention is not recommended.

In summary, both cholestatic and non-cholestatic types of liver disease may be complicated by HO, predominately osteoporosis. The prevalence of bone disease increases with the degree of cirrhosis. Accelerated bone loss is most severe after liver transplantation. Patients with advanced liver disease, in particular those awaiting transplantation, with poor nutritional status, or with low trauma fractures, should be investigated for HO. Grade C Low 25(OH)D_3 levels should be corrected and calcium supplementation given. Postmenopausal women should receive HRT if this therapy is not contraindicated, although only Grade B evidence is available to support this recommendation. If BMD fails to improve, or fragility fractures occur, the anti-resorptive bisphosphonates should be administered, based on the evidence from two small randomized trials. Grade A

INFLAMMATORY BOWEL DISEASE

Prevalence

The importance of metabolic bone disease in patients with IBD has been recognized for some time. However, the point prevalence of bone disease in this population varies greatly from one study to another, with estimates as low as 5%[50] to as high as 78%.[51] This variation reflects a number of factors, including definitions of bone disease used, the site of bone density measurement, and the heterogeneous nature of the IBD population. A list of potential factors that need to be considered when evaluating studies in this area is provided in Table 11.3.

In a well conducted study, Abitbol *et al*[52] evaluated the BMD of 84 consecutive patients with IBD (34 Crohn's disease, 50 ulcerative colitis, excluding proctitis). Overall, 43% of this population had osteopenia in the lumbar spine. Steroid users were at significantly greater risk of osteopenia (58% vs 28% in non-users, $P = 0.03$). Six patients with a mean

Table 11.3 Factors influencing interpretation of studies of bone disease in GI patients

Definition of osteopenia	Z scores of ≤ 1
Diagnostic method	X-ray, SPA, DPA, QCT, DXA
Results expressed	BMD, BMC, radiological fracture
Bone site studied	Spine, forearm or total hip
High risk patients	Included or excluded
Control of confounders	Smoking, steroid use

SPA, single photon absorptiometry; QCT, quantitative computed tomography; DPA, dual photon absorptiometry; DXA, dual energy X-ray absorptiometry; BMD, bone mineral density; BMC, bone mineral content.

age of 50 had vertebral crush fractures (mean Z score was −1.63). Five patients were found to have low 25(OH) vitamin D_3 levels; however, the cause of this deficiency was felt to be extraintestinal in all but one case. Multiple regression analysis of the lumbar Z score revealed a significant correlation between osteopenia and age, cumulative corticosteroid dose, inflammatory status as assessed by the erythrocyte sedimentation rate (ESR), and low osteocalcin levels ($r^2 = 0.76$, $P < 0.05$).

The rate of bone loss in IBD has been studied in several longitudinal studies.[53–56]. The annual rate of bone loss appears to be greater in the spine than at the radius, and varies from 3 to 6%. Corticosteroid use[56] and low body mass index[53] were found, in some studies, to negatively affect bone mass. Overall, metabolic bone disease is an important problem among patients with IBD, with an estimated prevalence in the range of 45%. However, there is no reliable documentation of the prevalence of fractures in subjects with IBD.

Malabsorption of calcium and vitamin D because of small bowel disease appears to play a minor role in the pathogenesis of the metabolic bone disease of IBD. Both low[57,58] and normal[59] vitamin D levels have been documented in patients with Crohn's disease (CD) and there is no clear correlation between vitamin D levels and bone mass. Osteomalacia appears to be much less common than osteoporosis.[52,59] Hessov *et al*[59] performed bone biopsy and serum vitamin D determinations on 36 randomly selected CD patients with previous surgical resections (mean length 105 cm). Only two patients were found to have below normal 25(OH) vitamin D_3 levels and/or osteomorphometric evidence of osteomalacia. However, the mean trabecular bone volume was reduced in this group compared to controls, suggestive of osteoporosis. This finding did not correlate with any of the measured clinical characteristics, including length of resection and serum vitamin D level.

Comparisons between CD and UC patients reveal that osteoporosis may be more prevalent in CD.[60–62] However, careful review of these publications suggests that the analysis may not have been fully controlled for the effects of disease activity and/or steroid use. Jahnsen *et al*,[60] in an age- and sex-matched cross-sectional study of 60 CD, 60 UC, and 60 controls, found no differences in BMD between UC patients and controls. However CD patients had significantly lower BMD. Overall 16% of UC and controls had Z scores ≤1 compared to 23% of CD patients. However, significantly more CD than UC patients used corticosteroids (72% vs 47%), and smoked (57% vs 28%). Although the disease activity was not specifically addressed in this study, 53% of the UC group had left-sided disease, with 40% having proctosigmoiditis or less. As well, the BMD of CD patients who were not using steroids was not significantly different from that of the other two groups. Ghosh *et al*[61] evaluated 30 IBD patients at the time of diagnosis and found that those with CD had significantly lower bone density than those with UC.

The mean lumbar spine Z score for CD patients was –1.06 vs –0.03 for those with UC. However, 7 of 15 UC patients had proctitis alone, and 1 had a "distal colitis". As well, the mean duration of disease before diagnosis (18.6 vs 12 weeks), and of steroid use (1.2 vs 0.5 weeks) before BMD, measurements are slightly longer in the Crohn's group, again suggesting that disease severity rather than diagnosis may be the important factor. Bernstein *et al*, in a study of 26 CD and 23 UC patients, also found a greater prevalence of osteopenia among CD patients.[62] However, using stepwise discriminant analysis, the authors found that steroid use rather than disease type was the most important predictive factor.

The study of metabolic bone disease in UC before and after restorative proctocolectomy also suggests that disease activity plays an important role, since BMD increases significantly with time after colectomy, with a mean annual increase of around 2%.[55,63]

Treatment

Clements *et al*, in an uncontrolled 2-year prospective study of hormone replacement therapy (HRT) in 47 postmenopausal women with IBD (25 UC, 22 CD), found that radial and spine BMD rose significantly over baseline with HRT.[63a] The authors found no differences in the responses between patients with UC and CD. Patients using corticosteroids also seemed to respond.

Vogelsang *et al*[64] randomized 75 CD patients, without short bowel syndrome, to vitamin D_3 + calcium or placebo. The BMC decreased in 80% of the control group versus 50% of the supplemented group at one year. BMD decreased less in calcium/vitamin D treated patients (median decrease in BMD treated 0.2%, interquartile range 3.8–(+14)%; control 7%, range 12.6–(+14)%; $P < 0.005$). The correlation between the change in vitamin D and change in BMC was low ($r = 0.19$).

Bernstein *et al*,[65] in a study of 17 IBD patients with a history of steroid use (14 men, 10 CD), assessed the efficacy of calcium supplementation (1000 mg/day) on BMD by DXA. The authors found that the dose of prednisone in the year prior to the study inversely correlated with bone density at the hip and Ward's triangle, but not at the spine. A statistically significant increase in bone density was not demonstrated after one year. However, there is a significant risk of a type 2 error in this small study.

Robinson *et al*[66] assessed the effect of low impact exercise in a randomized controlled trial. Although no statistically significant increase in BMD was observed in the exercise group, secondary analysis revealed that the number of exercise sessions correlated significantly with increased BMD at the hip and spine.

R Grade A

In summary, osteopenia is an important problem among patients with IBD, even at initial diagnosis. The risk appears to be greatest among those with the greatest disease activity and duration, and among those treated with corticosteroids. The risk of osteoporosis in UC is likely similar to that seen in CD, however after proctocolectomy the bone density of UC patients increases. There is evidence that IBD patients with low BMD benefit from a combination of vitamin D and calcium, and those on corticosteroids should be considered for the interventions discussed in the next section. If not contraindicated, postmenopausal women should be given HRT. Existing studies have used surrogate outcome measures, particularly measures of BMD. Further studies are needed to assess the true fracture risk among patients with IBD and low BMD, and to assess the impact of newer agents such as bisphosphonates on this clinically important outcome.

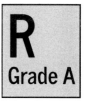

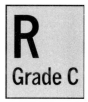

R Grade C

GLUCOCORTICOID-INDUCED BONE LOSS

Glucocorticoids are widely used in the treatment of inflammatory bowel disease, and as discussed earlier are a risk factor for bone loss. Cross-sectional studies have demonstrated a relationship between cumulative corticosteroid dose and bone loss, in multiple populations, but some prospective studies have failed to support this relationship, perhaps because of a beneficial effect of corticosteroids on disease activity.[67]

Data from cross-sectional studies of patients on corticosteroids estimate that the incidence of fractures varies from 30 to 50%.[67,68] In a study by Adinoff, 11% of asthma patients on oral steroids for one year developed vertebral fractures.[69] In a case–control study, Cooper *et al* found that use of oral steroids resulted in a relative risk of 1.16 (1.47–1.76) for hip fracture and 2.6 (2.31–2.92) for vertebral fracture.[70] There is also evidence that the relationship between bone density and fracture may underestimate the risk of fracture in patients on corticosteroids.[71]

Glucocorticoid-induced bone loss is greatest in the initial 6–12 months of treatment,[72,73] and involves areas of the skeleton which have the greatest turnover – in particular, the lumbar spine, cortical rim of the vertebral body, and Ward's triangle of the femoral neck. Hahn *et al* demonstrated that trabecular bone loss is greater than cortical bone loss in rheumatoid arthritis patients on prednisone (preferential loss at the distal metaphysis of the forearm).[74]

Pathogenesis

The mechanism of corticosteroid-induced osteoporosis (CSOP) is multifactorial and not well understood. CSOP differs from other forms of osteoporosis in that bone formation is greatly decreased at a time of increased bone resorption. This results in an imbalance between formation and resorption – "remodeling imbalance".[71] Corticosteroids cause a reduction in bone formation by increasing the apoptosis of osteoblasts.[64] Steroids stimulate osteoclastic activity through various growth factors such as insulin-like growth factor and transforming growth factor β (TGF-β). Steroids may also cause an inhibition of intestinal calcium absorption and an increase in urinary excretion of calcium, which in turn leads to an elevation of parathyroid hormone.[75] Secondary hyperparathyroidism causes increased osteoclast resorption and an increase in urinary phosphate excretion. Glucocorticoids also suppress the hypothalamic–pituitary–gonadal axis that leads to a functional hypogonadism and increased bone loss.[76] Women who are receiving steroids have adrenal suppression that results in decreased adrenal androgen secretion. Finally, steroids cause loss of muscle mass, and muscle strength is correlated with bone density.

Prevention and treatment

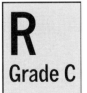

R
Grade C

A baseline bone density measurement is recommended for patients who are to remain on steroids for a prolonged period and in patients who are at risk of other types of osteoporosis, such as postmenopausal osteoporosis. The first principle of prevention is to minimize the dose of steroids. Maintenance of muscle mass through exercise is also beneficial. Supplemental calcium of 1000 mg per day and vitamin D 800 IU/day should be recommended if dietary deficiency is suspected.

A number of medications have been used for the prevention and treatment of CSOP. Tables 11.4–11.6 below summarize our results of those controlled trials of prevention and treatment of CSOP, which had vertebral fractures as an endpoint. These tables show results according to intention to treat analysis. Efficacy results are indicated.

Recent guidelines have been developed by a UK consensus group for the primary and secondary prevention of glucocorticoid osteoporosis, based on evidence from recent clinical trials.[71] This group recommends that patients be considered for therapeutic intervention if the BMD T score is below −1.5. Follow-up bone densitometry is recommended after one year and then every 1–3 years depending on the result.

CALCIUM AND VITAMIN D

Calcium and vitamin D have been used to prevent losses that occur from decreased calcium absorption, increased renal excretion of calcium, and secondary hyperparathyroidism.

Buckley *et al* conducted a 2-year RCT with calcium (1000 mg/day) and vitamin D_3 (500 IU/day) in rheumatoid arthritis patients on steroids and found that the loss of BMD in the lumbar spine and trochanter was prevented.[77] Adachi *et al* evaluated the efficacy of vitamin D (50 000 U per week) and 1000 mg calcium in patients on moderate to high dose corticosteroids and found that vitamin D and calcium prevented the early loss of bone but did not seem to be beneficial in the long term.[78] A Cochrane meta-analysis found that calcium and vitamin D prevented bone loss at the lumbar spine with a pooled weighted mean difference of 2.6% (95% CI 0.76–4.53).[79] Three trials using vitamin D and calcium have assessed vertebral fractures as an outcome (Table 11.4). Neither the individual trials nor a meta-analysis of the three trials demonstrated a statistically significant reduction in vertebral fractures (pooled relative risk 0.56, 95% CI 0.24–1.32). However, the number of patients included in these trials was small.[78,80,81]

R
Grade A

ANTIRESORPTIVE AGENTS

Since steroids increase bone resorption, antiresorptive agents such as bisphosphonates, calcitonin and hormone replacement have been used for the treatment and prevention of osteoporosis.

There have been six published RCTs of calcitonin (intranasal or subcutaneous) for prevention of osteoporosis in patients on corticosteroids.[81–86] These trials show a positive effect of calcitonin on lumbar spine bone density at 1 year. However, no statistically significant reduction in fractures was demonstrated in the five trials in which this was analyzed (Table 11.5). Meta analysis of these five trials did not demonstrate a reduction in fractures (pooled relative risk was 0.60, 95% CI 0.24–1.46).

HRT was compared to calcium supplementation in a 2-year RCT in 200 patients with rheumatoid arthritis, of whom 41 were receiving corticosteroids.[87] BMD in the spine fell by 1.19% (95% CI 2.29—0.09) in the control group, but increased in HRT treated patients (2.22%, 95% CI 0.72–3.72; P <0.001). Subgroup analysis of the steroid treated group also showed benefit of HRT treatment on spine BMD (3.75%, 95% CI 0.72–6.78). There are no published data on fracture reduction with hormone replacement therapy in CSOP. Similarly, there is little evidence to support the use of testosterone in men on corticosteroids. A small RCT of 15 men with asthma on oral glucocorticoids demonstrated that monthly testosterone injections were effective in preventing bone loss.[88]

Table 11.4 Randomized trials of calcium/vitamin D for prevention and treatment of steroid-induced osteoporosis and fractures[a]

Study	Disease (no. of patients)	Placebo (M : F)	Treatment (M : F)	Intervention (duration)	Control	Lumbar BMD (WMD)	Vertebral fractures RR (95% CI)
Sambrook, 1993[81]	PMR/RA 103	29 (7 : 22)	34 (7 : 27)	Calcitriol 0.5–1.0 μg 2 yr	Calcium 1000 mg	−1.3	Efficacy: 0.43 (0.04–4.47)
Adachi, 1996[78]	PMR/TA 62	31	31	50 000 U vitD 3 yr	Placebo	–0.7	ITT: 0.56 (0.24–1.32)
Dyckman, 1984[80]	Rheumatic disease 23	10 (1 : 9)	13 (3 : 10)	Calcium + 1,25 vitD 18 mth	Placebo + 500 mg calcium		Efficacy: 0.58 (0.17–2.01)

[a]Only studies in which vertebral fractures were included as an outcome measure have been listed.
ITT, Intention to treat analysis; PMR, polymyalgia rheumatica; RA, rheumatoid arthritis; TA, temporal arteritis.
WMD is a weighted average of the trials and the weight given to each study is the inverse of the variance. To calculate the WMD, the mean percentage change from baseline in the treatment and control groups was multiplied by the inverse of the associated variance.

Table 11.5 Randomized trials of calcitonin for prevention and treatment of steroid-induced osteoporosis and fractures[a]

Study	Disease (no. of patients)	Placebo (M : F)	Treatment (M : F)	Intervention	Control	Lumbar BMD (WMD)	Vertebral fractures RR (95% CI)
Sambrook, 1993[81]	RA, PMR 103	29 (7 : 22)	29 (6 : 23)	400 IU intranasal 2 yr	Calcium	1.1	Efficacy: 1.00 (0.15–6.63)
Ringe, 1987[82]	Lung disease 36	18 (4 : 14)	18 (3 : 15)	100 IU q 2 days sc 6 mth	Placebo + calcium		Efficacy: 0.14 (0.01–2.58)
Kotaniemi, 1996[83]	RA/all women 78	31	32	100 IU intranasal 1 yr	Placebo + calcium	10.9	ITT: 0.32 (0.01–7.65)
Healey, 1996[84]	PMR/TA 48	23 (3 : 20)	25 (9 : 16)	100 IU 3/wk sc 1 yr	Calcium/vitD vitD	–1.5	Efficacy: 0.74 (0.14–3.95)
Luengo, 1994[86]	Asthma 44	22 (3 : 19)	22 (3 : 19)	200 IU q2 days intranasal 1 yr	Placebo + calcium	10.6	ITT: 1.00 0.15–0.48)

[a]Only studies in which vertebral fractures were included as an outcome measure have been listed.
Abbreviations as in Table 11.4.

Bisphosphonates have been used for the treatment and prevention of CSOP. We identified 12 trials that used bisphosphonates for either treatment or prevention of corticosteroid osteoporosis. A Cochrane meta-analysis found that the weighted mean difference between bisphosphonates and placebo was 4% with a 95% CI of 2.5–5.5.[89] There was significant heterogeneity between trials. Five of these trials used fracture reduction in addition to BMD as an outcome measure (Table 11.6). Meta-analysis of these five trials demonstrated a significant reduction in vertebral fractures (pooled relative risk: 0.48, 95% CI 0.23–0.98).[90–94] For two of the trials, data were available to permit subgroup analysis by gender. Significant effects of treatment were not demonstrated in either gender, although a trend was apparent for benefit in females but not males.

R
Grade A

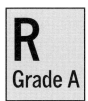

BONE FORMATION AGENTS

Monosodium fluoride has been shown to increase BMD at the lumbar spine.[95,96] However, efficacy of fluoride for vertebral fracture reduction has not been demonstrated for CSOP.[95–97] Other agents that hold promise for the future include injections of human parathyroid hormone 1-34 (hPTH 1-34) fragment. Lane *et al* compared daily injections of hPTH 1-34 along with estrogens with estrogen therapy alone in 51 osteoporotic postmenopausal women receiving glucocorticoids for rheumatic diseases, and

Table 11.6 Randomized trials of bisphosphonates for prevention or treatment of steroid-induced osteoporosis and fractures[a]

Study	Disease (no. of patients)	Placebo (M : F)	Treatment (M : F)	Intervention	Control	Lumbar BMD (WMD)	Vertebral fracture RR (95% CI)
Worth, 1994[94]	Asthma 40	20 (3/11)	20 (9/10)	Etidronate 400 mg 6 mth	Calcium	9.3	0.11 (0.01–1.94)
Adachi, 1997[90]	PMR/TA 116	74 (28/46)	67 (26/41)	Etidronate 400 mg 1 yr	Placebo + calcium	3.8	0.55 (0.20–1.53) Men: 1.44 (0.35–5.81) PM women: 0.15 (0.02–1.13)
Saag, 1998[91]	RA/PMR/ IBD/asthma 288	159 (52/107)	318 (89/229)	Alendronate 5 or 10 mg 48 wk	Placebo + calcium/vitD	2.5 —	0.60 (0.19–1.94) Men: 1.18 (0.35–4.01) PM women: 0.51 (0.14–1.83)
Boutsen, 1997[92]	PMR/TA 15	17	15	Pamidronate iv 1 yr	Placebo		0.38 (0.02–8.57)
Roux, 1997[93]	PMR/RA	58	59	Etidronate 400 mg 1 yr	Placebo + calcium	3.1	0.79 (0.22–2.78)

[a]Only studies in which vertebral fractures were included as an outcome measure have been listed.
PM, postmenopausal; other abbreviations as Table 11.4

demonstrated a 35% increase in trabecular bone mass as measured by QCT.[98] Fracture risk was not quantified.

CONCLUSION

Metabolic bone disease is an important problem in patients with liver disease and inflammatory bowel disease. In the latter condition the use of steroids is an important, but not precisely defined contributing factor. Few controlled trials have evaluated the efficacy of treatments in the absence of steroid therapy. In patients on corticosteroids, however, there is information from a number of RCTs about the efficacy of therapeutic agents in other groups of patients.

Patients at particular risk for osteoporosis include patients on glucocorticoids for IBD, those with end-stage liver disease and liver transplant patients, women who may already be osteopenic due to their postmenopausal state, and patients with vertebral abnormalities or radiographic evidence of osteopenia. In these individuals bone density measurement early in their treatment is recommended. Minimization of steroid use and use of therapeutic/preventive agents such as HRT, bisphosphonates and vitamin D are indicated in those who are already osteopenic.

While the evidence for prevention and treatment of steroid-induced osteoporosis is convincing, better designed trials of interventions for the bone disease of IBD and liver disease are needed. There is a need for evidence based guidelines for strategies to prevent osteoporosis in these populations.[99]

REFERENCES

1 World Health Organization. *Assessment of fracture risk and its application to screening for postmenopausal osteoporosis*. No 843; 1994.

2 Lindor KD. Management of osteopenia of liver disease with special emphasis on primary biliary cirrhosis. *Semin Liver Dis* 1993; **13**(4):367–73.

3 Eastell R, Boyle IT, Compston J *et al*. Management of male osteoporosis: report of the UK Consensus Group. *Q J Med* 1998; **91**: 71–92.

4 Melton LJ, Atkinson EJ, O'Fallon WM *et al*. Long term fracture prediction by bone mineral assessed at different skeletal sites. *J Bone Miner Res* 1993; **8**: 1227–33.

5 Hui SL, Slemenda CW, Johnston CC. Age and bone mass as predictors of fracture in a prospective study. *J Clin Invest* 1988; **81**: 1804–9.

6 Marshall D, Johnell O, Wedel H. Meta-analysis of how well measures of bone mineral density predict occurence of osteoporotic fractures. *Br Med J* 1996; **312**: 1254–9.

7 Lunt M, Felsenberg D, Adams J *et al*. Population-based geographic variations in DXA bone density in Europe: the EVOS study. *Osteoporos Int* 1997; **7**: 175–89.

8 Nguyen T, Sambrook P, Kelly P *et al*. Prediction of osteoporotic fractures by postural instability and bone density. *Br Med J* 1993; **307**: 1111–15.

9 Green CJ. *Bone mineral density testing: does the evidence support its selective use in well women?* Vancouver: British Columbia Office of Health Technology Assessment, The University of Ottawa, 1997 (BCOHTA 97: 2T).

10 Compston JE. Hepatic osteodystrophy: vitamin D metabolism in patients with liver disease. *Gut* 1986; **27**(9): 1073–90.

11 Eastell R, Dickson ER, Hodgson SF *et al*. Rates of vertebral bone loss before and after liver transplantation in women with primary biliary cirrhosis. *Hepatology* 1991; **14**(2): 296–300.

12 Hay JE, Lindor KD, Wiesner RH *et al*. The metabolic bone disease of primary sclerosing cholangitis. *Hepatology* 1991; Aug; **14**(2): 257–61.

13 Mobarhan SA, Russell RM, Recker RR *et al*. Metabolic bone disease in alcoholic cirrhosis: a comparison of the effect of vitamin D_2, 25-hydroxyvitamin D, or supportive treatment. *Hepatology* 1984; **4**(2): 266–73.

14 Chappard D, Plantard B, Fraisse H *et al*. Bone changes in alcoholic liver cirrhosis, a histomorphometrical analysis of 52 cases. *Pathol Res Pract* 1989; **184**(5): 480–5.

15 Stellon AJ, Webb A, Compston JE. Bone histomorphometry and structure in corticosteroid treated chronic active hepatitis. *Gut* 1988; **29** (3): 378–84.

16 Diamond T, Stiel D, Lunzer M *et al.* Osteoporosis and skeletal fractures in chronic liver disease. *Gut* 1990; **31**(1): 82–7.

17 Chen CC, Wang SS, Jeng FS *et al.* Metabolic bone disease of liver cirrhosis: is it parallel to the clinical severity of cirrhosis? *J Gastroenterol Hepatol* 1996; **11**(5): 417–21.

18 Gallego-rojo FJ. Bone mineral density, serum insulin-like growth factor I and bone turnover markers in viral cirrhosis. *Hepatology* 1998; **28**: 695–9.

19 Porayko MK, Wiesner RH, Hay JE *et al.* Bone disease in liver transplant recipients: incidence, timing, and risk factors. *Transplant Proc* 1991; **23**(1 Pt 2): 1462–5.

20 Park KM, Hay JE, Lee SG *et al.* Bone loss after orthotopic liver transplantation: FK 506 versus cyclosporine. *Transplant Proc* 1996; **28**(3): 1738–40.

21 Diamond TH, Stiel D, Lunzer M *et al.* Hepatic osteodystrophy. Static and dynamic bone histomorphometry and serum bone Gla-protein in 80 patients with chronic liver disease. *Gastroenterology* 1989; **96**(1): 213–21.

22 Hodgson SF, Dickson ER, Wahner HW *et al.* Bone loss and reduced osteoblast function in primary biliary cirrhosis. *Ann Intern Med* 1985; **103** (6 Pt 1): 855–60.

23 Whelton MJ, Kehayoglou AK, Agnew JE *et al.* 47 Calcium absorption in parenchymatous and biliary liver disease. *Gut* 1971; **12**(12): 978–83.

24 Krawitt EL, Grundman MJ, Mawer EB. Absorption, hydroxylation, and excretion of vitamin D_3 in primary biliary cirrhosis. *Lancet* 1977; **ii** (8051): 1246–9.

25 Davies M, Mawer EB, Klass HJ *et al.* Vitamin D deficiency, osteomalacia, and primary biliary cirrhosis. Response to orally administered vitamin D3. *Dig Dis Sci* 1983; **28**(2): 145–53.

26 Wagonfeld JB, Nemchausky BA, Bolt M *et al.* Comparison of vitamin D and 25-hydroxy-vitamin-D in the therapy of primary biliary cirrhosis. *Lancet* 1976; **ii**: 391–4.

27 Long RG, Varghese Z, Meinhard EA *et al.* Parenteral 1,25-dihydroxycholecalciferol in hepatic osteomalacia. *Br Med J* 1978; **1**: 75–7.

28 Dibble JB, Sheridan P, Hampshire R *et al.* Osteomalacia, vitamin D deficiency and cholestasis in chronic liver disease. *Q J Med* 1982; **51**: 89–103.

29 Cuthbert JA, Pak CYC, Zerwekh JE *et al.* Bone disease in primary biliary cirrhosis: increased bone resorption and turnover in the absence of osteoporosis or osteomalacia. *Hepatology* 1984; **4**: 1–8.

30 Guanabens N, Pares A, Monegal A *et al.* Etidronate versus fluoride for treatment of osteopenia in primary biliary cirrhosis: preliminary results after 2 years. *Gastroenterology* 1997; **113**(1): 219–24.

31 Maddrey WC. Bone disease in patients with primary biliary cirrhosis. *Prog Liv Dis* 1990; **9**: 537–54.

32 Herlong HF, Recker RR, Maddrey WC. Bone disease in primary biliary cirrhosis: histologic features and response to 25-hydroxyvitamin D. *Gastroenterology* 1982; **83**(1:Pt 1): 103–8.

33 Stellon AJ, Webb A, Compston J *et al.* Low bone turnover state in primary biliary cirrhosis. *Hepatology* 1987; **7**(1): 137–42.

34 Cuthbert JA, Pak CY, Zerwekh JE *et al.* Bone disease in primary biliary cirrhosis: increased bone resorption and turnover in the absence of osteoporosis or osteomalacia. *Hepatology* 1984; **4**(1): 1–8.

35 Peris P, Pares A, Guanabens N *et al.* Bone mass improves in alcoholics after 2 years of abstinence. *J Bone Miner Res* 1994; **9**(10): 1607–12.

36 Mitchison HC, Bassendine MF, Malcolm AJ *et al.* A pilot, double-blind, controlled 1-year trial of prednisolone treatment in primary biliary cirrhosis: hepatic improvement but greater bone loss. *Hepatology* 1989; **10**(4): 420–9.

37 Compston JE, Horton LW, Thompson RP. Treatment of osteomalacia associated with primary biliary cirrhosis with parenteral vitamin D_2 or oral 25-hydroxyvitamin D_3. *Gut* 1979; **20**(2): 133–6.

38 Reed JS, Meredith SC, Nemchausky BA *et al.* Bone disease in primary biliary cirrhosis: reversal of osteomalacia with oral 25-hydroxyvitamin D. *Gastroenterology* 1980; **78**(3): 512–1.

39 Camisasca M, Crosignani A, Battezzati PM *et al.* Parenteral calcitonin for metabolic bone disease associated with primary biliary cirrhosis. *Hepatology* 1994; **20**(3): 633–7.

40 Guanabens N, Pares A, Del R *et al.* Sodium fluoride prevents bone loss in primary biliary cirrhosis. *J Hepatol* 1992; **15**(3): 345–9.

41 Matloff DS, Kaplan MM, Neer RM *et al.* Osteoporosis in primary biliary cirrhosis: effects of 25-hydroxyvitamin D_3 treatment. *Gastroenterology* 1982; **83** (1): 97–102.

42 Floreani A, Zappala F, Fries W *et al.* A 3-year pilot study with 1,25-dihydroxyvitamin D, calcium, and calcitonin for severe osteodystrophy in primary biliary cirrhosis. *J Clin Gastroenterol* 1997; **24** (4): 239–44.

43 Neuhaus R, Lohmann R, Platz KP *et al.* Treatment of osteoporosis after liver transplantation. *Transplant Proc* 1995; **27**(1): 1226–7.

44 Riemens SC, Oostdijk A, van DJ *et al.* Bone loss after liver transplantation is not prevented by cyclical etidronate, calcium and alphacalcidol. The Liver Transplant Group, Groningen. *Osteoporos Int* 1996; **6**(3): 213–18.

45 Crippin JS, Jorgensen RA, Dickson ER *et al.* Hepatic osteodystrophy in primary biliary cirrhosis: effects of medical treatment. *Am J Gastroenterol* 1994; **89**(1): 47–50.

46 Epstein O, Kato Y, Dick R *et al.* Vitamin D, hydroxyapatite, and calcium gluconate in treatment of cortical bone thinning in postmenopausal women with primary biliary cirrhosis. *Am J Clin Nutr* 1982; **36**(3): 426–30.

47 Wolfhagen FH, van Buuren HR, den Ouden JW *et al.* Cyclical etidronate in the prevention of bone loss in corticosteroid-treated primary biliary cirrhosis. A prospective, controlled pilot study. *J Hepatol* 1997; **26**(2): 325–30.

48 Lindor KD, Janes CH, Crippin JS *et al.* Bone disease in primary biliary cirrhosis: does ursodeoxycholic acid make a difference? *Hepatology* 1995; **21** (2): 389–92.

49 Stellon A, Davies A, Webb A *et al.* Microcrystalline hydroxyapatite compound in prevention of bone loss in corticosteroid-treated patients with chronic active hepatitis. *Postgrad Med J* 1985; **61**(719): 791–6.

50 Silvennoinen JA, Karttunen TJ, Niemela SE *et al.* A controlled study of bone mineral density in patients with inflammatory bowel disease. *Gut* 1995; **37**(1): 71–6.

51 Bjarnason I, Macpherson A, Mackintosh C *et al.* Reduced bone density in patients with inflammatory bowel disease. *Gut* 1997; **40** (2): 228–33.

52 Abitbol V, Roux C, Chaussade S *et al.* Metabolic bone assessment in patients with inflammatory bowel disease. *Gastroenterology* 1995; **108** (2): 417–22.

53 Motley RJ, Crawley EO, Evans C *et al.* Increased rate of spinal trabecular bone loss in patients with inflammatory bowel disease. *Gut* 1988; **29** (10): 1332–6.

54 Ryde SJ, Clements D, Evans WD *et al.* Total body calcium in patients with inflammatory bowel disease: a longitudinal study. *Clin Sci* 1991; **80** (4): 319–24.

55 Roux C, Abitbol V, Chaussade S *et al.* Bone loss in patients with inflammatory bowel disease: a prospective study. *Osteoporos Int* 1995; **5** (3): 156–60.

56 Motley R. A four-year longitudinal study of bone loss in patients with inflammatory bowel disease. *Bone Miner* 1993; **23**: 95–104.

57 Driscoll RHJ, Meredith SC, Sitrin M *et al.* Vitamin D deficiency and bone disease in patients with Crohn's disease. *Gastroenterology* 1982; **83** (6): 1252–8.

58 Compston JE, Creamer B. Plasma levels and intestinal absorption of 25-hydroxyvitamin D in patients with small bowel resection. *Gut* 1977; **18**(3): 171–5.

59 Hessov I, Mosekilde L, Melsen F *et al.* Osteopenia with normal vitamin D metabolites after small-bowel resection for Crohn's disease. *Scand J Gastroenterol* 1984; **19**(5): 691–6.

60 Jahnsen J, Falch JA, Aadland E *et al.* Bone mineral density is reduced in patients with Crohn's disease but not in patients with ulcerative colitis: a population based study. *Gut* 1997; **40**: 313–19.

61 Ghosh S, Cowen S, Hannan WJ *et al.* Low bone mineral density in Crohn's disease, but not in ulcerative colitis, at diagnosis. *Gastroenterology* 1994; **107**(4): 1031–9.

62 Bernstein CN, Seeger LL, Sayre JW *et al.* Decreased bone density in inflammatory bowel disease is related to corticosteroid use and not disease diagnosis. *J Bone Miner Res* 1995; **10**(2): 250–6.

63 Abitbol V, Roux C, Guillemant S *et al.* Bone assessment in patients with ileal pouch-anal anastomosis for inflammatory bowel disease. *Br J Surg* 1997; **84**(11): 1551–4.

63a Clements D, Compston J, Evans W, Rhodes J. Hormone replacement therapy prevents bone loss in patients with inflammatory bone disease. *Gut* 1993; **34**: 1543–6.

64 Vogelsang H, Ferenci P, Resch H *et al.* Prevention of bone mineral loss in patients with Crohn's disease by long-term oral vitamin D supplementation. *Eur J Gastroenterol Hepatol* 1995; **7**(7): 609–14.

65 Bernstein CN, Seeger LL, Anton PA *et al.* A randomized, placebo-controlled trial of calcium supplementation for decreased bone density in corticosteroid-using patients with inflammatory bowel disease: a pilot study. *Aliment Pharmacol Ther* 1996; **10**(5): 777–86.

66 Robinson RJ, Krzywicki T, Almond L *et al.* Effect of a low-impact exercise program on bone mineral density in Crohn's disease – a randomized controlled trial. *Gastroenterology* 1998; **115** (1): 36–41.

67 Lane NE, Lukert B. The science and therapy of glucocorticoid-induced bone loss. *Endocrinol Metabol Clin North Am* 1998; **27**(2): 465–83.

68 Lukert B, Raisz LG. Glucocorticoid-induced osteoporosis: pathogenesis and management. *Ann Intern Med* 1990; **112**: 352–64.

69 Adinoff AD, Hollister JR. Steroid-induced fractures and bone loss in patients with asthma. *N Engl J Med* 1983; **309**: 265–8.

70 van Staa TP, Cooper C, Abenhaim L *et al.* Use of oral corticosteroids and risk of fractures. *J Bone Miner Res* 1998; **11**(Suppl 1): S202.

71 Eastell R, Reid DM, Compston J *et al.* A UK Consensus group on management of

glucocorticoid-induced osteoporosis: an update. *J Intern Med* 1998; **244**: 271–92.
72 Laan. Low-dose prednisone induces rapid reversible axial bone loss in patients with rheumatoid arthritis. A randomized, controlled study. *Ann Intern Med* 1993; **119**: 963–8.
73 Sambrook PN. Corticosteroid induced osteoporosis. *J Rheumatol* 1996; **45**(Suppl): 19–22.
74 Hahn TJ, Boiseau VC, Alviole LV *et al.* Effect of chronic corticosteroid administration on diaphyseal and metaphyseal bone mass. *J Clin Endrocrinol Metabol* 1974; **39**: 274–82.
75 Suzuki Y, Ichikawa Y, Saito E *et al.* Importance of increased urinary calcium excretion in the development of secondary hyperparathyroidism of patients under glucocorticoid therapy. *Metabolism* 1983; **32**: 151–6.
76 Macadams MR. Reduction in serum testosterone levels during chronic glucocorticoid therapy. *Ann Intern Med* 1998; **104**: 648–51.
77 Buckley LM, Leib ES, Cartularo KS *et al.* Calcium and vitamin D_3 supplementation prevents bone loss in the spine secondary to low-dose corticosteroids in patients with rheumatoid arthritis. A randomized double-blind, placebo controlled trial. *Ann Intern Med* 1996; **125** (12): 961–8.
78 Adachi JD, Bensen WG, Bianchi F *et al.* Vitamin D and calcium in the prevention of corticosteroid induced osteoporosis: a 3-year followup. *J Rheumatol* 1996; **23**: 995–1000.
79 Homik J, Suarez-Almazor ME, Shea B *et al.* Calcium and vitamin D for corticosteroid-induced osteoporosis (Cochrane Review). In: The Cochrane Library (database on disk and CD-ROM). Oxford: The Cochrane Collaboration. Update Software; 1999, issue 1.
80 Dykman TR, Haralson KM, Gluck OS *et al.* Effect of oral 1,25-dihydroxyvitamin D calcium on glucocorticoid-induced osteopenia in patients with rheumatic diseases. *Arthritis Rheum* 1984; **27**(12): 1336–43.
81 Sambrook P, Birmingham J, Kelly P *et al.* Prevention of corticosteroid osteoporosis. *N Engl J Med* 1993; **238**(24): 1747–52.
82 Ringe JD, Welzel D. Salmon calcitonin in the therapy of corticoid-induced osteoporosis. *Eur J Clin Pharmacol* 1987; **33**(1): 35–9.
83 Kotaniemi A, Piirainen H, Paimela L *et al.* Is continuous intranasal salmon calcitonin effective in treating axial bone loss in patients with active rheumatoid arthritis receiving low dose glucocorticoid therapy? *J Rheumatol* 1996; **23**: 1875–9.
84 Healey JH, Paget SA, Williams-Russo P *et al.* A randomized controlled trial of salmon calcitonin to prevent bone loss in corticosteroid-treated temporal arteritis and polymyalgia rheumatica. *Calcif Tissue Int* 1996; **58**: 73–80.
85 Luengo M, Picado C, Del R *et al.* Treatment of steroid-induced osteopenia with calcitonin in corticosteroid-dependent asthma. A one-year follow-up study. *Am Rev Respir Dis* 1990; **142**(1): 104–7.
86 Luengo M, Pons F, Martinez D *et al.* Prevention of further bone mass loss by nasal calcitonin in patients on long term glucocorticoid therapy for asthma: a two year follow up study. *Thorax* 1994; **49**(11): 1099–102.
87 Hall GM, Daniels M, Doyle DV *et al.* Effect of hormone replacement therapy on bone mass in rheumatoid arthritis patients treated with and without steroids. *Arthritis Rheum* 1994; **37** (10): 1499–505.
88 Reid IR, Wattie DJ, Evans MC *et al.* Testosterone therapy in glucocorticoid-treated men. *Arch Intern Med* 1996; **156**(11): 1173–7.
89 Homik J, Cranney A, Shea B *et al.* Bisphosphonates for steroid induced osteoporosis (Cochrane Review). In: The Cochrane Library (database on disk and CD-ROM). Oxford: The Cochrane Collaboration. Update Software; 1999, issue 1.
90 Adachi JD, Bensen WG, Brown J *et al.* Intermittent etidronate therapy to prevent corticosteroid-induced osteoporosis. *N Engl J Med* 1997; **337** (6): 382–7.
91 Saag KG. Alendronate for the prevention and treatment of glucocorticoid-induced osteoporosis. *N Engl J Med* 1998; **339**: 292–9.
92 Boutsen Y, Jamart J, Esselinckx W *et al.* Primary prevention of glucocorticoid-induced osteoporosis with intermittent intravenous pamidronate: a randomized trial. *Calcif Tissue Int* 1997; **61** (4): 266–71.
93 Roux C. Randomized trial of effect of cyclical etidronate in the prevention of corticosteroid-induced bone loss. *J Clin Endrocrinol Metabol* 1998; **83**: 1128–33.
94 Worth H, Stammen D, Keck E. Therapy of steroid-induced bone loss in adult asthmatics with calcium, vitamin D, and a diphosphonate. *Am J Respir Crit Care* 1994; **150**: 394–7.
95 Lems WF, Jacobs JW, Bijlsma JW *et al.* Is addition of sodium fluoride to cyclical etidronate beneficial in the treatment of corticosteroid induced osteoporosis? *Ann Rheum Dis* 1997; **56** (6): 357–63.
96 Lippuner K, Haller B, Casez JP *et al.* Effect of disodium monofluorophosphate, calcium and vitamin D supplementation on bone mineral density in patients chronically treated with glucocorticosteroids: a prospective, randomized, double-blind study. *Miner Electrolyte Metabol* 1996; **22**(4): 207–13.
97 Guaydier-Souquieres G, Kotzki P, Sabatier J *et al.* In corticosteroid-treated respiratory diseases,

monofluorophosphate increases lumbar bone density: a double-masked randomized study. *Osteoporos Int* 1996; **6**(2): 171–7.
98 Lane NE, Roe B, Genant HK. Parathyroid hormone can reverse glucocorticoid-induced osteoporosis: results of a randomized controlled trial. *J Clin Invest* 1998; **102**(8): 1627–33.
99 Scott EM, Scott BB. A strategy for osteoporosis gastroenterology. *Eur J Gastroenterol Hepatol* 1998; **10**: 689–98.

Colorectal cancer in ulcerative colitis: surveillance

12

BRET A LASHNER, ALASTAIR JM WATSON

EPIDEMIOLOGICAL INVESTIGATION

Many questions are posed by patients, clinicians, and investigators regarding the recommended methods of cancer surveillance in ulcerative colitis. In the absence of scientific rigor conferred by randomized clinical trials, answers to these questions only can be inferred from observational studies. The evidence from cohort studies, case–control studies, and studies of diagnostic testing coupled with surveillance theory and perceived patient preferences can be used to answer some of the more pressing questions and provide recommendations.

Cohort studies are epidemiological investigations that address specific "natural history" questions.[1] Groups of ulcerative colitis patients and controls are followed from the inception of disease until the development of specific outcomes, such as dysplasia or cancer, and incidence rates are compared between groups. Cohort studies are particularly useful for quantifying cancer risk as well as for identifying risk factors for disease outcome.[2–10] For example, recent cohort studies mostly have found primary sclerosing cholangitis to be a risk factor for dysplasia or cancer in patients with ulcerative colitis (Table 12.1).[11–16] However, incorrect conclusions related to prognosis can be made if cohort studies are performed without careful attention to issues of bias and confounding variables. Standards have been published delineating the scientific requirements for the performance of valid cohort studies on cancer risk in ulcerative colitis. These include assembly of an inception cohort, blind assessment of objective outcomes, complete follow-up, and a description of the referral pattern.[17]

Case–control studies can also be used to examine etiological associations.[1] Ulcerative colitis cases with cancer or dysplasia are compared to controls without neoplasia to test for differences in the odds of exposure to possible causative agents. Case–control studies are highly susceptible to bias and confounding variables. For a putative etiological factor to be considered valid it must be strong, consistent from study to study, occur before the effect, be biologically plausible, and exhibit a dose–response relationship to the event of interest. As an example, case–control studies are best for identifying agents such as folic acid that may prevent the development of cancer or dysplasia.[18–20]

Studies of diagnostic testing provide important insights into the optimization of parameters related to cancer surveillance.[1,21] Studies comparing the sensitivity and specificity of different diagnostic tests can help choose the best test. Studies examining the sensitivity–specificity tradeoff between different cut-points of the same test can help choose the optimal criterion for a positive test. Among surveillance tests examined in ulcerative colitis (such as DNA aneuploidy, salicyl-Tn expression, p53 suppressor gene

Table 12.1 Cohort studies of primary sclerosing cholangitis (PSC) as a risk factor for dysplasia or cancer in ulcerative colitis

Study	Center	Patients	Dysplasia or cancer	Relative risk (95% CI)
Broome, 1992[11]	Huddinge	5 PSC	4 (80%)	6.7 (2.6–17.4)
		67 controls	8 (12%)	
Gurbuz, 1995[12]	Baltimore	35 PSC	13 (37%)	Increased
Broome, 1995[13]	Huddinge	40 PSC	16 (40%)	3.2 (1.6–6.2)
		80 controls	10 (12%)	
Brentnall, 1996[14]	Seattle	20 PSC	9 (45%)	4.9 (1.4–17.7)
		25 controls	4 (16%)	
Loftus, 1996[15]	Rochester	143 PSC	8 (6%)	4.9 (0.1–27)
Marchesa 1997[16]	Cleveland	27 PSC	18 (67%)	10.4 (4.1–26.1)
		1185 controls	145 (12%)	

overexpression, and dysplasia), dysplasia is the best studied and the test with the best surveillance program performance.[22] When evaluating biopsy specimens for dysplasia, the optimal criterion for a positive test is low-grade dysplasia (a criterion with high sensitivity), rather than high-grade dysplasia (a criterion with high specificity).

AXIOMS

Many accepted practices related to cancer surveillance in ulcerative colitis have not been studied, but are assumed to be valid. Indeed, there are certain axiomatic statements that must be true for surveillance to be at all accepted by patients and physicians.

(1) *The cancer risk is elevated in ulcerative colitis patients and too high to ignore.* There have been many epidemiological studies investigating the cancer risk in ulcerative colitis.[3–10] These studies are usually from Northern Europe or North America where ulcerative colitis incidence is high and accurate and complete databases exist. From these studies, it is reasonable to assume that the lifetime incidence of colorectal cancer in a patient with panulcerative colitis is approximately 6%, since a risk of this magnitude has been established for the background risk in the American population,[23] and the risk of cancer-related mortality is approximately 3%. These figures are too high to ignore, assuming there is either effective surveillance available or acceptable prophylactic treatment. Furthermore, in some countries like the US, either prophylactic colectomy or cancer surveillance colonoscopy have become the standard of care for ulcerative colitis patients, especially those diagnosed at a young age. In older patients, especially those with severe co-morbidity or disability, the case for surveillance is much less clearcut since they may be more likely to die from other diseases and not be fit for proctocolectomy.

(2) *Most patients would rather not have prophylactic colectomy.* Colectomy prior to the development of dysplasia or cancer is sure to dramatically reduce, if not eliminate, the mortality from colorectal cancer.[24] The existence of cancer surveillance programs, whether or not they are effective, has convinced some patients that the excess cancer mortality risk with ulcerative colitis can be minimized, and that the minimized risk is preferred to the morbidity following proctocolectomy.

(3) *Patients would agree to proctocolectomy if the cancer risk is very high, as it is with a positive test from surveillance.* There is no point to performing surveillance colonoscopy if a

patient will refuse to have a proctocolectomy for a positive test. Clinicians need to counsel patients carefully so they understand that surveillance is meant to identify the patients at very high cancer risk for proctocolectomy and allow the remaining patients to continue in the cancer surveillance program. From that approach, a majority of patients, those without dysplasia, will not have a colectomy recommended.

In an optimally performing program, all cancer deaths will be averted through colectomy on high risk patients, and no cancer deaths will occur among patients not having colectomy. There has been no perfectly performing surveillance program reported. Program performance is likely to improve following the development of a diagnostic test with better sensitivity and specificity than the presence or absence of dysplasia and/or with more frequent testing than is currently done.

QUESTIONS

Existing evidence only can partially answer some of the questions related to cancer surveillance in ulcerative colitis. Understanding the limits of this evidence and identifying priorities for future investigation could improve technical aspects of surveillance and, ultimately, decrease cancer related mortality. Questions regarding expected outcomes, the method of surveillance, testing intervals, and the criterion for a positive test will be addressed.

(1) *How effective will a surveillance program be for reducing cancer related mortality?* The number of patients needed to be enrolled in a surveillance program who comply with all of its parameters (ie repeated testing with colectomy for a positive test) in order to avert one cancer death can be calculated using expected risk reductions. The number needed to treat (NNT) is the inverse of the absolute risk reduction.[1] Assuming the cancer related mortality in high risk patients is 3%, the NNT in a perfectly performing program in which colectomy for dysplasia is highly effective for prevention of death from cancer and results in the complete elimination of cancer related mortality is 1/0.03 or 33. For an absolute risk reduction from surveillance of 1% (ie 3% to 2%), the NNT is 100, and for an absolute risk reduction of 2% (ie 3% to 1%), the NNT is 50. It is reasonable to assume that surveillance will have some benefit and the NNT most likely will fall between 33 and 100. Therefore, for every 100 patients with panulcerative colitis who are entered into and faithfully comply with the parameters of a surveillance program, between 1 and 3 cancer deaths will be averted.

R
Grade C

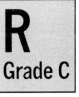

(2) *What is the best testing method for cancer surveillance?* Using colonoscopy with multiple biopsies of the colon as a testing method is problematical, but still the best and most accepted method of testing for cancer surveillance in ulcerative colitis. Since dysplasia can be present focally, and not necessarily diffusely, biopsies must be taken throughout the colon. The more biopsies taken, the better will be the sensitivity for detecting dysplasia. However, the more biopsies taken, the higher will be the pathology costs, the longer will be the time (and the associated costs) of the procedure, and the greater will be the morbidity of the colonoscopy. Even the most intensive sampling protocols sample less than 0.05% of the colon. While it has not been studied, it seems to be a reasonable tradeoff between sensitivity and cost/morbidity to sample the colon with two biopsies taken from each 10 cm colonic segment and of any lesion suspicious of a dysplasia-associated lesion or mass (DALM). DALMs can be suspected by an irregular, furry appearance that resembles a sessile adenoma, but can only be confirmed by detecting dysplasia histologically.[25]

Problematical issues involve pseudopolyps and strictures. A patient with multiple pseudo polyps that cannot be adequately biopsied could easily harbor dysplastic tissue that would not be biopsied. These patients need to be informed of the poor sensitivity of surveillance, and the benefits of prophylactic colectomy. Likewise, colonic strictures that do not allow passage of the colonoscope and adequate sampling could, and very often do, harbor dysplasia.[26] Once again, these patients should be considered for prophylactic colectomy since surveillance of these patients is insensitive.

While it does not appear that other tests will have adequate sensitivity or specificity to be used in the near future for cancer surveillance, research is progressing in the area of testing alternatives. Acquired genetic abnormalities such as DNA aneuploidy, p53 suppressor gene mutations, and salicyl-Tn expression could be used with dysplasia to improve sensitivity.[22] Patients would be considered to have a positive test if either dysplasia or a genetic abnormality is present. Of course, improved sensitivity will be at the cost of specificity and result in increased numbers of false positives. The penalty for lowering specificity is high – a proctocolectomy in a patient who might not have developed cancer. These alternative tests would be acceptable for use in a surveillance program if the cost were relatively low, the availability high, the gain in sensitivity great, and the loss of specificity minimal.

(3) *What is the best testing interval?* The more tests that are performed in a lifetime, the higher the likelihood that dysplasia will be detected and treated prior to the development of cancer and the lower the cancer related mortality. Of course, the more tests that are performed, the higher will be the cost, morbidity, and patient intolerance to colonoscopy. A balance between benefits and costs needs to be struck.

The approximate time between the development of low grade dysplasia and cancer, the lead time, is 3 years[27,28] While patients could progress at a slower or faster rate, the mean value for the lead time is 3 years. Therefore, testing at intervals longer than 3 years should be discouraged. A majority of patients who develop cancer would not have an opportunity to have dysplasia detected from surveillance examinations.

R
Grade C

The risk of developing cancer or dysplasia increases with increasing duration of disease. The benefits of frequent testing (short interval) also increase with increasing duration of disease. It can be concluded that uniform testing intervals over a lifetime of disease is not an efficient way to allocate the performance of costly and invasive test procedures. A decision analysis suggests that efficient testing is characterized by decreasing the testing interval with increasing duration of disease.[27] One reasonable method, which certainly can be adjusted according to patient and physician preferences, specifies testing every 3 years for the first 20 years of disease, every 2 years for the next 10 years of disease, and yearly thereafter. Such an approach would require at least 20 tests over a 40-year lifetime of disease, with most allocated in the later years when the risk is the highest.

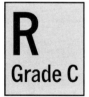

(4) *What is the best criterion for a positive test?* The type of dysplastic lesion to be used as a criterion for a positive test is best determined by weighing the tradeoff between sensitivity and specificity. Sensitivity is defined as the proportion of patients with disease who are positive for the test in question. Likewise, specificity is defined as the proportion of patients without disease who are negative for the test in question. A standard 2×2 contingency table for N patients (N =a+b+c+d) is shown in Figure 12.1.

In normally distributed populations, sensitivity (a/[a+c]) and specificity (d/[b+d]) are stable values that do not vary with prevalence of disease. Sensitivity and specificity will vary though, when the "cut-point" or the criterion for a positive test changes. For example, if the criterion for a positive test changes from high-grade dysplasia to

	Cancer	No cancer
Dysplasia	a	b
No dysplasia	c	d

$$\textbf{Sensitivity} = \frac{a}{a+b}$$

$$\textbf{Specificity} = \frac{d}{d+b}$$

Figure 12.1 Contingency table for calculating sensitivity and specificity of dysplasia for the diagnosis of cancer

low-grade dysplasia, the sensitivity will increase (more a's and less c's) and the specificity will decrease (more b's and less d's). As the criterion for a positive test changes, there is a tradeoff between sensitivity and specificity – as one increases the other decreases.

The sensitivity and specificity of screening for dysplasia to identify patients with asymptomatic cancer has been studied with remarkably consistent results. A blinded review from the University of Chicago of all regions in colectomy specimens in 22 ulcerative colitis patients with cancer identified dysplasia distant from the malignancy in 16 (73% sensitivity for any dysplasia).[29] Eleven patients had high grade dysplasia (50% sensitivity for high grade dysplasia). In a comparable group of 22 ulcerative colitis patients without cancer, 6 had dysplasia (73% specificity for any dysplasia) and 2 had high grade dysplasia (91% specificity for high grade dysplasia). Nearly identical results were found in a study from the Mayo Clinic, where 100 colectomy specimens from patients with ulcerative colitis, 50 of whom had cancer, were studied.[30] The sensitivity for any dysplasia was 74% (37/50) and the sensitivity for high grade dysplasia was 32% (16/50). The specificity of any dysplasia was 74% (37/50) and the specificity of high grade dysplasia was 98% (49/50). Both studies acknowledged that only a small minority of patients were followed in cancer surveillance programs. In a study from St Mark's Hospital, London, principally of ulcerative colitis patients participating in surveillance programs, 37 of 50 colectomy specimens with cancer had dysplasia distant from the malignancy (74% sensitivity for any dysplasia).[30] Sixteen of those patients had high grade dysplasia (32% sensitivity for high grade dysplasia). Therefore, both the sensitivity and specificity of testing for any dysplasia is approximately 74% (Table 12.2). If high grade dysplasia were to be used as a criterion for a positive test, the sensitivity would fall to less than 50% and the specificity would rise to greater than 90%.

Definitions for sensitivity and specificity for surveillance are somewhat different from these definitions for screening. The endpoint of interest in the former situation is death from colon cancer in distinction to its detection alone. Over the course of the disease, patients in a surveillance program will have several colonoscopic examinations with biopsies for dysplasia or cancer. The sensitivity of a surveillance program may be regarded as the proportion of patients with cancer who are successfully treated with colectomy. Those who die of colorectal cancer are false negative patients (group c in Figure 12.1) in whom surveillance has failed to prevent a cancer related death. This definition of sensitivity represents a conservative value, since there are patients who had a colectomy

Table 12.2 The sensitivity and specificity of dysplasia to diagnose colorectal cancer in ulcerative collitis patients stratified by degree of dysplasia

Study center	Sensitivity (%)	Specificity (%)
University of Chicago, 1985[29]		
Any dysplasia	73	73
High grade dysplasia	50	91
Mayo Clinic, 1992[30]		
Any dysplasia	74	74
High grade dysplasia	32	98
St Mark's Hospital, 1994[31]		
Any dysplasia	74	—
High grade dysplasia	32	—

12.3 The sensitivity and specificity of 11 large colorectal cancer surveillance programs in ulcerative colitis patients

Study center	No. of patients	Sensitivity	Specificity
Univ. of Leeds, 1980[32]	43	2/2 (100%)	34/41 (83%)
Cleveland Clinic, 1985[33]	248	6/7 (86%)	194/241 (80%)
Univ. of Chicago, 1989[34]	99	4/8 (50%)	73/91 (80%)
Karolinska Institute, 1990[35]	72	2/2 (100%)	54/70 (77%)
Lahey Clinic, 1991[36]	213	4/10 (40%)	171/203 (84%)
Helsinki Univ., 1991[37]	66	0/0 —	57/66 (86%)
Lennox Hill Hosp., 1992[38]	121	4/7 (57%)	91/114 (80%)
St Mark's Hosp., 1994[39]	284	13/17 (76%)	205/267 (77%)
Ornskoldsvik Hosp., 1994[40]	131	2/4 (50%)	103/127 (81%)
Tel Aviv Med. Center, 1995[41]	154	3/4 (75%)	141/150 (94%)
Univ. of Bologna, 1995[42]	65	4/4 (100%)	58/61 (95%)

for dysplasia in whom cancer would have developed if the colectomy had not been performed. Since it is impossible to know which patients with dysplasia would have developed cancer, these patients are not included in the calculations of sensitivity. The specificity of a surveillance program is the proportion of patients who do not develop cancer and who do not have dysplasia detected. Since cancer is rare in a surveillance program, specificity is very well estimated by the proportion of patients in the surveillance program who do not develop dysplasia ($[c+d]/N$). For the purposes of this review, sensitivity of surveillance is defined as the proportion of patients with cancer who survive following colectomy and specificity is defined as the proportion of patients without cancer who do not develop dysplasia. Using these definitions, estimates of sensitivity and specificity from 11 large surveillance programs are shown in Table 12.3.[32–42] Specificity from surveillance is approximately 85%. The estimate of sensitivity is much less stable from study to study due to the low number of cancers in each program, but is for the most part over 50%.

If high grade dysplasia is used as the criterion for a positive test, specificity will increase. The tradeoff between specificity and sensitivity is impossible to determine since patients with low grade dysplasia are often not observed for the development of cancer; rather colectomy or more intensive surveillance is recommended. The increase in specificity with

Table 12.4 Comparisons of specificity with low grade dysplasia or high grade dysplasia used as the criterion for a positive test in colorectal cancer surveillance from 11 large surveillance programs

Study center	Specificity using low grade dysplasia as a cut-point	Specificity using high grade dysplasia as a cut-point
Univ. of Leeds, 1980[32]	34/41 (83%)	40/41 (98%)
Cleveland Clinic, 1985[33]	194/241 (80%)	231/241 (96%)
Univ. of Chicago, 1989[34]	73/91 (80%)	87/91 (96%)
Karolinska Institute, 1990[35]	54/70 (77%)	64/70 (91%)
Lahey Clinic, 1991[36]	171/203 (84%)	182/203 (90%)
Helsinki Univ., 1991[37]	57/66 (86%)	58/66 (88%)
Lennox Hill Hosp., 1992[38]	91/114 (80%)	114/114 (100%)
St Mark's Hosp., 1994[39]	205/267 (77%)	255/267 (96%)
Ornskoldsvik Hosp., 1994[40]	103/127 (81%)	123/127 (97%)
Tel Aviv Med. Center, 1995[41]	141/150 (94%)	144/150 (96%)
Univ. of Bologna, 1995[42]	58/61 (95%)	61/61 (100%)

high grade dysplasia rather than low grade dysplasia as the criterion for a positive test is shown in Table 12.4. Specificity using high grade dysplasia as a criterion for a positive test is approximately 95%.

The optimal criterion for a positive test also depends on the consequences of false positive (group b, Figure 12.1) and false negative (group c, Figure 12.1) testing. Patients who have a false positive test have dysplasia but are not destined to develop malignancy. These are the patients who have a proctocolectomy without truly needing one. Unfortunately, there is currently no way to predict which patients will fall into this false positive category. In the future, alternative markers of malignancy, such as the presence of p53 suppressor gene mutations, may help in determining which patient with dysplasia is a true positive patient (group a) and which is a false positive patient (group b). Likewise, patients with false negative examinations die of cancer without having proctocolectomy recommended from the detection of dysplasia. In these patients, either the testing interval was too long or the imperfect specificity of testing (mostly due to the focality of dysplasia) led to a false negative test. While both false positive and false negative errors are difficult to accept, false negative errors are the more grievous and the category that should be minimized with the most vigor. Therefore, the criterion for a positive test should be the detection of any dysplasia, low grade or high grade, on any biopsy of any examination.

IMPROVING CANCER SURVEILLANCE PROGRAMS IN ULCERATIVE COLITIS

Evidence based recommendations can be made to improve and optimize cancer surveillance strategies using currently available techniques. Factors related to the disease, the test, and the treatment can be optimized based on the above discussion.

1 Preferentially test high risk patients, such as patients with panulcerative colitis of at least 8 years or patients with primary sclerosing cholangitis, with colonoscopy and extensive biopsy. Patients with lower cancer risk, such as ulcerative colitis patients with

left-sided ulcerative colitis or Crohn's colitis, should receive cancer surveillance if resources exist. Grade C

2 The testing interval should shorten with increasing duration of disease to maximize the efficiency of a surveillance program.

3 The criterion for a positive test should optimize sensitivity. A positive test is defined as the presence of any dysplasia on any biopsy on any examination. "Confirmatory" testing is unnecessary. A positive test places the patient at extremely high risk of dying from colorectal cancer and thus necessitates a strong recommendation for proctocolectomy. Grade C

REFERENCES

1 Sackett DL, Hayes RB, Guyatt GH *et al. Clinical epidemiology: a basic science for clinical medicine*, 2nd edn. Boston: Little, Brown, 1991.

2 Greenstein AJ, Sachar DB, Smith H *et al.* Cancer in universal and left-sided ulcerative colitis: factors determining risk. *Gastroenterology* 1979; **77**: 290–4.

3 Brostrom O, Lofberg R, Nordenvall B *et al.* The risk of colorectal cancer in ulcerative colitis: an epidemiologic study. *Scand J Gastroenterol* 1987; **22**: 1193–9.

4 Gyde SN, Prior P, Allen RN *et al.* Colorectal cancer in ulcerative colitis: a cohort study of primary referrals from three centers. *Gut* 1988; **29**: 206–17.

5 Gilat T, Fireman Z, Grossman A *et al.* Colorectal cancer in patients with ulcerative colitis: a population study in central Israel. *Gastroenterology* 1988; **94**: 870–7.

6 Lashner BA, Kane SV, Hanauer SB. Colon cancer surveillance in chronic ulcerative colitis: an historical cohort study. *Am J Gastroenterol* 1990; **85**: 1083–7.

7 Lennard-Jones JE, Melville DM, Morson BC *et al.* Precancer and cancer in ulcerative colitis: findings among 401 patients over 22 years. *Gut* 1990; **31**: 800–6.

8 Ekbom A, Helmick C, Zack M *et al.* Ulcerative colitis and colorectal cancer: a population-based study. *N Engl J Med* 1990; **323**: 1228–33.

9 Farmer RG, Easley KA, Rankin GB. Clinical patterns, natural history, and progression of ulcerative colitis: a long-term follow-up of 1,116 patients. *Dig Dis Sci* 1993; **38**: 1137–46.

10 Lashner BA, Provencher K, Bozdech JM *et al.* Worsening risk for the development of cancer or dysplasia in patients with ulcerative colitis. *Am J Gastroenterol* 1995; **90**: 377–80.

11 Broome U, Lindberg G, Lofberg R. Primary sclerosing cholangitis in ulcerative colitis – a risk factor for the development of dysplasia and DNA aneuploidy? *Gastroenterology* 1992; **102**: 1877–80.

12 Gurbuz AK, Giardiello FM, Bayless TM. Colorectal neoplasia in patients with ulcerative colitis and sclerosing cholangitis. *Dis Colon Rectum* 1995; **38**: 37–41.

13 Broome U, Lofberg R, Veress B *et al.* Primary sclerosing cholangitis and ulcerative colitis: evidence for increased neoplastic potential. *Hepatology* 1995; **22**: 1404–8.

14 Brentnall TA, Haggitt RC, Rabinovitch PS *et al.* Risk and natural history of colonic neoplasia in patients with primary sclerosing cholangitis and ulcerative colitis. *Gastroenterology* 1996; **110**: 331–8.

15 Loftus Jr EV, Sandborn WJ, Tremaine WJ III *et al.* Risk of colorectal neoplasia in patients with primary sclerosing cholangitis. *Gastroenterology* 1996; **110**: 432–40.

16 Marchesa P, Vazio VW, Lavery IC *et al.* The risk of cancer and dysplasia among ulcerative colitis patients with primary sclerosing cholangitis. *Am J Gastroenterol* 1997; **92**: 1285–8.

17 Sackett DL, Whelan G. Cancer risk in ulcerative colitis: scientific requirements for the study of prognosis. *Gastroenterology* 1980; **78**: 1632–5.

18 Lashner BA, Heidenreich PA, Su GL *et al.* Effect of folate supplementation on the risk of dysplasia and cancer in ulcerative colitis. *Gastroenterology* 1989; **97**: 255–9.

19 Lashner BA. Red blood cell folate is associated with cancer and dysplasia in ulcerative colitis. *J Cancer Res Clin Oncol* 1993; **119**: 549–54.

20 Lashner BA, Provencher KS, Seidner DL *et al.* The effect of folic acid supplementation on the risk for cancer or dysplasia in ulcerative colitis. *Gastroenterology* 1997; **112**: 29–32.

21 Cole P, Morrison AS. Basic issues in population screening for cancer. *J Natl Cancer Inst* 1980; **64**: 1263–72.

22 Shapiro BD, Lashner BA. Cancer biology in ulcerative colitis and potential use in endoscopic surveillance. *Gastrointest Clin North Am* 1997; **7**: 453–68.

23 Byers T, Levin B, Rothenberger D *et al.* American Cancer Society guidelines for screening and surveillance for early detection of colorectal polyps and cancer: Update 1997. *CA Cancer J Clin* 1997; **47**: 154–60.
24 Provenzale D *et al.* Prophylactic colectomy or surveillance for chronic ulcerative colitis? A decision analysis. *Gastroenterology* 1995; **109**: 1188–96.
25 Blackstone MO, Riddell RH, Rogers BHG *et al.* Dysplasia-associated lesion or mass (DALM) detected by colonoscopy in long-standing ulcerative coitis: an indication for colectomy. *Gastroenterology* 1981; **80**: 366–74.
26 Lashner BA, Turner BC, Bostwick DG *et al.* Dysplasia and cancer complicating strictures in ulcerative colitis. *Dig Dis Sci* 1990; **35**: 349–52.
27 Lashner BA, Hanauer SB, Silverstein MD. Optimal timing of colonoscopy to screen for cancer in ulcerative colitis. *Ann Intern Med* 1988; **108**: 274–8.
28 Shapiro BD, Goldblum JR, Husain A *et al.* The role of p53 mutations in colorectal cancer surveillance for ulcerative colitis. *Gastroenterology* 1997; **112**: A1089.
29 Ransohoff DF, Riddell RH, Levin B: Ulcerative colitis and colonic cancer: problems in assessing the diagnostic usefulness of mucosal dysplasia. *Dis Colon Rectum* 1985; **28**: 383–8.
30 Taylor BA, Pemberton JH, Carpenter HA *et al.* Dysplasia in chronic ulcerative colitis: Implications for colonoscopic surveillance. *Dis Colon Rectum* 1992; **35**: 950–6.
31 Connell WR, Talbot IC, Harpaz N *et al.* Clinicopathological characteristics of colorectal carcinoma complicating ulcerative colitis. *Gut* 1994; **35**: 1419–23.
32 Dickenson RJ, Dixon MF, Axon ATR. Colonoscopy and the detection of dysplasia in patients with longstanding ulcerative colitis. *Lancet* 1980; **2**: 620–2.
33 Rosenstock E, Farmer RG, Petras R *et al.* Surveillance for colonic carcinoma in ulcerative colitis. *Gastroenterology* 1985; **89**: 1342–6.
34 Lashner BA, Silverstein MD, Hanauer SB. Hazard rates for dysplasia and cancer in ulcerative colitis: results from a surveillance program. *Dig Dis Sci* 1989; **34**: 1536–41.
35 Lofberg R, Brostrom O, Karlen O *et al.* Colonoscopic surveillance in longstanding ulcerative colitis: a 15-year follow-up study. Gastroenterology 1990; **99**: 1021–31.
36 Nugent FW, Haggitt RC, Gilpin PA. Cancer surveillance in ulcerative colitis. *Gastroenterology* 1991; **100**: 1241–8.
37 Leidenius M, Kellokumpu I, Husa A *et al.* Dysplasia and carcinoma in longstanding ulcerative colitis: an endoscopic and histologic surveillance program. *Gut* 1991; **32**: 1521–5.
38 Woolrich AJ, DaSilva MD, Korelitz BI. Surveillance in the routine management of ulcerative colitis: the predictive value of low-grade dysplasia. *Gastroenterology* 1992; **103**: 431–8.
39 Connell WR, Lennard-Jones JE, Williams CD *et al.* Factors affecting the outcomes of endoscopic surveillance for cancer in ulcerative colitis. *Gastroenterology* 1994; **107**: 934–44.
40 Jonsson B, Ahsgren L, Andersson LO *et al.* Colorectal cancer survival in patients with ulcerative colitis. *Br J Surg* 1994; **81**: 689–91.
41 Rozen P, Baratz M, Fefer F *et al.* Low incidence of significant dysplasia in a successful endoscopic surveillance program of patients with ulcerative colitis. *Gastroenterology* 1995; **108**: 1361–70.
42 Biasco G, Brandi G, Paganelli GM *et al.* Colorectal cancer in patients with ulcerative colitis: a prospective cohort study in Italy. *Cancer* 1995; **75**: 2045–50.

13 Colorectal cancer: population screening and surveillance

THERESE BEVERS, BERNARD LEVIN

EPIDEMIOLOGY

Worldwide, colorectal cancer is the third most frequently occurring cancer in both sexes; however, it ranks second in developed countries. Although the developed world includes only about a quarter of the world's population, approximately two-thirds of the estimated world total of 572 000 new cases a year in 1980 occurred in this group.[1] In the United States, the cumulative lifetime risk of developing colorectal cancer is about 6%.[2] In spite of the advances in the treatment of this disease, the 5-year survival is only about 55%.[3] Studies have shown that survival improves with diagnosis at an earlier stage, thus providing a rationale for screening.[4]

THE BIOLOGY OF COLORECTAL CANCER

The adenoma–carcinoma sequence

An understanding of the biology of colorectal cancer is essential to guide the application of available screening tests. It is generally accepted that most colorectal cancers evolve from adenomatous polyps. Direct evidence supporting this belief is limited, since ethical concerns preclude observing the natural history of polyps. However, indirect studies have demonstrated that cancers rarely arise in the absence of adenomatous polyps, individuals with a history of adenomatous polyps are at increased risk of developing cancer[5] and removal of these premalignant lesions reduces the incidence of colorectal cancer.[6,7]

A series of genetic alterations appears to be the impetus from which normal colonic mucosa develops into an adenomatous polyp and ultimately transforms into a cancer.[8] The time required for the transformation of a small adenomatous polyp to localized cancer and ultimately to invasive cancer, the so-called 'polyp dwell time', is of great interest in colorectal cancer screening. Knowledge of the polyp dwell time can be utilized to determine the window of opportunity during which screening is effective in the prevention and early detection of colorectal cancer.

The average polyp dwell time is not precisely known. An interdisciplinary expert panel originally convened by the Agency of Health Care Policy and Research to establish colorectal cancer screening guidelines estimated that it takes an average of about 10 years for an adenomatous polyp to transform into invasive cancer.[4] Knowledge of this transformation time has been the basis on which the frequency of accepted screening tests is determined.

SCREENING FOR COLORECTAL CANCER

Five different tests for the screening of colorectal cancer are presented. Of all the modalities mentioned, the strongest evidence exists for fecal occult blood testing. Intermediate level evidence is available for flexible sigmoidoscopy and only indirect evidence supports the use of colonoscopy and double contrast barium enema.

Fecal occult blood test

Screening for the presence of blood in the stool is based on the fact that most cancers and some polyps bleed.[9] The bleeding is intermittent and blood is unevenly distributed throughout the stool. Additionally, the amount of bleeding is dependent on the size of the polyp or cancer. Screening for the presence of blood in the stool is far less sensitive for polyps than for cancers. Polyps, especially small ones, do not bleed or do so only infrequently.[10] However, screening by fecal occult blood testing may detect the presence of polyps because large polyps, those most likely to be precancerous, do bleed. Furthermore, false positive results lead to diagnostic testing that discovers polyps whether or not they have bled.

Guaiac-based tests for peroxidase activity are the most commonly used means of testing for blood in the stool. Dietary restrictions are important to eliminate the possibility of false positive results. False negative tests may result if the cancer or premalignant lesion did not bleed during the performance of the test. A positive test for occult blood does not confirm the presence of a cancer or polyp but only suggests its presence. Further diagnostic testing, preferably by colonoscopy, must be undertaken to ascertain the source of the occult blood.

Current recommendations are that testing be conducted on two samples from three different stool specimens on consecutive days as multiple, consecutive samplings increase the likelihood of detecting blood. The sensitivity of the test is improved if the test is performed as a part of a program of testing over a period of several years instead of a one-time test, as this offers several opportunities to detect intermittent bleeding.[4] The sensitivity of this test is also dependent on the hydration status of the developed sample cards. Rehydration of the samples with a few drops of distilled water prior to the addition of the developing reagent increases the sensitivity at the expense of the specificity and is not recommended.

To date, four randomized controlled studies have investigated fecal occult blood testing for colorectal cancer screening. Three of the trials have been completed and the fourth is still in progress.[11–13] These trials incorporate a program of screening with multiple, consecutive tests on an annual or biannual basis rather than a single test in time. In studies using non-rehydrated samples, sensitivities ranged from 72% to 78% with a specificity of 98% and a positive predictive value of 10–17%. The sensitivity increased to 88–92% when rehydrated samples were used; however, the specificity dropped to 90–92% and the positive predictive value fell to 2–6%.[4]

The Minnesota trial was initiated using non-rehydrated samples but slide processing was modified early in the trial to incorporate rehydration; ultimately, 83% of the slides were developed after rehydration. Participants were randomly assigned to annual or biannual screening or to a control group. After 13 years, the group receiving annual screening showed a 33% reduction in colorectal cancer mortality while the group receiving biennial screening showed a non-significant 5% reduction.[11] Combination of the annual and the biennial groups resulted in an overall reduction of 19% in the risk of colorectal cancer death with screening. Adverse events related to diagnostic colonoscopy, perforation or hemorrhage, were reported to occur at the rate of 12 complications per 10 000 colonoscopies. There is some question as to how much of the mortality reduction demonstrated in this trial is due to the high rate of colonoscopy performed as a result of the increased positivity of the rehydrated sample. In an analysis of the study by other authors, it was estimated that one-third to one-half of the mortality reduction was due to the increased number of colonoscopies done and not attributable to fecal occult blood testing alone.[14,15] The assumptions in that analysis have been disputed by the authors of the Minnesota study. Using actual data in a model, they concluded that 16–25% of the reduction in colorectal cancer deaths effected by fecal occult blood testing was due to chance detection.[16]

R Grade A

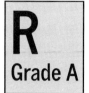

The question has been raised as to the effect that biannual screening, as opposed to the annual screening employed in this study, would have on colorectal cancer mortality. Two other prospective controlled trials offered biannual screening and did not perform rehydration of the fecal occult blood slides. Diagnostic evaluation of positive tests in both studies was performed by colonoscopic evaluation. Both studies had a low colonoscopy rate as compared to the Minnesota study. The Nottingham trial had a mean follow-up of 7.8 years and showed a 15% reduction in colorectal cancer mortality.[12] The Funen study showed an 18% reduction in mortality after 10 years.[13]

R Grade A

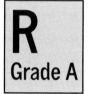

Unpublished results from the Goteborg trial, published in the Cochrane Review with information supplied by the principal investigator of that study, indicates that there is a 12% reduction in colorectal cancer mortality with biennial screening after 8 years of follow-up. The investigators reported a 0.3% complication rate (30 complications per 10 000 endoscopies), as evidenced by perforation and hemorrhage, out of 2298 endoscopies (colonoscopies and sigmoidoscopies).

R Grade A

Using data from these four randomized controlled studies, a systematic review including a meta-analysis was performed and published in the Cochrane Library[17] (Figure 13.1). This analysis showed an overall significant reduction in colorectal cancer mortality with screening by fecal occult blood testing of 16% (RR 0.84, CI 0.77–0.93). When the relative risk is adjusted for attendance for screening in individual studies, the mortality reduction is 23%. Overall, if 10 000 persons were offered screening and approximately two-thirds attended for at least one fecal occult blood test, there would be 8.5 deaths from colorectal cancer prevented over 10 years. Stating this another way, in order to prevent one death from colorectal cancer over 10 years, 1173 persons would need to be screened. However, the screening program would also result in 2800 participants having at least one colonoscopy. If harmful effects of screening from the Minnesota trial are considered, there would be 3.4 colonoscopy complications. If harmful effects of screening from the Goteborg trial are considered, approximately 600 participants would need at least one sigmoidoscopy and double contrast enema, resulting in 1.8 perforations or hemorrhage.

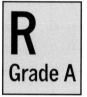

The estimate of mortality reduction from the randomized controlled trials of fecal occult blood tests is now well quantified and the confidence intervals are narrow enough to allow the conclusion that colorectal cancer screening is likely to be beneficial in a program of colorectal cancer screening. However, the wide range of mortality reduction seen in these studies and the overall modest mortality reduction indicates a need for continued improvement in fecal occult blood test technology. Detection of gene mutations or loss of heterozygositiy in DNA from stool samples may facilitate early diagnosis in the future.

Review: Screening for colorectal cancer using Hemoccult
Comparison: All Hemoccult screening programs vs Control
Outcome: Colorectal cancer mortality

Study	Expt n/N	Ctrl n/N	Peto OR (95%CI Fixed)	Weight %	Peto OR (95%CI Fixed)
Randomized controlled trials					
Funen	205 / 30967	249 / 30966		24.7	0.82 [0.66,0.99]
Goteborg	121 / 34144	138 / 34164		14.1	0.88 [0.69,1.12]
Minnesota	199 / 31157	121 / 15394		15.4	0.81 [0.64,1.02]
Nottingham	360 / 76466	420 / 76384		42.5	0.86 [0.74,0.99]
Subtotal (95%CI)	885 / 172734	928 / 156908		96.6	0.84 [0.77,0.92]
Chi-square 0.35 (df=3) Z=3.61					

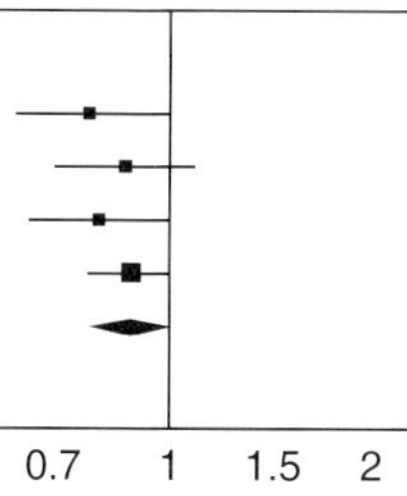

Figure 13.1 Meta-analysis of randomized controlled trials of hemoccult screening programs as an intervention for reducing mortality from colorectal cancer. (*Source*: Towler BP, Irwig L, Glasziou P *et al*. Screening for colorectal cancer using the faecal occult blood test, Hemoccult (Cochrane Review). In: *The Cochrane Library*, Issue 1, 1999. Oxford: Update Software)

Other benefits of fecal occult blood testing have yet to be definitively proven. Most notably, a reduction in the incidence of colorectal cancer may be observed as a result of detection and removal of colorectal adenomas. Additionally, treatment of early stage colorectal cancers may involve less invasive surgery.

In all three randomized studies evaluating the effectiveness of fecal occult blood testing, a favorable stage shift to earlier stage disease, which has better outcomes, was seen. In the Nottingham study, 90% of the screened group had Dukes A or B compared with 40% of the control group.[12] A similar stage shift was seen in the other two randomized controlled trials described.

Flexible sigmoidoscopy

The rationale for screening with sigmoidoscopy is that it provides direct visualization of the colon, and suspicious lesions can be biopsied. The most obvious disadvantage is that it examines only that portion of the distal colon within reach of the endoscope. Approximately 65–75% of adenomatous polyps and 40–65% of colorectal cancers are within the reach of a 60 cm flexible sigmoidoscope.[18–21] As with the fecal occult blood test, patients with a positive examination require further evaluation by colonoscopy . It has been well established that patients with an adenomatous polyp found on sigmoidoscopy have an increased probability of additional lesions located more proximally.[22–24]

The sensitivity of flexible sigmoidoscopy is 96.7% for cancer and large polyps and 73.3% for small polyps. The specificity is 94% for cancer and large polyps with a 92% specificity for small polyps.[4]

Only indirect evidence derived from several case–control studies using either rigid sigmoidoscopy or a combination of rigid with flexible sigmoidoscopy currently exists to support the effectiveness of flexible sigmoidoscopy.[25,26] The best designed trial, by Selby *et al*, avoided many of the biases inherent in case–control studies. The screening histories of persons who died of colorectal cancer were compared against controls and a 59% reduction in mortality from cancers of the rectum and distal colon was found in individuals who had undergone sigmoidoscopic evaluation.[25] Newcomb *et al* reported an

R
Grade B

80% reduction in mortality from cancer of the rectum and distal colon in persons who had ever undergone sigmoidoscopic examination compared to individuals who had never done so.[26] Several potential biases limit the applicability of this study; however, it does provide independent collaboration of the effectiveness of sigmoidoscopy in a colorectal cancer screening program.

Of great interest is the optimal interval for screening sigmoidoscopy. In the study by Selby *et al* described above, the effectiveness of screening sigmoidoscopy was found to be just as great for patients who had undergone the procedure 9–10 years before as compared to those who had just undergone the examination[27] A modeling study evaluating the optimal interval for sigmoidoscopic screening found that 90% of the effectiveness of annual screening was preserved with an interval of 10 years.[21] This model assumes that adenomatous polyps take 10–14 years to evolve into invasive cancers.

Double contrast barium enema

Evidence for the use of double contrast barium enema in screening is limited. The fact that detecting polyps and early cancers in other screening studies has resulted in a reduction in the incidence and mortality of colorectal cancer provides indirect evidence that double contrast barium enema, which detects many of these lesions, would be beneficial. The sensitivity of double contrast barium enema is 84% for cancer, 82% for large polyps, and 67% for small polyps. The specificity is 97.5% for cancer, 83.3% for large polyps, and 75% for small polyps.[4]

R Grade A

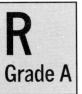

One randomized controlled trial investigated the addition of double contrast barium enema to sigmoidoscopy compared to colonoscopy. Colonoscopy was found to be more sensitive in detecting small polyps but no difference was found between the groups for large polyps and cancers.[28] Grade A

R Grade A/C

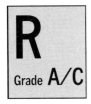

The frequency at which double contrast barium enema should be performed has not been well studied. An interval of 5–10 years has been suggested based on the estimated polyp dwell time of 10 years and the performance characteristics of the double contrast barium enema, which is known to be less sensitive in detecting small polyps. For this reason, a shorter time interval of 5 years is a part of the recommended screening procedure.[4] Grade A/C

Colonoscopy

R Grade B

Colonoscopy is the only technique that offers screening, diagnostic and, at times, therapeutic management all in one procedure. Most data available on the effects of colonoscopy are derived either from studies of colonoscopy in a diagnostic and surveillance setting or from indirect evidence as outlined above for double contrast barium enema. There are no studies currently available that evaluate colonoscopy as a screening test in terms of reduction of colorectal cancer mortality. However, to the extent that colonoscopy is a significant part of the fecal occult blood test program, these trials of occult blood testing also provide evidence of the effectiveness of colonoscopy.[11] Additional support is provided from one case–control study which showed that persons who had undergone colonoscopy had a 70–80% reduction in colorectal cancers.[7]

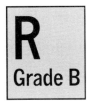

Colonoscopy can detect both polyps and cancers, although it is less accurate when the lesions are small. In studies evaluating the performance of colonoscopy, it has been demonstrated that 15% of small polyps but few large polyps are missed.[29] False positive

results are rare but about one-third of polyps removed are not adenomatous.[30] Colonoscopic sensitivity is 96.7% for cancers, 85% for large polyps, and 78.5% for small polyps; specificity is 98% for all lesions.[4]

No studies address the optimal frequency with which screening with colonoscopy should be carried out. Based on the natural history of the disease and the high accuracy of colonoscopy in the detection of polyps, it has been suggested that a screening interval of 10 years would be protective.[4] This is supported by the case–control study of Selby *et al* evaluating sigmoidoscopy, which suggests a protective effect for up to 10 years.[25]

R Grade B

The emerging technology of virtual colonoscopy (three-dimensional colography) is anticipated with enthusiasm in the hope that a non-invasive method of imaging the entire colon will increase compliance with colorectal cancer screening.

Digital rectal examination

Less than 10% of colorectal cancers are within the 7–8 cm reach of the examining finger.[31] Additionally, stool obtained during the course of a digital rectal examination is an inadequate sample upon which to screen for the presence or absence of blood and this type of fecal occult blood testing is not recommended. Finally, there is no evidence that digital rectal examination reduces morbidity or mortality from colorectal cancer, and it is not currently indicated as a screening test for the prevention or early detection of colorectal cancer.[4]

R Grade C

SCREENING RECOMMENDATIONS

Using the above evidence, the interdisciplinary Task Force, initially convened by the Agency for Health Care Policy and Research and completed with funding from seven professional societies, developed recommendations for the screening of colorectal cancer.[4] In 1997, the American Cancer Society published its recommendations for screening, which were based largely on, and nearly identical to those developed by the Agency for Health Care Policy and Research Task Force.[2] While the recommendations of these two entities are more liberal than the very conservative recommendations presented by the authors of the Cochrane review, they allow for tests or a combination of tests that may promote early detection of malignant or premalignant lesions.

The appropriate age at which to stop screening has not been well established; however, logic and indirect evidence suggest that screening would appropriately cease when significant comorbid conditions exist. In addition, consideration must be given to an individual's ability to tolerate the screening procedures as well as any further diagnostic evaluation that may be necessary.

Risk stratification

A key component of the American Cancer Society's Guidelines for Screening and Surveillance for Early Detection of Colorectal Polyps and Cancer (Table 13.1) is the stratification of individuals based on their risk profile. To better understand average risk, a definition of moderate and high risk must first be outlined.

Moderate risk individuals are those with a personal history of adenomatous polyps. In addition, a history of adenomatous polyps or colorectal cancer in a first degree relative

Table 13.1 ACS guidelines for screening and surveillance for early detection of colorectal polyps and cancer[a]

Risk category	Recommendation[b]	Age to begin	Interval
Average risk			
All people 50 years or older who are not in the categories below	One of the following: FOBT plus flexible sigmoidoscopy[c]	Age 50	FOBT every year and flexible sigmoidoscopy every 5 yr
	or TCE[d]	Age 50	Colonoscopy every 10 yr or DCBE every 5–10 yr
Moderate risk			
People with single, small (<1 cm) adenomatous polyps	Colonoscopy	At time of initial polyp diagnosis	TCE within 3 yr after initial polyp removal; if normal, as per average risk recommendations (above)
People with large (≥1 cm) or multiple adenomatous polyps of any size	Colonoscopy	At time of initial polyp diagnosis	TCE within 3 yr after initial polyp removal; if normal, TCE every 5 yr
Personal history of curative-intent resection of colorectal cancer	TCE[e]	Within 1 yr after resection	If normal, TCE in 3 yr; If normal, TCE every 5 yr
Colorectal cancer or adenomatous polyps in first-degree relative younger than 60 yr or in two or more first-degree relatives of any ages	TCE	Age 40 or 10 yr before the youngest case in the family, whichever is earlier	Every 5 yr
Colorectal cancer in other relatives (not included above)	As per average risk recommendations (above); may consider beginning screening before age 50		
High risk			
Family history of familial adenomatous polyposis	Early surveillance with endoscopy, counseling to consider genetic testing, and referral to a specialty center	Puberty	If genetic test positive or polyposis confirmed, consider colectomy; otherwise, endoscopy every 1–2 yr
Family history of hereditary non-polyposis colon cancer	Colonoscopy and counseling to consider genetic testing	Age 21	If genetic test positive or if patient has not had genetic testing, colonoscopy every 2 yr until age 40 yr, then every year
Inflammatory bowel disease	Colonoscopies with biopsies for dysplasia	8 yr after the start of pancolitis; 12–15 yr after the start of left-sided colitis	Every 1–2 yr

[a]Approximately 70–80% of cases are from average risk individuals, approximately 15–20% are from moderate risk individuals, and 5–10% are from high risk individuals.
[b]Digital rectal examination should be done at the time of each sigmoidoscopy, colonoscopy, or DCBE.
[c]Annual FOBT has been shown to reduce mortality from colorectal cancer, so it is preferable to no screening: however, the ACS recommends that annual FOBT be accompanied by flexible sigmoidoscopy to further reduce the risk of colorectal cancer mortality.
[d]TCE includes either colonoscopy or DCBE. The choice of procedure should depend on the medical status of the patient and the relative quality of the medical examinations available in a specific community. Flexible sigmoidoscopy should be performed in those instances in which the rectosigmoid colon is not well visualized by DCBE. DCBE would be performed when the entire colon has not been adequately evaluated by colonoscopy.
[e]This assumes that a perioperative TCE was done.
DCBE = double contrast barium enema; FOBT = fecal occult blood testing; TCE = total colon examination; yr = year.
Source: modified from *CA Cancer Journal for Clinicians* 1997;**47**:159–60.

younger than 60 years or in two first degree relatives of any age increases the risk of developing colorectal cancer. Approximately 15–20% of colorectal cancers occur in persons of moderate risk.

Persons at high risk of developing colorectal cancer fall into two categories. Those with one of two hereditary syndromes, familial adenomatous polyposis (FAP) and hereditary non-polyposis colorectal cancer (HNPCC) syndrome, and those with inflammatory bowel disease including both ulcerative colitis and Crohn's disease. Persons in the high risk category who develop colorectal cancer comprise approximately 5–10% of the colorectal cancers diagnosed.

Individuals in the average risk category are by definition those persons who do not meet the criteria for either the moderate or high risk categories. Approximately 70–80% of colorectal cancers diagnosed occur in this risk category. The proportions of hereditary and sporadic colorectal cancer in the population are depicted in Figure 13.2

Average risk screening recommendations

Persons at average risk should begin colorectal cancer screening at age 50 with either an annual fecal occult blood test in conjunction with flexible sigmoidoscopy every 5 years or total colonic examination either by colonoscopy every 10 years or double contrast barium enema every 5–10 years. The decision as to which screening modality to use should be made between the patient and clinician. Factors to consider are the availability of trained and competent clinicians to perform the examination as well as cost and patient acceptability. Any positive fecal occult blood test, abnormal flexible sigmoidoscopy or double contrast barium enema should usually be followed up by colonoscopy for diagnostic evaluation. Consideration should be given to performing a supplemental double contrast barium enema for those in whom colonoscopy is not complete, ie to the cecum.

R
Grade **A/B**

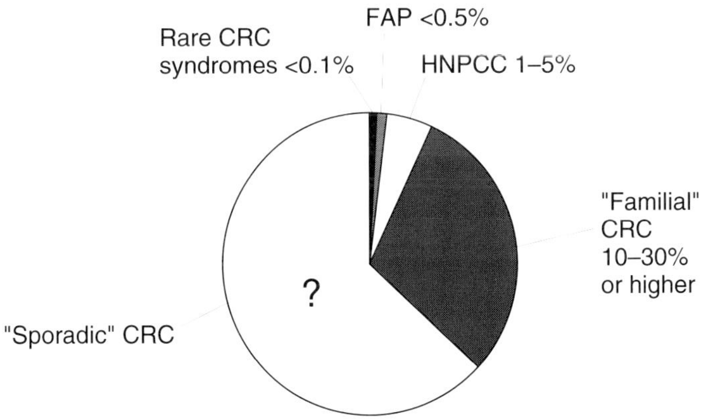

Figure 13.2 Familial causes of colorectal cancer. The rare colorectal cancer (CRC) syndromes include the hamartomatous polyposis conditions and other extremely rare disease. FAP accounts for about 0.5% of cases and HNPCC for 1–5%. Epidemiological studies suggest that familial CRC outside the well-defined syndromes involves adenomatous polyps and suggest that this proportion is much higher and that familial factors, probably inherited, may be present in the majority of colonic neoplasms. (Reproduced with permission from Burt RW, Petersen GM. Prevention and early detection of colorectal cancer. In: *Familial colorectal cancer; diagnosis and management.* London: WB Saunders, 1996, p 173)

Moderate risk screening recommendations

R
Grade A/B/C

Persons diagnosed with one or more adenomatous polyps on flexible sigmoidoscopy should undergo further evaluation of the entire colon by colonoscopy to complete the diagnostic evaluation for additional polyps. Interval screening, or surveillance, for individuals with a history of adenomatous polyps should be carried out by total colonic examination within 3 years of initial polyp removal. If this evaluation is normal, subsequent examinations can be carried out every 5 years unless the polyp was single and small (less than 1 cm), in which case screening can return to the average risk guidelines.

For persons with a family history of either colorectal cancer or adenomatous polyps in a first degree relative younger than 60 years of age or in more than one first degree relative of any age, screening should be carried out by total colonic examination every 5 years beginning at age 40 or 10 years prior to the index case, whichever is earlier.

High risk screening recommendations

Familial adenomatous polyposis is a hereditary syndrome in which persons expressing the gene develop hundreds of polyps early in life and have nearly 100% probability of developing colorectal cancer. Recommendations for individuals thought to be at risk for this condition include genetic counseling and testing in addition to endoscopic evaluation every 1–2 years beginning at puberty. Because the polyps are distributed throughout the colon, flexible sigmoidoscopy is considered to be as effective as colonoscopy to monitor for the initial development of polyps. Due to the vast number of polyps that develop in these individuals, it would be impossible to manage these patients by colonoscopic polypectomy. The only feasible preventive strategy at present in this group is colectomy, and the main decision to be made is the timing of this preventive measure. However, chemopreventive strategies are being developed aimed at preventing the development of adenomas or their malignant transformation.[32]

R
Grade A

The other major hereditary condition which places an individual in the high risk category is the HNPCC syndrome. Risk for colorectal cancer is increased by age 21 and is very high by age 40. Individuals suspected of having this syndrome should undergo genetic counseling and testing. Additionally, screening with colonoscopy, necessary because of the proximal distribution of the lesions, should be carried out every 2 years beginning at age 21 and yearly beginning at age 40. Because of the increased risk of endometrial cancer, consideration should be given to screening for this malignancy.

Persons with inflammatory bowel disease, comprising both ulcerative colitis and Crohn's disease of the colon, are at increased risk of developing colorectal cancer and this risk is related to the duration and extent of the disease. Recommendations are to begin screening with colonoscopy and perform random biopsies for dysplasia beginning 8 years after the onset of pancolitis and 15 years after the start of left sided colitis. While there is no direct evidence demonstrating a reduction in mortality for these individuals with this screening regimen, the rationale is that early detection of dysplasia would result in management that would lower the risk of developing an invasive cancer.

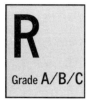

COST-EFFECTIVENESS OF COLORECTAL CANCER SCREENING

Increasingly, decisions about preventive services are being made after due consideration of the cost-effectiveness of the screening regimen. Cost analyses of colorectal cancer screening programs have been carried out to provide a basis from which legislation can be influenced and benefit plans can be constructed. While these analyses are limited by the assumptions that were made, they provide a means by which health care decisions can be made with the benefit of some economic input.

The cost-effectiveness of colorectal cancer screening is estimated to be approximately $40 000 per year of life gained.[33] This compares favorably with the costs of other preventive services; for example, annual breast screening with mammography would cost approximately $34 500 per year of life gained. In the analysis by the Congressional Office of Technology Assessment and the National Cancer Institute, it was demonstrated that the cost of missing an early curable cancer, or of failing to prevent cancers, is greater than the cost of screening.[33] As a result of this and other analyses, colorectal cancer screening services are now provided by law in the United States as a Medicare benefit.

In conclusion, there is sufficient evidence supporting the colorectal cancer screening recommendations discussed in this chapter. This evidence arises from both observed mortality reduction and from a calculated economic benefit. It is more cost-effective to treat early stage disease and even more cost-effective to prevent colorectal cancer than it is to treat it at an advanced stage.

REFERENCES

1 Coleman MP, Esteve J, Damiecki P *et al.* Colon and rectum. In: *Trends in cancer incidence and mortality*. Oxford: Oxford University Press, 1993.

2 Byers T, Levin B, Rothenberger D *et al.* American Cancer Society guidelines for screening and surveillance for early detection of colorectal polyps and cancer: Update 1997. *CA Cancer J Clin* 1997; **47**: 154–60.

3 Bond JH, Levin B. Screening and surveillance for colorectal cancer. *Am J Managed Care* 1998; **4**: 431–7.

4 Winawer SJ, Fletcher RH, Miller L *et al.* Colorectal cancer screening: clinical guidelines and rationale. *Gastroenterology* 1997; **112**: 594–642.

5 Atkin WS, Morson BC, Cuzick J. Long-term risk of colorectal cancer after excision of rectosigmoid adenomas. *N Engl J Med* 1992; **326**: 658–62.

6 Winawer SJ, Zauber AG, Ho MN *et al.* Prevention of colorectal cancer by colonoscopic polypectomy. The National Polyp Study Workgroup. *N Engl J Med* 1993; **329**: 1977–81.

7 Muller AD, Sonnenberg A. Prevention of colorectal cancer by flexible endoscopy and polypectomy. A case-control study of 32 702 veterans. *Ann Intern Med* 1995; **123**: 904–10.

8 Vogelstein B, Fearon ER, Hamilton SR *et al.* Genetic alterations during colorectal tumor development. *N Engl J Med* 1988; **319**: 525–32.

9 Simon JB. Occult blood screening for colorectal carcinoma: a critical review. *Gastroenterology* 1985; **88**: 820–37.

10 Macrae FA, St. John DJ. Relationship between patterns of bleeding and Hemoccult sensitivity in patients with colorectal cancers and adenomas. *Gastroenterology* 1982; **82**: 891–8.

11 Mandel JS, Bond JH, Church TR *et al.* Reducing mortality from colorectal cancer by screening for fecal occult blood. Minnesota Colon Cancer Control Study. *N Engl J Med* 1993; **328**: 1365–71.

12 Hardcastle JD, Chamberlain JO, Robinson MHE *et al.* Randomised controlled trial of faecal-occult-blood screening for colorectal cancer. *Lancet* 1996; **348**: 1472–7.

13 Kronberg O, Fenger C, Olsen J *et al.* Randomised study of screening for colorectal cancer with faecal-occult-blood test. *Lancet* 1996; **348**: 1467–71.

14 Ahlquist DA, Moertel CG, McGill DB. Screening for colorectal cancer (Letter). *N Engl J Med* 1993; **329**: 1351.

15 Lang, CA, Ransohoff DF. Fecal occult blood screening for colorectal cancer. Is mortality reduced by chance selection for screening colonoscopy. *JAMA* 1994; **271**: 1011–13.

16 Ederer, F, Church TR, Mandel JS. Fecal occult blood screening in the Minnesota study: role of chance detection of lesions. *J Natl Cancer Inst* 1997; **89**: 1423–8.

17 Towler BP, Irwig L, Glasziou P *et al.* Screening for colorectal cancer using the faecal occult blood test, Hemoccult (Cochrane Review). In: *The Cochrane Library*, Issue 3, 1998. Oxford: Update Software.

18 Tedesco JF, Wave JD, Avella JR *et al.* Diagnostic implications of the spatial distribution of colonic mass lesions (polyps and cancers): a prospective colonoscopic study. *Gastrointest Endosc* 1980; **26**: 95–7.

19 Shinya H, Wolff WI. Morphology, anatomic distribution and cancer potential of colonic polyps: an analysis of 7000 polyps endoscopically removed. *Ann Surg* 1979; **190**: 679–83.

20 Winawer SJ, Gottlieb LS, Stewart ET *et al.* First progress report of the National Polyp Study. *Gastroenterology* 1983; **84**: 1352.

21 Report of the US Preventive Services Task Force. *Guide to clinical preventive services*, 2nd edn. Baltimore, MD: Williams & Wilkins, 1996.

22 Winawer SJ, Zauber AG, O'Brien MJ *et al.* The National Polyp Study. 1. Design, methods and characteristics of patients with newly diagnosed polyps. The National Polyp Study Workgroup. *Cancer* 1992; **70**(Suppl 5): 1236–45.

23 Grossman S, Milos ML, Tekawa IS *et al.* Colonoscopic screening of persons with suspected risk factors for colon cancer. II. Past history of colorectal neoplasms. *Gastroenterology* 1989; **96**: 299–306.

24 Tripp MR, Morgan TR, Sampliner RE *et al.* Synchronous neoplasms in patients with diminutive colorectal adenomas. *Cancer* 1987; **60**: 1599–603.

25 Selby JV, Friedman GD, Quesenberry CP Jr *et al.* A case–control study of screening sigmoidoscopy and mortality from colorectal cancer. *N Engl J Med* 1992; **326**: 653–7.

26 Newcomb PA, Norfleet RG, Storer BE. Screening sigmoidoscopy and colorectal cancer mortality. *J Natl Cancer Inst* 1992; **84**: 1572–5.

27 Selby JV, Friedman GD, Quesenberry CP Jr *et al.* Effect of fecal occult blood testing on mortality from colorectal cancer. A case-control study. *Ann Intern Med* 1993; **118**: 1–6.

28 Rex DK, Weddle RA, Lehman GA *et al.* Flexible sigmoidoscopy plus air contrast barium enema versus colonoscopy for suspected lower gastrointestinal bleeding. *Gastroenterology* 1990; **98**: 855–61.

29 Hixson LJ, Femerty MB, Sampliner RE *et al.* Prospective study of the frequency and size distribution of polyps missed by colonoscopy. *J Natl Cancer Inst* 1990; **82**: 1769–72.

30 Bernstein MA, Feczko PJ, Halpert RD *et al.* Distribution of colonic polyps: increased incidence of proximal lesions in older patients. *Radiology* 1985; **155**: 35–38.

31 Winawer SJ. Surveillance overview. In: Cohen AM, Winawer SJ (eds), *Cancer of the colon, rectum and anus*. New York: McGraw-Hill,1995, pp 279–90.

32 Giardiello FM, Hamilton SR, Krush AJ *et al.* Treatment of colonic and rectal adenomas with sulindac in familial adenomatous polyposis. *N Engl J Med* 1993; **328**: 1313–16.

33 Wagner JL, Tunis S, Brown M *et al.* The cost-effectiveness of colorectal cancer screening in average-risk adults. In: Young G, Levin B, Rozen A (eds), *Prevention and early detection of colorectal cancer*. London: WB Saunders, 1996, pp 321–56.

Irritable bowel syndrome: diagnosis and treatment

14

JAROL B KNOWLES, DOUGLAS A DROSSMAN

INTRODUCTION

Patients with functional gastrointestinal (GI) disorders are commonly seen in medicine, comprising 12% of patient encounters in primary care practice[1] and 41% of those in a general GI practice.[2–4] These disorders account for an estimated 2.4–3.5 million physician visits per year in the United States.[5,6] The irritable bowel syndrome (IBS), the most common functional bowel disorder, is characterized by abdominal pain, bloating, and disturbed defecation. The functional GI disorders result in significant utilization of health care resources. A recent community based study showed that subjects with IBS incurred on average annual health care costs of $742 (1992 dollars) compared to $429 for patients without IBS.[7]

RATIONALE FOR SYMPTOM BASED DIAGNOSTIC CRITERIA

The first published account of IBS was made by Powell in 1818.[8] The syndrome remained poorly understood until recently, but there has been a substantial increase in research and publications since 1979.[9] The reasons for the increased interest in IBS relate to several historical factors. Newer investigative techniques in motility assessment initially implicated altered motility as the underlying pathophysiological basis for IBS. Yet, these early studies did not fully explain the symptom complex of IBS, and more recent studies have studied the role of visceral hypersensitivity.[10] The clinical observation that stress exacerbated the symptoms of IBS led to the hypothesis that there was a psychophysiological component to the illness.

In the late 1970s, George Engel developed the Biopsychosocial Model to provide a framework to reconcile the emerging data in the biomedical field that suggested that social environment could contribute to the clinical expression of a disease.[11] He advocated that illness is the product of biological, psychological and social subsystems interacting at multiple levels. This framework provided the conceptual basis for understanding GI symptoms not easily attributed to specific diseases. Using biopsychosocial research, we recognize that IBS is not caused by intestinal dysmotility, but may reflect dysregulation of the CNS–enteral nervous system linkages. The phenomenon of enhanced visceral sensitivity may amplify even subthreshold GI regulatory input to the brain, and cortical processes may regulate symptom perception either intrinsically or through descending influences on the spinal cord.[12]

The diagnostic criteria for defining functional GI disorders, first described by Manning,[13] were determined by discriminate function analysis, and were later refined. Arbitrary selection criteria in the Manning formulation (for example, combining patient groups with predominant diarrhea with those with predominant constipation) yielded mixed clinical populations that were difficult to study. The first international consensus conference on diagnostic criteria for IBS occurred at the 13th International Congress of Gastroenterology in 1988 in Rome.[14] The diagnostic criteria were subsequently referred to as the 'Rome Criteria'. They are now under revision and will soon be published as 'Rome II'. The functional GI disorders are subclassified into five regions (esophageal, gastroduodenal, bowel, biliary, and anorectal). Patients fulfilling the criteria for a particular subgroup of the 21 functional GI disorders tend to be more similar to each other with regard to the underlying pathophysiology and treatment methods than to those having other diagnoses. This presumption provides a framework for patient identification and investigation. The diagnostic criteria for irritable bowel syndrome are shown in Box 14.1.

IBS is the prototype functional bowel disorder. Functional abdominal bloating, functional constipation, and functional diarrhea are distinct bowel symptom patterns that have their own criteria. Chronic abdominal pain is placed in a different category since it occurs independent of known physiological activity in the gut. Diagnosis of each of these syndromes depends on the clinical features, and each syndrome has a unique differential diagnosis.

The Rome Criteria for IBS were derived from discriminant function analyses that differentiated the symptoms of IBS patients from normal subjects or patients with other GI disorders.[9] Two studies using factor analysis have been done that validate the Rome Criteria.[15,16] Palsson *et al* administered a questionnaire containing 85 questions that corresponded to 17 of the 21 functional GI disorders in 895 patients seen at the UNC Gastroenterology Clinic.[17] Using principal components factor analysis, 13 symptom clusters corresponded to the Rome Criteria items. Recently, further validation of the Rome Criteria was reported by Vanner *et al.*[18] In this study, 98 patients fulfilling at least one of

Box 14.1 Diagnostic criteria (Rome Criteria) for irritable bowel syndrome

At least 12 weeks, which need not be consecutive, in the preceding 12 months of abdominal discomfort or pain that has two out of three features:

(a) Relieved with defecation; and/or
(b) Onset associated with a change in frequency of stool; and/or
(c) Onset associated with a change in form (appearance) of stool.

The below is not officially part of the criteria

Symptoms that cumulatively support the diagnosis of irritable bowel syndrome

(a) Abnormal stool frequency (for research purposes "abnormal" may be defined as greater than 3 bowel movements per day and less than 3 bowel movements per week);
(b) Abnormal stool form (lumpy/hard or loose/watery stool);
(c) Abnormal stool passage (straining, urgency, or feeling of incomplete evacuation);
(d) Passage of mucus;
(e) Bloating or feeling of abdominal distension.

the Rome Criteria were studied with respect to diagnosis made by application of the criteria versus the gastroenterologist's diagnosis. The latter was considered to be the gold standard in this analysis. Using the Rome Criteria for diagnosis, there were no false positives and 16 false negatives, giving a sensitivity of 63% and a specificity of 100%. Furthermore, of the 30 true positives, follow-up over 2 years showed no errors in diagnosis.

EPIDEMIOLOGY

Prevalence data

IBS is a common condition in population surveys of adults. The prevalence rate varies depending on the specific population being surveyed. Many prevalence estimates were drawn from populations that are not representative of the general population. In large population based studies, such as the NCHS, the functional GI disorders are not given a specific diagnostic code, but are lumped into larger codes such as 'gastritis' or 'unspecified enteritis'. The true prevalence of IBS in the population cannot be determined from population based studies that do not include IBS as a diagnostic code. Five population based surveys have used diagnostic criteria specific for IBS and these provide the population prevalence rates of 14–24% of women and 5–19% of men.[19–23]

The first presentation to the physician usually occurs between the ages of 30 and 50 years, although children also have the illness.[24] The prevalence of cases decreases after age 60.[19] There is a strong gender difference in the prevalence rates, which varies with the clinical setting. In population surveys the female to male prevalence is 2–3 : 1, while in referral centers it is 4–5 : 1.[1] The data on racial differences in prevalence rates are scarce. Of the five randomly sampled surveys of American and European adults,[19–23] blacks were under-represented. One study of culturally diverse American college students,[25] however, showed a prevalence rate in blacks that was similar to whites. There are few data that address the prevalence of IBS in non-Western countries.

The symptoms of IBS tend to wax and wane, making point prevalences difficult to interpret. When the prevalence is examined in the same population at two different time points, the incidence of new cases at the second time point is approximately half of the prevalence noted at the first time point.[19,23] Once the diagnosis of IBS is made, it is considered to be a chronic disease, and approximately 75% of patients will continue to be symptomatic. In a study of 25 patients with IBS, symptoms were evaluated over 8 weeks using time series analysis. In these patients, IBS severity was predictable over more than 1 day, and symptoms tended to occur in clusters rather than randomly.[26]

Health care utilization

One of the notable features of patients with IBS is the increased rate of health care utilization for both GI and non-GI illnesses. Patients with IBS have other chronic diseases, including fibromyalgia, chronic fatigue syndrome, endometriosis, migraine headaches, and depression. In one study, patients with fibromyalgia and IBS had poorer health status than those with either disease alone.[27] In the US householder survey,[22] persons with IBS visited physicians for non-GI complaints 3.88 times in the previous year. These same persons visited a physician for GI complaints 1.64 times. The risk of abdominal surgery is increased in patients with IBS,[28] and women with IBS are three times more likely to receive a hysterectomy.[29]

One study in England evaluated the health care impact of 20 female patients with chronic functional abdominal pain, a subgroup of the functional GI disorders that is distinct from IBS because of the absence of motility disturbances. In this study, the patients were seen by an average of 5.7 consultants, underwent 6.4 endoscopic or radiological procedures, and had 2.7 major operations.[30] Similarly, patients with IBS have increased pain reporting with anxiety or acute stress. Although it may be assumed that more frequent visits are associated with greater disease activity or physiological dysfunction, several studies show that psychological distress and psychosocial disturbance independently influence who will seek health care.[31–34]

Prevalence of psychological disturbances

Psychological stress or emotional reactions to stress can affect GI function in both normals and IBS patients.[35] Because the effects of stress on gut function are universal, they have no diagnostic value. Yet, the degree of psychosocial impairment is usually greater in patients with IBS. Three psychiatric diagnoses are more frequently seen in patients with IBS: anxiety disorders (panic and generalized anxiety disorder), mood disorders (major depression and dysthymic disorder), and somatoform disorders (hypochondriasis and somatization disorder).[36]

The coexistence of a psychiatric disorder with IBS is seen more frequently in referral centers than in the community setting. In a review of the prevalence of psychiatric diagnoses, the coexistence of psychiatric disorder and IBS was present in 42–61% of patients seen in gastroenterology clinics.[37] The presence of a psychiatric disorder is even higher in studies from tertiary care centers, when lifetime psychiatric diagnosis is considered.[38] One study examined the difference in the prevalence of psychological disturbances between patients with IBS who had seen a doctor and those who had never seen a doctor and compared them to a control group of subjects without bowel symptoms. They found that the IBS non-patients were not psychologically different from normals and that the patients with IBS had greater psychological disturbances than the other two groups.[31] Thus, the psychological difficulties in IBS relate primarily to patients who see physicians.

Although psychological disturbance is not part of the IBS *per se*, it influences health seeking behavior. The increased utilization of health care services in patients with IBS may be influenced by cultural factors, family role modeling, illness behavior, coping mechanisms, and the tendency towards somatization. A series of studies[31–34] have shown that individuals who seek care for functional GI disorders have more psychological distress, a higher proportion of abnormal personality patterns, and greater illness behaviors than those who do not.

With patients with unexplained, severe or refractory symptoms and a high health care use rate, the documentation of the contributing psychosocial factors is an important diagnostic feature. Psychosocial stressors, such as a history of physical or sexual abuse, major loss (eg death or divorce), and other major trauma, influence the development of IBS.[39] The loss of an intimate relationship is closely associated with the onset of symptoms of IBS.[40] In another study, severely stressful life events or chronic social difficulties was associated with the onset of symptoms.[41] Stressful life events also had a significant impact on health care visits and disability days.[42]

Additionally, sexual and physical abuse history is more common in IBS patients with severe symptoms. Drossman *et al*[43] reported a prevalence of abuse history in 44% of patients seen at a GI referral center. In another study comparing IBS patients to healthy controls, the prevalence of sexual abuse was 31.6% in the IBS group compared to 7.6% in the controls.[44] An abuse history does not determine that IBS will occur, since it is also associated with other chronic syndromes (pelvic pain, headaches, fibromyalgia, bulimia, substance abuse).[45] The importance of a history of abuse relates to the tendency of persons with abuse histories to communicate psychological distress through physical symptoms. In GI patients with abuse histories, there is more severe pain and poorer daily function, and there are three times as many days spent in bed, and 30% more physician visits and surgeries.[46,47]

Over time, the changes in GI function that result from stress modify the person's appraisal of bodily symptoms and lead to unwarranted feelings of guilt. These factors can produce a chronic state of symptom amplification originating at the CNS (hypervigilance to body sensations) or the gut level (visceral hypersensitivity and conditioned hypermotility). Eventually a vicious cycle of health care seeking, refractoriness, and repeated referral develops.[48]

DIAGNOSIS OF IBS

The use of symptom based criteria

Although the error rate of classifying patients with symptoms of IBS falsely with a diagnosis of IBS is approximately 3% (0–10%), the use of the Rome Criteria has improved clinical decision making. The Rome Criteria were derived by a team of international experts brought together to produce consistency in opinion by the "Delphi method".[49] These criteria categorize patients by symptom clusters into five anatomical regions: esophageal, gastroduodenal, bowel, biliary, and anorectal. The symptom clusters are based on disturbances in sensory or motor function by target organ, and the approach to treatment varies depending on the target organ involved. Patients having symptoms in one anatomical region are presumed to be similar to each other with regard to their pathophysiology and treatment effects, compared to patients who do not fulfill the symptom based criteria.

The primary argument against the use of symptom based criteria is that they have no external validation, ie no structural, biochemical or physiological markers that confirm their existence.[50] Yet, most common medical symptoms, like nausea, headache, and fatigue, do not have external validation, yet are recognized as clinical entities. Until valid physiological measures are developed to explain the functional GI disorders, the use of symptom based criteria provides the best basis for standardized research and clinical care.

Diagnostic approaches for the diagnosis of IBS

The interview process has been identified as the cornerstone of determining the presence of IBS. The high association of psychosocial problems in patients with IBS requires that physicians perform an effective interview that identifies the symptoms, and the events that may affect them. It is important to try to make the diagnosis and explain it to the patient at the initial visit.[51]

There is no single diagnostic test that confirms the presence of IBS. Careful interpretation of abdominal pain sensations and abnormal defecation patterns is the cornerstone of diagnosing IBS. Although the exacerbation of GI symptoms by stress factors is an important observation in persons with IBS, it is not a diagnostic criterion. However, this observation can be helpful in planning treatment. The relief of pain with a bowel movement is important to identify that the pain relates to the intestine. The interview process obtains history through non-directive, non-judgemental interview, determines the patient's concerns, responds to the patient's expectations, involves the patient in the treatment plan, and establishes a long term relationship with the primary care provider.

Use of diagnostic tests

The clinical diagnosis of IBS includes ruling out organic disease. IBS can mimic other diseases, and specific diagnostic tests are indicated for selected patients, particularly when they do not precisely fulfill the Rome Criteria. Demographic features, the duration of symptoms and change over time are important to distinguish organic disease from IBS. Previous diagnostic tests help determine the need for further investigation. A history of colon cancer or IBD in a family member may lead to further studies. The minimum screening diagnostic tests recommended for patients suspected of having IBS include a CBC and ESR, stool for ova and parasites, occult blood, and white blood cells, and a flexible sigmoidoscopy (colonoscopy is recommended in patients over age 55). These unvalidated recommendations are guidelines based on a technical review intended to assist practising physicians in the absence of evidence.[1] The majority of otherwise healthy patients who fulfill criteria for IBS will have a normal screening evaluation.

Targeted investigation based on symptoms

When further evaluation is needed, the studies should be targeted toward the predominant symptoms. For *diarrhea*, a determination of stool volume should be made. Patients with IBS typically have frequent, but small volume stools (<300 ml/day) which does not usually require additional studies. If large stool volume is present, osmolality and stool electrolytes can differentiate between osmotic and secretory causes of diarrhea. A laxative screen is often helpful to identify surreptitious laxative abuse.

If *constipation* is the predominate symptom, a radio-opaque Sitzmark study[52] will determine whole gut transit time for the diagnosis of colonic inertia. Symptoms of dyschezia or incomplete evacuation are evaluated by anorectal manometry or pelvic floor EMG. The balloon expulsion test or defecography is indicated in cases of possible obstructive defecation. Patients with hypothyroidism or medication induced constipation should be identified before the diagnosis of IBS is made.

When *pain and bloating* symptoms predominate, an abdominal plain X-ray can be helpful to exclude aerophagia, increased stool retention, or less commonly, an overlooked small bowel obstruction. If *vomiting* is the predominate symptom, EGD is useful to diagnose organic obstructive pathology in the stomach or duodenum. A barium small bowel series should be done to exclude partial small bowel obstruction or other small bowel disease. A gastric emptying scan is useful to determine gastric emptying time. In extreme cases, a small bowel motility study will measure the migrating motor complexes in the small intestine and be helpful in the diagnosis of intestinal pseudo-obstruction.

The impulse to investigate in an effort to rule out organic disease is understandable. The individual symptoms of IBS have a long list of rare causes that can be responsible for that individual symptom. When the symptom is long-standing and previous evaluations have been negative, follow-up studies of adults yield specific etiologies in less than 10% of patients.[53] It is important to remember that the individual symptoms of IBS need to be evaluated in the context of the Rome Criteria, with a focus on the psychosocial factors that contribute to the perception and reporting of symptoms. If the diagnosis is in doubt, it is best to re-evaluate the clinical features over one or more visits.

With patients with unexplained, severe or refractory symptoms and a high health care use rate, the documentation of the contributing psychosocial factors is an important diagnostic feature. Changes in GI function resulting from stress can modify the person's appraisal of bodily symptoms over time, and, as described above, can lead to feelings of guilt, a chronic state of symptom amplification, and the development of a repeating care seeking–refractoriness–referral cycle.[54]

TREATMENT

Validity of clinical trials

The validity of clinical trials of interventions for IBS must be evaluated within a framework that recognizes the following considerations:

1 Long term efficacy of various treatments is unknown. A wide variety of interventions have been developed to treat patients with IBS, yet most of the relevant clinical trials have been seriously flawed.[55] Since 1966, there have been 58 randomized, double-blind, placebo controlled studies. The trials were generally of short duration, ranging from 3 days to 24 weeks. Only 16 trials evaluated an intervention for 12 weeks or longer. Careful analysis of the duration of response after treatment is important to determine the efficacy of various treatments in IBS.
2 The therapeutic relationship affects prognosis in IBS patients. The value of the therapeutic relationship is supported by the observation that 30–88% of patients with IBS respond to a placebo in clinical trials.[56] In one retrospective study, the establishment of a long term relationship with a primary care provider was associated with a reduction in health care visits.[57] Reassurance has therapeutic value, since IBS tends to be chronic and characterized by exacerbations and remissions.
3 Recruitment for clinical trials of patients who satisfy the Rome Criteria results in more homogeneous groups of patient. Patients with IBS tend to fluctuate from one symptom subtype to another, yet patients with diarrhea-predominant IBS are clinically distinct from those with constipation-predominant IBS. Trials that separate IBS patients into symptom subgroups by application of the Rome Criteria are more clinically useful than trials where the patients are lumped into one group. Trials that exclude patients with mild, irregular or intermittent IBS symptoms have a similar advantage.
4 The severity of the IBS also affects prognosis and treatment. Patients with mild IBS require a different treatment approach than patients with severe symptoms. A Functional Bowel Disorder Severity Index has been developed by Drossman *et al*[58] and has been used by clinicians to rate and stratify patients into mild, moderate or severe categories. One validation study confirmed that a patient self-administered rating was highly correlated with a physician severity rating.[58] Another severity index developed

by Francis *et al* incorporated pain, distension, bowel dysfunction, and quality of life/global wellbeing into a severity index.[59] Very few published studies of treatment trials include an analysis of the severity of the disorder in the study population, making generalizability of the treatment results uncertain.

5 Treatment trials without a placebo group are uninterpretable, since the placebo response in patients with IBS may be higher than 70%.[56] Since there is no accepted standard treatment for IBS, all treatment trials of IBS should be placebo controlled.

OUTCOME MEASURES

A plethora of outcome measures have been used to assess efficacy of interventions for IBS.[56] Abdominal pain is the most commonly employed outcome measure (83% of trials), followed by alternating diarrhea and constipation (50% of trials). Other outcome measures include abdominal distension, urgency/frequency of bowel movements, and assessment of symptom severity using any of the following: adjectival scales, visual analogue scales, overall assessment of wellbeing, or physician's global assessment. Outcome measures that have proved to be useful in clinical trials of patients with IBS are symptom based. Talley[55] recommends three domains to be considered for outcome assessment, pain, disturbed defecation, and global wellbeing, because they are reproducible and respond to change.

PAIN

Pain is the most important symptom in IBS patients that predicts physician visits and patient distress.[31] No specific disease measures for IBS exist, and most trials have used standard pain indices to evaluate the response to pain. The Rome Committee has recommended 7- to 10-step adjectival ordinal scales or a 10 cm visual analogue scale (VAS) to increase sensitivity in the measurement of pain in IBS trials.[56]

BOWEL HABITS

A change in bowel habits is a prominent feature of IBS, and patients should be questioned about the form and appearance of their stools. The Bristol Stool Form Scale is the most commonly used instrument in clinical trials, and describes the stool in seven categories ranging from separate, hard lumps to watery. It has been shown to correlate with transit time in patients with IBS.[60] Yet, stool form does not evaluate the other features of disturbed defecation seen in IBS patients. Symptoms often reported by IBS patients include: urgency, unproductive calls to stool, anal pain during defecation, excessive straining at stool, feeling of incomplete evacuation, altered stool frequency, and passage of mucus. Measuring defecation symptoms is important, yet no valid objective assessment exists that is reproducible.

HEALTH RELATED QUALITY OF LIFE

The lack of clearly defined structural and biochemical indices for persons with IBS has led to the development of health related quality of life outcome measures. The most commonly used instrument, the IBS-QOL, was developed to evaluate the patient's perceptions, illness experience, and functional status of patients with IBS. This instrument has 34 questions and assesses dysphoria, interference with activity, body image, health worry, food avoidance, social reaction, sexual function, and relationships. The internal consistency reliability of the summed score was 0.95, and the intraclass correlation coefficient 0.86.[61] The convergent and discriminant validity of the IBS-QOL was compared to the SF-36 and SCL-90R. Correlations were strongest with bodily pain, social functioning, somatization, and obsessive-compulsiveness.[61] Persons with diarrhea-predominant symptoms reported the lowest overall quality of life. The IBS-QOL is recommended as one of the outcome measures that is sensitive to change in clinical trials.[62]

APPROACHES TO TREATMENT

General approach

Both diagnostic and treatment strategies for IBS depend on a biopsychosocial approach that incorporates both physiological and psychosocial information.[54] The first step is determination of the type and severity of the symptoms followed by individualized treatment plans. Patients with IBS can be classified as mild, moderate or severe based on the constancy of symptoms, presence of altered gut physiology, psychosocial difficulties, recognition of stress, and the frequency of health care use.

The therapeutic relationship plays an important role in the approach to treatment. Empathy has been shown to be correlated with the patient's evaluation of physician competence, compliance with medical visits, and an overall positive effect on patient's coping.[63] A therapeutic relationship implies a non-judgemental approach, the ability to offer warmth and genuineness, addressing fears, providing explanations, and involving the patient in management decisions.[64] When IBS is severe, the therapeutic relationship has been shown to affect outcome by promoting a sense of control or mastery over the symptoms.[51]

R
Grade C

The three symptom groups – abdominal pain and bloating, diarrhea, and constipation – have very different approaches to therapy. Each symptom will be considered individually. In cases where the predominant symptom is not determined, a symptom diary is helpful. The patient is asked to record the time and severity of the symptoms and the presence of associated factors that aggravate or alleviate the symptoms. After 2–3 weeks, the physician can review the diary and consider diet, lifestyle, or behavioral modifications with the patient. This approach has the additional benefit of encouraging active patient engagement in the treatment approach. Many patients take a passive attitude towards their illness, and feel that the illness is controlling them. A symptom diary allows patients to feel they are collaborators in their care.

Dietary approach

LACTOSE RESTRICTION

Dietary modification has not been well studied, except for the role of lactose and of fiber in patients with IBS. The symptoms of lactose malabsorption are nearly identical to those of IBS. In one study, almost 25% of patients with a diagnosis of IBS had evidence of lactose malabsorption by hydrogen breath tests.[65] In a population based study, subjective

Table 14.1 Double-blind placebo controlled trials of fiber supplementation in patients with IBS

Study (mth)	Study type	Grams of fiber daily	Duration (mth)	Difference between treatment groups	Symptom response
Soltoft, 1976[68]	Crossover	14.4	1.5	NS	None
Manning, 1977[69]	Parallel group	7.0	1.5	NS	Pain improved
Ornstein, 1981[70]	Crossover	7.0	4	NS	Constipation improved
Longstreth, 1981[71]	Crossover	9.8	2	NS	None
Cann, 1984[72]	Crossover	9.6	1	NS	Constipation improved
Arrfman, 1985[73]	Crossover	9.6	1.5	NS	Constipation improved
Lucey, 1987[74]	Crossover	12.8	3	NS	None
Cook, 1990[75]	Crossover	20	7	NS	Improvement with time, not fiber
Badiali, 1995[76]	Crossover	24	1	NS	Increased transit time with fiber

NS = P>0.05.

intolerance to lactose and the prevalence of symptoms determined by questionnaire, were studied and formal lactose tolerance testing was performed in 580 subjects.[66] In this population, 24% were lactose maldigesters with no known organic gastrointestinal disease. In the population of both lactose maldigesters and lactose digesters, 15% of the subjects met the Rome Criteria for IBS. Using logistic regression analysis, subjective lactose intolerance was strongly associated with IBS with an odds ratio of 4.6 (CI 2.1–10.1). The symptoms of IBS tend to improve after a lactose *restricted* diet is introduced,[67] but the co-mingling of subjective lactose intolerance and IBS tends to confound the clinical response. Only patients with a positive lactose intolerance test should eliminate lactose from the diet. In patients with subjective lactose intolerance who fulfill the Rome Criteria for IBS, symptom based and psychological treatment may be more effective.

FIBER SUPPLEMENTATION

An increase in dietary fiber is recommended in both constipation-predominant and diarrhea-predominant IBS patients with mild or moderate symptoms, but not for those with severe or refractory symptoms. Table 14.1 evaluates the randomized trials of fiber supplementation in patients with IBS.[68–76] The response rate to added fiber was 31–75%, in these trials, while the response rate to placebo was 38–71%. These trials were flawed by inadequate sample size, short duration of treatment (median 8 weeks), ill-defined inclusion criteria, other design flaws, and a high withdrawal rate. Despite these pitfalls, addition of bran to the diet is a very common recommendation of physicians because it is cheap and unlikely to cause harm. Quantitative analysis of the trials is not possible. However, perusal of the data suggests that the symptoms more likely to benefit from fiber supplementation are the passage of hard stools, constipation, and urgency.

R
Grade C

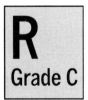

Approach to abdominal pain

Since abdominal pain is one of the diagnostic features of IBS, recent research has focused on the pathways that modulate pain. The stimulus that generates the experience of pain (nocioception) initiates neuronal discharges that involves the enteric nervous system (ENS), its vagal and sympathetic connections to the CNS, and the ascending pathways in the spinal cord to centers in the hindbrain and midbrain before reaching consciousness in the cerebral cortex. Altered afferent receptor and spinal neuron function may produce long term sensitization of pathways involved in the transmission of visceral sensation. Several studies suggest that visceral hypersensivity is an enteric neural occurrence that is influenced by, but independent of, abnormal motility and psychological factors.[77–88]

ANTICHOLINERGIC AGENTS

R Grade A

The most frequently prescribed class of medications for abdominal pain in the United States is anticholinergics. The rationale for the use of these drugs lies in their ability to reduce postprandial colonic motor activity through inhibition of cholinergic receptors. Older anticholinergics inhibit both nicotinic and muscarinic receptors and have been associated with more adverse effects than the newer antimuscarininc agents (hyoscyaminc). A recent meta-analysis of smooth muscle relaxants/antispasmodics included 26 randomized controlled trials that studied these preparations in IBS.[89] The analysis showed that these medications were significantly better than placebo for treatment of abdominal pain.

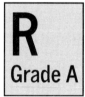

OTHER NEUROACTIVE DRUGS

Neuropeptides that act on the gut–brain axis include: 5-hydroxytryptamine, bradykinin, tachykinins, calcitonin gene-related peptide (CGRP), and the enkephalins, to name a few. The 5-hydroxytryptamine ($5HT_3$) receptor antagonists which may be useful for the treatment of IBS are presently under investigation in clinical trials. Preliminary data suggests that the $5HT_4$ agonists are prokinetic (for constipation predominant IBS) and may also have anti-nociceptive effects while the $5HT_3$ antagonists are primarily antidiarrheal. Although these agents seem to be promising tools for the treatment of visceral hyperalgesia and its consequences (abdominal pain and disturbed reflexes), their clinical efficacy remains to be shown. Other substances, such as somatostatin, opioid peptides, cholecystokinin, oxytocin, and adenosine, modulate the transmission of nociceptive inputs from the gut to the brain and are of clinical interest. Narcotic analgesics in the control of abdominal pain are contraindicated as they may lead to narcotic bowel syndrome.[90]

Approach to diarrhea

R Grade A

When the predominant symptom is diarrhea, the opioid derivatives (loperamide and diphenoxylate) are useful. Loperamide exerts an opioid effect on colonic muscle tone. Diphenoxylate exerts an antisecretory effect at the mucosal level and delays intestinal transit by inhibiting the opiate receptor in the myenteric plexus. Loperamide has been shown to be effective in reducing the number of stools in IBS patients in placebo controlled clinical trials, but no controlled trials have been performed for diphenoxylate.[91] One recent study suggested that bile acid malabsorption is responsible for 30% of diarrhea-like symptoms in IBS.[92] For patients who have suspected bile acid malabsorption, cholestryamine was an effective treatment in one study reported in abstract form.[92]

Approach to constipation

Severe constipation that is unresponsive to fiber supplementation requires more aggressive therapy. Surfactants (ducosate sodium) have been associated with impairment of small intestinal water absorption[93] and disruption of intestinal epithelium.[94] Stimulant laxatives, such as phenolphthalein, cascara, senna, and bisacodyl, are not recommended for chronic use. Long term use of these laxatives have been associated with a 'cathartic colon'.[95,96] Cisapride is a substituted benzamide compound that stimulates motor activity in all segments of the gastrointestinal tract by enhancing the release of acetylcholine from the enteric nervous system. It was compared to placebo in one controlled trial and improved stool consistency and frequency.[97] In another placebo controlled trial, cisapride was not superior to placebo in the treatment of constipation and abdominal discomfort, although there was a trend towards improving the difficulty of stool passage.[98] Severe cases of slow transit constipation seem refractory to cisapride.

R Grade A

R Grade C

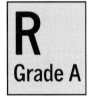

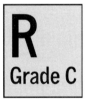

The most effective therapies for severe constipation are osmotic laxatives, colonic lavage with PEG, and bowel retraining. Lactulose and sorbitol have been shown to increase intraluminal bulk and stimulate peristalsis in placebo controlled trials.[99–101] The use of an oral isotonic solution containing PEG is safe and not associated with net ion absorption or loss. In one randomized placebo controlled trial, PEG ingestion was associated with an improvement in stool frequency and consistency.[102] Bowel retraining involves sitting on the commode for a distraction free period of 15 or 20 minutes each day without the obligation to perform, in addition to using a high fiber diet and an osmotic laxative. If no bowel movement occurs, an enema every 2–3 days is added to the bowel retraining. An uncontrolled study showed an improvement in bowel regularity using this method in 50–75% of affected children.[103] No controlled clinical trials of bowel retraining have been published for adults with IBS, yet clinical experience has shown an improvement in bowel regularity by this behavioral technique. Subtotal colectomy should be performed only in selected patients with severe colonic inertia, who have failed medical therapy.[104,105]

Psychological interventions

Five types of psychological interventions have been studied in the treatment of IBS: relaxation therapy, hypnosis, biofeedback, cognitive behavior therapy, and psychodynamic therapy. *Relaxation* methods reduce sympathetic nervous system activity and produce skeletal muscle relaxation. *Hypnosis* may be effective for IBS by reducing pain perception in the gut.[106] *Biofeedback* uses audio or visual instruments to reduce skeletal muscle activity. *Cognitive behavioral therapy* (CBT) involves identifying stressors, recognizing thoughts that increase distress, and learning new ways to cope with the stress by restructuring the personal reactions to them. Interpersonal or brief *psychodynamic therapy* helps patients to modify interpersonal conflicts that contribute to symptoms. The choice of psychological intervention depends on the ability of the patient to perceive it as part of a treatment plan.

Randomized controlled trials of psychological interventions have usually used conventional pharmacotherapy as the control intervention[106–112] (Table 14.2). There appears to be no difference in outcome based on the specific psychological technique. Post hoc subgroup analysis of these studies has identified the patients who are more likely to respond to psychological interventions: patients who have insight about the role of

Table 14.2 Randomized trials of psychological interventions vs medical therapy for IBS

Study	Psychological intervention compared to medical therapy	Treatment effect	Follow-up period (mth)	Comments
Svedlund, 1983[111]	Psychodynamic	Psychodynamic better	12	Improvement sustained
Whorwell, 1984[112]	Hypnotherapy	Psychodynamic better	18	Improvement sustained
Bennett, 1985[106]	CBT	NS		CBT better for anxiety
Guthrie, 1993[108]	Psychodynamic	Psychodynamic better		Reduced number of physician visits
Shaw, 1991[110]	CBT	CBT better	12	Improvement sustained
Rumsey, 1991[109]	CBT	Medical better	6	CBT better for depression and anxiety
Corney, 1991[107]	CBT	CBT better	9	Improvement in GI symptoms correlated with improvement in psychological scores

CBT, cognitive behavioral therapy.
Medical therapy = antispasmodics, general medical therapy.

stressors, patients who are under 50 years of age, and patients with lower levels of trait anxiety.[113]

ANTIDEPRESSANT MEDICATIONS

It is now recognized that the antidepressants have neuromodulatory and analgesic properties, independent of their psychotropic effect. Antidepressants have been used successfully in other chronic pain syndromes such as neuropathic pain (60% response rate) and chronic headaches (75% response rate).[114] The analgesic effects are similar in depressed and non-depressed patients.[115] Both tricyclic antidepressants (amitriptyline, imipramine, desimpramine) and selective serotonin reuptake inhibitors (fluoxetine, sertraline, paroxetine, fluvoxamine) are frequently used to treat patients with IBS. The decision to use the SSRIs versus the tricyclics is based on the specific subgroup of IBS symptoms, and the profile of adverse effects of the particular drug. The patient with diarrhea, nausea, and abdominal pain is a candidate for tricyclic antidepressant therapy, while the SSRIs are more appropriate for the patient with constipation-predominant IBS. A patient with considerable anxiety might do better on an antidepressant that tends to be more sedating, for example, trazadone or doxepin.

R Grade C

Of eight randomized trials of tricylic antidepressants, six[116–122] showed a significant improvement in symptoms (Table 14.3). The SSRIs have begun to play a larger role in the therapy of IBS, since up to 30% of patients experience adverse reactions to tricyclics.[123] The adverse effects profile of the various antidepressants is shown in Table 14.4. The lower incidence of adverse effects and rapid onset of efficacy with the use of SSRIs provide rationale for their use in IBS. However, there are no randomized controlled trials demonstrating efficacy of SSRIs in IBS. One case series showed efficacy of fluoxetine in controlling abdominal pain in IBS[124] Grade C but this study was not a randomized controlled trial. The prokinetic effects of the SSRIs make them particularly useful in patients with constipation and/or abdominal bloating.

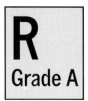

R Grade A

Table 14.3 Placebo controlled trials of tricyclic antidepressants in IBS

Author	Treatment	Clinical outcome	Comments
Heefner, 1978[116]	Desipramine vs placebo	No difference between groups	Combined constipation and diarrhea patients
Greenbaum, 1987[117]	Desipramine vs placebo	Diarrhea and pain improved with drug	Constipation patients did not improve
Myren, 1984[118]	Trimipramine vs placebo	Vomiting and mucous content of stool improved on drug	Depression improved on drug
Ritchie, 1980[120]	Nortriptyline and fluphenazine	Improved pain and diarrhea on drug	Constipation patients did not improve. No placebo group
Lancaster-Smith, 1982[122]	Nortriptyline and fluphenazine vs placebo	Improved pain and diarrhea on drugs	
Tripathi, 1989[121]	Trimipramine vs placebo	Improved pain on drug	

Table 14.4 Antidepressant drugs: effects on CNS receptor sites and adverse effects

Antidepressant	Anticholinergic effect	5HT receptor uptake	Histaminic effects	Daily dosage range	Adverse effects
TCAs					
Amitriptyline	++++	+++	++++	50–300 mg	Sedation, orthostasis, dry mouth, constipation
Desipramine	+	+++	+	50–300 mg	Diaphoresis, dry mouth, orthostasis
Doxepin	++	+++	++++	50–300 mg	Sedation, dry mouth
Maprotiline	+	Nil	++++	100–150 mg	Orthostasis, dry mouth, seizure, sedation
Nortriptyline	++	+	++	75–150 mg	Dry mouth
SSRIs					
Fluoxetine	Nil	++++	Nil	10–60 mg	N+V, bruxism, HA, diarrhea
Fluvoxamine	Nil	+++	Nil	50–300 mg	N+V, bruxism, HA, diarrhea
Paroxetine	Nil	++++	Nil	20–60 mg	N+V, bruxism, HA, diarrhea
Sertraline	Nil	++++	Nil	50–200 mg	N+V, bruxism, HA, diarrhea
Comipramine	++++	+++	+	25–250 mg	Sedation
ATYP					
Bupropion		Nil	Nil	200–450 mg	Seizures (>450 mg/day), Parkinsonian symptoms
Trazodone	Nil	+++	+++	50–600 mg 100–150 mg	Sedation, priapism
Nefazodone	Nil	++	+++	200–600 mg 20–60 mg 50–200 mg	Sedation
Venlafaxine	Nil	+++	Nil	50–200 mg	N+V, diarrhea

N+V, nausea and vomiting; HA, headache.
Antidepressant classes: TCA, tricyclic antidepressants; SSRI, selective serotonin reuptake inhibitors; NE/5HT, mixed adrenergic/serotonergic antidepressants; ATYP, atypical antidepressants.
Source: Psych Working Team Report for the Rome II Committee (1999; in press)

PROGNOSIS

The functional GI disorders differ from other gastrointestinal diseases, in that the organic pathology is not well defined. Because there are no biological markers to define IBS, symptom based criteria have been validated for the diagnosis.[53] Clinical expertise is needed to individualize therapy for these patients. The nature of symptoms, predisposing factors, altered physiology, psychosocial modifiers, and illness behavior, all interact to influence clinical decision making and the ultimate prognosis.

IBS is a chronic disease, with over 75% of patients continuing to have fluctuating symptoms. The goal should be judicious use of medical testing, within an atmosphere of an empathetic patient–doctor relationship. Recurrences should be treated by a symptom based approach, with careful attention to the psychosocial triggers that contribute to exacerbation. In a cohort study reported by Harvey *et al*[24] 104 patients with IBS were studied prospectively to determine their prognosis over a 5-year period. The response to treatment was better in men than in women, in patients with predominant constipation rather than diarrhea, in patients whose symptoms had initially been triggered by an episode of acute diarrhea, and in patients with a relatively short history. With a few simple investigations, sympathetic explanation and appropriate treatment, most patients with IBS have a good prognosis.

CONCLUSION

IBS is one of the most common medical conditions seen in clinical practice and patients with IBS comprise 40–50% of gastroenterology practice. It is responsible for a considerable economic burden because of the high frequency of physician visits and work absenteeism. After consideration of demographic features, the nature of the symptoms, and the severity index, only limited investigations to rule out organic disease are indicated. The variety of symptoms, the lack of understanding of the pathophysiology, the complex interaction of the CNS and ENS and their receptors, suggest that no single drug will cure IBS. A strong physician–patient relationship helps control health care utilization.

REFERENCES

1 Drossman DA, Whitehead WE, Camilleri M (Patient Care Committee AGA). Irritable bowel syndrome: a technical review for practice guideline development. *Gastroenterology* 1997; **112**(6): 2120–37.

2 Switz DM. What the gastroenterologist does all day. A survey of a state society's practice. *Gastroenterology* 1976; **70**: 1048.

3 Ferguson A, Sircus W, Eastwood MA. Frequency of "functional' gastrointestinal disorders. Lancet 1977; **2**: 613.

4 Mitchell CM, Drossman DA. Survey of the AGA membership relating to patients with functional gastrointestinal disorders. *Gastroenterology* 1987; **92**: 1282.

5 Sandler R. Epidemiology of irritable bowel syndrome in the United States. *Gastroenterology* 1990; **99**: 409.

6 Everhart JE, Renault PF. Irritable bowel syndrome in office-based practice in the United States. *Gastroenterology* 1991; **100**: 998–1005.

7 Talley NJ, Gabriel SE, Harmsen WS *et al*. Medical costs in community subjects with irritable bowel syndrome. *Gastroenterology* 1995; **109**(6): 1736–41.

8 Powell R. On certain painful afflictions of the intestinal canal. *Med Trans R Coll Phys* 1818; **6**: 106.
9 Drossman DA, Chairmen WTC. The functional gastrointestinal disorders and their diagnosis: a coming of age. In: Drossman DA (ed), *The functional gastrointestinal disorders: diagnosis, pathophysiology, and treatment*. Boston: Little, Brown and Company, 1994, pp 1–23.
10 Mayer EA, Gebhart GF. Basic and clinical aspects of visceral hyperalgesia. *Gastroenterology* 1994; **107**: 271–93.
11 Engel GL. The need for a new medical model: a challenge for biomedicine. *Science* 1977; **196**: 129–36.
12 Drossman DA. Presidential Address: Gastrointestinal Illness and the Biopsychosocial Model. *Psychosom Med* 1998; **60**: 258–67.
13 Manning AP, Thompson WG, Heaton KW *et al.* Towards positive diagnosis of the irritable bowel. *Br Med J* 1978; **2**: 653–4.
14 Thompson WG, Dotevall G, Drossman DA *et al.* Irritable bowel syndrome: guidelines for the diagnosis. *Gastroenteorology Int* 1989; **2**: 92.
15 Whitehead WE, Cromwell MD, Bosmajian L *et al.* Existence of irritable bowel syndrome supported by factor analysis of symptoms in two community samples. *Gastroenterology* 1990; **98**: 336–40.
16 Talley NJ, Phillips SF, Melton LJ *et al.* A patient questionnaire to identify bowel disease. *Ann Intern Med* 1989; **111**: 671–4.
17 Palsson OS, Taub E, Cook E, III *et al.* Validation of Rome Criteria for functional gastrointestinal disorders by factor analysis. *Am J Gastroenterol* 1996; **91**: 2000.
18 Vanner S, Glenn D, Paterson W *et al.* Diagnosing irritable bowel syndrome: predictive value of Rome Criteria. *Gastroenterology* 1997; **112** (abstract).
19 Kay L, Jorgensen T, Jensen KH. The epidemiology of irritable bowel syndrome in a random population: prevalence, incidence, natural history and risk factors. *J Intern Med* 1994; **236**: 23–30.
20 Jones R. Irritable bowel syndrome. *Practitioner* 1991; **235**: 811–14.
21 Heaton KW. Epidemiology of irritable bowel syndrome. *Eur J Gastroenterol Hepatol* 1994; **6**: 465–9.
22 Drossman DA, Li Z, Andruzzi E *et al.* US householder survey of functional gastrointestinal disorders. Prevalence, sociodemography, and health impact. *Dig Dis Sci* 1993; **38**(9): 1569–80.
23 Talley NJ, O'Keefe EA, Zinsmeister AR *et al.* Prevalence of gastrointestinal symptoms in the elderly: a population-based study. *Gastroenterology* 1992; **102**: 895–901.
24 Harvey RF, Mauad EC, Brown AM. Prognosis in the irritable bowel syndrome: a five-year prospective study. *Lancet* 1987; **i**: 963–5.
25 Taub E, Cuevas JL, Cook E, III *et al.* Irritable bowel syndrome defined by factor analysis. Gender and race comparisons. *Dig Dis Sci* 1995; **40**(12): 2647–55.
26 Stevens JA, Wan CK, Blanchard EB. The short-term natural history of irritable bowel syndrome: a time-series analysis. *Behav Res Ther* 1997; **35**(4): 319–28.
27 Sivri A, Cindas A, Dincer F *et al.* Bowel dysfunction and irritable bowel syndrome in fibromyalgia patients. *Clin Rheumatol* 1996; **15**(3): 283–6.
28 Burns DG. The risk of abdominal surgery in irritable bowel syndrome. *South Afr Med J* 1986; **70**: 91.
29 Whitehead WE, Cheskin LJ, Heller BR *et al.* Evidence for exacerbation of irritable bowel syndrome during menses. *Gastroenterology* 1990; **98**: 1485–9.
30 Maxton DG, Whorwell PJ. Use of medical resources and attitudes to health care of patients with "chronic abdominal pain". *Br J Med Econ* 1992; **2**: 75–9.
31 Drossman DA, McKee DC, Sandler RS *et al.* Psychosocial factors in the irritable bowel syndrome. A multivariate study of patients and nonpatients with irritable bowel syndrome. *Gastroenterology* 1988; **95**: 701–8.
32 Smith RC, Greenbaum DS, Vancouver JB *et al.* Psychosocial factors are associated with health care seeking rather than diagnosis in irritable bowel syndrome. *Gastroenterology* 1990; **98**: 293–301.
33 Whitehead WE, Bosmajian L, Zonderman AB *et al.* Symptoms of psychologic distress associated with irritable bowel syndrome. Comparison of community and medical clinic samples. *Gastroenterology* 1988; **95**: 709–14.
34 Drossman DA. Illness behaviour in the irritable bowel syndrome. *Gastroenterol Int* 1991; **4**: 77–81.
35 Holtmann G, Enck P. Stress and gastrointestinal motility in humans: a review of the literature. *J Gastrointest Motil* 1991; **3**(4): 245–54.
36 Lydiard RB, Fossey MD, March W *et al.* Prevalence of psychiatric disorders in patients with irritable bowel syndrome. *Psychosomatics* 1993;**34**: 229–34.
37 Drossman DA, Creed FH, Fava GA *et al.* Psychosocial aspects of the functional gastrointestinal disorders. *Gastroenterol Int* 1995; **8**: 47–90.
38 Walker EA, Gelfand AN, Gelfand MD *et al.* Psychiatric diagnoses, sexual and physical victimization, and disability in patients with irritable bowel syndrome or inflammatory

bowel disease. *Psychol Med* 1995; **25**(6): 1259–67.

39 Drossman DA, Talley NJ, Leserman J *et al.* Sexual and physical abuse and gastrointestinal illness. Review and recommendations. *Ann Intern Med* 1995; **123**(10): 782–94.

40 Craig TKJ, Brown GW. Goal frustration and life events in the aetiology of painful gastrointestinal disorder. *J Psychosom Res* 1984; **28**: 411–21.

41 Creed F, Craig T, Farmer R. Functional abdominal pain, psychiatric illness, and life events. *Gut* 1988; **29**(2): 235–42.

42 Whitehead WE, Crowell MD, Robinson JC *et al.* Effects of stressful life events on bowel symptoms: subjects with irritable bowel syndrome compared to subjects without bowel dysfunction. *Gut* 1992; **33**: 825–30.

43 Drossman DA, Leserman J, Nachman G *et al.* Sexual and physical abuse in women with functional or organic gastrointestinal disorders. *Ann Intern Med* 1990; **113**: 828–33.

44 Delvaux M, Denis P, Allemand H. Sexual abuse is more frequently reported by IBS patients than by patients with organic digestive diseases or controls. Results of a multicentre inquiry. French Club of Digestive Motility. *Eur J Gastroenterol Hepatol* 1997; **9**(4): 345–52.

45 Laws A. Does a history of sexual abuse in childhood play a role in women's medical problems? A review. *J Women's Hlth* 1993; **2**: 165–72.

46 Drossman DA, Li Z, Leserman J *et al.* Health status by gastrointestinal diagnosis and abuse history. *Gastroenterology* 1996; **110**(4): 999–1007.

47 Longstreth GF, Wolde-Tsadik G. Irritable bowel-type symptoms in HMO examinees. Prevalence, demographics, and clinical correlates. *Dig Dis Sci* 1993; **38**: 1581–9.

48 Drossman DA. Irritable bowel syndrome and sexual/physical abuse history. *Eur J Gastroenterol Hepatol* 1997; **9**(4): 327–30.

49 Milholland AV, Wheeler SG, Heieck JJ. Medical assessment by a Delphi group opinion technique. *N Engl J Med* 1973; **298**: 1272–5.

50 Christensen J. Defining the irritable bowel syndrome. *Perspect Biol Med* 1994; **38**: 21–35.

51 Drossman DA. Diagnosing and treating patients with refractory functional gastrointestinal disorders. *Ann Intern Med* 1995;**123**(9):688–97.

52 Metcalf AM, Phillips SF, Zinsmeister AR *et al.* Simplified assessment of segmental colonic transit. *Gastroenterology* 1987; **92**: 40–7.

53 Drossman DA, Richter JE, Talley NJ *et al* (eds). *Functional gastrointestinal disorders: diagnosis, pathophysiology and treatment*, volume 1. McLean, VA: Degnon Associates, 1994.

54 Drossman DA. Presidential Address: Gastrointestinal Illness and the Biopsychosocial Model. *Psychosom Med* 1998; **60**: 258–67.

55 Talley NJ, Nyren O, Drossman DA *et al.* The irritable bowel syndrome: toward optimal design of controlled treatment trials. *Gastroenterol Int* 1993; **4**: 189–211.

56 Talley NJ. Optimal design of treatment trials. In: Drossman DA, Richter JE, Talley NJ *et al* (eds), *Functional gastrointestinal disorders: diagnosis, pathophysiology and treatment*, volume 1. McLean, VA: Degnon Associates, 1994, pp. 265–309.

57 Owens DM, Nelson DK, Talley NJ. Irritable bowel: it helps to have a friendly physician – or so it would seem. *Gastroenterology* 1995; **109**: 1711–13.

58 Drossman DA, Li Z, Toner BB *et al.* Functional bowel disorders. A multicenter comparison of health status and development of illness severity index. *Dig Dis Sci* 1995; **40**(5): 986–95.

59 Francis CY, Morris J, Whorwell PJ. The irritable bowel severity scoring system: a simple method of monitoring irritable bowel syndrome and its progress. *Aliment Pharmacol Ther* 1997; **11**(2): 395–402.

60 Heaton KW, Ghosh S, Braddon FE. How bad are the symptoms and bowel dysfunction of patients with the irritable bowel syndrome? A prospective, controlled study with emphasis on stool form. *Gut* 1991; **32**(1): 73–9.

61 Patrick DL, Drossman DA, Frederick IO. *A quality of life measure for persons with irritable bowel syndrome (IBS-QOL). User's manual and scoring diskette*, volume 1. Seattle: University of Washington, 1997.

62 Drossman DA, Patrick DL, Whitehead,WE *et al.* Responsiveness of the IBS-QOL: further validation of a disease specific quality of life measure for IBS. *Gastroenterology* 1999; **116** (abstract).

63 DiMatteo MR, DiNicola DD. *Achieving patient compliance*. New York, NY: Pergamon Press, 1982.

64 Lipkin MJ. The medical interview and related skills. In: Branch WT (ed), *Office practice of medicine*, volume 3. Philadelphia: WB Saunders, 1993, pp 35–45.

65 Bohmer CJ, Tuyman HA. The clinical relevance of lactose malabsorption in irritable bowel syndrome. *Eur J Gastroenterol Hepatol* 1996; **8**(10): 1013–16.

66 Vesa TH, Seppo LM, Marteau PR *et al.* Role of irritable bowel syndrome in subjective lactose intolerance. *Am J Clin Nutr* 1998; **67**: 710–15.

67 Vernia P, Ricciardi MR, Frandian C *et al.* Lactose malabsorption and irritable bowel syndrome. Effect of a long-term lactose-free diet. *Ital J Gastroenterol* 1995; **27**(3): 117–21.

68 Soltoft J, Gudmund-Hoyer AG, Krag B *et al.* A double-blind trial of the effects of wheat bran on symptoms of irritable bowel syndrome. *Lancet* 1976: **i**: 270–2
69 Manning AP, Heaton KW, Harvey RF *et al.* Wheat bran and irritable bowel syndrome. *Lancet* 1977; **ii**: 417–18
70 Ornstein MH, Littlewood ER, Baird IM *et al.* Are fibre supplements really necessary in diverticular disease of the colon? Controlled clinical trial. *Br Med J* 1981; **282**: 1353–6.
71 Longstreth GF, Fox DD, Youkeles L *et al.* Psyllium therapy in the irritable bowel syndrome. A double-blind trial. *Ann Intern Med* 1981; **95**: 53–6.
72 Cann PA, Read NWH, Holdsworth CD. What is the benefit of coarse bran in patients with irritable bowel syndrome? *Gut* 1984; **25**: 168–71.
73 Arrfman S, Andersen JR, Hegnoj J *et al.* The effect of coarse wheat bran in the irritable bowel syndrome. A double-blind cross-over study. *Scand J Gastroenterol* 1985; **20**: 295–8.
74 Lucey MR, Clark ML, Lowndes JO *et al.* Is bran efficacious in irritable bowel syndrome? A double-blind placebo-controlled study. *Gut* 1987; **21**: 221–5.
75 Cook IJ, Irvine EJ, Campbell D *et al.* Effect of dietary fiber on symptoms and rectosigmoid motility in patients with irritable bowel syndrome. A controlled crossover study. *Gastroenterology* 1990; **98**(1): 66–72.
76 Badiali D, Corazziari E, Habib FI *et al.* Effect of wheat bran in treatment of chronic nonorganic constipation. A double-blind controlled trial. *Dig Dis Sci* 1995; **40**(2): 349–56.
77 Ritchie J. Pain from distension of the pelvic colon by inflating a balloon in the irritable bowel syndrome. *Gut* 1973; **6**: 105–12.
78 Whitehead WE, Engel BT, Schuster MM. Irritable bowel syndrome: physiological and psychological differences between diarrhea-predominant and constipation-predominant patients. *Dig Dis Sci* 1980; **25**: 404–13.
79 Moriarty KJ, Dawson AM. Functional abdominal pain: further evidence that whole gut is affected. *Br Med J* 1982; **284**: 1671–2.
80 Prior A, Colgan SM, Whorwell PJ. Changes in rectal sensitivity after hypnotherapy in patients with irritable bowel syndrome. *Gut* 1990; **31**: 896–8.
81 Mertz H, Naliboff B, Munakata J *et al.* Altered rectal perception is a biological marker of patients with irritable bowel syndrome. *Gastroenterology* 1995; **109**: 40–52.
82 Sun WM, Read NW, Prior A *et al.* Sensory and motor responses to rectal sensation vary according to rate and pattern of balloon inflation. *Gastroenterology* 1990; **99**: 1008–15.
83 Bradette J, Delvaux M, Staumont G *et al.* Evaluation of colonic sensory thresholds in IBS patients using a barostat: definition of optimal conditions and comparison with healthy subjects. *Dig Dis Sci* 1994; **39**: 449–57.
84 Hasler WL, Soudah HC, Owyang C. Somatostatin analog inhibits afferent response to rectal distension in diarrhea-predominant irritable bowel patients. *J Pharmacol Exp Ther* 1994; **268**: 1206–11.
85 Lembo T, Munakata J, Mertz H *et al.* Evidence for the hypersensitivity of the lumbar splanchnic afferents in irritable bowel syndrome. *Gastroenterology* 1994; **107**: 1686–96.
86 Hammer J, Phillips SF, Talley NJ *et al.* Effect of a $5HT_3$-antagonist (ondansetron) on rectal sensitivity and compliance in health and the irritable bowel syndrome. *Aliment Pharmacol Ther* 1993; **291**: 2079.
87 Whitehead WE, Holtkotter B, Enck P *et al.* Tolerance for rectosigmoid distension in irritable bowel syndrome. *Gastroenterology* 1990; **98**: 1187–92.
88 Slater BJ, Plusa SM, Smith AN *et al.* Rectal hypersensitivity in the irritable bowel syndrome. *Int J Colorectal Dis* 1997; **12**(1): 29–32.
89 Poynard T, Naveau S, Mory B *et al.* Meta-analysis of smooth muscle relaxers in the treatment of irritable bowel syndrome. *Aliment Pharmacol Ther* 1994; **8**: 499–510.
90 Sandgren JE, McPhee MS, Greenberger NJ. Narcotic bowel syndrome treated with clonidine. *Ann Intern Med* 1984; **101**: 331–4.
91 Pace F, Coremans G, Dapoigny M *et al.* Therapy of irritable bowel syndrome – an overview. *Digestion* 1995; **56**(5): 433–42.
92 Smith M, Cherian P, Raju GS. Bile acid malabsorption (BAM)-related diarrhea: common, easily diagnosed and treatable (abstract). *Gastroenterology* 1998; (Suppl): G0170.
93 Rachmilowitz D, Marmeli F. Effect of bisacodyl and dioctyl sodium sulphosuccinate on rat intestinal prostaglandin E2, Na-K-ATPase, adenyl cyclase and phosphodiesterase activities. *Gastroenterology* 1979; **76**: 1221.
94 Saunders PR, Kosecka U, McKay DM *et al.* Acute stressors stimulate ion secretion and increase epithelial permeability in rat intestine. *Am J Physiol* 1994: G794–G799.
95 Smith B. Effect of irritant purgatives on the myenteric plexus in man and the mouse. *Gut* 1968; **9**: 139.
96 Cummings JH, Sladen GE, James OFW *et al.* Laxative-induced diarrhoea: a continuing clinical problem. *Br Med J* 1974; 537–41.
97 Van Outryve M, Milo R, Toussaint J *et al.* "Prokinetic" treatment of constipation-

predominant irritable bowel syndrome: a placebo-controlled study of cisapride. *J Clin Gastroenterol* 1991; **13**: 49–57.

98 Schutze K, Brandstatter G, Dragosics B *et al.* Double-blind study of the effect of cisapride on constipation and abdominal discomfort as components of the irritable bowel syndrome. *Aliment Pharmacol Ther* 1997; **11**(2): 387–94.

99 Lederle FA, Busch DL, Mattox KM *et al.* Cost-effective treatment of constipation in the elderly: a randomized double-blind comparison of sorbitol and lactulose. *Am J Med* 1990; **89**: 597–601.

100 Wessalius-DeCasparis A. Treatment of chronic constipation with lactulose syrup: results of a double blind study. *Gut* 1969; **9**: 84–6.

101 Brown RL. Effects of lactulose and other laxatives on ileal and colonic pH as measured by a radiotelemetry device. *Gut* 1974; **15**: 999–1004.

102 Andorsky RI, Goldner F. Colonic lavage solution (polyethylene glycol electrolyte lavage solution) as a treatment for chronic constipation: a double-blind, placebo-controlled study. *Am J Gastroenterol* 1990; **85**(3): 261–5.

103 Sarahan T, Weintraub WH, Coran A *et al.* The successful management of chronic constipation in infants and children. *J Pediatr Surg* 1982; **17**: 171–4.

104 Leon SH, Krishnamurthy S, Schuffler MD. Subtotal colectomy for severe idiopathic constipation: a follow up study of 13 patients. *Dig Dis Sci* 1987; **32**: 1249–54.

105 Gasslander T, Larsson J, Wetterfors J. Experience of surgical treatment for chronic idiopathic constipation. *Acta Chir Scand* 1987; **153**: 553–5.

106 Bennett P, Wilkinson S. A comparison of psychological and medical treatment of the irritable bowel syndrome. *Br J Clin Psychol* 1985; **24**: 215–16.

107 Corney RH, Stanton R, Newell R *et al.* Behavioral psychotherapy in the treatment of irritable bowel syndrome. *J Psychosom Res* 1991; **35**: 461–9.

108 Guthrie E, Creed F, Dawson D *et al.* A randomised controlled trial of psychotherapy in patients with refractory irritable bowel syndrome. *Br J Psychiatry* 1993; **163**: 315–21.

109 Rumsey N. *Group stress management programmes vs pharmacological treatment in the irritable bowel syndrome.* Lyme Regis: Lyme Regis Printing Co., 1991

110 Shaw G, Srivastava ED, Sadlier M *et al.* Stress management for irritable bowel syndrome: a controlled trial. *Digestion* 1991; **50**: 36–42.

111 Svedlund J. Psychotherapy in irritable bowel syndrome: a controlled outcome study. *Acta Psychiatr Scand* 1983; **67**(306): 1–86.

112 Whorwell PJ, Prior A, Faragher EB *et al.* Controlled trial of hypnotherapy in the treatment of severe refractory irritable bowel syndrome. *Lancet* 1984; **2**: 1232–3.

113 Talley NJ, Owen BK, Boyce P *et al.* Psychological treatments for irritable bowel syndrome: a critique of controlled treatment trials. *Am J Gastroenterol* 1996; **91**(2): 277–83.

114 Egbunike IG, Chaffee BJ. Antidepressants in the management of chronic pain syndromes. *Pharmacotherapy* 1990; **10**(4): 262–70.

115 McQuay H, Carroll D, Jadad AR *et al.* Anticonvulsant drugs for management of pain: a systematic review. *Br Med J* 1995; **311**(7012): 1047–52.

116 Heefner JD, Wilder RM, Wilson JD *et al.* Irritable colon and depression. *Psychosomatics* 1978; **19**: 540–7.

117 Greenbaum DS, Mayle JE, Vanegeren LE *et al.* The effects of desipramine on IBS compared with atropine and placebo. *Dig Dis Sci* 1987; **32**: 257–66.

118 Myren J, Lovland B, Larssen SE *et al.* A double-blind study of the effect of trimipramine in patients with the irritable bowel syndrome. *Scand J Gastroenterol* 1984; **19**: 835–43.

119 Myren J, Groth J, Larssen SE *et al.* The effect of trimipramine in patients with irritable bowel syndrome. *Scand J Gastroenterol* 1982; **17**: 871–5.

120 Ritchie JA, Truelove SC. Comparison of various treatments for irritable bowel syndrome. *Br Med J* 1980; **281**: 257–66.

121 Tripathi BM, Misra NP, Gupta AK. Evaluation of tricyclic compound (trimipramine) vis-à-vis placebo in irritable bowel syndrome (double-blind randomized study). *J Assoc Phys India* 1989; **31**: 201–3.

122 Lancaster-Smith MJ, Prout BJ, Pinto T *et al.* Influence of drug treatment on the irritable bowel syndrome and its interaction with psychoneurotic morbidity. *Acta Psychiatr Scand* 1982; **66**: 33–41.

123 Cannon RO, Quyyumi AA, Mincemoyer R *et al.* Imipramine in patients with chest pain despite normal coronary angiograms. *N Engl J Med* 1994; **20**: 1411–17.

124 Eisendrath SJ, Kodama KT. Fluoxetine management of chronic abdominal pain. *Pscychosomatics* 1992; **33**: 229–31.

15 Gallstone disease: surgical treatment

CALVIN HL LAW, VÉD R TANDAN

INTRODUCTION

Surgical therapy for gallstones can be associated with morbidity and mortality which has led to debate on its use, especially in asymptomatic and mildly symptomatic patients. These issues have been further clouded by the introduction of laparoscopic cholecystectomy with its touted benefits of decreased morbidity and improved recovery times. The evidence concerning the benefits and risks of surgical therapy for gallstone disease and its complications is discussed.

ELECTIVE CHOLECYSTECTOMY

Asymptomatic cholelithiasis in the general population

There are no controlled studies comparing prophylactic surgery with expectant management in asymptomatic patients with cholelithiasis. However, a number of cohort studies have been performed to assess the probability of developing biliary pain and biliary complications in asymptomatic persons with gallstones.

Through the 1980s, a series of cohort studies were conducted by Gracie and Ransohoff,[1] McSherry *et al*[2] and Friedman *et al*.[3] Gracie's study had complete follow-up on 123 persons for 11 to 24 years.[1] The cumulative probability of the development of biliary pain was 10% at 5 years, 15% at 10 years, and 18% at 20 years. However, 89% of the study population were white American males and all were faculty members of the University of Michigan, a factor which limits the generalizability of this study. McSherry's study retrospectively identified 135 patients with asymptomatic cholelithiasis who were subscribers to the Health Insurance Plan of Greater New York, a mainly middle income population of diverse ethnic origin.[2] Over a mean follow-up of 46 months 10.4% of patients developed symptoms, yielding a 2.7% annual rate of developing symptoms. Similarly, the study by Friedman followed 123 ethnically diverse patients with asymptomatic gallstones in the Kaiser Permanenete Medical Care Program (San Francisco) for 16–25 years.[3] There was a 3–4% annual rate of biliary events in the initial 10 years, and a 1–2% annual rate in the following 10 years. At 5 years, 18% of patients had developed biliary symptoms. One death was attributable to gallstones (cholangitis). A more detailed examination of Gracie's data showed that though three patients eventually had biliary complications (2.4% of the population), all had presented with pain first. In McSherry's study, 10% of the population eventually developed symptoms and 71% of these patients had biliary colic as their only indication for elective cholecystectomy. The remaining patients had biliary complications prior to surgery (3% of the study population) but it is unclear if they presented with pain first. Overall, these studies estimate an annual rate of 1–2% of developing symptoms, and that 90% will present with pain prior to developing a biliary complication, while only 10% will present with a biliary complication as the first manifestation of their biliary tract disease.[4,5]

The Group for Epidemiology and Prevention of Cholelithiasis (GREPCO) in Italy[6] prospectively followed 118 patients with asymptomatic cholelithiasis. The cumulative probability of developing biliary colic was 12% at 2 years, 17% at 4 years, and 26% at 10 years. The cumulative probability of biliary complications was 3% at 10 years. One patient died of a gallbladder carcinoma. This represents a higher rate of symptoms, but not complications, than the studies from the 1980s.

Ransohoff *et al* performed a decision analysis[7] on data first published by Gracie.[1] Using cholecystectomy mortality rates up to 1983, they found prophylactic cholecystectomy slightly decreased survival, while economic analysis did not favor prophylactic cholecystectomy.

Considering the current evidence, expectant management rather than prophylactic cholecystectomy is indicated for the typical patient with asymptomatic gallstones. However, certain populations who are more at risk for complications of gallstone disease need to be considered separately.

R
Grade B

Asymptomatic cholelithiasis in the diabetic

More liberal thresholds for elective cholecystectomy in asymptomatic diabetics have been suggested,[8] citing a higher incidence of gallstone disease and biliary complications, and poorer outcomes for emergency surgery for biliary complications. Only Grade B evidence is available, which supports expectant management of asymptomatic cholelithiasis in this population rather than a more aggressive approach.

In 1952, Lieber studied 26 895 autopsies, revealing an overall incidence of cholelithiasis of 11.6%; among diabetics the rate of cholelithiasis was 30.2%.[9] Since then, the belief that cholelithiasis is more common in diabetics has become widely held.[10] More recently, Chapman reviewed 308 diabetics and 318 non-diabetic controls.[11] The incidence of cholelithiasis was higher in the diabetic population (32.7% vs 20.8%, $P<0.001$). When the data were subjected to multiple regression analysis, however, diabetes did not correlate strongly with the incidence of cholelithiasis except in a subgroup of females with non-insulin dependent diabetes.

Del Favero[12] prospectively studied the natural history of cholelithiasis in the diabetic by following a cohort of 47 diabetic patients with asymptomatic cholelithiasis. After 5 years, seven patients (15%) had developed symptoms or complications. Of this group, five had presented with pain as their first symptom. One patient presented with cholecystitis and one with jaundice. These data compare favorably with the data available from the studies of the general population.

Higher complication rates with emergent surgery for biliary complications in the diabetic have been observed. Hickman[13] studied 72 diabetic patients who underwent cholecystectomy for cholecystitis and matched them for age, gender and date of operation with 72 non-diabetic patients. Morbidity for diabetics was 38.9% compared to 20.8% in the non-diabetic population. Mortality only occurred in the diabetic population in 4.2% and was attributed to sepsis. The septic complication rate was higher in the diabetics (19.4%) than in the non-diabetic group (6.9%). This higher rate was maintained whether the diabetic patients had concurrent medical illness or not.

The apparent higher incidence of cholelithiasis in diabetics is likely related to factors other than diabetes itself. The natural history of asymptomatic cholelithiasis in diabetics appears similar to that in the general population. Nevertheless, diabetics who have biliary complications may have increased morbidity with emergency cholecystectomy, though this has not been well studied to date. Individualized considerations such as concurrent illness must be considered in deciding whether to recommend prophylactic cholecystectomy in this population, and recommendations will often have to be made without good supporting evidence.

Asymptomatic cholelithiasis and the risk of cancer

Autopsy data reveal that greater than 80% of patients with gallbladder cancer will have concomitant cholelithiasis.[14] Maringhini followed 2583 patients with known gallstones in the Rochester, Minnesota area. Only five patients (0.2%) developed gallbladder carcinoma.[15] In the previously discussed cohorts of patients with asymptomatic cholelithiasis, only one patient (of a total of 499 patients followed for up to 25 years) was found to have gallbladder carcinoma.

The incidence of gallbladder cancer varies widely with different populations, even in the presence of gallstone disease. Lowenfels reported a case–control study of 131 patients with gallbladder carcinoma and 2399 subjects without gallbladder carcinoma.[16] The 20-year cumulative risk for gallbladder cancer ranged from 0.13% in the black male to 1.5% in the native American female. They calculated that 769 cholecystectomies were required to prevent one gallbladder cancer in a low risk population; however, only 67 cholecystectomies would be necessary to prevent one gallbladder cancer in a high risk population.

Patients with gallstones greater than 3 cm in diameter may be at increased risk for the development of gallbladder carcinoma. Diehl reported this in a case–control study in 1983[17] and it was confirmed by Lowenfels in 1989.[18] These studies indicated a 9–10-fold increase in relative risk of developing gallbladder carcinoma between patients with stones greater than 3 cm in diameter and those patients with stones less than 1 cm in diameter.

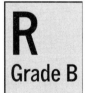

R
Grade B

Grade B evidence supports the view that the risk of developing gallbladder cancer may be higher in patients with cholelithiasis. However, the increased risk appears to be insufficient to recommend for prophylactic cholecystectomy.[5,19] Although some subsets of the population (especially the native American Indian female) and patients with stones greater than 3 cm may be at sufficient risk to justify prophylactic cholecystectomy, further evidence would be needed to support a firm recommendation.

Symptomatic cholelithiasis

R
Grade B

Grade B evidence supports the current approach to patients with symptomatic cholelithiasis. Patients with uncomplicated biliary colic should be offered surgery as an option to controlling symptoms. Patients with complications of cholelithiasis should have surgery to prevent future complications. The previously discussed natural history studies of McSherry *et al*[2] and Friedman *et al*[3] included a group of patients with symptomatic cholelithiasis. Additional data are also available from the National Cooperative Gallstone Study (NCGS).[20] McSherry followed 556 patients with symptomatic cholelithiasis.[2] During an average follow-up of 83 months, 169 (30%) patients reported worsened or continued severe symptoms, nine (1.6%) patients developed jaundice, and 47 (8.5%) patients developed acute cholecystitis. These data indicate a 4.3% annual rate of worsening or persistently severe symptoms and a 1.5% annual rate of biliary complications arising from symptomatic cholelithiasis. Friedman followed 298 patients with mild or non-specific symptoms and cholelithiasis for 16–25 years.[3] The annual rate of developing cholecystitis or jaundice was 1%.

The NCGS was designed as a double-blind randomized controlled trial of chenodiol.[21] The group of patients who had received placebo provided another opportunity to study the natural history of symptomatic cholelithiasis. One hundred and twelve patients receiving placebo had symptomatic cholelithiasis.[20] Seventy-seven patients presented with worsening symptoms of biliary colic or prolonged biliary pain in 2 years of follow-up. Seven patients "required cholecystectomy" during the follow-up as well. This represents a 34% annual incidence of worsening symptoms and a 3% annual incidence of "requiring a cholecystectomy". The patients with symptomatic cholelithiasis in these studies did not suffer any greater mortality during the follow-up period than was experienced by patients in the asymptomatic population.

The rate of complications secondary to symptomatic cholelithiasis appears to be higher than that in the general population with asymptomatic cholelithiasis. Recurrent or worsening symptoms may develop but there is no increased mortality from observation, at least in the short term. Therefore, "the subjective experience of the patient should be the principal determinant of whether and when the procedure should be performed".[22] The exceptions to this recommendation are the special populations discussed above. Once cholelithiasis is complicated by acute cholecystitis, choledocholithiasis, cholangitis, or pancreatitis, early surgicial treatment is indicated.

R
Grade B

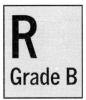

Elective laparoscopic versus open cholecystectomy

Supporters of laparoscopy point out improved cosmesis, faster recovery times, and decreased postoperative stay as major advantages. Others note that since the introduction of laparoscopic cholecystectomy the rate of bile duct injury has increased and the claimed benefits of the procedure need to be more closely examined.[23] Despite the ongoing debate, laparoscopic cholecystectomy has had a significant impact on the management of gallstone disease as evidenced by markedly increasing rates of elective cholecystectomy since its introduction.[24]

Grade A evidence from four randomized controlled trials comparing elective laparoscopic cholecystectomy and mini-laparotomy cholecystectomy is available (Table 15.1).[25–28] There is no statistically significant difference in the incidence of biliary tract injuries, although in McMahon's study, the only major biliary injury occurred in the laparoscopic group. Quality-of-life data were obtained by both Barkun[25] and McMahon.[26] The laparoscopic group experienced a faster improvement in quality of life, but the two treatment groups were equal in this respect at 3 months. Similarly, there was better satisfaction with scarring in the laparoscopic group, but both groups were equally satisfied with their result at 3 months. The data from Majeed[28] revealed no difference in time off work or time to return to full activity. A cost-minimization economic analysis was performed by McMahon.[26] Laparoscopic cholecystectomy was more costly after considering both perioperative and hospitalization costs (£1486 compared to £1090, $P<0.001$).

Further data comparing laparoscopic to open cholecystectomy are available from Shea *et al* in a large analysis of 78 747 patients undergoing laparoscopic cholecystectomy and

Table 15.1 Randomized, controlled trials of laparoscopic cholecystectomy (LC) and mini-cholecystectomy (MC)

		Study (reference number)		
		Barkun *et al* (25)	McMahon *et al* (26)	McGinn *et al* (27)
Number of patients	LC	37	151	155
	MC	25	148	155
Operative time (min)	LC	85.9	57*	74*
	MC	73.1	71*	50*
Conversion to standard open cholecystectomy	LC	1 (3%)	15 (10%)	20 (13%)
	MC	0 (0%)	14 (10%)	6 (4%)
Time to oral intake	LC	1.1 days*	N/A	N/A
	MC	1.7 days*	N/A	N/A
Hospital stay (days)	LC	3*	2*	2[a]
	MC	4*	4*	3[a]
Non-biliary complications	LC	1 (3%)	30 (20%)[b]	12 (7.7%)*
	MC	1 (4%)	26 (17%)[b]	2 (1.3%)*
Biliary complications	LC	0 (0%)	5 (3%)[c]	1 (0.6%)
	MC	1 (4%)	3 (2%)[c]	2 (1.3%)
Mortality	LC	0 (0%)	0 (0%)	1 (0.6%)
	MC	0 (0%)	1 (0.7%)	0 (0%)

N/A, data not available.
*Indicates difference reached statistical significance.
[a]This was statistically significant but did not include patients who were converted to standard cholecystectomy. If included, there was no statistical difference in length of hospital stay.
[b]Total complications.
[c]This included 1 (0.7%) major biliary injury in the LC group and no major biliary injuries in the MC group.

R
Grade B

12 973 patients undergoing open cholecystectomy.[29] Mortality rates were lower for laparoscopic cholecystectomy than for open cholecystectomy, while common bile duct injury was higher for laparoscopic cholecystectomy than for open cholecystectomy. The data for common duct injury were re-analyzed by group-level logistic regressions to identify the differences in rates among the studies. A pattern of infrequent common duct injury in early studies, an increased incidence in studies initiated in early 1990, followed by a subsequent decrease in rate was revealed. However, the data were quite variable in terms of reporting of results and length of follow-up. The authors conceded that "there still are some considerable uncertainties that need to be addressed by better-designed studies and more complete reporting".

Considering the current evidence, in the elective setting, laparoscopic cholecystectomy appears to be as safe as open cholecystectomy and provides a short term improvement in quality of life. There is a lack of convincing evidence of its touted beneficial effect on length of stay or recovery time (and thus possibly economic benefit) from the randomized trials. The potential for more hazardous injuries to the common bile duct may have been related to a learning curve, but longer term studies will be needed to answer this critical question definitively.

Acute cholecystitis

Acute cholecystitis, inflammation secondary to obstruction of the cystic duct, is the most common complication of cholelithiasis. There is little disagreement that treatment of acute cholecystitis should involve cholecystectomy. The areas of controversy are the timing of cholecystectomy and the use of laparoscopic versus open cholecystectomy.

In the prelaparoscopic era, the question of early versus delayed cholecystectomy was heavily debated. Evidence from five randomized trials performed in the 1970s to 1980s is available.[30–34] The results are summarized in Table 15.2. The studies demonstrated that cholecystectomy could be carried out at the acute stage with shorter hospital stay, decreased mortality, and fewer operative complications. However, with the introduction of laparoscopic cholecystectomy and increased concern about bile duct injury, there was a movement to return to delayed cholecystectomy for acute cholecystitis. Two randomized controlled trials studying early versus delayed laparoscopic cholecystectomy have been carried out[35,36] (Table 15.3). Once again, the data show that early cholecystectomy, even if carried out with the laparoscopic approach, is safe and better for patients in terms of shorter illness and hospital stay compared to delayed surgery. Laparoscopic cholecystectomy appears to be at least as safe as open cholecystectomy when the results of Tables 15.2 and 15.3 are analyzed. However, two further randomized trials have been published which compared laparoscopic versus open cholecystectomy for acute cholecystitis.[37,38] Grade A Those results are summarized in Table 15.4. The laparoscopic approach did not increase

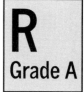

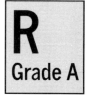

R
Grade A

R
Grade A

Table 15.2 Controlled, prospective trials comparing early versus delayed open cholecystectomy for acute cholecystitis

		Study (reference number)			
		McArthur *et al* (30)	Lahtinen *et al* (31)[a]	van der Linden *et al* (32)[a]	Jarvinen *et al* (33)[a]
Number of patients	Early	15	47	70	80
	Delayed	13	44	58	75
Operative time (min)	Early	N/A	76.7	N/A[b]	93
	Delayed	N/A	98.0	N/A[b]	85
Hospital stay (days)	Early	13.1	13.0	10.1	10.7
	Delayed	24.2	25.0	10.9 + 8[c]	18.2
Biliary complications	Early	1 (6.7%)	1 (2.1%)	0	3 (3.8%)
	Delayed	0	3 (6.8%)	0	2 (2.7%)
Non-biliary complications	Early	3 (20%)	12 (25.5%)	10 (14.3%)	11 (13.8%)
	Delayed	5 (38.4%)	16 (36.4%)	2 (3.4%)	13 (17.3%)
Mortality	Early	0	0	0	0
	Delayed	0	4 (9.1%)	0	1 (1.3%)
Failure of delayed treatment[d]		3 (23.1%)	7 (15.9%)	0	10 (13.3%)

N/A, data not available.
[a]Also showed decreased insurance payments (for time off work) for the patients treated with early cholecystectomy.
[b]No average or mean time for surgery was given but the distributions of operative times were similar.
[c]The mean stay for initial conservative management was 10.9 days followed by a mean stay of 8.0 days at the time of the delayed cholecystectomy.
[d]Patients randomized to conservative treatment initially who failed and required urgent cholecystectomy.

Table 15.3 Randomized prospective controlled trials comparing early versus delayed laparoscopic cholecystectomy for acute cholecystitis

		Study (reference number)	
		Lo *et al* (35)	Lai *et al* (36)
Number of patients	Early	45	53
	Delayed	41	51
Operative time (min)	Early	135	122.8
	Delayed	105	106.6
Conversion	Early	5 (11%)	(21%)
	Delayed	9 (23%)	(24%)
Hospital stay (days)	Early	6	7.6
	Delayed	11	11.6
Biliary complications	Early	1 (2.2%)	
	Delayed	3 (7.3%)	
Non-biliary complications	Early	5	(11.1%)
	Delayed	9 (22.0%)	
Mortality	Early	0	
	Delayed	0	
Failure of delayed treatment[a]		8 (19.5%)	

[a]Patients randomized to conservative treatment initially who failed and required urgent cholecystectomy.

Table 15.4 Randomized, prospective, controlled trials comparing open (OC) versus laparoscopic (LC) cholecystectomy for acute cholecystitis

		Study (reference number)	
		Kiviluoto *et al* (37)	Lujan *et al* (38)
Number of patients	OC	31	110
	LC	32	114
Operative time (min)	OC	99.8	77
	LC	108.2	88
Conversion	LC (only)	5 (16%)	17 (15%)
Hospital stay (days)	OC	6	8.1
	LC	4	3.3
Biliary complications	OC	0	1 (0.9%)
	LC	0	4 (3.5%)[a]
Non-biliary complications	OC	7 (minor) (23%) 6 (major) (19%)	28 (25.5%)
	LC	1 (minor) (3%)	14 (12.3%)
Mortality	OC	0	0
	LC	0	0

[a]2 out of 4 were retained CBD stones.

mortality or morbidity compared to the open approach and offered the benefit of shorter hospital stay. Both studies found that the rate of conversion to the open procedure was slightly higher than the average observed in elective cholecystectomy series.

Considering the current evidence, acute cholecystitis should be treated with early laparoscopic cholecystectomy with a reasonable threshold for conversion to open surgery. Grade A

GALLSTONE PANCREATITIS

Early ERCP

Three randomized controlled trials have studied early endoscopic retrograde cholangiopancreatography (ERCP) with stone extraction as a therapy for biliary pancreatitis.[39–41] In patients with severe pancreatitis or with evidence of biliary obstruction or cholangitis, early ERCP within 72 hours of presentation probably decreases morbidity and mortality rates. In patients without these criteria, early ERCP has no benefit and may increase morbidity and mortality. See Chapter 16 for further discussion.

R
Grade A

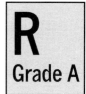

Preoperative ERCP or cholecystectomy with cholangiogram?

Gallstone pancreatitis is considered an indication for imaging of the biliary tree with either ERCP or intraoperative cholangiogram (IOC). Because of the possibility of common bile duct stones, no studies have evaluated cholecystectomy without imaging of the biliary tree. Seven case series, two with controls, have assessed the optimal approach to imaging the biliary tree following an attack of gallstone pancreatitis.[42–48] Gallstone pancreatitis does not appear to be a strong predictor of common bile duct stones without evidence of a dilated common bile duct, persistently abnormal alkaline phosphatase or bilirubin, or evidence of cholangitis. Patients with these features may be considered for preoperative ERCP and others should undergo IOC. In one retrospective study,[42] the incidence of procedure-induced pancreatitis was 19% in the ERCP group and 6% in the surgical/IOC group. The other retrospective study demonstrated similar results with pancreatic-biliary complications in 24% of the ERCP group and 6% in the surgical/IOC group.[48] These data suggest that preoperative ERCP may in fact increase overall morbidity over cholecystectomy with IOC, further supporting the approach of performing ERCP only selectively in this group of patients.

R
Grade B

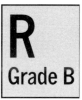

R
Grade B

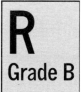

Timing of surgery

A number of studies have evaluated early versus delayed cholecystectomy in patients with gallstone pancreatitis. Burch *et al*[49] evaluated patients who underwent surgery after recovering from the acute pancreatitis either during the same hospital admission or following discharge and scheduling for elective surgery. Although surgical complication rates were the same in both groups, total hospital stay was significantly longer in the delayed group (14 vs 17 days, $P = 0.01$). Furthermore, in the delayed group only 60% returned for surgery and 29% of the original cohort required emergency treatment for recurrent pancreatitis or biliary disease prior to elective surgery. Kelly *et al*[50] randomized patients to early (less than 48 hours) and delayed (more than 48 hours) surgery. With

R
Grade B

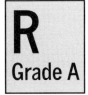

R Grade A

early surgery, the morbidity and mortality rates were 30.1% and 15.1%, as compared with 5.1% and 2.4% in the delayed group ($P<0.005$). When patients were stratified for disease severity based on Ranson's criteria, the differences in morbidity and mortality rates between early and delayed surgery were not statistically significant in patients with three or fewer Ranson's criteria. In patients with severe pancreatitis (more than three Ranson's criteria), the differences remained significant.

Based on these data, it is recommended that patients with acute gallstone pancreatitis undergo cholecystectomy following resolution of the acute episode but during the initial hospital stay. Grade A/C

CHOLEDOCHOLITHIASIS

There are three approaches to the management of common bile duct stones (CBDS): open common bile duct exploration (OCBDE), ERCP and sphincterotomy (ERCP), and laparoscopic common bile duct exploration (LCBDE). There is evidence to support the approach of LCBDE over preoperative ERCP in patients with known or suspected CBDS. In centers where LCBDE is unavailable OCBDE appears to be superior to ERCP, although the data are somewhat conflicting.

R Grade A

Five randomized trials have compared OCBDE with ERCP in the management of CBDS.[51–55] In the two smaller studies,[52,53] with 52 and 34 patients respectively, no differences in morbidity or mortality were seen. OCBDE was more successful at clearing stones than ERCP in one study[48] (88% vs 65%). The two larger studies, with 228 and 120 patients respectively,[51,54] demonstrated statistically significant increases in morbidity with ERCP, with the latter study also showing an increase in mortality with ERCP. The fifth study[55] (83 patients) also demonstrated a trend to increased morbidity with ERCP, but the difference was not statistically significant.

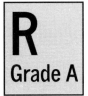

R Grade A

Two randomized trials have compared LCBDE with ERCP[56,57] and showed no difference in morbidity and mortality between the two approaches. One study[56] demonstrated a statistically significant decrease in hospital stay for LCBDE (1 day vs 3.5 days), and the other[57] demonstrated a similar trend that was not statistically significant.

It should be noted that the rates of complications with ERCP in these studies are relatively high (11–28%). In a recent series of 2347 ERCP,[58] the rate of complications in patients who underwent the procedure for removal of CBDS was 4.9%.

R Grade A/C

LCBDE and ERCP are highly operator dependent techniques with a steep learning curve. The approach to CBD stones should be individualized and based on the type of expertise available.

REFERENCES

1 Gracie WA, Ransohoff DF. The natural history of silent gallstones: the innocent gallstone is not a myth. *N Engl J Med* 1982; **307**(13): 798–800.

2 McSherry CK, Ferstenberg H, Calhoun WF *et al.* The natural history of diagnosed gallstone disease in symptomatic and asymptomatic patients. *Ann Surg* 1985; **202**(1): 59–63.

3 Friedman GD, Raviola CA, Fireman B. Prognosis of gallstones with mild or no symptoms: 25 years of follow-up in a health maintenance organization. *J Clin Epidemiol* 1989; **42**(2): 127–36.

4 Ransohoff DF, Gracie WA. Treatment of gallstones. *Ann Intern Med* 1993; **119**(7): 606–19.

5 Friedman GD. Natural history of asymptomatic and symptomatic gallstones. *Am J Surg* 1993; **165**(4): 399–404.

6 Attili AF, De Santis A, Capri R *et al.* The natural history of gallstones: the GREPCO experience. The GREPCO Group. *Hepatology* 1995; **21**(3): 655–60.

7 Ransohoff DF, Gracie WA, Wolfenson LB *et al.* Prophylactic cholecystectomy or expectant

management for silent gallstone? A decision analysis to assess survival. *Ann Intern Med* 1983; **99**(2): 199–204.
8 Gibney EJ. Asymptomatic gallstones. *Br J Surg* 1990; 77(4): 368–72.
9 Lieber MM. The incidence of gallstones and their correlation with other diseases. *Ann Surg* 1952; **135**: 394–405.
10 Ikard RW. Gallstones, cholecystitis and diabetes. *Surg Gynecol Obstet* 1990; **171**(6): 528–32.
11 Chapman BA, Wilson IR, Frampton CM *et al.* Prevalence of gallbladder disease in diabetes mellitus. *Dig Dis Sci* 1996; **41**(11): 2222–8.
12 Del Favero G, Meggiato CA, Volpi A *et al.* Natural history of gallstones in non-insulin dependent diabetes mellitus. A prospective 5-year follow-up. *Dig Dis Sci* 1994; **39**(8): 1704–7.
13 Hickman MS, Schwesinger WH, Page CP. Acute cholecystitis in the diabetic. A case-control study of outcome. *Arch Surg* 1988; **123**(4): 409–11.
14 Cubertafond P, Gainant A, Cucchiaro G. Surgical treatment of 724 carcinomas of the gall-bladder. Results of the French Surgical Association Survey. *Ann Surg* 1994; **219**(3): 275–80.
15 Maringhini A, Moreau JA, Melton LJ *et al.* Gallstones, gallbladder cancer and other gastrointestinal malignancies: an epidemiologic study in Rochester, Minnesota. *Ann Intern Med* 1987; **107**(1): 30–5.
16 Lowenfels AB, Lindstron CG, Conway MJ *et al.* Gallstones and risk of gallbladder cancer. *J Natl Cancer Inst* 1985; **75**(1): 77–80.
17 Diehl AK. Gallstone size and the risk of gallbladder cancer. *JAMA* 1983; **250**(17): 2323–6
18 Lowenfels AB, Walker AM, Althaus DP *et al.* Gallstone growth, size, and risk of gallbladder cancer: an interracial study. *Int J Epidemiol* 1989; **18**(1): 50–4.
19 Gibney EJ. Asymptomatic gallstones. *Br J Surg* 1990; **77**(4): 368–72.
20 Thistle JL, Cleary PA, Lachin JM *et al.* The natural history of cholelithiasis: the National Cooperative Gallstone Study. *Ann Intern Med* 1984; **101**(2): 171–5.
21 Way LW. The National Cooperative Gallstone Study and chenodiol. *Gastroenterology* 1983; **84**(3): 648–51.
22 Wetter LA, Way LW. Surgical therapy of gallstone disease. *Gastroenterol Clin North Am* 1991; **20**(1): 157–69.
23 Windsor JA, Pong J. Laparoscopic biliary injury: more than a learning curve problem. *Aust NZ J Surg* 1998; **68**(3): 186–9.
24 Steinle EW, VanderMolen RL, Silbergleit A *et al.* Impact of laparoscopic cholecystectomy on indications for surgical treatment of gallstones. *Surg Endosc* 1997; **11**: 933–5.
25 Barkun JS, Barkun AN, Sampalis JS *et al.* Randomised controlled trial of laparoscopic versus mini cholecystectomy. *Lancet* 1992; **340**(8828): 1116–19.
26 McMahon AJ, Russell IT, Baxter JN *et al.* Laparoscopic versus minilaparotomy cholecystectomy: a randomised trial. *Lancet* 1994; **343**(8890): 135–8
27 McGinn FP, Miles AJ, Ulgalow M *et al.* Randomized trial of laparoscopic cholecystectomy and mini-cholecystectomy. *Br J Surg* 1995; **82**(10): 1347–77.
28 Majeed AW, Troy G, Nicholl JP *et al.* Randomised, prospective, single blind comparison of laparoscopic versus small incision cholecystectomy. *Lancet* 1996; **347**(9007): 989–94.
29 Shea JA, Healey MJ, Berlin JA *et al.* Mortality and complications associated with laparoscopic cholecystectomy. A meta-analysis. *Ann Surg* 1996; **224**(5): 690–720.
30 McArthur P, Cuschieri A, Sells RA *et al.* Controlled clinical trial comparing early with interval cholecystectomy for acute cholecystitis. *Br J Surg* 1975; **62**(10): 850–2.
31 Lahtinen J, Alhava EM, Aukee S. Acute cholecystitis treated by early and delayed surgery. A controlled clinical trial. *Scand J Gastroenterol* 1978; **13**(6): 673–8.
32 van der Linden W, Sunzel H. Early versus delayed operation for acute cholecystitis. A controlled clinical trial. *Am J Surg* 1970; **120**(1): 7–13.
33 Jarvinen HJ, Hastbacka J. Early cholecystectomy for acute cholecystitis: a prospective randomized study. *Ann Surg* 1980; **191**(4): 501–5.
34 Norrby S, Herlin P, Holmin T *et al.* Early or delayed cholecystectomy in acute cholecystitis? A clinical trial. *Br J Surg* 1983; **70**(3): 163–5.
35 Lo CM, Liu CL, Fan ST *et al.* Prospective randomized study of early versus delayed laparoscopic cholecystectomy for acute cholecystitis. *Ann Surg* 1998; **227**(4): 461–7.
36 Lai PB, Kwong KH, Leung KL *et al.* Randomized trial of early versus delayed laparoscopic cholecystectomy for acute cholecystitis. *Br J Surg* 1998; **85**(6): 764–7.
37 Kiviluoto T, Siren J, Luukkonen P *et al.* Randomised trial of laparoscopic versus open cholecystectomy for acute and gangrenous cholecystitis. *Lancet* 1998; **351**(9099): 321–5.
38 Lujan JA, Parrilla P, Robles R *et al.* Laparoscopic cholecystectomy vs open cholecystectomy in the treatment of acute cholecystitis: a prospective study. *Arch Surg* 1998; **133**(2): 173–5.
39 Neoptolemos JP, Carr-Locke DL, London NJ *et al.* Controlled trial of urgent endoscopic retrograde cholangiopancreatography and endoscopic sphincterotomy versus conservative treatment for acute pancreatitis due to gallstones. *Lancet* 1988; **2**(8618): 979–83.

40 Fan ST, Lai EC, Mok FP *et al.* Early treatment of acute biliary pancreatitis by endoscopic papillotomy. *N Engl J Med* 1993; **328**(4): 228–32.
41 Folsch UR, Nitsche R, Ludtke R *et al.* Early ERCP and papillotomy compared with conservative treatment for acute biliary pancreatitis. The German Study Group on Acute Biliary Pancreatitis. *N Engl J Med* 1997; **336**(4): 237–42.
42 Sees DW, Martin RR. Comparison of preoperative endoscopic retrograde cholangiopancreatography and laparoscopic cholecystectomy with operative management of gallstone pancreatitis. *Am J Surg* 1997; **174**(6): 719–22.
43 Lin G, Halevy A, Girtler O *et al.* The role of endoscopic retrograde cholangiopancreatography in management of patients recovering from acute biliary pancreatitis in the laparoscopic era. *Surg Endosc* 1997; **11**(4): 371–5.
44 Robertson GS, Jagger C, Johnston PR *et al.* Selection criteria for preoperative endoscopic retrograde cholangiopancreatography in the laparoscopic era. *Arch Surg* 1996; **131**(1): 89–94.
45 Scapa E. To do or not to do an endoscopic retrograde cholangiopancreatography in acute biliary panceatitis? *Surg Laparosc Endosc* 1995; **5**(6): 453–4.
46 De Virgilio C, Verbin C, Chang L *et al.* Gallstone pancreatitits. The role of preoperative endoscopic retrograde cholangiopancreatography. *Arch Surg* 1994; **129**(9): 909–13.
47 Leitman IM, Fisher ML, McKinley MJ *et al.* The evaluation and management of known or suspected stones of the common bile duct in the era of minimal access surgery. *Surg Gynecol Obstet* 1993; **176**(6): 527–33.
48 Srinathan SK, Barkun JS, Mehta SN *et al.* Evolving management of mild-to-moderate gallstone pancreatitis. *J Gastrointestinal Surg* 1998; **2**(4): 385–90.
49 Burch JM, Feliciano DV, Mattox KL *et al.* Gallstone pancreatitis: the question of time. *Arch Surg* 1990; **125**(7): 853–9.
50 Kelly TR, Wagner DS. Gallstone pancreatitis: a prospective randomized trial of the timing of surgery. *Surgery* 1988; **104**(4): 600–5.
51 Neoptolemos JP, Carr-Locke DL, Fossard DP. Prospective randomised study of preoperative endoscopic sphincterotomy versus surgery alone for common bile duct stones. *Br Med J (Clin Res Ed)* 1987; **294**(6570): 470–4.
52 Stain SC, Cohen H, Tsuishoysha M *et al.* Choledocholithiasis. Endoscopic sphincterotomy or common bile duct exploration? *Ann Surg* 1991; **213**(6): 627–33.
53 Stiegmann GV, Goff JS, Mansour A *et al.* Precholecystectomy endoscopic cholangiography, and common bile duct exploration. *Am J Surg* 1992; **163**(2): 227–30.
54 Suc B, Escat J, Cherqui D *et al.* Surgery versus endoscopy as primary treatment in symptomatic patients with suspected common bile duct stones: a multi-centre randomised trial. *Arch Surg* 1998; **133**(7): 702–8.
55 Hammarstrom LE, Holmin T, Stridbeck H *et al.* Long-term follow-up of a prospective randomised study of endoscopic versus surgical treatment of bile duct calculi in patients with gallbladder in situ. *Br J Surg* 1995; **82**(11): 1516–21.
56 Rhodes M, Sussman L, Cohen L *et al.* Randomised trial of laparoscopic exploration of common bile duct versus postoperative endoscopic retrograde cholangiography for common bile duct stones. *Lancet* 1998; **351**(9097): 159–61.
57 Cuschieri A, Croce E, Faggioni A *et al.* EAES ductal stone study. Preliminary findings of multi-centre prospective randomised trial comparing two-stage vs single-stage management. *Surg Endosc* 1996; **19**(12): 1130–5.
58 Freeman M, Nelson D, Sherman S *et al.* Complications of endoscopic biliary sphincterotomy. *N Engl J Med* 1996; **335**(13): 909–18.

Acute pancreatitis: prognosis and treatment

16

JONATHON SPRINGER, HILLARY STEINHART

INTRODUCTION

Acute pancreatitis is a common admission diagnosis on gastroenterology and general surgical services. The incidence varies based on the geographical location but is reported at between 20 and 40/100 000 per year.[1,2] In 1987, it accounted for 108 000 hospitalizations (not including VA hospitals) in the United States, with 2251 deaths.[3] The term acute pancreatitis encompasses a wide spectrum of clinical and pathological findings arising from many different causes. Despite extensive research in the area, the underlying pathophysiology of acute pancreatitis still remains speculative.

Most patients with acute pancreatitis will have a mild form and ultimately follow a benign clinical course, but up to 20% will develop severe pancreatitis with all its inherent morbidity and risk of mortality. Despite the many advances in the treatment and diagnosis of acute pancreatitis, the mortality rate remains between 5 and 15%.

Unfortunately, acute pancreatitis generally has an unpredictable course and prognosis. This has prompted a search for the ideal prognostic tools (single or multiple laboratory or clinical variables) that might predict severe disease and morbid complications early in the course when potential therapeutic interventions may alter the natural history. However, the variable nature of the disease, its many different causes, and potential complications make it a difficult disease to treat and one for which a universally effective treatment is unlikely to be achievable. At the present time there is no single, simple, universally accepted prognostic instrument or treatment protocol for those with acute pancreatitis.

This chapter will critically review the evidence available from the literature that examines the use of various prognostic instruments and the medical, surgical and endoscopic treatment options available for acute pancreatitis.

A review of the literature was conducted by performing a computerized search of the Medline database for the years 1974 to 1998. The search included all English language articles indexed under the MeSH heading "pancreatitis" and the text words "acute pancreatitis". Review articles and articles of special interest in the area were reviewed and their bibliographies were searched for additional references. The articles dealing with prognosis or treatment of acute pancreatitis were then critically reviewed but a formal meta-analysis was not conducted.

PROGNOSIS

Some patients with acute pancreatitis may go on to develop life-threatening complications while others will have a brief illness and recover uneventfully. It is important to be able to accurately identify which patients are at greater risk for potential complications, including death, if an efficient and effective use of resources is to be achieved. Most studies have suggested that a basic clinical assessment at the time of admission is quite poor for identifying these patients.[4–6] Corfield *et al* found in their prospective study of 418 patients that 60% who went on to develop severe pancreatitis were not predicted to do so by a basic clinical assessment at the time of admission.[5] With this knowledge in mind, various methods have been used in an attempt to predict the severity of acute pancreatitis. This has included the use of multiple clinical scoring systems, individual laboratory tests, invasive procedures (paracentesis), and imaging techniques (CT scanning). However, none of these prognostic tools is both highly sensitive and specific and therefore all have limited application for the individual patient. We will review some of the variables that have been investigated more extensively and shown some promise.

Multiple variable scoring systems

Ranson's criteria, the Glasgow score, and the APACHE-II score are three common clinical scoring systems used to predict the severity of acute pancreatitis. Ranson's criteria is the most widely used clinical scoring system for the prediction of severity (Table 16.1). Ranson's initial study was retrospective, looked at 43 variables in 100 patients and identified 11 variables with prognostic capabilities.[7] The presence of three or more clinical signs predicted a significant risk of death or severe illness. These findings were weakened by the retrospective nature of the study and the disproportionately large number of variables studied for the sample size. However, Ranson's criteria were subsequently validated by several large studies[4,6,8–14] (Table 16.2). Drawbacks associated with the use of Ranson's criteria include the 48-hour observation period required for a prediction to be made, the maximum "one-time" assessment and its original derivation from a population of patients with mostly alcoholic pancreatitis. It is also cumbersome to remember all the

Table 16.1 Ranson criteria

	Non-gallstone pancreatitis	Gallstone pancreatitis
On admission		
Age (yr)	>55	>70
WBC (/mm^3)	>16 000	>18 000
Glucose (mmol/l)	11.1	12.2
LDH (IU/l)	>200	>400
AST (IU/l)	>350	>250
Within 48 h		
Hct decreases (%)	>10	>10
BUN increases (mg/dl)	>5	>2
Calcium (mmol/l)	<2.0	<2.0
Po_2 (mmHg)	<60	—
Base deficit (mmol/l)	>4	>5
Fluid (litres)(I–O)	>6	>4

Table 16.2 Ranson criteria prognostic ability

Study	Sample size	Endpoint	Sensitivity	Specificity	Criticisms
Ranson[7]	100	D/ICU stay >7 days	46%	99%	See text
Ranson[8] subjective	200	D/ICU stay >7 days	96%	92%	Endpoint
Larvin[6]	290	OF/PC	75%	68%	
McMahon[4]	79	14 day hospitalization OF/PC	82%	79%	
Wilson[9]	160	OF/PC/D	87%	71%	
Gross[10]	75	D/comp. >2	Ppv 80%	Npv 68%	
Dominguez-Munoz[11]	182	D/OF/PC	77%	70%	
Agarawal[12] Retrospective,	76	OF/PC	40%	90%	
					Ranson >2
Banks[13]	75		74%	71%	
Wilson[14]	72		88%	79%	

D, death; PC, pancreatic collection; OF, organ failure; comp., complication; Ppv, positive predictive value; Npv, negative predictive value.

Table 16.3 APACHE-II prognostic ability

Study	Sample size	Endpoint	Sensitivity	Specificity	Criticisms
Larvin[6] (score >9)	290	OF/PC	63% (0 h) 75% (48 h)	81% (0 h) 92%(48 h)	Variable dependent on endpoint
Wilson[9]	160	PC/OF/D	95% (>5) 82% (>9)	54% (>5) 74% (>9)	

D, death; PC, pancreatic collection; OF, organ failure.

criteria and often some of the laboratory tests required to establish the score are not done routinely.

The Glasgow criteria were created because of the concern that Ranson's criteria were formulated on a population of mostly alcoholic pancreatitis and, as a result, might not hold the same prognostic value in other populations.[15] The Glasgow criteria have subsequently been modified on several occasions but the comparative studies have shown no added benefit for one scoring system over another. The Glasgow criteria have nine clinical variables but still require 48 hours of observation and do not allow for continuous monitoring. The sensitivity and specificity are comparable to Ranson's criteria and have been reported as 55–85% and 75–90% respectively.[4–6,9,11,14,16]

More recently, the APACHE-II scoring system has been used as a prognostic index in acute pancreatitis because of the perceived limitations of the Glasgow and Ranson scoring systems. Unlike the other scoring systems, it allows early assessment of prognosis and continuous monitoring and reassessment. Comparative studies have shown that an APACHE-II score >5 or a peak score >9 provides operating characteristics similar to or slightly better than the other multiple variable scoring systems.[6,9] The operating characteristics for the APACHE-II score are shown in Table 16.3.

There are several problems with the studies that have examined the use of scoring systems as a prognostic tool in acute pancreatitis. The retrospective nature of some studies or the lack of consecutive accrual of study patients in prospective trials may lead to selection bias but likely does not impact the results significantly. However, the lack of complete data in some studies makes interpretation of the results very difficult. Finally, the differences in the definition of severe pancreatitis make comparison between trials questionable. The definition of severe pancreatitis as major organ failure biases the prognostic ability of an APACHE-II score and inflates its accuracy, because the calculation of the score is directly dependent on inclusion of at least part of the endpoint. Overall, these scoring systems are helpful but only provide a slight improvement from a basic clinical assessment performed at 48 hours. In general, they do not adequately identify patients at risk of severe pancreatitis (low positive predictive value) but can identify those patients who experience only mild pancreatitis (high negative predictive value).[17]

More recently, the Hong Kong criteria were formulated in an attempt to simplify the previous prognostic scoring systems. Fan *et al* have shown that a urea level above 7.4 mmol/l and a blood glucose level above 11.0 mmol/l predicted severity of disease with a sensitivity of 79% and a specificity of 67%.[18] However, their results were not reproduced by Heath *et al*, who compared the Hong Kong criteria to the Glasgow criteria in 125 European patients and found a sensitivity of only 33% and a specificity of 86%, much lower than the operating characteristics for the Glasgow criteria.[19] This discrepancy may be explained by differences in study populations but this characteristic limits its general application.

Computed tomography

The limited usefulness of the scoring systems and the cumbersome nature of calculating them has stimulated further investigation into other potential tools. Contrast enhanced CT scanning has been investigated extensively because of its ability to identify local complications (pseudocyst, abscess, phlegmon, peripancreatic fluid) and necrotizing pancreatitis, both of which are thought to lead to increased morbidity and mortality.[20–26]

Table 16.4 CT scan prognostic ability

Study	Sample size	Endpoint	Sensitivity	Specificity	Criticisms
Balthazar[20] Grade D+E	83	PC/D	89%	71%	
Balthazar[21] Grade D+E	88	PC/D	90%	73%	
Hjelmqvist[22]	47	PC/14 day hospitalization	71%	80%	
London[23]	32	D/PC/20 day hospitalization	83%	65%	Selection bias, criteria
London[24]	126	D/PC	71%	77%	
Clavian[25]	176	D/PC	66%	97%	
Poulakkainen[26]	88		66%	100%	

D, death; PC, pancreatic collection; OF, organ failure.

Table 16.5 Peritoneal tap prognostic ability

Study	Sample size	Endpoint	Sensitivity	Specificity	Criticisms
McMahon[4] (10 ml)	79	14 day hospitalization/ PC/OF/D	72%	95%	Selection bias, 68 patients excluded for mild disease
Corfield[5]	253		53%		155 n.a.
Mayer[27]	231		60%	87%	

PC, pancreatic collection; OF, organ failure; D, death; n.a., not assessed.

The sensitivity and specificity of CT findings for the prediction of severe pancreatitis from several prospective studies is shown in Table 16.4. Although the presence of necrosis did correlate with a more complicated course, the extent of necrosis did not provide any additional prognostic value. Unfortunately, comparison between studies is problematical because of the lack of a standardized CT staging system, variations in the definitions of clinical disease severity, dissimilar inclusion criteria, and the timing of the CT scan. However, based on the evidence available, contrast enhanced CT scans which can detect pancreatic necrosis and local complications, can serve a valuable role in the management of these patients but the exact timing of the scan remains controversial. It is probably best utilized between 48 and 96 hours after onset of the symptoms in patients without improvement.

Paracentesis

The color and volume of peritoneal fluid obtained by means of percutaneous drainage from a patient shortly after diagnosis have been shown to predict the severity of pancreatitis to the same extent as non-invasive techniques but also provide information on possible alternative diagnoses (eg bowel perforation).[1,4,5,27] However, the procedure is invasive and carries a 0.8% risk of complications.[1] The operating characteristics of a paracentesis for prognosis in acute pancreatitis are shown in Table 16.5. The application of the results of these studies and their interpretation are hindered by the selection criteria used for inclusion. Patients selected for the procedure tended to be those with more severe disease because of the invasive nature of the procedure. Thus, a broad spectrum of disease severity and presentations were not assessed.

Individual laboratory tests

In an attempt to simplify the prognostic indices and provide a non-invasive early assessment of disease severity, many studies have examined individual laboratory tests. Only tests that have been studied extensively or shown some promise in this area will be reviewed below.

C-reactive protein is an acute phase reactant that rises in many inflammatory conditions, including acute pancreatitis. Several studies have measured C-reactive protein in acute pancreatitis and found a correlation between the height of C-reactive protein and

Table 16.9 Gabexate clinical trials

Study	Study design/intervention	Patients (no.)	Conclusion
Yang[64]	RCT gabexate vs placebo	42	No benefit
Valderrama[65]	Multicenter RCT gabexate vs placebo	100	No benefit
Pederzoli[66]	RCT gabexate vs aprotinin	182	Reduction in systemic complications
Buchler[67]	Multicenter RCT/gabexate vs placebo	223	No benefit

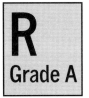

R Grade A

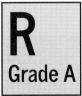

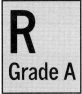

(>150 patients) found no reduction in morbidity or mortality. An earlier study had suggested a reduction in mortality, particularly in the elderly, but these results have not been reproduced.[63]

R Grade A

Gabexate mesylate, a potent lower molecular weight protease inhibitor thought to enter pancreatic acinar cells and inhibit intracellular proteases, has been studied in several RCTs (Table 16.9).[64–67] Despite initiation of treatment early in the course (within 12 hours of symptoms in one study[65]), a reduction in morbidity or mortality was not seen. One study,[66] which compared gabexate with aprotinin in patients with severe pancreatitis (at least two Ranson criteria), found a reduction in systemic and total complications in those treated with gabexate. However, the study lacked a placebo arm and the treatment groups differed in some important baseline characteristics such as the proportion with necrotizing pancreatitis.

R Grade A

The use of fresh frozen plasma (FFP) to replenish the levels of naturally occurring antiproteases has also been examined. Leese *et al* conducted a RCT on 202 patients and found no difference in mortality or morbidity between those who received FFP and those who received colloid.[68]

Anti-inflammatory therapy

R Grade A

More recently, as our knowledge of the pathophysiology of acute pancreatitis has evolved, the focus of treatment has changed. Platelet activating factor (PAF), a proinflammatory lipid mediator released by macrophages, neutrophils, and endothelial cells, plays a significant role in acute inflammation. There have been two RCTs which have examined the use of lexipafant, a platelet activating factor (PAF) antagonist, in the treatment of acute pancreatitis.[69,70] Both studies, despite their small size (<100 patients), found a significant reduction in organ failure scores. This was seen in all patients irrespective of the severity of pancreatitis. The studies were not designed to detect a change in mortality or local complications but a trend toward lower mortality was seen in one of the studies.[70] Although there is insufficient evidence presently available to advocate the use of PAF inhibitors, the results to date are encouraging and should lead to further research. If these agents are to have any role it will likely be in reducing the risk of early systemic complications in those patients predicted to have severe disease.

Antibiotics

The close association between infection and increased morbidity and mortality in severe pancreatitis (particularly necrotizing pancreatitis) has led to studies of the use of antibiotic prophylaxis. Initial studies in the early 1970s were disappointing and the concept was dropped until recently. On further review, it was recognized that these early studies were not designed in a manner that could adequately address the effect of antibiotic prophylaxis. The three randomized trials had small sample sizes and all compared ampicillin with placebo.[71–73] The mortality in the control groups was zero, indicating that the study population had mild disease with a negligible risk of pancreatic infection. Given that the incidence of infection in the control groups was only 7%, it would have been virtually impossible to achieve a clinically or statistically significant result with the sample sizes studied. In addition, the choice of antibiotic has now been recognized as inappropriate, because ampicillin is not effective against many of the organisms commonly seen in pancreatic infection and as it has poor penetration into pancreatic tissue.

With this in mind, three further randomized studies have been conducted. Pederzoli and colleagues randomized 74 patients with necrotizing pancreatitis to receive a 14-day course of imipenem, a broad-spectrum antibiotic with good pancreatic penetration, or placebo within 72 hours of onset.[74] All pancreatic infections were confirmed microbiologically by tissue culture from aspiration or surgical debridement. The unblinded study found that the incidence of both pancreatic sepsis (30% vs 12%, $P<0.01$) and non-pancreatic sepsis (49% vs 15%, $P<0.01$) were decreased in patients on imipenem. However, there were no differences in the number of operations for pancreatic sepsis (33% vs 29%), the incidence of organ failure (39% vs 29%), or death (12% vs 7%).

R
Grade A

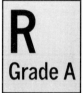

Sainio and colleagues conducted a similar randomized study in Finland comparing cefuroxime (4.5 g/day for 14 days) versus placebo in 60 patients with alcohol-induced necrotizing pancreatitis.[75] The mean Ranson score was 5.5 and the degree of pancreatic necrosis was over 30% in 80% of the patients. The total number of infectious complications was higher in the placebo group (54 vs 30, $P<0.01$) but this was largely due to a higher rate of urinary tract infections (17 vs 6, $P = 0.0073$). The incidence of pancreatic infections was similar in the two groups (40% vs 30%). Although the overall incidence of infection was lower in the antibiotic treated group, there were no differences in length of hospital stay or need for pancreatic drainage or debridement. However, prophylaxis with cefuroxime reduced overall mortality (23% vs 3%, $P<0.03$, NNT = 5). Since three deaths in the placebo group were associated with pancreatic cultures positive for *Staphylococcus epidermidis* the authors suggest that cefuroxime may reduce severe infectious complications and prevent secondary *S. epidermidis* infections.

R
Grade A

The finding that most bacteria in pancreatic infection are enteric flora has led to the presumption that most such organisms migrate from the intestine by bacterial translocation. Luiten and colleagues[76] performed a randomized study in 102 patients with severe pancreatitis (Imrie score >2 or Balthazar grade D or E on CT scan) comparing selective bowel decontamination using topical pharyngeal (paste), rectal (enema), and oral preparations of colistin sulfate, amphotericin, and norfloxacin with placebo. The patients in the treatment arm also received cefotaxime intravenously every 8 hours until cultures of the rectum and pharynx were free of Gram-negative bacteria. The overall mortality was similar in the two groups in an intention-to-treat analysis (35% vs 22%, $P = 0.19$). When corrected for disease severity by a multivariate analysis, a modest survival benefit was evident ($P = 0.048$) owing to a reduction in late mortality (>2 weeks)

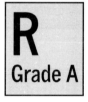

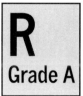

R
Grade A

R Grade A

the primary endpoint of the study was the incidence of the systemic inflammatory response syndrome, with sepsis, organ failure, hospital stay, and mortality as secondary endpoints. All the patients randomized to the enteral feeding group tolerated this form of nutritional support. The median amount of non-protein energy delivered was 5.02 MJ in the enterally fed patients and 7.52 MJ in the parenterally fed patients ($P<0.0004$). However, the nitrogen delivery was 9.24 and 9.4 g/patient per day in the two groups respectively (P = NS). Clinical outcome measures all improved in the enterally fed patients when compared with the parenterally fed patients. However, only the reduction in systemic inflammatory response syndrome (SIRS) was statistically significant, with 11 patients in the enterally fed group fulfilling the criteria prior to nutritional support but only two patients meeting the criteria after enteral nutrition ($P<0.05$). On the other hand, in the parenterally fed group, there was no significant change (12 versus 10) in the incidence of SIRS. Hospital stay and mortality were not statistically significantly different between the two groups.

R Grade A

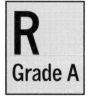

Collectively, these studies, although small, suggest that enteral nutrition is safe and at least as efficacious as parenteral nutrition in patients with mild and severe pancreatitis. As the cost is much less and there is a potential for improved clinical outcome, enteral nutrition should supplant parenteral nutrition as the standard of care for patients in whom nutritional support is indicated. However, large scale trials examining the role of enteral nutrition and different formulations for patients with severe pancreatitis are needed before more specific recommendations can be made. Certainly, it would be reasonable to attempt to provide nutritional supplementation enterally in most patients, using clinical judgement to determine whether individual patients are unable to tolerate this method.

ENDOSCOPIC RETROGRADE CHOLANGIOPANCREATOGRAPHY (ERCP)

Several studies (Table 16.10) have examined the benefit of early endoscopic intervention in patients with pancreatitis of presumed biliary origin in the belief that endoscopic sphincterotomy (ES) and removal of stones impacted in the ampulla of Vater or floating in the common bile duct will reduce subsequent morbidity and mortality.

R Grade A

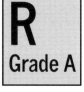

The first RCT of urgent endoscopic retrograde cholangiopancreatography (ERCP) for acute biliary pancreatitis was published in 1988 by Neoptolemos and colleagues.[101] Within 72 hours of presentation they randomized 121 patients, stratified according to disease severity, to undergo ERCP (and ES if appropriate) or to receive conventional treatment. They found a significant reduction in the complication rate, the primary outcome measure of the trial, in ERCP treated patients (ERCP 17% vs control 34%, $P = 0.03$; NNT = 6). This difference in morbidity appeared to be accounted for by a difference in the severe disease stratum (ERCP 24% vs control 61%; $P<0.01$), while no benefit from the intervention was demonstrated in the mild disease stratum. Although not statistically significant, there was a trend toward reduced mortality in the ERCP group (2% vs 8%).

In 1993, Fan and colleagues published the results of a randomized controlled trial of early ERCP in 195 patients with acute pancreatitis, approximately two-thirds of whom were eventually considered to have biliary pancreatitis. Patients were randomized within 24 hours of presentation to undergo ERCP (and ES if appropriate) or conventional therapy. Treatment of the latter group included ERCP electively after the acute attack subsided or

Table 16.10 Randomized controlled trials of early ERCP in acute pancreatitis (AP)

Study	Patients (no.)	Outcome meaures	Rate in ERCP group (%)	Rate in control group (%)	ARR (%)	NNT	*P*
Neoptolemos[101]	121	Complications					
	Presumed gallstone	Severe stratum	24	61	17	6	<0.01
	pancreatitis	All patients	17	34	37	3	0.03
		Mortality	2	8			ns
Fan[102]	195	Local and systemic					
	Acute pancreatitis	complications	18	29			0.07
		Biliary sepsis	0	13	13	8	0.001
		Mortality	5	9			ns
Folsch[10]	238	Overall mortality	11	6.2			ns
	Gallstone pancreatitis	Mortality due to					
	without biliary	pancreatitis	7.9	3.6			ns
	obstruction or	Complications	46	57			ns
	cholangitis						

selectively at an earlier time for those patients whose condition deteriorated.[102] The rate of local or systemic complications (including sepsis), the primary outcome measure of the trial, was 18% in the early ERCP group and 29% in the control group ($P = 0.07$). The mortality rates were 5% and 9% (P = NS), respectively. Subgroup analysis of the results in patients with proven gallstones also revealed that morbidity was significantly reduced in the ERCP group (16% vs 33%, $P = 0.03$) and there was a trend toward lower mortality (2% vs 8%, $P = 0.09$). Additional subgroup analysis revealed no significant difference in the local or systemic complications, but the incidence of subsequent biliary sepsis was significantly lower in the ERCP group (0% vs 13%, $P = 0.001$). The latter results should be interpreted with caution, since it appears that no corrections were applied to the statistical analysis to account for the use of multiple subgroup analyses.

R Grade A

More recently, Folsch and colleagues conducted a multicenter study in which they randomized 126 patients with biliary pancreatitis without significant biliary obstruction or cholangitis to early ERCP (within 72 hours) or conventional therapy.[103] Forty-eight per cent of the invasive group had biliary stones at ERCP. Eleven per cent in the invasive treatment group and 6% in the conservative treatment group died ($P = 0.10$). The overall rate of complications was similar in the two groups but patients in the invasive treatment group appeared to have more severe complications, particularly respiratory failure (12% vs 4%, $P = 0.03$). These results were not analyzed according to the severity of pancreatitis in the affected patients.

R Grade A

Collectively, these three studies suggest that early ERCP is generally a safe procedure in the setting of acute pancreatitis. In two of three trials the complication rate was reduced by this intervention and in the same trials there was a trend toward a reduction in mortality. In a third trial there was no significant effect on complications, although respiratory failure was more common in the early intervention group and there was a trend toward increased mortality in this group. Patients with severe biliary pancreatitis appear to be more likely to benefit from early intervention. Larger studies on patients with severe disease would be required to demonstrate a significant beneficial effect of early ERCP on mortality, if indeed one exists.

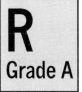

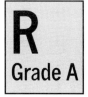

SURGICAL MANAGEMENT

Early vs delayed surgery for biliary pancreatitis

The surgical management of acute pancreatitis has evolved considerably over the past 30 years. In the 1960s and 1970s early surgical management was considered for the treatment of biliary pancreatitis to remove stones impacted in the distal common bile duct (CBD), to remove the gallbladder and stones contained within it, and to resect, debride or drain a necrotic pancreas or fluid collection. However, several uncontrolled retrospective studies[104–106] suggested that early intervention is potentially hazardous and appeared to increase mortality. The observations led to the recommendation that definitive biliary surgery should be avoided until the acute pancreatitis resolves, but performed prior to discharge from hospital.[104] Kelly and Wagner confirmed the wisdom of this approach when they conducted a randomized study in 165 patients comparing early definitive biliary surgery (within 48 hours) to delayed surgery (after the pancreatitis subsided 4–10 days later).[107] They found a significant overall reduction in morbidity and mortality in the group who underwent the delayed surgery, with most of the observed benefit derived in those patients with severe pancreatitis, as defined by having more than three Ranson criteria. In the overall population of patients with mild and severe pancreatitis the morbidity rates were 30% and 5.1% ($P<0.005$) for the early and delayed surgery groups, respectively, and the mortality rates were 15.1% and 2.4% ($P<0.005$). In patients with severe pancreatitis the morbidity rates were 82.6% and 17.6% ($P<0.001$) for those with early and delayed surgery respectively and the mortality rates were 47.8% and 11% ($P<0.025$). From these data the NNT, the number of patients needed to be treated by early surgery to cause one additional death, is approximately eight overall and approximately three for patients with severe pancreatitis. Although these data are convincing, the more widespread use of ERCP since the time that these studies were conducted has shifted this question to the possible benefits of early ERCP and has made the question of a role for early definitive biliary surgery much less relevant. The current recommendation is for cholecystectomy not to be performed until the acute pancreatitis has subsided. This is based on very strong evidence. It is also recommended that it is performed as soon as possible after the pancreatitis has subsided, although the evidence supporting this recommendation is somewhat less convincing.

R Grade A/B

Peritoneal lavage

More recently, early surgical intervention has been limited to early peritoneal lavage and the treatment of infected pancreatic necrosis or peritonitis. However, there still remains considerable controversy as to the method and timing of surgical intervention in the setting of necrotizing pancreatitis and the use of peritoneal lavage in the non-operative setting. Several small controlled studies have examined the effectiveness of continuous peritoneal lavage. Ranson and colleagues[8] randomized 10 patients with severe pancreatitis to receive continuous lavage for 48–96 hours or standard therapy. They found no statistically significant differences in the duration of ICU care, rapidity of resumption of oral intake, or duration of hospitalization, although there was a trend favoring lavage for each of these outcomes. Stone and colleagues[108] randomized 70 patients with severe alcoholic pancreatitis to 24 hours of peritoneal lavage or supportive treatment followed by 24 hours of peritoneal lavage for those who worsened. They found a "decided improvement in the overall condition" in 29 of 34 patients in the treatment group compared to 13 of 36 in the control group ($P = 0.001$). However, the method of determining this improvement was not discussed, and the mortality rate was not significantly different between the two groups. In addition, 17 of 36 patients in the control group were crossed over to peritoneal lavage after worsening in 24 hours, making interpretation of the results problematical. Subsequently, two larger randomized studies by Mayer *et al* ($n = 91$)[109] and Ihse *et al* ($n = 39$)[110] have failed to show benefit from peritoneal lavage. Teerenhovi and colleagues[111] randomized 24 patients with necrotizing pancreatitis to undergo lesser sac lavage for 7 days or drainage, following laparotomy and choledochostomy or cholecystostomy. They were unable to identify any benefit for lavage over drainage as the mortality and morbidity were similar in both groups (36% vs 17% mortality). However, neither group underwent necrosectomy, and the onset of symptoms before operation was 4.1 ± 3.6 days for the lavage group, a pretreatment interval which is much longer than previously advocated for lavage alone.

R
Grade A

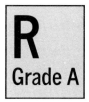

All the studies listed above examined short courses of peritoneal lavage with durations less than 4 days and may have overlooked a beneficial time/response relationship. Therefore, Ranson and colleagues[112] randomized 29 patients with severe pancreatitis to long peritoneal lavage (7 days) or short lavage (2 days). They found no statistically significant difference between the groups with respect to either pancreatic sepsis (long lavage 22% vs short lavage 40%) or death from sepsis (long lavage 0% vs short lavage 20). Grade A However, in the subgroup of patients with five or more prognostic signs, pancreatic sepsis occurred in 30% of the long lavage group vs 57% of the short lavage group and death from sepsis occurred in 0% and 43%, respectively ($P = 0.05$). Grade C These promising results must be interpreted with caution since they are the result of post hoc subgroup analysis of a rather small trial. However, they suggest that longer duration of peritoneal lavage might benefit those with the most severe forms of acute pancreatitis. Larger studies would be needed to confirm this result before peritoneal lavage can be advocated as part of the standard treatment of severe pancreatitis.

Early pancreatic resection without documented infection

The management of necrotizing pancreatitis in the absence of documented infection remains the most controversial surgical issue in acute pancreatitis. Early pancreatic resection for severe acute pancreatitis has been examined in small retrospective studies that have generally shown high mortality and morbidity.[113] Grade B Only two studies have compared resection with alternative forms of management. Kivilaakso and colleagues[114] randomized 35 patients with severe pancreatitis to subtotal pancreatic resection and T-tube placement or operative peritoneal lavage and T-tube placement for 7–12 days. Twenty-two per cent died in the resection group and 47% in the lavage group (NS). Grade A The septic complication rate and duration of hospital stay were similar, but 6/14 patients who underwent resection developed diabetes while none did in the lavage group. This study suggested that resection might benefit a select group of patients, but in addition to the lack of a statistically significant result, the study design, without a true control group in which patients were not exposed to the usual surgical risks, prevented any definite conclusions. In addition, the degree of pancreatitis in the randomized patients was not severe, with a mean number of prognostic signs of less than four. A second small study by the same group re-examined this question using an improved study design.[115] They randomized 21 patients with severe pancreatitis to non-operative peritoneal lavage or pancreatic resection. There was no statistically significant difference in mortality (27% for resection and 10% for lavage) or in morbidity or hospital stay between the groups. These studies together with the previous retrospective data suggest that early pancreatic resection offers no benefit over non-operative management for severe acute pancreatitis. Grade A/B

Management of infected pancreatic necrosis

While there is considerable controversy regarding the use of surgical management for severe acute pancreatitis without sepsis, there is no disagreement about the need for surgical intervention or drainage for infected necrosis. However, the timing and surgical method in this setting remain controversial. Three main patterns of surgical management of infected necrosis have developed over the past 20 years. They include: conventional treatment with necrosectomy followed by simple drainage of the peripancreatic bed, closed procedures with necrosectomy followed by continuous closed lavage, or open management with necrosectomy and subsequent scheduled reoperations or continued open abdominal management. The evidence for or against these treatment modalities is based on case series either followed prospectively or retrospectively but there is a paucity of randomized studies.

R Grade B

Warshaw and Gongliang[116] retrospectively reviewed their experience in 45 patients with pancreatic abscesses. Their patients had a 24% mortality with conventional treatment and 84% had further complications. Allardyce[117] performed a retrospective review and found that 14 of 17 patients with infected necrosis or abscess died with the conventional treatment. Both groups advocated a more aggressive debridement of necrotic tissue and adequate drainage.

R Grade B

Wertheimer and Norris[118] reported their results in 10 consecutive patients with persistent infected necrosis treated with necrosectomy and packing with continued open abdominal management in the intensive care unit. Their 20% mortality rate was much lower than expected for the patient population and, as a result, this approach has gained some popularity. Bradley and Allen[119] prospectively followed 27 patients with infected necrosis treated with debridement, open drainage, and scheduled reoperation. Mortality was 15% in this group, again lower than expected, but no concurrent control group was available for comparison.

Necrosectomy with continuous closed lavage has also gained favor over conventional treatment of infected necrosis. Gebhardt and Gall[120] retrospectively reviewed their surgical results for necrotizing pancreatitis and found a mortality of 37% for those treated with necrosectomy, drainage and lavage compared to 54% for those treated earlier in their experience with surgery alone without drainage or lavage. Larvin and colleagues[121] prospectively followed 14 patients with necrotizing pancreatitis who underwent pancreatic debridement, closed drainage and lavage. Their mortality rate was 3/14 with only 2 patients requiring reoperation. Bassi and colleagues[122] retrospectively reviewed their experience with surgically treated patients with acute and chronic pancreatitis and intra-abdominal sepsis. Fifty-five patients had infected necrosis and were treated with necrosectomy and closed lavage. The mortality rate in this cohort was 24% but the severity of their pancreatitis as represented by a conventional multiple scoring system was not discussed, making interpretation of the results difficult. Finally, Farkas and colleagues[123] retrospectively reviewed their results with necrosectomy and closed lavage for infected necrosis in 123 patients with severe pancreatitis (mean Ranson score = 6.2).

Their mortality rate was only 7%, with a 17% reoperation rate. However, 46% had another surgical procedure performed at the time of the necrosectomy (distal pancreatectomy, splenectomy, colonic resection, cholecystectomy, or sphincteroplasty). Nevertheless, the results of this study, albeit retrospective, suggest a benefit in widespread necrosectomy, lavage with multiple drains, and additional surgery when necessary. Collectively, these studies, although limited by their retrospective study designs and use of historical controls, suggest that the treatment of infected necrosis should involve necrosectomy and long term lavage or open management instead of the previous conventional surgical management. It is unlikely that large randomized studies of this approach will be undertaken, and as a result, recommendations are based on the relatively weak evidence which is available.

R
Grade B

CONCLUSION

Medical management continues to remain the mainstay of treatment for patients with acute pancreatitis. Further research identifying patients at risk for severe pancreatitis at an earlier stage is needed if a dramatic decrease in the mortality rate is to be achieved. Early reduction in the systemic response to pancreatitis might be achieved with pharmacotherapy, but this has not been proven to be effective with the agents available to date. Antibiotic prophylaxis is likely to become part of the standard therapy for those with necrotizing pancreatitis. While TPN is of little benefit for those with severe pancreatitis, early enteral feeding shows promise and should become the standard method of nutritional supplementation in these patients. Early ERCP for those patients with jaundice or cholangitis has proven to be beneficial when used by experienced individuals, but its role beyond that remains unclear. The role of peritoneal lavage remains controversial and the patient population who may benefit from this intervention is not well defined. Early pancreatic resection or necrosectomy with closed drainage appears to contribute to increased complications without overall benefit. As such, early surgical management of acute pancreatitis should be limited to those patients with *infected necrosis*. The surgical approach still remains controversial but, based on the evidence available, widespread necrosectomy and lavage, or necrosectomy and open management probably results in a better overall outcome than the conventional surgical approach.

REFERENCES

1 Thompson SR, Hendry WS, Mcfarlane GA *et al.* Epidemiology and outcome of acute pancreatitis. *Br J Surg* 1987; **74**: 398–401.

2 Halvorsen FA, Ritland S. Acute pancreatitis in Buskerud County, Norway. Incidence and etiology. *Scand J Gastroenterol* 1996; **31**: 411–14.

3 Steinberg W, Tenner S. Acute pancreatitis. *N Engl J Med* 1994; **330**: 1198–209.

4 McMahon MJ, Playforth MJ, Pickford IR. A comparative study of methods for the prediction of severity of attacks of acute pancreatitis. *Br J Surg* 1980; **67**: 22–5.

5 Corfield AP, Williamson RCN, McMahon MJ *et al.* Prediction of severity in acute pancreatitis: prospective comparison of three prognostic indices. *Lancet* 1985; **ii**: 403–7.

6 Larvin M, McMahon MJ. APACHE-II score for assessment and monitoring of acute pancreatitis. *Lancet* 1989; **ii**: 201–5.

7 Ranson JHC, Rifkind KM, Roses DF *et al.* Prognostic signs and the role of operative management in acute pancreatitis. *Surg Gynecol Obstet* 1974; **139**: 69–81.

8 Ranson JHC, Rifkind KM, Turner JW. Prognostic signs and nonoperative peritoneal lavage. *Surg Gynecol Obstet* 1976; **143**: 209–19.

9 Wilson C, Heath DI, Imrie CW. Prediction of outcome in acute pancreatitis: a comparative study of APACHE-II, clinical assessment and multiple factor scoring systems. *Br J Surg* 1990; **77**: 1260–4.

10 Gross V, Scholmerich J, Leser HG *et al.* Granulocyte elastase in assessment of severity of acute pancreatitis. *Dig Dis Sci* 1990; **35**: 97–105.

11 Dominguez-Munoz JE, Carballo F, Carcia MJ *et al.* Clinical usefulness of polymorphonuclear elastase in predicting the severity of acute pancreatitis: results of a multicentre study. *Br J Surg* 1991; **78**: 1230–4.

12 Agarwal N, Pitchumoni CS. Simplified prognostic criteria in acute pancreatitis. *Pancreas* 1986; **1**: 69–73.

13 Bank S, Wise L, Gersten M. Risk factors in acute pancreatitis. *Radiol Clin North Am* 1989; **78**: 637–40.

14 Wilson C, Heads A, Shenkin A *et al.* C-reactive protein, antiproteases and complement factors as objective markers of severity in acute pancreatitis. *Br J Surg* 1989; **76**: 177–81.

15 Imrie CW, Benjamin IS, Ferguson JC *et al.* A single-centre double-blind trial of Trasylol therapy in primary acute pancreatitis *Br J Surg* 1978; **65**: 337–41.

16 Blamey SL, Imrie CW, O'Neill J *et al.* Prognostic factors in acute pancreatitis. *Gut* 1984; **25**: 1340–6.

17 Steinberg WM. Predictors of severity of acute pancreatitis. *Gastroentrol Clin North Am* 1990; **19**: 849–61.

18 Fan ST, Lai E, Mok F. Prediction of the severity of acute pancreatitis. *Am J Surg* 1993; **166**: 262–9.

19 Heath DI, Imrie CW. The Hong Kong Criteria and severity prediction in acute pancreatitis. *Int J Pancreatol* 1994; **15**: 1–7.

20 Balthazar EJ, Ranson JHC, Naidich DP *et al.* Acute pancreatitis: prognostic value of CT. *Radiology* 1985; **156**: 767–72.

21 Balthazar EJ, Robinson DL, Megibow AJ *et al.* Acute pancreatitis: value of CT in establishing prognosis. *Radiology* 1990; **174**: 331–6.

22 Hjelmqvist B, Wattsgard C, Borgstrom A *et al.* Early diagnosis and classification in acute pancreatitis. *Digestion* 1989; **44**: 177–83.

23 London NJM, Leese T, Lavelle JM *et al.* Rapid-bolus contrast-enhanced dynamic computed tomography in acute pancreatitis: a prospective study. *Br J Surg* 1991; **78**: 1452–6.

24 London NJM, Neoptolemos JP, Lavelle J *et al.* Contrast-enhanced abdominal computed tomography scanning and prediction of severity of acute pancreatitis: A prospective study. *Br J Surg* 1989; **76**: 268–72.

25 Clavien PA, Hauser H, Meyer P *et al.* Value of contrast-enhanced computerized tomography in the early diagnosis and prognosis of acute pancreatitis. *Am J Surg* 1988; **155**: 457–66.

26 Puolakkainen PA. Early assessment of acute pancreatitis. A comparative study of computed tomography and laboratory tests. *Acta Chir Scand* 1989; **155**: 25–30.

27 Mayer AD, McMahon MJ. The diagnostic and prognostic value of peritoneal lavage in patients with acute pancreatitis. *Surg Gynecol Obstet* 1985; **160**: 597–612.

28 Buchler M, Malfertheiner P, Schoetensack D *et al.* Sensitivity of antiproteases, complement factors and C-reactive protein in detecting pancreatic necrosis. Results of a prospective clinical study. *Int J Pancreatol* 1986; **1**: 227–35.

29 Leese T, Shaw D, Holliday M. Prognostic markers in acute pancreatitis: can pancreatic necrosis be predicted? *Ann R Coll Surg Engl* 1988; **70**: 227–32.

30 Puolakkainen P, Valtonen V, Paanenen A *et al.* C-reactive protein (CRP) and serum phospholipase A2 in the assessment of the severity of acute pancreatitis. *Gut* 1987; **28**: 764–71.

31 Gudgeon AM, Heath DI, Hurley P *et al.* Trypsmogen activation peptides assay in the early prediction of severity of acute pancreatitis. *Lancet* 1990; **i**: 4–8.

32 Paajanen H, Laato M, Jaakkola M *et al.* Serum tumor necrosis factor compared with C–reactive protein in the early assessment of severity of acute pancreatitis. *Br J Surg* 1995; **82**: 271–73.

33 Leser HG, Gross V, Scheibenbogen C *et al.* Elevation of serum interleukin 6 concentration precedes acute-phase response and reflects severity in acute pancreatitis. *Gastroenterology* 1991; **101**: 782–85.

34 Viedma JA, Perez-Mateo M, Agullo J *et al.* Inflammatory response in the early prediction of severity in human acute pancreatitis. *Gut* 1994; **35**: 822–7.

35 Kaufmann P, Tilz GP, Lueger A *et al.* Elevated plasma levels of soluble tumor necrosis factor receptor (sTNFRp60) reflect severity of acute pancreatitis. *Int Care Med* 1997; **23**: 841–8.

36 Hedstrom J, Sainio V, Kemppainen E *et al.* Serum complex of trypsin 2 and alpha$_1$ antitrypsin as diagnostic and prognostic marker of acute pancreatitis: clinical study in consecutive patients. *Br Med J* 1996; **313**: 333–7.

37 Kemppainen E, Sand J, Puolakkainen P *et al.* Pancreatitis associated protein as an early marker of acute pancreatitis. *Gut* 1996; **39**: 675–8.

38 Lankisch PG, Koop H, Otto J *et al.* Evaluation of methaemalbumin in acute pancreatitis. *Scand J Gastroenterol* 1978; **13**: 975–8.

39 Lankisch PG, Schirren CA, Otto J. Methemalbumin in acute pancreatitis: an evaluation of its prognostic value and

comparison with multiple prognostic parameters. *Am J Gastroenterol* 1989; **84**: 1391–5.
40 Loiudice TA, Lang J, Mehta H *et al.* Treatment of acute alcoholic pancreatitis: the role of cimetidine and nasogastric suction. *Am J Gastroenterol* 1984; **79**: 553–8.
41 Naeije R, Salingret E, Clumeck N *et al.* Is nasogastric suction necessary in acute pancreatitis? *Br Med J* 1978; **2**: 659–60.
42 Levant JA, Secrist D, Resin H *et al.* Nasogastric suction in the treatment of alcoholic pancreatitis. *JAMA* 1974; **229**: 51–2.
43 Lange P, Pedersen T. Initial treatment of acute pancreatitis. *Surg Gynecol Obstet* 1983; **157**: 332–4.
44 Broe PJ, Zinner MJ, Cameron JL. A clinical trial of cimetidine in acute pancreatitis. *Surg Gynecol Obstet* 1982; **154**: 13–16.
45 Meshkinpour H, Molinaari MD, Gardner L *et al.* Cimetidine in the treatment of acute alcoholic pancreatitis: a randomized, double blind study. *Gastroenterology* 1979; **77**: 687–90.
46 Waterworth MW, Barbezat GO, Bank S. Glucagon in treatment of acute pancreatitis. *Lancet* 1974; **i**: 1231.
47 Medical Research Council of the United Kingdom. Death from acute pancreatitis: multicentre trial of glucagon and aprotinin. *Lancet* 1977; **ii**: 632–5.
48 Olazabal A, Fuller R. Failure of glucagon in the treatment of alcoholic pancreatitis. *Gastroenterology* 1978; **74**: 489–91.
49 Durr HK, Maroske D, Zelder O *et al.* Glucagon therapy in acute pancreatitis. Report of a double blind trial. *Gut* 1978; **19**: 175–9.
50 Debas HT, Hancock RJ, Soon-Shiong P *et al.* Glucagon therapy in acute pancreatitis: prospective randomized double blind study. *Can J Surg* 1980; **23**: 578–80.
51 Kronborg O, Bulow S, Jowrgensen PM *et al.* A randomized double-blind trial of glucagon in treatment of first attack of severe acute pancreatitis without associated biliary disease. *Am J Gastroenterol* 1980; **73**: 423–5.
52 Goebell H, Ammann R, Herfarth CH *et al.* A double-blind trial of synthetic salmon calcitonin in the treatment of acute pancreatitis. *Scand J Gastroenterol* 1979; **14**: 881–9.
53 Paul F, Ohnhaus E, Hesch RD. Einfluss von salmcalcitonin auf der verlauf der akuten pancreatitis. *Dtsch Med Wochenschr* 1979; **104**: 615–22.
54 Schwedes M, Althoff PM, Klempa L. Effects of somatostatin on bile induced acute haemorrhagic pancreatitis in the dog. *Horm Metabol Res* 1979; **11**: 655–61.
55 Baxter JN, Jenkins SA, Day DW *et al.* Effects of somatostatin and a long acting somatostatin analogue on the prevention and treatment of experimentally induced acute pancreatitis in the rat. *Br J Surg* 1985; **72**: 382–5.
56 Paran H, Neufeld D, Mayo A *et al.* Preliminary report of a prospective randomized study of octreotide in the treatment of severe acute pancreatitis. *J Am Coll Surg* 1995; **182**: 121–4.
57 Planas M, Perez A, Iglesia R *et al.* Severe acute pancreatitis: treatment with somatostatin. *Intens Care Med* 1998;**24**:37–9.
58 Choi TK, Mok F, Zhan WH *et al.* Somatostatin in the treatment of acute pancreatitis: a prospective randomized controlled trial. *Gut* 1989; **30**: 223–7.
59 Binder M, Uhl W, Friess H *et al.* Octreotide in the treatment of acute pancreatitis: results of a unicenter prospective trial with three different octreotide dosages. *Digestion* 1994; **55**(S1): 20–3.
60 D'Amico D, Favia G, Biasiato R *et al.* The use of somatostatin in acute pancreatitis: results of a multicenter trial. *HepatoGastroenterology* 1990; **37**: 92–8.
61 Gjorup I, Roikjaer O, Andersen B *et al.* A double-blinded multicenter trial of somatostatin in the treatment of acute pancreatitis. *Surg Gynecol Obstet* 1992; **175**: 397–400.
62 McKay C, Baxter J, Imrie C. A randomized, controlled trial of octreotide in the management of patients with acute pancreatitis. *Int J Pancreatol* 1997; **21**: 13–19.
63 Trapnell JE, Rigby CC, Talbot CH *et al.* A controlled trial of Trasylol in the treatment of acute pancreatitis. *Br J Surg* 1974; **61**: 177–82.
64 Yang CH, Chang-Chien CS, Liaw YF. Controlled trial of protease inhibitor gabexelate mesilate (Foy) in the treatment of acute pancreatitis. *Pancreas* 1987; **2**: 698–700.
65 Valderrama R, Perez-Mateo M, Navarro S *et al.* Multicenter double-blind trial of gabexate mesylate (Foy) in unselected patients with acute pancreatitis. *Digestion* 1992; **51**: 65–70.
66 Pederzoli P, Cavallini G, Falconi M *et al.* Gabexate mesilate vs aprotinin in human acute pancreatitis (GA.ME.P.A.). *Int J Pancreatol* 1993; **14**: 117–24.
67 Buchler M, Malfertheiner P, Uhl W *et al* and the German Pancreatitis Study Group. Gabexate mesilate in human acute pancreatitis. *Gastroenterology* 1993; **104**: 1165–70.
68 Leese T, Holliday M, Heath D *et al.* Multicentre clinical trial of low volume fresh frozen plasma therapy in acute pancreatitis. *Br J Surg* 1987; **74**: 907–11.
69 Kingsnorth AN, Galloway SW, Formela LJ. Randomized, double-blind phase II trial of lexipafant, a platelet-activating factor

antagonist, in human acute pancreatitis. *Br J Surg* 1995; **82**: 1414–20.
70 Mckay CJ, Curran F, Sharples C *et al.* Prospective placebo-controlled randomized trial of lexipafant in predicted severe acute pancreatitis. *Br J Surg* 1997; **84**: 1239–43.
71 Craig RM, Dordal E, Myles L. The use of ampicillin in acute pancreatitis. *Ann Intern Med* 1975; **83**: 831–2.
72 Howes R, Zuidema GD, Cameron JL. Evaluation of prophylactic antibiotics in acute pancreatitis. *J Surg Res* 1975; **18**: 197–200.
73 Finch WTK, Sawyers JL, Schenker S. A prospective study to determine the efficacy of antibiotics in acute pancreatitis. *Ann Surg* 1976; **183**: 667–71.
74 Pederzoli P, Bassi C, Vesentini S *et al.* A randomized multicenter clinical trial of antibiotic prophylaxis of septic complications of acute necrotizing pancreatitis with Imipenem. *Surg Gynecol Obstet* 1993; **176**: 480–3.
75 Sainio V, Kemppainen E, Puolakkainen P *et al.* Early antibiotic treatment in acute necrotising pancreatitis. *Lancet* 1995; **346**: 663–7.
76 Luiten EJT, Hop WCJ, Lange JF *et al.* Controlled clinical trial of selective decontamination for the treatment of severe acute pancreatitis. *Ann Surg* 1995; **222**: 57–65.
77 Van Gossum A, Lemoyne M, Greig PD *et al.* Lipid-associated total parenteral nutrition in patients with severe acute pancreatitis. *J Parent Ent Nutr* 1988; **12**: 250–5.
78 Robin AP, Campbell R, Palani CK *et al.* Total parenteral nutrition in severe pancreatitis: clinical experience with 156 patients. *World J Surg* 1990; **14**: 572–9.
79 Buch A, Buch J, Carlsen A *et al.* Hyperlipidemia and pancreatitis. *World J Surg* 1980; **4**: 307–14.
80 Silberman H, Dixon NP, Eisenberg D. The safety and efficacy of a lipid-based system of parenteral nutrition in acute pancreatitis. *Am J Gastroenterol* 1982; **77**: 494.
81 Grant JP, James S, Grabowski V *et al.* Total parenteral nutrition in pancreatic disease. *Ann Surg* 1984; **200**: 627.
82 Leibowitz AB, O'Sullivan P, Iberti TJ. Intravenous fat emulsions and the pancreas: a review. *Mt Sinai J Med* 1992; **59**: 38–42.
83 Sitzman JV, Steinborn PA, Zinner MJ *et al.* Total parental nutrition and alternate energy substrates in the treatment of severe acute pancreatitis. *Surg Gynecol Obstet* 1989; **168**: 311–17.
84 Kalfarentzos FE, Karavias DD, Karatzas TM *et al.* Total parenteral nutrition in severe acute pancreatitis. *J Am Coll Nutr* 1991; **10**: 156–62.
85 Sax HC, Warner BW, Talamini MA *et al.* Early total parenteral nutrition in acute pancreatitis: lack of beneficial effects. *Am J Surg* 1987; **153**: 117–24.
86 DiMagno EP, Vay LW, Summerskill HJ. Intraluminal and post-absorptive effects of amino acids on pancreatic enzyme. *J Lab Clin Med* 1971; **82**: 241–8.
87 Ragins H, Levenson SM, Singer R *et al.* Intrajejunal administration of an elemental diet at neutral pH avoids pancreatic stimulation. *Am J Surg* 1973; **126**: 606–14.
88 Keith RG. Effect of a low fat elemental diet on pancreatic secretion during pancreatitis. *Surg Gynecol Obstet* 1980; **151**: 337–43.
89 Cassim MM, Allardyce DB. Pancreatic secretion in response to jejunal feeding of elemental diet. *Ann Surg* 1974; **180**: 228–31.
90 Grant JP, Davey-McCrae J, Snyder PJ. Effect of enteral nutrition on human pancreatic secretions. *J Parent Ent Nutr* 1987; **11**: 302–4.
91 Alverdy JC, Aoys E, Moss GS. Total parenteral nutrition promotes bacterial translocation from the gut. *Surgery* 1988; **104**: 185–90.
92 Purandare S, Offenbartl K, Westerom B *et al.* Increased permeability to fluorescein isothiocyanate–dextran after total parenteral nutrition in the rat. *J Gastroenterol* 1989; **24**: 678–82.
93 Li J, Gocinski Bj, Henken B *et al.* Effects of parenteral nutrition on gut-associated lymphoid tissue. *J Trauma* 1995; **39**: 44–52.
94 Kudsk KA, Campbell SM, O'Brien T *et al.* Postoperative jejunal feedings following complicated pancreatitis. *Nutr Clin Pract* 1990; **5**: 14–17.
95 Parekh D, Lawson HH, Segal I. The role of total enteral nutrition in pancreatic disease. *S Afr J Surg* 1993; **31**: 57–61.
96 Voitk A, Brown RA, Echave V *et al.* Use of an elemental diet in the treatment of complicated pancreatitis. *Am J Surg* 1973; **125**: 223–7.
97 Simpson WG, Marsano L, Gates L. Enteral nutritional support in acute alcoholic pancreatitis. *J Am Coll Nutr* 1995; **14**: 663–5.
98 McClave, SA, Greene LM, Snider HL *et al.* Comparison of the safety of early enteral vs parenteral nutrition in mild acute pancreatitis. *J Parent Ent Nutr* 1997; **21**: 14–20.
99 Kalfarentzos FE, Kehagias J, Mead N *et al.* Enteral nutritition is superior to parenteral nutrition in severe acute pancreatitis: results of randomized prospective trial. *Br J Surg* 1997; **84**: 1665–9.
100 Windsor ACJ, Kanwar S, Li AGK *et al.* Compared with parenteral nutrition, enteral feeding attenuates the acute phase response and improves disease severity in acute pancreatitis. *Gut* 1998; **42**: 431–5.

101 Neoptolemos JP, London NJ, James D *et al.* Controlled trial of urgent endoscopic retrograde cholangiopancreatography and endoscopic sphincterotomy versus conservative treatment for acute pancreatitis due to gallstones. *Lancet* 1988; **ii**: 979–83.
102 Fan ST, Lai ECS, Mok FPT *et al.* Early treatment of acute biliary pancreatitis by endoscopic papillotomy. *N Engl J Med* 1993; **328**: 228–32.
103 Folsch UR, Nitsche R, Ludtke R *et al* and the German Study Group on Acute Biliary Pancreatitits. Early ERCP and papillotomy compared with conservative treatment for acute biliary pancreatitis. *N Engl J Med* 1997; **336**: 237–42.
104 Ranson JHC. The timing of biliary surgery in acute pancreatitis *Ann Surg* 1978; **189**: 654–62.
105 Kelly TR. Gallstone pancreatitis: the timing of surgery. *Surgery* 1980; **88**: 345–50.
106 Osborne DH, Imrie CW, Carter DC. Biliary surgery in the same admission for gallstone-associated acute pancreatitis. *Br J Surg* 1981; **68**: 758–61.
107 Kelly TR, Wagner DS. Gallstone pancreatitis: a prospective randomized trial of the timing of surgery. *Surgery* 1988; **104**: 600–5.
108 Stone HH, Fabian TC. Peritoneal dialysis in the treatment of acute alcoholic pancreatitis. *Surg Gynecol Obstet* 1980; **150**: 878–882.
109 Mayer AD, Mcmahon MJ, Corfield AP *et al.* Controlled clinical trial of peritoneal lavage for the treatment of severe acute pancreatitis. *N Engl J Med* 1985; **312**: 399–404.
110 Ihse I, Evander A, Holmberg JT *et al.* Influence of peritoneal lavage on objective prognostic signs in acute pancreatitis. *Ann Surg* 1986; **204**: 122–7.
111 Teerenhovi O, Nordback I, Eskola J. High volume lesser sac lavage in acute necrotizing pancreatitis. *Br J Surg* 1989; **76**: 370–3.
112 Ranson JHC, Berman RS. Long peritoneal lavage decreases pancreatic sepsis in acute pancreatitis. *Ann* Surg1990; **211**: 708–16.
113 Alexandre JH, Guerrari MT. Role of total pancreatectomy in the treatment of necrotizing pancreatitis. *World J Surg* 1981; **5**: 369–77.
114 Kivilaakso E, Lempinen M, Makelainen A *et al.* Pancreatic resection versus peritoneal lavation for acute fulminant pancreatitis. *Ann Surg* 1984; **199**: 426–31.
115 Schroder T, Sainio V, Kivisaari L *et al.* Pancreatic resection versus peritoneal lavage in acute necrotizing pancreatitis. *Ann Surg* 1991; **214**: 663–6.
116 Warshaw AL, Gongliang J. Improved survival in 45 patients with pancreatic abscess. *Ann Surg* 1985; **202**: 408–15.
117 Allardyce DB. Incidence of necrotizing pancreatitis and factors related to mortality. *Am J Surg* 1987; **154**: 295–9.
118 Wertheimer MD, Norris CS. Surgical management of necrotizing pancreatitis. *Arch Surg* 1986; **121**: 484–7.
119 Bradley EL, Allen K. A prospective longitudinal study of observation versus surgical intervention in the management of necrotizing pancreatitis. *Am J Surg* 1991; **161**: 19–24.
120 Gebhardt C, Gall FP. Importance of peritoneal irrigation after surgical treatment of hemorrhagic, necrotizing pancreatitis. *World J Surg* 1981; **5**: 379–85.
121 Larvin M, Chalmers AG, Robinson PJ *et al.* Debridement and closed cavity irrigation for the treatment of pancreatic necrosis. *Br J Surg* 1989; **76**: 465–71.
122 Bassi C, Vesentini S, Nifosi F *et al.* Pancreatic abscess and other pus-harboring collections related to pancreatitis: a review of 108 cases. *World J Surg* 1990; **14**: 505–12.
123 Farkas G, Marton J, Mandi Y *et al.* Surgical strategy and management of infected pancreatic necrosis. *Br J Surg* 1996; **83**: 930–3.

17 Hepatitis C: diagnosis and treatment

Patrick Marcellin

Hepatitis C is characterized by its propensity to chronicity. Since chronic hepatitis C is generally silent, its diagnosis is often fortuitous. Systematic screening should be recommended in subjects who have a history of blood transfusion or intravenous drug addiction. The ELISA is the appropriate test for screening. In ELISA positive subjects, the presence of chronic infection is established by the detection of serum HCV RNA by polymerase chain reaction (PCR). A liver biopsy is recommended in patients who are HCV RNA positive with increased ALT levels in order to assess the severity of the liver disease and determine whether there is an indication for therapy. Combination therapy with interferon and ribavirin is now standard therapy, which results in a sustained response in approximately 40% of patients. Genotyping of the virus and the measure of baseline viral load are useful to assess the probability of sustained response and to determine the appropriate duration of combination therapy.

INTRODUCTION

Hepatitis C is a relatively common disease. An estimated 3% of the world population is chronically infected with hepatitis C virus (HCV), and HCV accounts for approximately 20% of cases of acute hepatitis and 70% of cases of chronic hepatitis.[1,2] Chronic hepatitis C is a major cause of cirrhosis and hepatocellular carcinoma. Moreover, HCV related endstage liver disease is the most frequent indication for liver transplantation.[2]

Many controlled studies have shown the efficacy of alpha-interferon (IFNα) therapy in a subgroup of patients. Recent studies have shown that the efficacy of therapy was significantly improved by the combination of interferon with ribavirin. Predictors of response to therapy have been identified.

ACUTE HEPATITIS

HCV is mainly transmitted by the blood. Post-transfusion acute hepatitis has almost disappeared, and most subjects are now infected by intravenous drug use. The average incubation period is 7–8 weeks.[3] Prodromic symptoms are rare. Acute hepatitis C is icteric in a minority of cases (20%) and anicteric with no or few symptoms in most cases (80%). Symptoms are non-specific (malaise, nausea, and right upper quadrant pain followed by dark urine and jaundice) and similar to those in other types of acute viral hepatitis. Thus, the clinical diagnosis of acute hepatitis C is rarely made and the diagnosis is based on the presence of viral markers. Severe acute hepatitis is rare, and whether fulminant hepatitis is caused by HCV is controversial.[4] When it is clinically apparent, the illness generally lasts for 2–12 weeks.

The first marker of HCV infection is serum HCV RNA detectable by PCR, as early as 1 week after exposure.[5–7] Anti-HCV antibodies become detectable at the acute phase of hepatitis in most cases but in some cases seroconversion is delayed up to several weeks. Serum alanine aminotransferase (ALT) levels begin to increase shortly before clinical symptoms appear. Peak levels are generally mildly or moderately increased, less than in acute hepatitis A or B.

In 15% of patients hepatitis resolves spontaneously, serum ALT levels return to normal, and serum HCV RNA becomes undetectable; anti-HCV antibodies remain detectable for many years . In 85% of patients, chronic infection develops and serum ALT levels can either normalize or remain elevated .[3,8,9] However, serum HCV RNA remains detectable, with the exception of a transient period of being negative in some cases.

CHRONIC HEPATITIS

There are three patterns of chronic hepatitis C: chronic hepatitis with normal serum ALT, mild chronic hepatitis, and moderate to severe chronic hepatitis.

Chronic hepatitis with normal ALT levels

About 25% of patients with chronic HCV infection have normal serum ALT levels despite detectable HCV RNA in serum.[10–15] These patients are often identified after donating blood or by systematic screening. The definition of this patient population includes the presence of anti-HCV, HCV RNA detectable by PCR, and persistently normal ALT levels (measured at least three times in 6 months). These patients are usually asymptomatic and histological lesions in the liver are generally mild.[2,16] Virological features (genotype and viral load) do not seem to be different in these patients as compared with those with increased serum ALT levels.[17,18] The long term outcome of this group of patients is not known. Monitoring is recommended, but the prognosis is probably good. A liver biopsy is not recommended for these patients.

Mild chronic hepatitis

About 50% of patients have mild liver disease with detectable serum HCV RNA and mildly elevated or fluctuating serum ALT levels. These patients are usually asymptomatic but may complain of fatigue. Liver histology shows mild necroinflammatory lesions and no or mild fibrosis. This type of chronic hepatitis C generally progresses very slowly and the long term risk of developing cirrhosis is low. However, a minority of these patients may eventually develop more progressive liver disease.[19]

Moderate or severe chronic hepatitis

About 25% of patients have moderate to severe chronic hepatitis. These patients are difficult to distinguish from those with mild chronic hepatitis. Clinically, most are asymptomatic; the intensity of fatigue, if present, is not correlated with the severity of liver disease. Clinical examination is generally normal. Although these patients generally have higher serum ALT levels, serum ALT levels are not a good prognostic factor on an individual basis. Increased serum gamma-glutamyl-transpeptidase, ferritin or gamma-globulin levels, or thrombocytopenia usually indicate severe liver disease but are not always present, ie they are fairly specific but not highly sensitive markers of severity. Ultrasonographic abnormalities are useful when present. However, a liver biopsy is the most accurate way to distinguish mild from moderate or severe chronic hepatitis and thus assess the prognosis. Liver histology shows marked necroinflammatory lesions and extensive fibrosis (or unexpected cirrhosis). This pattern of chronic hepatitis is more common in older patients and in those with aggravating factors such as alcohol or immune deficiency. These patients have a high risk of developing cirrhosis in 5 to 10 years.[9,19]

CIRRHOSIS AND HEPATOCELLULAR CARCINOMA

For many years HCV related cirrhosis may be silent. Thus, asymptomatic cirrhosis is often discovered at liver biopsy. In other cases, cirrhosis is diagnosed because of a complication (variceal hemorrhage, ascites, jaundice or hepatocellular carcinoma). Clinical examination, ultrasonography, and biochemistry may help to predict the presence of cirrhosis.

In patients with HCV related cirrhosis, mortality related to portal hypertension, hepatic failure or hepatocellular carcinoma is 2–5% per year. Endstage HCV related cirrhosis is the most prevalent indication for liver transplantation.[2] The incidence of hepatocellular carcinoma is high (3–4% per year).[20] Although the rationale for the systematic monitoring with ultrasonography and α-fetoprotein is not clearly demonstrated, it is usually recommended.[20]

EXTRAHEPATIC MANIFESTATIONS

Many extrahepatic manifestations have been described in association with HCV infection.[21,22] Some are well demonstrated, while others may be fortuitous (Table 17.1).

Table 17.1 Extrahepatic manifestations associated with hepatitis C

Manifestations	Evidence of association
Mixed cryoglobulinemia	+++
Glomerulonephritis	+++
Porphyria cutanea tarda	+
Autoimmune thyroiditis	±
Lichen planus	±
Low grade malignant lymphoma	±
Sjögren's syndrome	–
Aplastic anemia	–
Polyarteritis nodosa	–
Erythema nodosum	–
Idiopathic pulmonary fibrosis	–

The disorder which is most clearly, and most frequently, associated with HCV is mixed cryoglobulinemia.[23,24] Although detectable cryoglobulinemia is common in chronic hepatitis C (30–50%), it is usually asymptomatic. The clinical syndrome of cryoglobulinemia with arthralgias, Raynaud's disease, and purpura is rare (1–3%). Glomerulonephritis or neuropathy are rare but may be severe.

TREATMENT

The objective of therapy in patients with chronic hepatitis C is to inhibit viral replication in order to decrease the activity of the liver disease. Decreased activity is believed to be associated with a decreased risk of occurrence of cirrhosis.

Effects of alpha-interferon

In chronic hepatitis C, the antiviral effect of IFNα is well demonstrated, with a rapid decrease of serum HCV RNA within the first weeks of therapy, and a parallel decrease of serum ALT.[25]

The response to therapy is defined by the normalization of serum ALT and the loss of detectable serum HCV RNA by PCR. The response should be evaluated at the end of treatment (end of treatment response) and 6 months after treatment (sustained response).

Patients who have a sustained response with persistently normal ALT levels and undetectable HCV RNA 6 months after treatment will maintain a sustained biochemical and virological response.[26,27]

In a study of 80 patients with a sustained response, with a follow-up of 1–7.6 years (4.0 ± 2.0 years, mean ± SD) after IFNα treatment, 93% of patients had persistently normal serum ALT levels and 96% had undetectable serum HCV RNA.[28] A comparison of liver histological findings before and 1–6.2 years after IFNα treatment showed a clear improvement in 94% of patients; in 62% of patients the last biopsy done showed normal or nearly normal histological findings. Liver HCV RNA was undetectable 1–5 years after treatment in all 27 patients tested.

In non-responders, a partial biochemical or histological improvement can be observed. Furthermore, an antifibrogenesis effect of IFNα has been shown.[29,30] However, the long term benefit of maintaining therapy in non- or partial responders has not been proven.

Therapeutic schedule

R
Grade A

The first controlled studies established the dose of 3 million units (MU), three times weekly, as the recommended regimen for IFNα therapy in chronic hepatitis C[31–37] (Table 17.2). Higher doses (5–10 MU) did not show significantly higher rates of sustained response in most studies and were associated with poor tolerability. Further controlled studies demonstrated improvement in sustained response rates by prolonging therapy from 6 months to 12 months[38–40] (Table 17.3). No advantage for 18 or 24 months, as compared with 12 months was demonstrated.[41,42] Therefore, the therapeutic regimen currently recommended is 3 MU for 12 months. This schedule gives a good efficacy/tolerability ratio, with about 20% of patients experiencing a sustained response, 30% an end of treatment response followed by relapse, and 50% of patients fail to respond.[25,43]

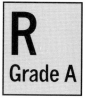

Table 17.2 Randomized controlled trials of alpha-interferon in patients with chronic hepatitis C: alpha-interferon vs no treatment or placebo – comparison of doses

			Response	
Study	No. of patients	Schedule	End of treatment (%)	Sustained (%)
Davis, 1989[31]	166	3 MU 6 mth	38	10
		1 MU 6 mth	16	10
		No treatment	4	
Di Bisceglie, 1989[32]	41	2 MU 6 mth	33	10
		Placebo 6 mth	4	
Marcellin, 1991[33]	60	3 MU 6 mth	39	25
		1 MU 6 mth	45	22
		No treatment	0	0
Causse, 1991[34]	90	3 MU 6 mth	43	13
		1 MU 6 mth	20	3
		Placebo 6 mth	7	3
Hakozaki, 1995[35]	91	10 MU 6 mth	67	43
		6 MU 6 mth	68	37
		3 MU 6 mth	50	23
Lin, 1995[36]	230	5 MU 6 mth	61	20
		3 MU 6 mth	64	17
Marcellin, 1995[37]	75	3, 5, 10 MU 6 mth	48	19
		3 MU 6 mth	51	17

Table 17.3 Randomized controlled trials of alpha-interferon in patients with chronic hepatitis C: comparison of durations

			Response	
Study	No. of patients	Schedule	End of treatment (%)	Sustained (%)
Jouët, 1994[38]	108	3, 2,1 MU 12 mth	45	29
		3 MU 6 mth	40	13
Kasahara, 1995[39]	93	5 MU 12 mth	59	50
		5 MU 6 mth	60	32
Chemello, 1995[40]	174	6, 3 MU 12 mth	76	49
		3 MU 12 mth	65	31
		6 MU 6 mth	74	28
Poynard, 1995[41]	303	3 MU 18 mth	45	22
		3 MU 6 mth	30	8
Lin[36]	230	3 MU 24 mth	55	32
		3 MU 6 mth	61	20

Treatment of patients with cirrhosis

In patients with cirrhosis, IFNα therapy is relatively ineffective (about 5% sustained response) and is associated with more frequent adverse effects.[44,45] This observation may justify not treating these patients. However, recent studies have suggested that IFNα therapy may decrease the risk of complications or the incidence of hepatocellular carcinoma.[46,47] This benefit remains controversial, and other studies have not found a significant difference between treated patients and untreated patients.[45,48] Most of the studies are uncontrolled, and retrospective and more controlled trials or cohort studies are needed to evaluate whether IFNα is beneficial for patients with cirrhosis.

Treatment of patients with normal ALT

In small, uncontrolled trials of IFNα in this group of patients, the rates of response are not different from those reported in patients with abnormal ALT levels.[16] Importantly, in most studies, serum ALT levels became abnormal during therapy in approximately half of affected patients. These findings suggest that IFNα therapy is not usually beneficial and may be harmful in these patients. The efficacy of combination therapy has not been evaluated and should not be used in this group of patients.

Treatment of special groups

In patients with hemophilia, kidney disease requiring hemodialysis, mixed cryoglobulinemia or HIV infection, the decision to treat should be taken on an individual basis. Current data and clinical experience demonstrate that IFNα therapy may be considered in these patients.[49,50] In patients undergoing renal or liver transplantation who develop hepatitis C virus infection, IFNα therapy is contraindicated because of the risk of precipitating allograft rejection.

COMBINATION THERAPY

Preliminary studies showed higher rates of sustained response with the combination of IFNα and ribavirin, as compared with interferon alone.[51–53] Two recent large controlled trials demonstrated that combination therapy was more effective than interferon alone for either 24 or 48 weeks[54,55] (Table 17.4). The rates of sustained response with the combined therapy for 48 weeks were 43% and 38% in these two trials, compared to responses with interferon therapy alone of 19% and 13% (ARR = 24 and 25). The NNT, the number of patients needed to treat for 48 weeks with combined therapy rather than interferon alone

R
Grade A

Table 17.4 End of treatment (ETR) and sustained (SR) virological response to interferon–ribavirin combination therapy and interferon therapy in two randomized controlled trials

Study	ETR IFN/placebo 48 wk	ETR IFN/ribavirin 24 wk	ETR IFN/ribavirin 48 wk	SR IFN/placebo 48 wk	SR IFN/ribavirin 24 wk	SR IFN/ribavirin 48 wk
Poynard, 1998[54] (*n* = 832)	93/278 (33%)	157/277 (57%)	145/277 (52%)	53/278 (19%)	96/277 (35%)	118/277 (43%)
McHutchison, 1998[55] (*n* = 681)	54/225 (24%)	121/228 (53%)	115/228 (50%)	29/225 (13%)	70/228 (31%)	87/228 (38%)
Total (*n* = 1513)	147/503 (29%)	278/505 (55%)	260/505 (51%)	82/503 (16%)	166/505 (33%)	205/505 (41%)

to obtain one additional sustained response, is 4. These results indicate that combination therapy should be standard for chronic hepatitis C.[56] Ribarivin is a nucleoside analog which has no or little antiviral effect on HCV. The mechanisms responsible for the improved efficacy of interferon in combination with ribavirin are not known. It is believed that the beneficial effect of ribavirin is related to immunomodulatory properties.[57]

PREDICTORS OF RESPONSE

The probability of sustained response to therapy depends on host related factors, biochemical factors, histological factors, and virological factors. Among the host related factors, young age and female gender are predictors of good response to therapy. Biochemical factors, such as high levels of gamma-glutamyl transpeptidase and ferritin are predictive of poor response to therapy. Extensive fibrosis or presence of cirrhosis decreases the probability of response. However, the virological characteristics (genotype and baseline viral load) are the main predictors of sustained response.

Unfortunately, genotype 1 (1a or 1b) which is associated with a poor response to therapy, is in the majority in Western Europe and the USA: the proportion of patients infected with genotype 1 ranges from 60% to 80% of cases in the different countries.[58,59] Genotypes 2 and 3, which are associated with a good response to therapy, are seen in a minority of cases: the proportion of patients infected with genotype 2 or genotype 3 ranges from 15% to 35%. Furthermore about half of the patients infected with genotype 1 have a relatively high viral load (serum HCV RNA above 2×10^6 Eq genome/ml) which further decreases the probability of sustained response. Finally, one may estimate that roughly one-third of the patients have genotype 1 with high viral load.

With interferon therapy, the overall sustained response rate is about 30% in patients with HCV genotype 2 or 3 and 5% in those with genotype 1 (1a or 1b).[60] With combination therapy, the overall sustained response rate is roughly doubled, with 64% in patients with HCV genotype 2 or 3, whatever the baseline viral load is, and 35% in patients with genotype 1 and low viral load. In patients with genotype 1 and high viral load, the sustained response rate depends on the duration of therapy: 28% and 8% with 12 months and 6 months, respectively[54] (Table 17.5).

Table 17.5 Sustained virological response to combination therapy according to genotype and viral load

	IFNα+ribavirin 48 wk (%)	IFNα+ribavirin 24 wk (%)	IFNα+placebo 48 wk (%)
Genotype 2 or 3			
HCV RNA $<2.10^6$	64	60	33
HCV RNA $>2.10^6$	64	67	34
Genotype 1, 4 or 5			
HCV RNA $<2.10^6$	36	35	29
HCV RNA $>2.10^6$	28	8	4

Source: Poynard *et al.*[54]

ADVERSE EFFECTS

Adverse effects of interferon

A wide array of adverse effects has been described.[61] The influenza-like adverse effects are common, but are usually ameliorated by acetaminophen and are acceptable. The most severe adverse effects are depression (with risk of suicide) and autoimmune thyroid disease, which account for discontinuation of treatment in 2–10% of the patients.

Adverse effects of ribavirin

The main adverse effect of ribavirin is hemolytic anemia, which is related to direct toxicity on red cells. It is responsible for a mean decrease of 3 g/dl, occurring usually during the first month of treatment.[54,55] This anemia may necessitate **a** decrease of the dose (rarely discontinuation) of ribavirin in approximately 20% of patients. A cardiac assessment is recommended in patients older than 50 years prior to therapy. Because of the teratogenic risk, women of childbearing potential and their partners should each use an effective contraceptive.

INDICATIONS FOR TREATMENT

In patients with acute hepatitis C, interferon therapy is indicated since it decreases the risk of chronicity from 85% to about 50%.[43]

R Grade A

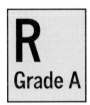

In patients with chronic hepatitis C, the decision to treat is a complex issue, which must take into consideration numerous variables: age of the patient, general state of health, risk of cirrhosis, likelihood of response, other medical conditions that may decrease life expectancy or contraindicate use of interferon or ribavirin. Also, impairment of quality of life during treatment should be taken into account.[62] The decision whether to initiate treatment is mainly based on the result of the liver biopsy. A recent Consensus Conference on Hepatitis C organized by the European Association for the Study of the Liver (EASL) recommended "treatment for the patients with moderate or severe chronic hepatitis" and stated that "the benefits of treating patients with histologically mild disease are uncertain".[56] Genotype and viral load are useful to assess the probability of sustained response to therapy. However, the virological characteristics should not be used as a reason to deny treatment since the decision to treat is mainly based on liver histology. Naive patients should be treated with combination therapy (interferon at the dose of 3 MU three times weekly, ribavirin at the dose of 1000–1200 mg daily). The duration of treatment should be 12 months in patients with genotype 1 and high viral load, 6 months for the others.

R Grade A

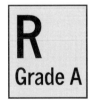

In patients who relapse after interferon therapy, retreatment should be considered: interferon (higher dose for 12 months) or combination of interferon with ribavirin for 6 months.[63,64] In patients who fail to respond to interferon therapy, there is currently no effective treatment.[63]

R Grade C

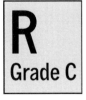

NEW STRATEGIES

Despite significant advances in the treatment of chronic hepatitis C, there are still roughly two-thirds of patients who do not have a sustained response after combination therapy with interferon and ribavirin. Thus, improved therapy is needed. Recombinant IFNα 2a or IFNα 2b give similar results. Lymphoblastoid or consensus interferon showed roughly similar rates of sustained response.[65,66] Current trials are assessing more intensive schedules of IFNα therapy, using higher dose (5–10 MU daily), or new types of IFNα (conjugated with polyethylene glycol (PEG), or triple therapy with interferon, ribavirin, and amantadine. Future strategies include the use of protease and helicase inhibitors, antisense oligonucleotides, and ribozymes.

REFERENCES

1 Alter MJ. Epidemiology of hepatitis C in the West. *Semin Liver Dis* 1995; **15**: 5–14.
2 Hoofnagle JH. Hepatitis C: the clinical spectrum of disease. *Hepatology* 1997; **26** (Suppl 1): 15S–20S.
3 Dienstag JL. NANB hepatitis I. Recognition, epidemiology and clinical features. *Gastroenterology* 1993; **85**: 439–62.
4 Hoofnagle JH, Carithers RL, Shapiro C *et al.* Fulminant hepatic failure: summary of a workshop. *Hepatology* 1995; **21**: 240–52.
5 Farci P, Alter HJ, Wong D *et al* A long term study of hepatitis C virus replication in non-A, non-B hepatitis. *N Engl J Med* 1991; **325**: 98–104.
6 Puoti M, Zonaro A, Ravaggi A *et al.* Hepatitis C virus RNA and antibody response in the clinical course of acute hepatitis C infection. *Hepatology* 1992; **16**: 877–81.
7 Hino K, Sainokami S, Shimoda K *et al.* Clinical course of acute hepatitis C and changes in HCV markers. *Dig Dis Sci* 1994; **39**: 19–27.
8 Alter HJ, Purcell RH, Shih JW *et al.* Detection of antibody to hepatitis C virus in prospectively followed transfusion recipients with acute and chronic non-A, non-B hepatitis. *N Engl J Med* 1989; **321**: 1494–500.
9 Mattsson L, Sönnerborg A, Weiland O. Outcome of acute symptomatic non-A, non-B hepatitis: a 13-year follow-up study of hepatitis C virus markers. *Liver* 1993; **13**: 274–8.
10 Esteban JI, Lopez-Talavera JC, Genescà J *et al.* High rate of infectivity and liver disease in blood donors with antibodies to hepatitis C virus. *Ann Intern Med* 1991; **115**: 443–9.
11 Alberti A, Morsica G, Chemello L *et al.* Hepatitis C viremia and liver disease in symptom-free individuals with anti-HCV. *Lancet* 1992; **340**: 697–8.
12 Prieto M, Olaso V, Verdu C *et al.* Does the healthy hepatitis C virus carriers state really exist? An analysis using polymerase chain reaction. *Hepatology* 1995; **22**: 413–17.
13 Shakil AO, Conry-Cantilena C, Alter HJ *et al.* Volunteer blood donors with antibody to hepatitis C virus: clinical, biochemical, virologic and histologic features. *Ann Intern Med* 1995; **123**: 330–7.
14 Serfaty L, Nousbaum JB, Elghouzzi MH *et al.* Prevalence, severity, and risk factors of liver disease in blood donors positive in a second-generation anti-hepatitis C virus screening test. *Hepatology* 1995; **21**: 725–9.
15 Conry-Cantilena C, Van Raden M, Gibble J *et al.* Routes of infection, viremia, and liver disease in blood donors found to have hepatitis C infection. *N Engl J Med* 1996; **334**: 1691–6.
16 Marcellin P, Lévy S, Erlinger S. Therapy of hepatitis C : patients with normal aminotransferase levels. *Hepatology* 1997; **26** (Suppl 1): 133S–137S.
17 Martinot-Peignoux M, Marcellin P, Gournay J *et al.* Detection and quantitation of serum hepatitis C virus (HCV) RNA by branched DNA amplification in anti-HCV positive blood donors. *J Hepatol* 1994; **20**: 676–8.
18 Silini E, Bono F, Cividini A *et al.* Differential distribution of hepatitis C virus genotypes in patients with and without liver function abnormalities. *Hepatology* 1995; **21**: 285–90.
19 Takahashi M, Yamada G, Miyamoto R *et al.* Natural course of chronic hepatitis C. *Am J Gastroenterol* 1993; **14**: 969–74.
20 Di Bisceglie AM. Hepatitis C and hepatocellular carcinoma. *Seminar Liver Dis* 1995; **15**: 64–9.
21 Marcellin P, Benhamou JP. Autoimmune disorders associated with hepatitis C. In Boyer JL, Ockner RK (eds), *Progress in liver diseases*, Volume XIII. Philadelphia: WB Saunders, 1995, pp 247–67.
22 Koff RS, Dienstag JL. Extrahepatic manifestations of hepatitis C and the association with alcohol liver disease. *Semin Liver Dis* 1995; **15**: 101–9.
23 Pawlotsky JM, Ben Hayia M, André C *et al.* Immunological disorders in C virus chronic active hepatitis: a prospective case–control study. *Hepatology* 1994; **19**: 841–8.
24 Lunel F, Musset L, Franjeul L *et al.* Cryoglobulinemia in chronic liver diseases: role of hepatitis C virus and liver damage. *Gastroenterology* 1994; **106**: 1291–300.

25 Hoofnagle JH, Di Bisceglie AM. The treatment of chronic viral hepatitis. *N Engl J Med* 1997; **226**: 347–56.
26 Chemello L, Cavalletto L, Casarin C *et al* and the TriVeneto Viral Hepatitis Group. Persistent hepatitis C viremia predicts late relapse after sustained response to interferon-a in chronic hepatitis C. *Ann Intern Med* 1996; **124**: 1058–60.
27 Barnes E, Webster G, Jacobs R *et al*. Long term efficacy of treatment of chronic hepatitis C with alpha interferon or alpha interferon and ribavirin. *J Hepatol*, in press.
28 Marcellin P, Boyer N, Gervais A *et al*. Long term histologic improvement and disappearance of intra hepatic HCV RNA after alpha interferon therapy in patients with chronic hepatitis C. *Ann Intern Med* 1997; **127**: 875–81.
29 Manabé N, Chevallier M, Chossegros P *et al*. Interferon-alpha2b therapy reduces liver fibrosis in chronic non-A, non-B hepatitis: a quantitative histological evaluation. *Hepatology* 1993; **8**: 1344–9.
30 Duchatelle V, Marcellin P, Giostra E *et al*. Changes in liver fibrosis at the end of alpha interferon therapy and 6 to 18 months later in patients with chronic hepatitis C: quantitative assement by a morphometric method. *J Hepatol* 1998; **29**: 20–8.
31 Davis GL, Balart LA, Schiff ER, Treatment of chronic hepatitis C with recombinant interferon alfa. A multicenter randomized controlled trial. *N Engl J Med* 1989; **321**: 1501–6.
32 Di Bisceglie AM, Martin P, Kassianides C *et al*. Recombinant interferon alfa therapy for chronic hepatitis C: a randomized, double-blind, placebo-controlled trial. *N Engl J Med* 1989; **321**: 1506–10.
33 Marcellin P, Boyer N, Giostra E *et al*. Recombinant human alpha interferon in patients with chronic non-A, non-B hepatitis: a multicenter randomized controlled trial from France. *Hepatology* 1991; **13**: 393–7.
34 Causse X, Godinot H, Chevallier M *et al*. Comparison of 1 or 3 MU of interferon alfa–2b and placebo in patients with chronic non-A, non B hepatitis. *Gastroenterology* 1991; **101**: 497–502.
35 Hakozaki Y, Shirahama T, Katou M *et al*. A controlled study to determine the optimal dose regimen of interferon-alpha 2b in chronic hepatitis C. *Am J Gastroenterol* 1995; **90**: 1246–9.
36 Lin R, Roach E, Zimmerman M *et al* for the Australia Hepatitis C Study Group. Interferon alfa-2b for chronic hepatitis C: effects of dose increment and duration of treatment on response rates. Results of the first multicenter Australian trial. *J Hepatol* 1995; **23**: 487–96.
37 Marcellin P, Pouteau M, Martinot-Peignoux M *et al*. JP. Lack of benefit of escalating dosage of interferon alfa in patients with chronic hepatitis C. *Gastroenterology* 1995; **109**: 156–65.
38 Jouet P, Roudot-Thoraval F, Dhumeaux D and the Groupe Français pour l'Etude et le Traitement des Hépatites Chroniques. Comparative efficacy of interferon alfa in cirrhotic and non-cirrhotic patients with non-A, non-B, C hepatitis. *Gastroenterology* 1994; **106**: 686–90.
39 Kasahara A, Hayashi N, Hiramatsu N *et al*. Ability of prolonged interferon treatment to supress relapse after cessation of therapy in patients with chronic hepatitis C: a multicenter randomized controlled trial. *Hepatology* 1995; **21**: 291–7.
40 Chemello L, Bonetti P, Cavalletto L *et al*. Randomized trial comparing three different regimens of alpha-2a interferon in chronic hepatitis C. *Hepatology* 1995; **22**: 700–6.
41 Poynard T, Bedossa P, Chevallier M *et al* and the Multicenter Study Group. A comparison of three interferon alfa-2b regimens for the long term treatment of chronic non-A, non-B hepatitis. *N Engl J Med* 1995; **322**: 1457–62.
42 Carithers RL, Emerson SS. Therapy of hepatitis C: meta-analysis of interferon alfa–2b trials. *Hepatology* 1997; **26** (Suppl 1): 83S–88S.
43 Poynard T, Leroy V, Cohard M *et al*. Meta-analysis of interferon randomized trials in the treatment of viral hepatitis C: effects of dose and duration. *Hepatology* 1996; **24**: 778–89.
44 Schalm SW, Fattovich G, Brouwer JT. Therapy of hepatitis C: patients with cirrhosis. *Hepatology* 1997; **26** (Suppl. 1): 128S–132S.
45 Valla D, Chevallier M, Marcellin P *et al*. Treatment of hepatitis C virus-related cirrhosis. A randomized controlled trial of interferon alpha-2b versus non treatment. *Hepatology* 1999; **29**: 1870–5.
46 Nishiguchi S, Kuroki T, Nakatani S *et al*. Randomised trial of effects of interferon-a on incidence of hepatocellular carcinoma in chronic active hepatitis C with cirrhosis. *Lancet* 1995; **346**: 1051–5.
47 Brunetto MR, Oliverti F, Koehler M *et al*. Effect of interferon-α on progression of cirrhosis to hepatocellular carcinoma: a retrospective cohort study. *Lancet* 1998; **351**: 1535–9.
48 Fattovich G, Giustina G, Degos F *et al*. Morbidity and mortality in compensated cirrhosis type C: a retrospective follow-up study of 384 patients. *Gastroenterology* 1997; **112**: 463–72.
49 Zoulim F. Hepatitis C virus infection in special groups. *J Hepatol* 1999, in press.
50 Pol S, Zylberberg H, Fontaine H *et al*. Treatment of chronic hepatitis C in other populations. *J Hepatol* 1999, in press.

51 Brillanti S, Garson J, Foli M *et al*. A pilot study of combination therapy with ribarivin plus interferon alfa for interferon alfa-resistant chronic hepatitis C. *Gastroenterology* 1994; **107**: 812–17.

52 Lai MY, Kao JH, Yang PM *et al*. Long term efficacy of ribavirin plus interferon alfa in the treatment of chronic hepatitis C. *Gastroenterology* 1996; **111**: 1307–12.

53 Reichard O, Norkrans G, Fryden A *et al* for the Swedish Study Group. Randomised, double-blind, placebo-controlled trial of interferon α2b with and without ribavirin for chronic hepatitis C. *Lancet* 1998; **351**: 83–7.

54 Poynard T, Marcellin P, Lee SS *et al*. Randomised trial of interferon α2b plus ribavirin for 48 weeks or for 24 weeks versus interferon α2b plus placebo for 48 weeks for treatment of chronic infection with hepatitis C virus. *Lancet* 1998; **352**: 1426–32.

55 McHutchison JG, Gordon SC, Schiff ER *et al*. Interferon alfa-2b alone or in combination with ribavirin as initial treatment for chronic hepatitis C. N Engl J Med 1998; **339**: 1485–92.

56 EASL International Consensus Conference on Hepatitis C. Consensus Statement. *J Hepatol* 1999, **30**: 956–61.

57 Thomas HC, Török ME, Fortin DM *et al*. Possible mechanisms of action and reasons for failure of antiviral therapy in chronic hepatitis C. *J Hepatol* 1999, in press.

58 Martinot-Peignoux M, Roudot-Thoraval F *et al* and the Groupe d'Etude Moléculaire des HEPatites. Hepatitis C virus genotypes in France: relationship with epidemiology, pathogenicity and response to interferon therapy. *J Viral Hepatitis* 1999, in press.

59 Mondelli MU, Silini E. Clinical significance of hepatitis C virus genotypes. *J Hepatol* 1999, in press.

60 Martinot-Peignoux M, Boyer N, Pouteau M *et al*. Predictors of sustained response to alpha interferon therapy in chronic hepatitis C. *J Hepatol* 1998; **29**: 214–23.

61 Dusheiko G. Side effects of alpha interferon in chronic hepatitis C. *Hepatology* 1997; **26** (Suppl. 1): 112S–121S.

62 Foster GR. Hepatitis C virus infection: side effects and quality of life. *J Hepatol* 1999, in press.

63 Alberti A, Chemello L, Noventa F *et al*. Therapy of hepatitis C: re-treatment with alpha interferon. *Hepatology* 1997; **27** (Suppl 1): 137S–142S.

64 Davis GL, Esteban-Mur R, Rustgi V *et al*. Interferon alfa-2b alone or in combination with ribavirin for the treatment of relapse of chronic hepatitis C. *N Engl J Med* 1998; **339**: 1493–9.

65 Keeffe EB, Hollinger FB and the Consensus Interferon Study Group. Therapy of hepatitis C: consensus interferon trials. *Hepatology* 1997; **26** (Suppl 1): 101S–107S.

66 Lindsay KL. Different types of interferon. Comparative virological response rates among the different interferons. *J Hepatol* 1999, in press.

Hepatitis B: prognosis and treatment

18

PIERO ALMASIO, CALOGERO CAMMÀ, MARCO GIUNTA, ANTONIO CRAXÌ

BACKGROUND

Hepatitis B virus (HBV) infection, together with hepatitis C and alcohol abuse, is among the leading causes of cirrhosis and hepatocellular carcinoma (HCC) worldwide.[1,2] Despite the availability of highly efficient vaccines and a decreased circulation of HBV among homosexual men and health care workers, in the Western world the incidence of HBV infection has remained rather high, since a substantial proportion of new cases of infection occurs in high risk heterosexuals and in iv drug users.[2,3] Chronic HBV infection may progress to cirrhosis, irreversible liver failure, and HCC. It thus represents an important cause of morbidity and mortality,[4–6] and induces substantial direct and indirect social costs. Estimates on the rate of progression of disease are contradictory, making it difficult to apply the Markov model, proposed for estimation of the long term costs of chronic hepatitis B.[7] An important confounding effect stems from the inclusion in some earlier studies,[8,9] of subjects with human immunodeficiency virus (HIV) infection, a known modifier of the immune response to HBV. HIV infection is by itself a cause of reduced life expectancy and has an adverse effect on the course of HBV related liver disease.[9] Since α-interferon (IFN) is now in widespread use as the first line therapy for chronic hepatitis B,[10,11] no additional prospective long term studies on the course of untreated disease will be feasible. Long term prospective cohort studies to evaluate the benefits of IFN therapy on clinically important endpoints, ie prevention of cirrhosis, liver failure, HCC, and death, are difficult to perform due to the prolonged course of the disease. Two long term studies from Western countries,[12,13] have shown that clearance of HBV replicative markers in patients undergoing IFN therapy is frequent and longlasting. Termination of viral replication, either spontaneous or treatment induced, occurs less often in Asian patients.[14]

A long term benefit of IFN treatment in patients with chronic HBeAg positive hepatitis (wild type HBV) has been theoretically affirmed by Wong,[7] using a mathematical simulation model. This benefit has been subsequently confirmed by Niederau[15] in a cohort of 103 treated patients. No sound evidence is available to support a disease-modifying effect of IFN in subjects with anti-HBe positive, HBV-DNA positive chronic hepatitis (HBeAg minus mutant) or in HBV carriers coinfected with other viruses (HDV, HCV).

EVALUATION OF AVAILABLE EVIDENCE

Progression to cirrhosis and HCC and mortality from chronic hepatitis B

Older studies[4,16] suggest that the yearly rate of development of cirrhosis in patients with chronic hepatitis B ranges from 0.4% to 14.2%. Subjects with normal liver histology and no evident viral replication (healthy HBV carriers) usually maintain normal aminotransferases and do not show histological evolution of liver disease over 10 or more years of follow-up.[17] When reactivation of viral replication occurs in these patients, it is accompanied by a peak of liver necroinflammation and is associated with evolution of disease towards cirrhosis.[18] Further evidence from prospective cohort studies[5,6,15,19] shows that the annual probability that patients with cirrhosis will develop decompensation (ascites, jaundice, encephalopathy, portal hypertensive bleeding, HCC) ranges from 3.8% to 9.5%. In a multicenter European study,[6] persistence of HBV-DNA or HBeAg positivity was not associated with decompensation of cirrhosis. Active viral replication in the late phases of HBV related liver disease is, however, distinctly uncommon among Europid patients. This is at variance with the Asian experience,[20] possibly because of different racial backgrounds and mode of acquisition of infection.

In the Western world, the annual rate of development of HCC among patients with chronic hepatitis and cirrhosis ranges from 0.2% to 7.8%.[5,6,15,19] Coinfection with the hepatitis C virus increases the rate of development of HCC.[21]

In Southern Europe, an area where HBV infection was acquired up to a few years ago almost exclusively by vertical or early horizontal transmission[22] and where HDV or HCV coinfection are not uncommon,[23] patients with chronic hepatitis B have a fivefold excess in mortality in comparison to the general population.[19] Subjects without cirrhosis at presentation remain asymptomatic for many years after diagnosis, but their life expectancy is reduced (standardized mortality rate (SMR) 6.2; 95% CI 2.98–11.4). When cirrhosis is already present, the prognosis is even worse (SMR 18.6; 95% CI 12–27).

The data on the incidence of cirrhosis and of HCC and on mortality emerging from longitudinal studies with prolonged follow-up must be considered with caution. The following factors may introduce errors in the estimates:

- low number of follow-up biopsies in patients with chronic hepatitis;
- high mortality from non-hepatic causes;
- selection and increased surveillance for cases with more severe disease and unfavourable course;
- progressive shift over the years of the global spectrum of the disease due to the introduction of new diagnostic tests and screening programs and new treatments.

SUMMARY

In summary, the rate of progression of chronic hepatitis B to cirrhosis ranges between 10 and 40% over a period of ≥10 years, with a huge variability between different countries. The rate of neoplastic transformation of HBV related cirrhosis is on average between 3 and 6% per year, and the annual death rate is 4–10%.

Factors predicting progression to cirrhosis, development of HCC, and liver related mortality

Studies on natural history of HBV infection conclusively show that the risk of progression of chronic hepatitis to cirrhosis increases with age, with the persistence of abnormal aminotransferases, and with a higher Hepatic Activity Index (HAI) score for grade and stage in the first liver biopsy.[24] Severe liver necroinflammation is an indication to start treatment, but a high grade is an uncommon finding in chronic hepatitis B, except during reactivation[18] or during the phase of HBeAg clearance.[18]

Insufficient data are available to evaluate the impact of infection with the HBe minus mutant, of HDV superinfection and of HCV coinfection on the clinical course of the disease. Viral replication as assessed by HBV-DNA positivity predicts worsening of chronic hepatitis and development of cirrhosis.[5,14,25] Data on the influence of alcohol consumption on progression of disease are inconclusive, due to the small numbers of patients evaluated. It has been suggested that ethanol abuse reduces the immune response to HBV,[26] thus possibly modifying the disease course. Although alcoholism is a definite modifier of the natural history of hepatitis C, this relationship has not been confirmed for HBV,[27] at least in terms of development of cirrhosis. There is, however, sound evidence of a relationship between alcohol consumption and risk of developing HCC among HBsAg positive subjects.[28,29] Male sex also strongly influences the likelihood of development of HCC.[6]

An important source of bias in the estimates of incidence of cirrhosis and HCC in chronic hepatitis B is the variable duration of pre-clinical disease. The prolonged, clinically silent course of chronic hepatitis B allows for decades of infection at the time of recruitment to studies, and may lead to marked heterogeneity of patients in clinical trials. The rate of progression from chronic hepatitis to cirrhosis has been reported in different studies to be between 10% and 40% within 10 years. Because of selection bias, the lower figure is probably more accurate. In patients with low HAI grades, the rate of progression to cirrhosis is low, but not negligible.

In a recent study[19] performed in order to evaluate clinical and virological factors that may predict liver related mortality, we assessed a prospective cohort of 302 HBsAg positive subjects with chronic hepatitis (86 with cirrhosis) with a median follow-up of 94 months. Independent predictive factors for decompensation of liver were old age, presence of cirrhosis at baseline, no sustained normalization of aminotransferases during follow-up, and no treatment (Table 18.1). Overall mortality in the entire cohort of patients with chronic hepatitis B was higher than in the general population (SMR 5.25; 95% CI 3.66–7.30; 35 deaths observed, 6.7 expected; $P < 0.0001$). Table 18.2 shows the SMRs of patients with chronic hepatitis B according to baseline liver histology, virological classes, and IFN treatment. Chronic HBV infection significantly increased mortality both in cirrhotics (SMR 18.6; 95% CI 12–27) and in patients without cirrhosis (SMR 6.20; 95% CI 2.98–11.4). The highest risk of death, assessed by SMRs, occurs in patients with dual HBV/HCV replicative infection, followed by HDV infection, wild type HBV, and HBe minus HBV.

SUMMARY

In summary, factors predicting progression from chronic hepatitis to cirrhosis are persistent HBV replication, ongoing moderate or severe liver necroinflammation (ALT;

Table 18.1 Factors predicting decompensation of liver disease in 302 patients with chronic hepatitis B

Variable	Variable code	β	SE	*P*	RR (95% CI)
Age	Continuous	0.034	0.012	0.005	1.034 (1.010–1.059)
Cirrhosis	0 = Absent 1 = Present	1.071	0.348	0.002	2.917 (1.475–5.768)
IFN treatment	0 = Yes 1 = No	–1.169	0.451	0.01	0.311 (0.128–0.752)
ALT normalization	0 = No 1 = Yes	–1.405	0.451	0.0020	245 (0.101–0.594)

Table 18.2 Effects of type of viral replication and coinfection, baseline liver histology, and IFN therapy on mortality from hepatitis B(SMR compared to general population)

Group	No. of patients	Observed deaths	Expected deaths	SMR	95% CI
Cirrhosis	86	25	1.34	18.6	12.03–27.53
No cirrhosis	216	10	1.60	6.20	2.98–11.41
Wild type HBV	86	8	0.47	17.0	7.33–33.49
HBeAg minus HBV	80	6	1.15	5.20	1.91–11.34
HDV infection	76	14	0.51	27.0	14.74–45.36
HCV infection	23	0	0.37	—	—
Dual HBV/HCV	20	7	0.14	49.0	19.65–100.94
All replicative markers negative	17	2	0.32	6.20	0.75–22.38
IFN treated	109	7	0.80	8.60	3.45–17.72
Untreated	193	28	1.47	18.90	12.57–27.41

HAI grade), and multiple viral infections. Factors predicting progression of cirrhosis to HCC are age and duration of infection, male gender, alcohol consumption, and coinfection with HCV.

Effects of IFN therapy on "surrogate" markers of response

R
Grade A

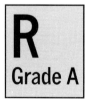

Meta-analyses[10,11] of randomized clinical trials of IFN for chronic hepatitis B conclusively prove its effectiveness for normalizing alanine aminotransferases (ALT) and clearing HBeAg and HBV-DNA from serum in 25–40% of patients. No data are available from these reviews on improvement of liver histology. Standardized response criteria have been set by the use of these "surrogate" markers of cure,[30,31] on grounds of clinical and biological plausibility. "True" clinically relevant disease endpoints (ie progression to cirrhosis, to hepatocellular carcinoma, and death) have not been assessed in RCTs of antiviral therapy because of the prolonged clinical course of chronic hepatitis B. Another major issue is that RCTs of antiviral therapy for chronic hepatitis B have been performed mainly in patients with wild type HBV infection (HBeAg and HBV-DNA positive). The generalizability of results to the whole spectrum of subjects with chronic liver disease due to HBV, mainly those infected by the HBe minus mutant, is questionable.

Many antiviral drugs with different characteristics have been tried for treating chronic hepatitis B. The only two classes of drugs for which sufficient experience is available for a critical review of effectiveness are the α-interferons and some nucleoside analogs. IFN was historically the first agent to be used, and considerable experience has been gained on a very large number of treated patients.[30,31] Nucleoside analogs have been studied mainly in experimental models of Hepadnavirus infection over the past decade. An excellent review of their modes of action and possible use has been recently published by Zoulim and Trèpo.[32]

We have reviewed 28 clinical trials recovered by Medline search (1985–98) which compared IFN to no treatment in adult patients with chronic hepatitis B due to wild type or HBe minus HBV,[33–60] excluding those with dual HBV/HDV or HBV/HCV coinfection. Surrogate endpoints considered were:

- stable normalization of ALT at 6–18 months of follow-up (for patients with wild type and HBe minus HBV);
- sustained loss of HBV-DNA at 6–18 months of follow-up (for patients with wild type and HBe minus HBV);
- clearance of HBeAg (for patients with wild type HBV).

Data on biochemical and virological responses were extracted from the intention to treat analyses of the RCTs, and the DerSimonian and Laird method (risk difference) was used to pool the results. The 28 RCTs included a total of 1065 patients, of whom 445 were not receiving any active treatment. IFN treatment had a favourable, statistically significant effect on all three endpoints compared to no treatment. Meta-analysis shows the following absolute risk reduction associated with IFN therapy:

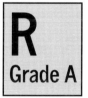

R
Grade A

- Persistent ALT normalization (Figure 18.1): 28% (95% CI 22–34%, $P < 0.0001$).
- Sustained loss of HBV-DNA (Figure 18.2): 25% (95% CI 21–30%, $P < 0.0001$).
- Clearance of HBeAg (Figure 18. 3): 24% (95% CI 1929%, $P < 0.0001$).

The NNT, the number of patients with chronic hepatitis B needed to treat with IFN to achieve one of the selected endpoints (eg sustained suppression of HBV replication) is 4.

R
Grade A

A separate evaluation of treatment efficacy of IFN on HBV-DNA clearance and sustained ALT normalization was performed by a second meta-analysis of five RCTs[41,52,53,55,60] which included only patients infected by the HBe minus mutant. All these RCTs were performed in centers from the Mediterranean area, indirectly confirming the high geographical prevalence of this mutation. Pooled data from the five studies (Figure 18.4), totalling 190 subjects, showed a significant effect of IFN therapy on the combined outcome of reduction of HBV replication and suppression of necroinflammation (absolute risk reduction 28%, 95% CI 11–42%, $P < 0.0002$).

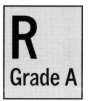

R
Grade A

IFN therapy was associated with an increase in the rate of clearance of HBsAg of 11% (95% CI 3–18%, $P < 0.001$). HBsAg clearance was observed mostly among subjects infected in adulthood, among those with more active disease at onset, and on average after 2–4 years from the moment of HBeAg/HBV-DNA clearance. It was almost never reported in patients infected by HBe minus HBV.

Significant histological improvement was usually observed among patients in whom ALT was normalized and serum HBV-DNA was cleared, but complete healing of liver

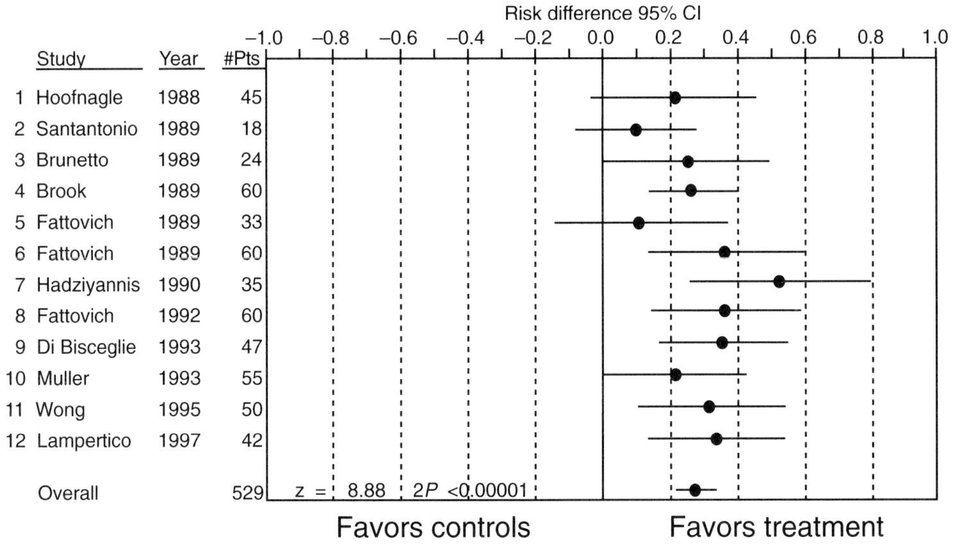

Figure 18.1 Meta-analysis of IFN therapy for chronic hepatitis B (all RCTs): effect of treatment (ARR) on sustained ALT normalization

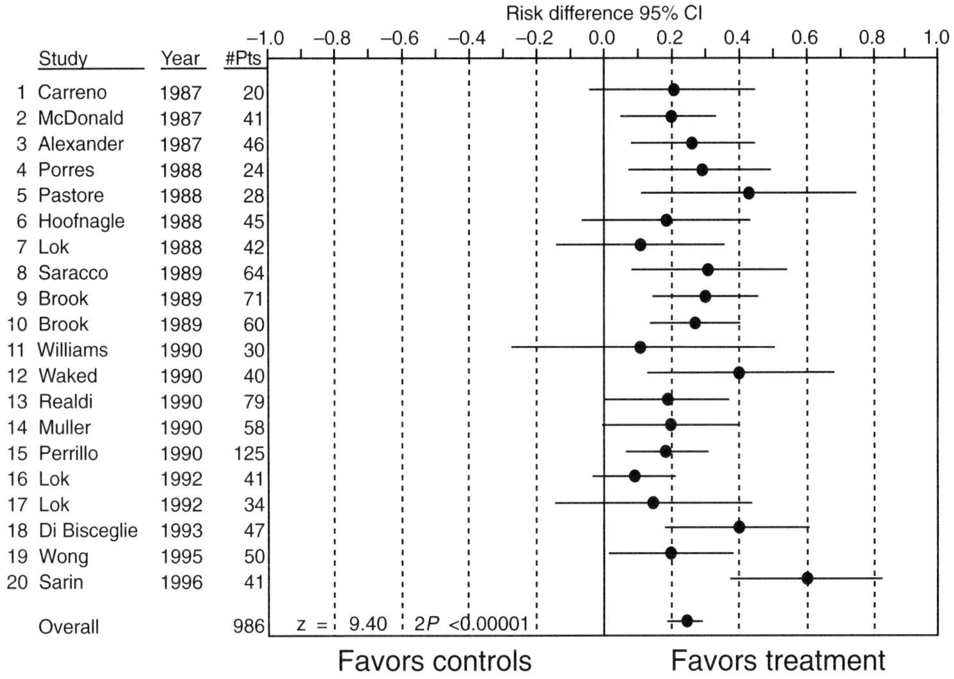

Figure 18.2 Meta-analysis of IFN therapy for chronic hepatitis B (all RCTs): effect of treatment (ARR) on sustained HBV-DNA loss

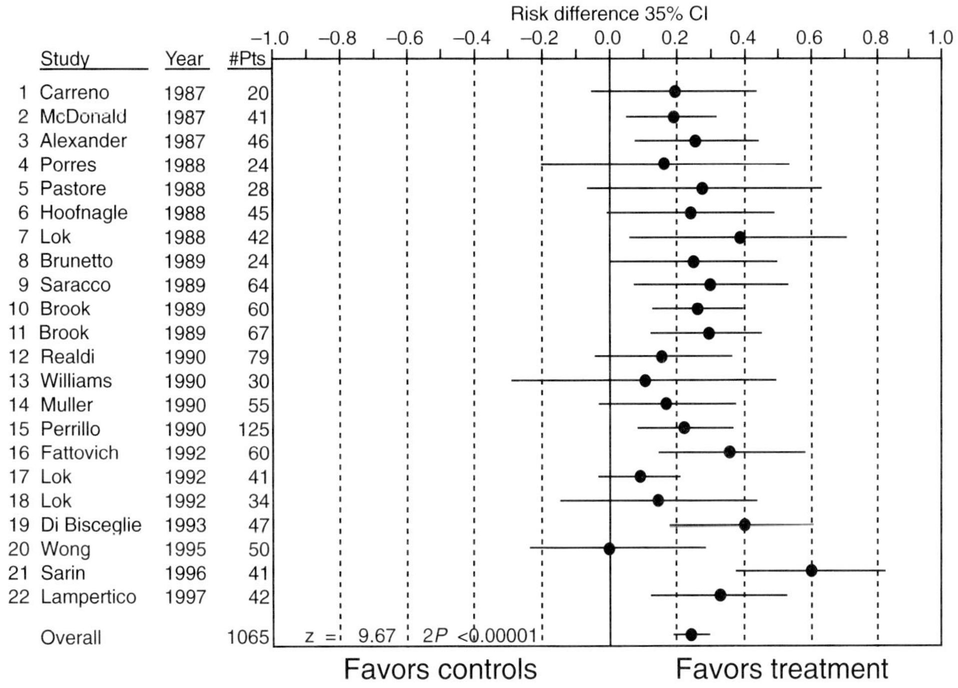

Figure 18.3 Meta-analysis of IFN therapy for chronic hepatitis B (RCTs on wild type HBV): effect of treatment (ARR) on HBeAg clearance

lesions was only seen among subjects rebiopsied many years after seroconversion.[61–63] Many of these patients had also lost serum HBsAg.

The total dose of IFN used appeared to influence the response. For subjects receiving a total dose of <200 MU the odds ratio was 1.37 (95% CI 0.95–1.98) compared to controls, while for those who had received >200 MU the odds ratio was 2.05 (95% CI 1.5–2.78).[64,65]

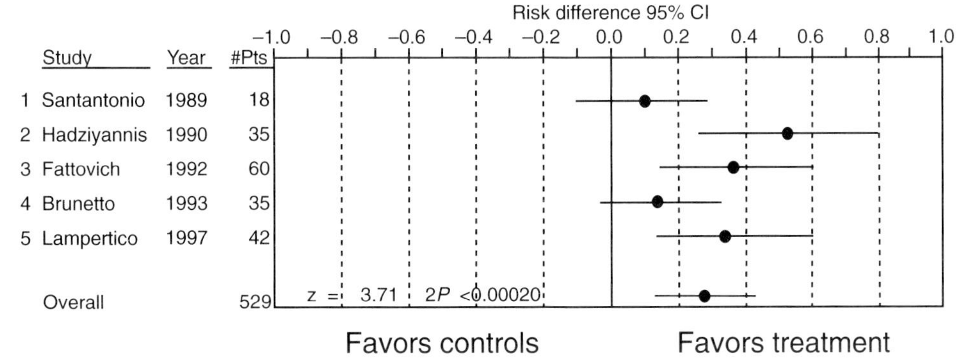

Figure 18.4 Meta-analysis of IFN therapy in chronic hepatitis B (RCTs on HBe minus HBV): effect of treatment (ARR) on sustained ALT normalization and HBV-DNA loss

Factors which predict a favourable response[10,11,49,54, 66–68,69] are:

- low serum HBV-DNA (<100 pg/ml);
- low amounts of HBcAg in the liver;
- high levels of ALT;
- high HAI grade at biopsy;
- infection during adulthood and/or a history of acute hepatitis;
- non-Asian ethnic origin.

There is no clearcut evidence that sex, presence of cirrhosis or other disease features affect the responsiveness to IFN.

R Grade A

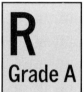

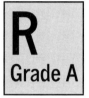

An alternative approach to chronic HBV infection is based on the induction of a brief period of immunosuppression by steroids,[69-70] followed by withdrawal to provoke an abrupt ALT elevation due to the host immune reconstitution, and a subsequent decline of HBV-DNA titer. IFN administration is then started 4 weeks after stopping steroids. The sequential schedule has been studied in several RCTs and the results have been subjected to a meta-analysis.[71] The cumulative rate of clearance of HBeAg in seven RCTs was similar for the sequential prednisone-IFN and IFN monotherapy groups (sequential therapy 41%, monotherapy 35%, OR 1.20; 95% CI 0.8–1.7). Similar results were observed for the endpoint of sustained ALT normalization (sequential therapy 44.5%, monotherapy 38%; OR 1.19; 95% CI 0.6–2.0). Subgroup analysis showed that sequential prednisone–IFN therapy was more effective than IFN monotherapy for HBeAg clearance (sequential therapy 47.9%, monotherapy 18.4%, ARR = 29.5%, NNT = 4, $P < 0.01$) for patients in whom serum ALT was low before starting therapy. There is thus a potential advantage in pretreatment with steroids for this subset of patients. This must be balanced against the possible risk of reactivation of HBV related liver disease after steroid withdrawal. A severe, often fatal "seroconversion hepatitis" has been reported in subjects with pre-existing cirrhosis.[72,73]

R Grade A

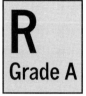

Children chronically infected by HBV have a silent course of liver disease, characterized by a low frequency of disease events during childhood[74–76] with subsequent appearance of clinically evident liver disease in adulthood.[19] Treatment of children with chronic hepatitis B with IFN alone[77–80] or in combination with the immunostimulant drug levamisole[81] has been assessed in RCTs and two meta-analyses have been performed.[82,83] The effectiveness of IFN therapy is rather comparable to that observed in adult patients, but is somewhat less due to the high number of children with high level HBV replication and low necroinflammatory indexes. The percentage of subjects clearing HBV-DNA at the end of therapy is higher in IFN treated children than in untreated controls (IFN 35.5%, control 11.4%, ARR = 24.1%, NNT = 4, $P = 0.0001$). This benefit persisted at the end of follow-up for clearance of HbV-DNA (IFN 28.6%, control 15%, ARR = 13.6%, $P = 0.014$) and HBeAg (IFN 23.0%, control 11.5%, ARR = 11.5%, NNT = 9, $P = 0.026$).

R Grade A

Data on the efficacy of IFN therapy in HIV infected patients with chronic hepatitis B[43,84–92] are scanty and in some respects conflicting. In the largest series[85] of 25 HBsAg positive, HIV infected subjects treated with IFN, compared to a non-randomized control group of 18 patients, there was a 2.15-fold increase in the rate of stable HBV-DNA clearance in patients receiving IFN (36% vs 16.7%). Other reports[86–91] are less optimistic concerning the effectiveness of IFN in eradicating HBV infection in immunocompromised patients. There is a consensus that IFN does not worsen the clinical course of the HIV disease. There is anecdotal evidence of a direct relationship between the immune status of

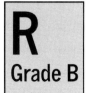

R Grade B

the patient, expressed by CD4 counts, and the likelihood of HBV-DNA clearance. The reduction of HIV viral load and the ensuing immune reconstitution obtained by highly active antiretroviral therapy apparently improve the spontaneous and post-therapeutic course of HCV related liver disease in HIV infected patients.[93] Similar evidence is not yet available for HBV. The use of direct antiviral agents, such as lamivudine or famciclovir, holds further promise for the treatment of these immunodeficient patients, in whom IFN effectiveness is impaired.

SUMMARY

Overall experience suggests that the most cost-effective strategy, as judged by surrogate endpoints is 9– 10 MU IFN three times weekly for 4–6 months for HBeAg positive patients, and 6 MU IFN three times weekly for 24 months (stopping after 6 months if ALT levels are still abnormal) for HBeAg negative, HBV-DNA positive patients. Effectiveness of treatment for HBe minus patients is still questionable.

Predictors of treatment effectiveness are ongoing moderate or severe liver necro-inflammation (ALT levels; HAI grade), low serum HBV-DNA, absence of HIV infection and European racial origin.

HBsAg clearance is uncommon and occurs years after HBV-DNA clearance.

Effects of nucleoside analog therapy on "surrogate" markers of response

Strong evidence for the effectiveness of the more recently introduced nucleoside analogs is not yet available. A number of trials of lamivudine (3-thiacytidine) have appeared over the past few years. Some evidence is also available for effectiveness of ganciclovir (mostly in the setting of immunosuppressed patients) and of famciclovir. Large scale clinical testing of another analog (adefovir dipivoxil) has started, while lobucavir trials have been stopped due to evidence of carcinogenicity in rats. Most of these drugs are used by the oral route and display a powerful inhibitory effect on the HBV-DNA polymerase.[32] Their action is often jeopardized by the appearance of mutations in specific regions of the polymerase-encoding HBV gene (so-called YMDD mutant and others).[32,94–96] These mutants, which often display cross-insensitivity to drugs,[97] cause reappearance of high level viral replication but tend to subside after stopping lamivudine.

The original observations on the anti-HBV efficacy of lamivudine came from the treatment of HIV infected subjects who were also HBsAg positive.[98–101] Effectiveness of lamivudine in reducing dramatically HBV replication has been exploited also in subjects with iatrogenic immune suppression, mostly recipients of organ tranplants.[102–117] or patients receiving antineoplastic chemotherapy.[118]

The majority of published clinical studies of lamivudine in immune-competent HBV patients[119–141]are pilot or dose-finding trials, or pharmacokinetic and virological studies, without appropriate control groups. Formal meta-analysis of these data is inappropriate, since there are only a small number of placebo controlled trials.[127,128,140] We have analyzed the results of nine clinical studies including 642 patients treated with different doses (25–300 mg daily) of lamivudine for periods of 12 weeks to 1 year. The optimal dosage, found by a dose-ranging study[128] and confirmed by an RCT,[140] is 100 mg daily. The median probability of response, in terms of ALT normalization under lamivudine, was

R
Grade B

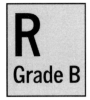

48.6% (range 0–100) and, in terms of clearance of HBV-DNA was 41% (range 12–100). All studies reporting a sufficient follow-up showed a relapse rate, both for ALT and HBV-DNA, above 90% over a 6-month period. The average rate of occurrence of the YMDD mutant was 15–22% at 1 year and 28–34% at 2 years (also Lai CL, unpublished data). Appearance of the YMDD mutant was usually, but not always, associated with an ALT relapse, but usually both the mutant and the necroinflammation peak subsided rapidly upon stopping lamivudine.

The inability of lamivudine to obtain a sustained virological and biochemical response has led to evaluation of combination therapy. The combination with IFN has been tested in a preliminary study[142] and is undergoing evaluation in ongoing RCTs. There are as yet no firm data available to suggest an increase in effectiveness over lamivudine alone. There is experimental evidence [143,144] to suggest that the appearance of lamivudine-induced HBV-mutants may be circumvented by the use of other nucleoside analogs. The potential benefits of these combinations has not yet been evaluated in clinical trials. Concerns have been raised about the possibility of enhanced toxicity.

Lamivudine has been registered in the USA and in other countries as an antiviral active against HBV.

SUMMARY

Available information is sufficient to make the following conclusions:

R
Grade B/C

R
Grade B/C

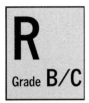

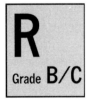

- HBeAg positive immunocompetent patients should receive lamivudine as a second-line drug (100 mg daily) only when IFN has failed.
- HBeAg negative, HBV-DNA positive patients can be treated with lamivudine as first-line therapy (100 mg daily), as an alternative to IFN. Lamivudine should be continued over an extended period of time (24 or more months). Its long term effectiveness in HBe minus patients is still unproven.
- Lamivudine is effective in reducing and sometimes clearing HBV replication in heavily immunosuppressed patients and can be safely administered to patients with advanced liver disease.

Long term benefits of IFN treatment

It has been suggested from retrospective and prospective studies that IFN treatment may have a protective effect against HCC development in patients with chronic HBV infection independent of viral clearance or resolution of necroinflammation.[145] We reviewed studies comparing the incidence of HCC in 356 IFN treated and 650 untreated subjects with HBV related cirrhosis followed for periods of 32–94 months.[19,146–150] No randomized trials have been performed. Some studies attempted to control for confounding variables using historical control patients matched for the principal known prognostic factors, or by the use multivariate analysis. Only one study[148] demonstrates a possible effect of IFN on the risk of HCC in HBV related cirrhosis. The other studies do not suggest a clinically important effect of therapy on this outcome.

Any protection against HCC appears to be mediated by prevention of cirrhosis due to reduction of HBV replication and of the ensuing necroinflammation in patients with pre-cirrhotic chronic hepatitis B

Summary

There is no sound evidence to support a recommendation for widespread use of IFN to prevent HCC in HBV related cirrhosis.

CONCLUSIONS

Data from studies of natural history and RCTs or non-randomized studies of antiviral treatment give sufficient data to conclude that:

- The natural history of chronic hepatitis B is variable, according to phenotypic and ethnic background, and is also influenced by viral coinfections and toxic cofactors. At least 20% of patients develop clinically significant liver disease in the long term.
- Presence of markers of HBV replication and of continuing liver necroinflammation predict an adverse outcome.
- Interferon therapy results in stable clearance of HBeAg in 25% of all patients chronically infected by wild type HBV, but only rarely results in HBsAg clearance.
- Interferon therapy results in stable clearance of HBV-DNA in 25% of all patients chronically infected by HBe minus HBV.
- Lamivudine is effective in clearing HBV-DNA and normalizing ALT during therapy in 65% of patients but its long term effectiveness is unknown.
- There is no acceptable evidence for a protective effect of IFN against development of HCC in HBV related cirrhosis.

REFERENCES

1 Margolis HS, Alter MJ, Hadler SC. Hepatitis B: evolving epidemiology and implications for control. *Semin Liver Dis* 1991; **11**: 84–92.
2 Shapiro CN. Epidemiology of hepatitis B. *Pediatr Infect Dis J* 1993; **12**: 433–7.
3 Grob P. Introduction to epidemiology and risk of hepatitis B. *Vaccine* 1995; **13**(Suppl 1): S14–15.
4 Liaw YF, Tai DI, Chu CM *et al*. The development of cirrhosis in patients with chronic type B hepatitis: a prospective study. *Hepatology* 1988; **8**: 493–6.
5 De Jongh FE, Janssen HLA, De Man RA *et al*. Survival and prognostic indicators in hepatitis B surface antigen-positive cirrhosis of the liver. *Gastroenterology* 1992; **103**: 1630–5.
6 Fattovich G, Giustina G, Schalm SW *et al*. Occurrence of hepatocellular carcinoma and decompensation in western European patients with cirrhosis type B. *Hepatology* 1995; **21**: 77–82.
7 Wong JB, Koff RS, Tiné F *et al*. Cost-effectiveness of interferon-alpha 2b treatment for hepatitis B e antigen-positive chronic hepatitis B. *Ann Intern Med* 1995; **122**: 664–75.
8 Perrillo RP, Aach RD. The clinical course and chronic sequelae of hepatitis B virus infection. *Semin Liver Dis* 1981; **1**: 15–25.
9 Gilson, RJC, Hawkins AE, Beecham MR *et al*. Interactions between HIV and hepatitis B virus in homosexual men: effects on the natural history of infection. *AIDS* 1997; **11**: 597–606.
10 Tiné F, Liberati A, Craxì A *et al*. Interferon treatment in patients with chronic hepatitis B: a meta-analysis ofthe published literature. *J Hepatol* 1993; **18**: 154–62.
11 Wong DK, Cheung AM, O'Rourke K *et al*. Effect of alpha-interferon treatment in patients with hepatitis B e antigen-positive chronic hepatitis B. A meta-analysis. *Ann Intern Med* 1993; **119**: 312–23.
12 Korenman J, Baker B, Waggoner J *et al*. Long-term remission of chronic hepatitis B after alpha-interferon therapy. *Ann Intern Med* 1991; **114**: 629–34.
13 Carreño V, Castillo I, Molina J *et al*. Long-term follow-up of hepatitis B chronic carriers who responded to interferon therapy. *J Hepatol* 1992; **15**: 102–6.
14 Lok AS, Chung HT, Liu VW *et al*. Long-term follow-up of chronic hepatitis B patients treated with interferon alfa. *Gastroenterology* 1993; **105**: 1833–8.

15 Niederau C, Heintges T, Lange S *et al.* Long-term follow-up of HBeAg-positive patients treated with interferon alfa for chronic hepatitis B. *N Engl J Med* 1996; **334**: 1422–7.
16 Realdi G, Alberti A, Rugge M *et al.* Seroconversion from hepatitis B e antigen to anti-HBe in chronic hepatitis B virus infection. *Gastroenterology* 1980; **79**:195–9.
17 De Franchis R, Meucci G, Vecchi M *et al.* The natural history of asymptomatic hepatitis B surface antigen carriers. *Ann Intern Med* 1993; **118**: 191–4.
18 Gupta S, Govindarajan S, Fong T-L *et al.* Spontaneous reactivation in chronic hepatitis B: patterns and natural history. *J Clin Gastroenterol* 1990; **12**: 562–8.
19 Di Marco V, Lo Iacono O, Cammà C *et al.* The long term course of chronic hepatitis B. *Hepatology* 1999; **30**(1): 257–64.
20 Lok ASF. Natural history and control of perinatally acquired hepatitis B virus infection. *Dig Dis Sci* 1992; **10**: 46–52.
21 Donato F, Boffetta P, Puoti M. A meta-analysis of epidemiological studies on the combined effect of hepatitis B and C virus infections in causing hepatocellular carcinoma. *Int J Cancer* 1998; **75**: 347–54.
22 Craxì A, Tinè F, Vinci M *et al.* Transmission of hepatitis B and hepatitis delta viruses in the households of chronic hepatitis B surface antigen carriers. A regression analysis of indicators of risk. *Am J Epidemiol* 1991; **134**: 641–50.
23 De Bac C, Clementi C, Duca F *et al.* Liver cirrhosis. Epidemiological aspects in Italy. *Res Virol* 1997; **148**: 139–42.
24 Fattovich G, Brollo, Giustina G. Natural history and prognostic factors for chronic hepatitis type B. *Gut* 1991; **32**; 294–8.
25 Schlichting P, Christensen E, Andersen PK *et al.* Prognostic factors in cirrhosis identified by Cox's regression model. *Hepatology* 1983; **3**: 889–95.
26 Geissler M, Gesien A, Wands JR. Chronic ethanol effects on cellular immune responses to hepatitis B virus envelope protein: an immunologic mechanism for induction of persistent viral infection in alcoholics. *Hepatology* 1997; **26**: 764–70.
27 Rosman AS, Waraich A, Galvin K *et al.* Alcoholism is associated with hepatitis C but not hepatitis B in an urban population. *Am J Gastroenterol* 1996; **91**: 498–505.
28 Miyakawa H, Izumi N, Marumo F *et al.* Roles of alcohol, hepatitis virus infection and gender in the development of hepatocellular carcinoma in patients with liver cirrhosis. *Alcoholism: Clin Exper Res* 1996; **20** (Suppl): 91A–94A.
29 Donato F, Tagger A, Chiesa R *et al.* Hepatitis B and C virus infection, alcohol drinking, and hepatocellular carcinoma:A case–control study in Italy. *Hepatology* 1997; **26**: 579–84.
30 Evans AA, London WT. Interferon for chronic hepatitis B. *Ann Intern Med* 1996; **124**: 276.
31 Carithers RL Jr. Effect of interferon on hepatitis B. *Lancet* 1998; **351**:157.
32 Zoulim F, Trépo C. Drug therapy for chronic hepatitis B: antiviral efficacy and influence of hepatitis B virus polymerase mutations on the outcome of therapy. *J Hepatol* 1998; **29**:151–68.
33 Lok ASF, Lai CL, Wu PC *et al.* α-Interferon treatment in Chinese patients with chronic hepatitis B. *J Hepatol* 1990; **11**(Suppl 1): S121–5.
34 Carreño V, Porres JC, Mora I *et al.* A controlled study of treatment with recombinant interferon alpha in chronic hepatitis B virus infection: induction and maintenance schedules. *Antiviral Res* 1987; **3**: 125–37.
35 Alexander GJ, Brahm J, Fagan EA *et al.* Loss of HBsAg with interferon therapy in chronic hepatitis B virus infection. *Lancet* 1987; **8550**: 66–9.
36 McDonald JA, Caruso L, Karayiannis P *et al.* Diminished responsiveness of male homosexual chronic hepatitis B virus carriers with HTLV-III antibodies to recombinant alpha-interferon. *Hepatology* 1987; **7**(4): 719–23.
37 Porres JC, Carreño V, Mora I *et al.* Different doses of recombinant alpha interferon in the treatment of chronic hepatitis B patients without antibodies against the human immunodeficiency virus. *Hepatogastroenterology* 1988; **6**: 300–3.
38 Pastore G, Santantonio T, Monno L *et al.* Permanent inhibition of viral replication induced by low dosage of human leukocyte interferon in patients with chronic hepatitis B. *Hepatogastroenterology* 1988; **35**(2): 57–61.
39 Lok AS, Lai CL, Wu PC *et al.* Long-term follow-up in a randomised controlled trial of recombinant alpha 2-interferon in Chinese patients with chronic hepatitis B infection. *Lancet* 1988; **2**: 298–302.
40 Hoofnagle JH, Peters M, Mullen KD *et al.* Randomized, controlled trial of recombinant human alpha-interferon in patients with chronic hepatitis B. *Gastroenterology* 1988; **95**: 1318–25.
41 Pastore G, Santantonio T, Milella M *et al.* Anti-HBe-positive chronic hepatitis B with HBV-DNA in the serum response to a 6-month course of lymphoblastoid interferon. *J Hepatol* 1992; **14**: 221–5.

42 Brunetto MR, Oliveri F, Rocca G *et al.* Natural course and response to interferon of chronic hepatitis B accompanied by antibody to hepatitis B e antigen. *Hepatology* 1989; **10**: 198–202.
43 Brook MG, McDonald JA, Karayiannis P *et al.* Randomised controlled trial of interferon alfa 2A (rbe) (Roferon-A) for the treatment of chronic hepatitis B virus (HBV) infection: factors that influence response. *Gut* 1989; **30**: 1116–22.
44 Brook MG, Chan G, Yap I *et al.* Randomised controlled trial of lymphoblastoid IFN alfa in Europid men with chronic hepatitis B virus infection. *Br Med J* 1989; **299**: 652–6.
45 Fattovich G, Brollo L, Boscaro S *et al.* Long-term effect of low dose recombinant interferon therapy in patients with chronic hepatitis. *Br J Hepatol* 1989; **9** (3): 331–7
46 Saracco G, Mazzella G, Rosina F *et al.* A controlled trial of human lymphoblastoid interferon in chronic hepatitis B in Italy. *Hepatology* 1989; **10**: 336–41.
47 Williams SJ, Craig PI, Cooksley WG *et al.* Randomised controlled trial of recombinant human interferon -alpha A for chronic active hepatitis B. *Aust N Z J Med* 1990; **20**: 9–19.
48 Waked I, Amin M, Abd el Fattah S *et al.* Experience with interferon in chronic hepatitis B in Egypt. *J Chemother* 1990; **2**: 310–18.
49 Realdi G, Fattovich G, Pastore G *et al.* Problems in the management of chronic hepatitis B with interferon: experience in a randomized, multicentre study. *J Hepatol* 1990; **11** (Suppl 1): S129–32.
50 Müller R, Baumgarten R, Markus R *et al.* Treatment of chronic hepatitis B with interferon alfa-2b. *J Hepatol* 1990; **11** (Suppl 1): S137–40.
51 Perrillo RP, Schiff ER, Davis GL *et al.* A randomized, controlled trial of interferon alfa-2b alone and after prednisone withdrawal for the treatment of chronic hepatitis B. The Hepatitis Interventional Therapy Group. *N Engl J Med* 1990; **323**: 295–301.
52 Hadziyannis S, Bramou T, Makris A *et al.* Interferon alfa-2b treatment of HBeAg negative/serum HBV DNA positive chronic active hepatitis type B. *J Hepatol* 1990; **11** (Suppl 1): S133–6.
53 Fattovich G, Farci P, Rugge M *et al.* A randomized controlled trial of lymphoblastoid interferon-α in patients with chronic hepatitis B lacking HBeAg. *Hepatology* 1992; **15**: 584–9.
54 Lok AS, Wu PC, Lai CL *et al.* A controlled trial of interferon with or without prednisone priming for chronic hepatitis B. *Gastroenterology* 1992; **102**(6): 2091–7.
55 Brunetto MR, Giarin M, Saracco G *et al.* Hepatitis B virus unable to secrete e antigen and response to interferon in chronic hepatitis B. *Gastroenterology* 1993; **105**: 845–50.
56 Di Bisceglie AM, Fong TL, Fried MW *et al.* A randomized, controlled trial of recombinant alpha-interferon therapy for chronic hepatitis B. *Am J Gastroenterol* 1993; **88**: 1887–92.
57 Müller R, Baumgarten R, Markus R *et al.* Low dose alpha interferon treatment in chronic hepatitis B virus infection. *Gut* 1993; **34**(Suppl): S97–8.
58 Wong DK, Yim C, Naylor CD *et al.* Interferon alfa treatment of chronic hepatitis B: randomized trial in a predominantly homosexual male population. *Gastroenterology* 1995; **108**: 165–71.
59 Sarin SK, Guptan RC, Thakur V *et al.* Efficacy of low-dose alpha interferon therapy in HBV-related chronic liver disease in Asian Indians: a randomized controlled trial. *J Hepatol* 1996; **24**: 391–6.
60 Lampertico P, Del Ninno E, Manzin A *et al.* A randomized, controlled trial of a 24-month course of interferon alfa 2b in patients with chronic hepatitis B who had hepatitis B virus DNA without hepatitis B e antigen in serum. *Hepatology* 1997; **26**: 1621–5.
61 Korenman J, Baker B, Waggoner J *et al.* Long-term remission of chronic hepatitis B after alpha-interferon therapy. *Ann Intern Med* 1991; **114**: 629–34.
62 Lok ASF, Ma OCK, Lau JYN. Interferon alfa therapy in patients with chronic hepatitis B virus infection.Effects on hepatitis B virus DNA in the liver. *Gastroenterology* 1991; **100**: 756–61.
63 Di Bisceglie AM. Long-term outcome of interferon-alpha therapy for chronic hepatitis B. *J Hepatol* 1995; **22** (Suppl 1): 65–7.
64 Krogsgaard K, Bindslev N, Christensen E *et al.* The treatment effect of alpha interferon in chronic hepatitis B is independent of pre-treatment variables.Results based on individual patient data from 10 clinical controlled trials. *J Hepatol* 1994; **21**: 646–55.
65 Krogsgaard K, Christensen E, Bindslev N *et al.* Relation between treatment efficacy and cumulative dose of alpha interferon in chronic hepatitis B. *J Hepatol* 1996; **25**: 795–802.
66 Perrillo RP. Factors influencing response to interferon in chronic hepatitis B: Implications for Asian and Western populations. *Hepatology* 1990; **12**: 1433–5.
67 Thomas HC, Karayiannis P, Brook G. Treatment of hepatitis B virus infection with interferon. Factors predicting response to interferon. *J Hepatol* 1991; **13** (Suppl.1): S4–7.

68 Carreño V, Castillo I, Molina J *et al.* Long-term follow-up of hepatitis B chronic carriers who responded to interferon therapy. *J Hepatol* 1992; **15**: 102–6.
69 Krogsgaard K. Does corticosteroid pretreatment enhance the effect of alfa interferon treatment in chronic hepatitis B. *J Hepatol* 1994; **20**: 159–62.
70 Krogsgaard K, Marcellin P, Trepo C *et al.* Prednisolone withdrawal therapy enhances the effect of human lymphoblastoid interferon in chronic hepatitis B. *J Hepatol* 1996; **25**: 803–13.
71 Cohard M, Poynard T, Mathurin P *et al.* Prednisone-interferon combination in the treatment of chronic hepatitis B: direct and indirect metanalysis. *Hepatology* 1994; **20**: 1390–8.
72 Perrillo R, Tamburro C, Regenstein F *et al.* Low-dose, titratable interferon alfa in decompensated liver disease caused by chronic infection with hepatitis B virus. *Gastroenterology* 1995; **109**: 908–16.
73 Perrillo RP. Chronic hepatitis B: problem patients (including patients with decompensated disease). *J Hepatol* 1995; **22** (Suppl 1): 45–8.
74 Ruíz-Moreno M. Chronic hepatitis B in children. Natural history and treatment. *J Hepatol* 1993; **17** (Suppl.3): S64–6.
75 Bortolotti F, Jara P, Crivellaro C *et al.* Outcome of chronic hepatitis B in Caucasian children during a 20-year observation period. *J Hepatol* 1998; **29**: 184–90.
76 Bortolotti F. Chronic hepatitis B acquired in childhood: Unanswered questions and evolving issues. *J Hepatol* 1994; **21**: 904–9.
77 Barbera C, Bortolotti F, Crivellaro C *et al.* Recombinant interferon-$_{2a}$ hastens the rate of HBeAg clearance in children with chronic hepatitis B. *Hepatology* 1994; **20**: 287–90.
78 Ruiz-Moreno M, Camps T, Jimenez J *et al.* Factors predictive of response to interferon therapy in children with chronic hepatitis B. *J Hepatol* 1995; **22**: 540–4.
79 Sokal EM, Conjeevaram HS, Roberts EA *et al.* Interferon alfa therapy for chronic hepatitis B in children: a multinational randomized controlled trial. *Gastroenterology* 1998; **114**: 988–95.
80 Ruiz-Moreno M, Rua MJ, Molina J *et al.* Prospective, randomized controlled trial of interferon-α in children with chronic hepatitis B. *Hepatology* 1991; **13**: 1035–9.
81 Ruiz-Moreno M, García R, Rua MJ *et al.* Levamisole and interferon in children with chronic hepatitis B. *Hepatology* 1993; **18**: 264–9.
82 Vajro P, Migliaro F, Fontanella A *et al.* Interferon: a meta-analysis of published studies in pediatric chronic hepatitis B. *Acta Gastroenterol Belg* 1998; **15**: 219–23.
83 Torre D, Tambini R. Interferon-alpha therapy for chronic hepatitis B in children: a meta-analysis. *Clin Infect Dis* 1996; **23**: 131–7.
84 Di Martino V, Lunel F, Cadranel JF *et al.* Long-term effects of interferon-alpha in five HIV-positive patients with chronic hepatitis B. *J Viral Hepatol* 1996; **3**: 253–60.
85 Zylberberg H, Jiang J, Pialoux G *et al.* Alpha-interferon for chronic active hepatitis B in human immunodeficiency virus-infected patients. *Gastroenterol Clin Biol* 1996; **3**: 968–71.
86 Wong DK, Yim C, Naylor CD *et al.* Interferon alfa treatment of chronic hepatitis B: randomized trial in a predominantly homosexual male population. *Gastroenterology* 1995; **3**: 165–71.
87 Pizarro Portillo A, Novella Arribas B, Sanz Sanz J. Treatment with interferon of chronic active hepatitis in patients with HIV infection. *Ann Med Intern* 1997; **13**: 297–8.
88 Miura T, Meguro T, Takayama S *et al.* Interferon therapy for Japanese hemophiliacs with chronic hepatitis C. *Acta Paediatr Jpn* 1997; **39**: 556–8.
89 Lidman C, Magnius L, Norder H *et al.* Interferon alpha-2b treatment in an HIV-infected patient with hepatitis B virus. *Scand J Infect Dis* 1993; **25**: 133–5.
90 Marcellin P, Boyer N, Colin JF *et al.* Recombinant alpha interferon for chronic hepatitis B in anti-HIV positive patients receiving zidovudine. *Gut* 1993; **34** (Suppl 2): S106.
91 Hess G, Rossol S, Voth R *et al.* Treatment of patients with chronic type B hepatitis and concurrent human immunodeficiency virus infection with a combination of interferon alpha and azidothymidine: a pilot study. *Digestion* 1989; **43**: 56–9.
92 Visco G, Alba L, Grisetti S *et al.* Zidovudine plus interferon alfa-2b treatment in patients with HIV and chronic active viral hepatitis. *Gut* 1993; **34** (Suppl): S107–8.
93 Rutschmann OT, Negro F, Hirschel B *et al.* Impact of treatment with human immunodeficiency virus (HIV) protease inhibitors on hepatitis C viremia in patients coinfected with HIV. *J Infect Dis* 1998; **177**: 783–5.
94 Atkins M, Gray DF. Lamivudine resistance in chronic hepatitis B. *J Hepatol* 1998; **28**: 169.
95 Allen MI, Deslauriers M, Andrews CW *et al.* Clinical Investigation Group: Identification and characterization of mutations in hepatitis B virus resistant to lamivudine. *Hepatology* 1998; **27**: 1670–7.

96 Chayama K, Suzuki Y, Kobayashi M *et al.* Emergence and takeover of YMDD motif mutant hepatitis B virus during long-term lamivudine therapy and re-takeover by wild type after cessation of therapy. *Hepatology* 1998; **27**: 1711–16.
97 Pichoud C, Seignères B, Wang ZR *et al.* Transient selection of a hepatitis B virus polymerase gene mutant associated with a decreased replication capacity and famciclovir resistance. *Hepatology* 1999; **29**: 230–7.
98 Benhamou Y, Dohin E, Lunel-Fabiani F *et al.* Efficacy of lamivudine on replication of hepatitis B virus in HIV-infected patients. *Lancet* 1995; **345**: 396–7.
99 Benhamou Y, Katlama C, Lunel F *et al.* Effects of lamivudine on replication of hepatitis B virus in HIV-infected men. *Ann Intern Med* 1996; **125**: 705–12.
100 Schnittman SM, Pierce PF. Potential role of lamivudine (3TC) in the clearance of chronic hepatitis B virus infection in a patient coinfected with human immunodeficiency virus type 1. *Clin Infect Dis* 1996; **23**: 638–9.
101 Altfeld M, Rockstroh JK, Addo M *et al.* Reactivation of hepatitis B in a long-term anti-HBs-positive patient with AIDS following lamivudine withdrawal. *J Hepatol* 1998; **29**: 306–9.
102 Bain VG, Kneteman NM, Ma MM *et al.* Efficacy of lamivudine in chronic hepatitis B patients with active viral replication and decompensated cirrhosis undergoing liver transplantation. *Transplantation* 1996; **62**: 1456–62.
103 Grellier L, Mutimer D, Ahmed M *et al.* Lamivudine prophylaxis against reinfection in liver transplantation for hepatitis B cirrhosis. *Lancet* 1996; **348**: 1212–15.
104 Ling R, Mutimer D, Ahmed N *et al.* Selection of mutations in the hepatitis B virus polymerase during therapy of transplant recipients with lamivudine. *Hepatology* 1996; **24**: 711–13.
105 Al Faraidy K, Yoshida EM, Davis JE *et al.* Alteration of the dismal natural history of fibrosing cholestatic hepatitis secondary to hepatitis B virus with the use of lamivudine. *Transplantation* 1997; **64**: 926–8.
106 Ben-Ari Z, Shmueli D, Mor E *et al.* Beneficial effect of lamivudine in recurrent hepatitis B after liver transplantation. Transplantation 1997; 63: 393–6.
107 Ben-Ari Z, Shmueli D, Mor E *et al.* Beneficial effect of lamivudine pre- and post-liver transplantation for hepatitis B infection. *Transplant Proc* 1997; **29**: 2687–8.
108 Rostaing L, Henry S, Cisterne JM *et al.* Efficacy and safety of lamivudine on replication of recurrent hepatitis B after cadaveric renal transplantation. *Transplantation* 1997; **64**: 1624–7.
109 Andreone P, Caraceni P, Grazi GL *et al.* Lamivudine treatment for acute hepatitis B after liver transplantation. *J Hepatol* 1998; **29**: 985–9.
110 De Man RA, Bartholomeusz AI, Niesters HGM *et al.* The sequential occurrence of viral mutations in a liver transplant recipient re-infected with hepatitis B: hepatitis B immune globulin escape, famciclovir non-response, followed by lamivudine resistance resulting in graft loss. *J Hepatol* 1998; **29**: 669–75.
111 Goffin E, Horsmans Y, Cornu C *et al.* Lamivudine inhibits hepatitis B virus replication in kidney graft recipients. *Transplantation* 1998; **66**: 407–9.
112 Herrero JI, Quiroga J, Sangro B *et al.* Effectiveness of lamivudine in treatment of acute recurrent hepatitis B after liver transplantation. *Dig Dis Sci* 1998; **43**: 1186–9.
113 Jung YO, Lee YS, Yang WS *et al.* Treatment of chronic hepatitis B with lamivudine in renal transplant recipients. *Transplantation* 1998; **66**: 733–7.
114 Markowitz JS, Martin P, Conrad AJ *et al.* Prophylaxis against hepatitis B recurrence following liver transplantation using combination lamivudine and hepatitis B immune globulin. *Hepatology* 1998; **28**: 585–9.
115 Marzano A, Debernardi-Venon W, Condreay L *et al.* Efficacy of lamivudine re-treatment in a patient with hepatitis B virus (HBV) recurrence after liver transplantation and HBV-DNA breakthrough during the first treatment. *Transplantation* 1998; **65**: 1499 500.
116 Nery JR, Weppler D, Rodriguez M *et al.* Efficacy of lamivudine in controlling hepatitis B virus recurrence after liver transplantation. *Transplantation* 1998; **65**: 1615–21.
117 Picardi M, Selleri C, De Rosa G *et al.* Lamivudine treatment for chronic replicative hepatitis B virus infection after allogeneic bone marrow transplantation. *Bone Marrow Transplant* 1998; **21**: 1267–9.
118 Ter Borg F, Smorenburg S, De Man RA *et al.* Recovery from life-threatening, corticosteroid-unresponsive, chemotherapy-related reactivation of hepatitis B associated with lamivudine therapy. *Dig Dis Sci* 1998; **43**: 2267–70.
119 Dienstag JL, Perrillo RP, Schiff ER *et al.* A preliminary trial of lamivudine for chronic hepatitis B infection. *N Engl J Med* 1995; **333**: 1657–61.
120 Honkoop P, De Man RA, Heijtink RA *et al.* Hepatitis B reactivation after lamivudine. *Lancet* 1995; **346**: 1156–7.

121 Nowak MA, Bonhoeffer S, Hill AM *et al.* H. Viral dynamics in hepatitis B virus infection. *Proc Natl Acad Sci* 1996; **93**: 4398–402.
122 Tipples GA, Ma MM, Fischer KP *et al.* Mutation in HBV RNA-dependent DNA polymerase confers resistance to lamivudine in vivo. *Hepatology* 1996; **24**: 714–17.
123 Heijtink RA, Kruining J, Honkoop P *et al.* Serum HBeAg quantitation during antiviral therapy for chronic hepatitis B. *J Med Virol* 1997; **53**: 282–7.
124 Honkoop P, De Man RA, Scholte HR *et al.* Effect of lamivudine on morphology and function of mitochondria in patients with chronic hepatitis B. *Hepatology* 1997; **26**: 211–15.
125 Honkoop P, Niesters HGM, De Man RAM *et al.* Lamivudine resistance in immunocompetent chronic hepatitis B – incidence and patterns. *J Hepatol* 1997; **26**: 1393–5.
126 Jaeckel E, Manns MP. Experience with lamivudine against hepatitis B virus. *Intervirology* 1997; **40**: 322–36.
127 Lai CL, Ching CK, Tung AKM *et al.* Lamivudine is effective in suppressing hepatitis B virus DNA in Chinese hepatitis B surface antigen carriers: A placebo-controlled trial. *Hepatology* 1997; **25**: 241–4.
128 Nevens F, Main J, Honkoop P *et al.* Lamivudine therapy for chronic hepatitis B: a six-month randomized dose-ranging study. *Gastroenterology* 1997; **113**: 1258–63.
129 Schalm SW. Clinical implications of lamivudine resistance by HBV. *Lancet* 1997; **349**: 3–4.
130 Schiano TD, Lissoos TW, Ahmed A *et al.* Lamivudine–stavudine-induced liver failure in hepatitis B cirrhosis. *Am J Gastroenterol* 1997; **92**: 1563–4.
131 Zeuzem S, De Man RA, Honkoop P *et al.* Dynamics of hepatitis B virus infection in vivo. *J Hepatol* 1997; **27**: 431–6.
132 Allen MI, Deslauriers M, Andrews CW *et al* and Lamivudine Clinical Investigation Group. Identification and characterization of mutations in hepatitis B virus resistant to lamivudine. *Hepatology* 1998; **27**: 1670–7.
133 Atkins M, Gray DF. Lamivudine resistance in chronic hepatitis B. *J Hepatol* 1998; **28**: 169.
134 Bernasconi E, Battegay M. Lamivudine for chronic hepatitis B. *N Engl J Med* 1998; **339**: 1786.
135 Boni C, Bertoletti A, Penna A *et al.* Lamivudine treatment can restore T cell responsiveness in chronic hepatitis B. *J Clin Invest* 1998; **102**: 968–75.
136 Buti M, Jardi R, Cotrina M *et al.* Transient emergence of hepatitis B variants in a patient with chronic hepatitis B resistant to lamivudine. *J Hepatol* 1998; **28**: 510–13.
137 Chayama K, Suzuki Y, Kobayashi M *et al.* Emergence and takeover of YMDD motif mutant hepatitis B virus during long-term lamivudine therapy and re-takeover by wild type after cessation of therapy. *Hepatology* 1998; **27**: 1711–16.
138 Honkoop P, De Man RA, Niesters HGM. Quantitative assessment of hepatitis B virus DNA during a 24-week course of lamivudine therapy. *Ann Intern Med* 1998; **128**: 697.
139 Honkoop P, De Man RA, Niesters HGM *et al.* Clinical impact of lamivudine resistance in chronic hepatitis B. *J Hepatol* 1998; **29**: 510–11.
140 Lai CL, Chien RN, Leung NWY *et al* and Asia Hepatitis Lamivudine Study Group. A one-year trial of lamivudine for chronic hepatitis B. *N Engl J Med* 1998; **339**: 61–8.
141 Niesters HGM, Honkoop P, Haagsma EB *et al.* Identification of more than one mutation in the hepatitis B virus polymerase gene arising during prolonged lamivudine treatment. *J Infect Dis* 1998; **177**: 1382–5.
142 Mutimer D, Naoumov N, Honkoop P *et al.* Combination alpha-interferon and lamivudine therapy for alpha-interferon-resistant chronic hepatitis B infection: results of a pilot study. *J Hepatol* 1998; **28**: 923–9.
143 Xiong XF, Flores C, Yang H *et al.* Mutations in hepatitis B DNA polymerase associated with resistance to lamivudine do not confer resistance to adefovir in vitro. *Hepatology* 1998; **28**: 1669–73.
144 Marques AR, Lau DTY, McKenzie R *et al.* Combination therapy with famciclovir and interferon-α for the treatment of chronic hepatitis B. *J Infect Dis* 1998; **178**: 1483–7.
145 Benvegnù L, Chemello L, Noventa F *et al.* Retrospective analysis of the effect of interferon therapy on the clinical outcome of patients with viral cirrhosis. *Cancer* 1998; **83**: 901–9.
146 Mazzella G, Accogli E, Sottili S *et al.* Alpha interferon treatment may prevent hepatocellular carcinoma in HCV-related liver cirrhosis. *J Hepatol* 1996; **24**(2): 141–7.
147 Fattovich G, Giustina G, Degos F *et al.* Effectiveness of interferon alfa on incidence of hepatocellular carcinoma and decompensation in cirrhosis type C. European Concerted Action on Viral Hepatitis (EUROHEP). *J Hepatol* 1997; **27**: 201–5.
148 Ikeda K, Saitoh S, Suzuki Y *et al.* Interferon decreases hepatocellular carcinogenesis in patients with cirrhosis caused by the hepatitis B virus: a pilot study. *Cancer* 1998; **82**: 827–35.
149 Fattovich G, Giustina G, Sanchez Tapias J *et al.* Delayed clearance of serum HBsAg in compensated cirrhosis B: relation to interferon alpha therapy and disease prognosis. European

Concerted Action on Viral Hepatitis (EUROHEP). *Am J Gastroenterol* 1998; **93**: 896–900.

150 Bonino F, Oliveri F, Colombatto P *et al.* Impact of interferon-alpha therapy on the development of hepatocellular carcinoma in patients with liver cirrhosis: results of an international survey. *J Viral Hepatol* 1997; **4**(Suppl 2): 79–82.

19 Alcoholic liver disease: screening and treatment

PHILIPPE MATHURIN, THIERRY POYNARD

SCREENING

In heavy drinkers, liver related mortality is mainly attributed to cirrhosis and hepatocellular carcinoma (HCC). Therefore, the main objectives of screening are: (a) to identify patients with significant liver injury; (b) to characterize the main risk factors for HCC; and (c) to perform an early diagnosis of HCC. In this chapter we focus on the non-invasive screening of cirrhosis and on the screening of HCC.

NON-INVASIVE SCREENING FOR CIRRHOSIS

Assessment of stage and severity of liver injury requires liver biopsy. Percutaneous transhepatic (standard) liver biopsy is an invasive procedure associated with severe complications leading to death in 0.015 % of patients.[1] Less than 30% of heavy drinkers have some features of significant liver injury, such as extensive fibrosis, alcoholic hepatitis, or cirrhosis.[2] As routine liver biopsy is non-essential in 70% of heavy drinkers, indirect diagnosis tests for cirrhosis are clearly necessary to avoid screening with routine liver biopsy.

Several serum proteins have been widely evaluated for their use as a non-invasive test for liver fibrosis: (a) extracellular matrix (procollagen I, procollagen III propeptide (PIIIP), laminin, transforming growth factor (TGF) β1, hyaluronate); (b) prothrombin time; (c) apolipoprotein A-I (ApoA-I); and (d) alpha–2-macroglobulin. The number of studies evaluating the diagnostic accuracy of procollagen I, laminin, and TGF β1 is clearly insufficient for reaching a conclusion. For PIIIP and hyaluronate, previous studies yield interesting results, although some data are still controversial.

Serum PIIIP did not provide any significant improvement in assessing the degree of fibrosis in two studies, whereas one study observed that PIIIP could be useful in detecting patients with cirrhosis in progress.[3–5] Recently, two studies observed the ability of PIIIP to correctly identify patients with fibrosis or cirrhosis.[6,7] In Teare's study, the receiver operating curve observed that at a cut-off of 0.7 U/ml, the sensitivity was 94% and the specificity 81% (positive predictive value 85%, negative predictive value 92%). A major problem, in addition to the wide heterogeneity of the assays used in the studies, is that the PIIIP screening cut-off is still unknown, even with a particular assay.

Hyaluronate, an unbranched polysaccahride, is a component of extracellular matrix. One study has observed that hyaluronate may be useful for the diagnosis of cirrhosis.[8] Serum hyaluronate concentrations were significantly higher in alcoholic patients with cirrhosis (467 μg/l, range 205–800 μg/l) than in alcoholic patients without cirrhosis (53 μg/l, range 14–78 μg/l). The diagnostic accuracy of serum hyaluronate for the evaluation of cirrhosis was confirmed in patients with primary biliary cirrhosis.[9–10] The screening cut-off for the diagnosis of cirrhosis in routine practice has been analyzed.[6] Hyaluronate concentration of ≥60 μg/l had a sensitivity of 97% and a specificity of 73% for the diagnosis of cirrhosis. In terms of applicability, the diagnostic accuracy of this cut-off should be confirmed in other patient populations.

Prothrombin time was initially designed to assess hepatocellular dysfunction. Recent improvement in the determination of the prothrombin index has rendered it more useful in this regard. Indeed, prothrombin time seemed to predict liver fibrosis and to be inversely correlated with the area of fibrosis measured by image analysis.[6,11,12]

Apolipoprotein A-I, the major component of high density lipoprotein cholesterol, was significantly correlated with liver injury.[13] In a study of 581 alcoholic patients, ApoA-I had an independent and discriminate value for the diagnosis of fibrosis versus steatosis (P <0.001) and for the diagnosis of cirrhosis versus non-cirrhotic fibrosis (P <0.001), or versus alcoholic hepatitis without alcoholic cirrhosis (P <0.001).[14] Conversely, serum apolipoprotein B was not correlated with hepatic fibrosis. We analyzed the mechanisms involved in the decrease of serum ApoA-I in heavy drinkers with fibrosis.[15–18] Those studies observed that: (a) an increase of ApoA-I mRNA may explain, at least in part, the increase of serum ApoA-I in heavy drinkers with steatosis; (b) fibrosis is associated with decreased serum ApoA-I, probably due to post-transcriptional mechanisms; and (c) severe alcoholic cirrhosis is associated with a non-specific decrease in ApoA-I mRNA. However, with regard to the wide overlap of serum ApoA-I in patients with different stages of liver fibrosis, the diagnostic accuracy of ApoA-I for the evaluation of cirrhosis was insufficient. Therefore we analyzed the diagnostic accuracy of a simple index called PGA that combines prothrombin index (P), gamma-glutamyl transpeptidase concentration (G) and apolipoprotein A-I (A).[12] The PGA value ranged from 0 to 12 (Table 19.1). When the PGA was <2, the probability of cirrhosis was 0% and the probability of a normal liver was 83%. Conversely, when the PGA was >9, the probability of cirrhosis was 86%. One study has suggested that the combination of PGA and PIIIP concentration may be useful to reduce the need for liver biopsy.[7]

Serum alpha–2-macroglobulin, a proteinase inhibitor, has been evaluated as a marker of cirrhosis. The serum level of this protein was higher in patients with cirrhosis than in patients without cirrhosis.[19,20] Based on those results, we assessed whether serum alpha–2-macroglobulin could improve the diagnostic accuracy of PGA.[21] We showed that addition of alpha–2-macroglobulin to the PGA index (PGAA index) could be useful in the detection of cirrhosis.

Table 19.1 PGA index

Score	Prothrombin time % of normal (seconds over control)	GGT (IU/l)	Apolipoprotein AI (mg/dl)
0	≥80% (<1)	<20	≥200
1	70–79% (1–2)	20–49	175–199
2	60–69% (2–3)	50–99	150–174
3	50–59% (3–4)	100–199	125–149
4	<50% (≥4)	≥200	<125

The PGA score ranges from 0 to 12.

The diagnostic accuracy of non-invasive serum markers (PIIIP, hyaluronate, laminin, TGF β1, prothrombin time, alpha–2-macroglobulin, PGA and PGAA) were compared.[6] The authors observed that hyaluronate concentration and prothrombin index were the most sensitive variables for screening.

In summary, prothrombin time, PGA and PGAA scores, PIIIP, and serum hyaluronate may be used in screening for cirrhosis in heavy drinkers. However, controversy surrounding the use of serum markers persists. The methods for the quantification of serum markers of extracellular matrix and the unit of quantification vary widely. The discrepancies between assays contributed to the wide heterogeneity of the cut-off levels between the studies. Therefore, additional studies are required to determine the screening cut-off level of PIIIP and hyaluronate before the application of these measurements to routine practice.

SCREENING FOR HEPATOCELLULAR CARCINOMA

In cirrhotic patients, the probability of developing HCC at 5 years is approximately 20%, with a yearly incidence rate of 3%. The identification of the subgroup of patients with higher risk for HCC and the early detection of HCC constitute two of the main challenges for hepatologists in the near future. In heavy drinkers, presence of cirrhosis, age >50 years, male sex, serum AFP ≥15 ng/ml, HBsAg and anti-HCV antibodies were independently associated with the occurrence of HCC.[22–24] A clinicobiological score has been developed which identified two groups at low (3-year cumulative incidence, 0%) and high (3-year cumulative incidence, 24%) risk of HCC.[25] In addition to these factors, the preneoplastic role of liver large cell dysplasia has been suggested.[26] In one study the estimated cumulative incidence of HCC at 3 years was 38% and 10% in patients with and without large cell dysplasia, respectively.[25] Another group confirmed that large cell dysplasia, detected in 24 % of patients, was a major risk factor for HCC.[27] Liver biopsy is necessary for the identification, utlizing this approach, of patients with a higher risk for HCC.

Screening for HCC is usually performed with ultrasonography and the determination of serum AFP. However, contrasting data have been reported on the effectiveness of ultrasonography for early detection of HCC. A French center observed that an initial diagnosis of tumor less than 3 cm in diameter was performed in only 21% of cases.[28] Conversely, in two studies, ultrasonography allowed the detection of small HCC in 76% of cases.[29,30] Regardless of those contrasting data, most liver units recommend a regular ultrasonography in the screening of HCC.

In conclusion, for heavy drinkers, in routine practice the following strategy of screening for HCC would be recommended. Screening for cirrhosis might be performed using serum markers such as PGA, PIIIP, or serum hyaluronate. Liver biopsy will be necessary in patients with a PGA score ≥9, a PIIIP ≥0.7 U/ml or serum hyaluronate ≥60 μg/l to confirm the diagnosis of cirrhosis and to detect the presence of large cell dysplasia. However, additional studies are needed to validate this strategy. Among the subgroup of patients at high risk for HCC, further studies will be needed to determine the effectiveness of intensive screening and preventive measures. Cost-effectiveness will be a major concern.

TREATMENT

In heavy drinkers, pharmacological treatments and liver transplantation have been tested to improve survival in those with severe liver injury such as alcoholic hepatitis or cirrhosis. However, the usefulness of pharmacological treatments for controlling the alcohol induced liver injury is still unsettled and controversies persist with regard to the selection of alcoholic patients for liver transplantation.[31,32]

Pharmacological treatments

To determine which pharmacological treatments are effective we have searched the literature for randomized controlled trials and performed meta-analysis[33] when a therapeutic modality was evaluated in two or more published randomized controlled trials (published in article form) using the same endpoint survival (short term or long term survival).

COLCHICINE

In the first RCT evaluating colchicine effect on long term survival in patients with alcoholic cirrhosis, 5- and 10-year survival rates were significantly higher in the colchicine group (75 and 56%, respectively) than in the placebo group (34% and 20%, $P < 0.001$).[34] However, in patients with alcoholic hepatitis, two other studies did not observe any effect of colchicine on short term survival.[35,36] Additional RCTs evaluating colchicine effect on long term survival will be necessary.

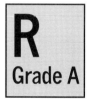

R Grade A

PROPYLTHIOURACIL

Two RCTs did not observe any effect of propylthiouracil on short term survival.[37,38] The meta-analysis of these RCTs confirms the lack of benefit on short term survival, with a mean difference of 1% (CI –7 to 9%). Grade A

The effect of propylthiouracil on long term survival was analyzed in a RCT with 310 alcoholic patients who received propylthiouracil (n= 157) or a placebo (n = 153) for 2 years.[39] The 2-year mortality rate was lower in the propylthiouracil group than in the placebo group: 13% vs 26% ($P < 0.05$, NNT = 8). Propylthiouracil treatment, prothrombin time, hemoglobin levels and mean daily urinary alcohol levels were independent prognostic factors. However, this study has two important limitations (a) the statistical analysis was performed using "per protocol analysis" and (b) the cumulative drop-out rates in both groups were approximately 60%. The authors stated that it was justified to use a "per protocol analysis" since compliance was accurately quantified using elaborate monitoring with a fluorescent compound detectable in the urine.[40] However, in randomized controlled trials intention to treat analysis is usually recommended, and the observed high drop-out rates also should be taken into account. Therefore any long term survival effect of propylthiouracil is controversial and additional RCTs evaluating propylthiouracyl on long term survival would be necessary before firm conclusions could be drawn.

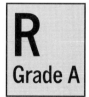

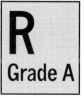

R Grade A

OTHER DRUGS

D-penicillamine, vitamin E, (+)-cyanidanol-3, thioctic acid, malotilate, and the calcium antagonist amlodipine have been evaluated in randomized trials, but none has been shown to decrease mortality.[41–47]

R Grade A

SYLIMARIN

The first RCT suggested that sylimarin would improve long term survival of patients with cirrhosis.[48] However, a recent RCT did not confirm any effect of sylimarin on survival.[49]

COMBINED TREATMENT WITH INSULIN AND GLUCAGON

R Grade A

The infusion of insulin and glucagon was tested in five RCTs (three published in article form and two in abstract form) in patients with alcoholic hepatitis.[50–54] Only one study reported a significant effect on short term survival.[50] Meta-analysis of these RCTs did not show any significant survival effect of insulin–glucagon association on short term survival, with a mean difference of 5% (CI −11 to 23%).

ANABOLIC–ANDROGENIC STEROIDS

R Grade A

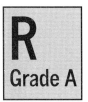

Five RCTs evaluating anabolic steroids reported negative results.[55–59] In one study, a sensitivity analysis suggested that anabolic steroids were effictive in the subgroup of patients with moderate malnutrition.[58] Meta-analysis of these five RCTs did not observe any effect of anabolic steroids on long term survival, with a mean difference of −10% (−20 to 1.0%). Based on these results, anabolic steroids are not indicated in patients with alcoholic liver disease. Furthermore, the use of anabolic–androgenic drugs is questionable when considering the potential risk of development of HCC associated with these drugs.

CORTICOSTEROIDS

Thirteen RCTs tested corticosteroids in patients with alcoholic hepatitis.[57,60–71] Only four trials observed a survival benefit in treated patients.[62,65,66,68] The wide variability of disease severity between the studies, the lack of histological analysis before enrolment of patients, the small sample size, and confounding factors prior to randomization such as renal insufficiency or gastrointestinal bleeding explained, at least in part, these contradictory results.[72,73]

R Grade A

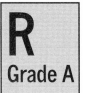

The Maddrey criterion is now used for identifying a subgroup of patients with a high risk of mortality.[67] Corticosteroid therapy has been shown to significantly decrease short term mortality in patients with severe alcoholic hepatitis (spontaneous encephalopathy or a Maddrey function ≥32) in two randomized controlled trials. Observed mortality rates were: steroid 65%, placebo 94% at 28 days (NNT = 3, $P = 0.006$) in a 28-day trial[62] and steroid 45%, placebo 88% (NNT = 2, $P = 0.001$) in a 66-day trial.[68]

R Grade A

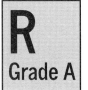

The meta-analysis of the 13 RCTs showed a significant short term survival effect of corticosteroids, with a mean difference of 15% (CI 6–24%, $P < 0.01$). The short term survival effect of corticosteroids was higher in the subgroup of patients with encephalopathy, with a mean difference of 27% (CI 11–44%, $P < 0.0001$).

In a recent study of 122 alcoholic patients with severe biopsy-proven alcoholic hepatitis we showed that: (1) corticosteroids are associated with short term survival benefit; (2) young patients with marked neutrophil infiltrate or neutrophilia obtained much stronger benefits from corticosteroid treatment; and (3) survival benefit due to corticosteroid treatment persisted for at least 1 year and disappeared at 2 years.[74]

NEW DRUGS

Pentoxyfilline, phosphatidylcholine, and S-adenosylmethionine

R Grade A

A RCT evaluating pentoxyfilline in patients with severe alcoholic hepatitis observed a significant difference between the pentoxyfilline group and the placebo group: 58% vs 42% ($P = 0.05$).[75] In the future, evaluation of pentoxyfilline will require further studies evaluating this drug versus corticosteroids. The effectiveness of phosphatidylcholine is being evaluated in a multicenter randomized trial in human (Veterans Administration Study 391). A recent RCT reported that adenosylmethionine might improve survival of patients with alcoholic cirrhosis.[76] Overall survival in the adenosylmethionine group (90%) was significantly better than in the placebo group (73%, $P = 0.04$). The authors observed that adenosylmethionine effect is restricted to the subgroup of patients with moderate liver disease (Child–Pugh A or B). This promising result will have to be confirmed in further RCTs.

R Grade A

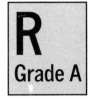

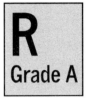

DRUG TREATMENT: SUMMARY

In summary, only corticosteroids are associated with a benefit of short term survival in patients with severe alcoholic hepatitis (Maddrey discriminant function >32 or presence of encephalopathy). The corticosteroid effect is higher in young patients with neutrophilia or marked neutrophil infiltrate. Future studies evaluating the effect of colchicine and propylthiouracil on long term survival are recommended. Recent studies report interesting data concerning new drugs such as pentoxyfilline, S-adenosylmethionine and phosphatidylcholine. Randomized controlled trials are ongoing for some of these drugs.

LIVER TRANSPLANTATION

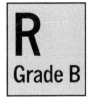

R Grade B

Liver transplantation is a highly effective therapeutic option for endstage liver disease. In patients with alcoholic cirrhosis, liver transplantation leads to survival rates which are similar to those of patients with non-alcoholic cirrhosis.[77–79] Due to the scarcity of donor organs, controversies surrounding liver transplantation in alcoholic patients have been focused on the identification of the subgroup with survival benefit, the validity of the abstinence criterion for patient selection and the societal issue of the high cost of treatment of a self-inflicted illness.

To assess the efficacy of liver transplantation in patients with alcoholic cirrhosis, we compared 2-year survival of 169 transplanted patients to survival of matched control patients and simulated control patients.[80] Simulated control group survival was given by a prognostic model (Beclere model) using the natural history of alcoholic cirrhosis. The final Beclere model combined four variables to obtain a risk score (R) for each patient in the following equation: $R = (0.0484 \times (\text{age in years}) + 0.469 \times (\text{encephalopathy}) + 0.537 \times \text{Loge}\ (\text{bilirubin in } \mu\text{mol/l}) - 0.052 \times (\text{albumin in g/l})$. Encephalopathy was rated 0 if absent and 1 if asterixis, confusion, or coma was present. Survival function for the Beclere model was S_1 at 1 year and S_2 at 2 years: $S_1 = 0.7334\text{exp.}\ (R - 3.058)$ and $S_2 = 0.643\text{exp.}\ (R - 3.058)$. Two-year survival of transplanted patients (73%, CI 67–79%) was similar to survival of matched patients (67%, CI 63–71%) and simulated patients (67%, CI 63–70%). In a sensitivity analysis of data for patients with severe liver disease, the 2-year survival of transplanted patients was significantly higher (64%, CI 42–86%) than that of

Table 19.2 Operating characteristics of the criterion of 6 months' abstinence pretransplantation as a test of alcoho recidivism after liver transplantat on

Study	Status post-transplant	Patients abstinent pretransplant <6 mth	Patients abstinent pretransplant ≥6 mth	Sensitivity (%)	Specificity (%)	Positive predict ve value (%)	Negative predictive value (%)
Bird, 1990[85]				100	92	75	100
	Abstinent	1	11				
	Not abstinent	3	0				
Kumar, 1990[86]				50	91	43	93
	Abstinent	4	42				
	Not abstinent	3	3				
Osario, 1994[87]				28	100	100	86
	Abstinent	0	30				
	Not abstinent	2	5				
Foster, 1997[84]				30	76	25	80
	Abstinent	12	38				
	Not abstinent	4	9				

Sensitivity: proportion of patients with a positive test (abstinent <6 months pretransplantation) who have the disease (are not abstinent after transplant). Specificity: proportion of patients with a negative test (abstinent ≥6 months pretransplantaion) who do not have the disease (are abstinent following transplant). Positive predictive value: proportion of patients who have the disease (were not abstinent from alcohol after transplant) with a positive test (abstinent <6 months pretransplant). Negative predictive value: proportion of pat ents who do not have the disease (were abstinent from alcohol post-transplant) and who had a negative test (abstinent ≥6 months pretransplant).

matched patients (41%, CI 23–59%) and simulated patients (23%, CI 19–27%). We concluded that: (1) efficacy of liver transplantation is limited to the subgroup of patients with severe liver disease; and (2) the Beclere model might be useful in the selection of alcoholic patients. However, a recent study observed that this model seems to overestimate the risk of death for patients specifically referred for transplantation.[81]

The selection practices of 14 transplant centers have been evaluated.[82] Eight of the centers reported that they would accept candidates with less than 1 year of alcoholic abstinence, four centers with less than 6 months of abstinence, one center with less than 1 month of abstinence, and one program would accept candidates who currently continued to drink alcohol. Most programs reported recommending a 6-month abstinence criterion for listing patients with alcoholic liver disease. However, the validity of the 6-month criterion has been recently called into question. Yates *et al* observed that the use of the 6-month abstinence criterion forces a significant number of patients with a low risk of relapsing to wait for transplant listing.[83] In a study of 84 transplanted patients, the receiver operating curve showed that 7–9 months' pretransplant abstinence provided the best cut-off for predicting subsequent abstinence, and 6 months' abstinence was a poor predictor of post-transplantation abstinence (Table 19.2).[84] Five variables were independently associated with post-transplant abstinence: the psychosocial inclusion criteria; absence of previous illicit drug use; presence of personal life insurance policy; number of alcoholic sisters; and the length of pretransplant abstinence. The pooling of the previous studies showed that the sensitivity of the 6-month abstinence criterion in predicting post-transplant abstinence ranged from 28 to 100% and the specificity ranged from 76 to 92%.[84–87]

A major objection to liver transplantation in alcoholic patients was the concern about the risk of alcoholism recidivism. In previous studies, the risk of recidivism ranged from 10 to 30%.[84,88–90] However, the authors did not observe any difference between abstinent and non-abstinent patients for survival and for compliance with immunosuppressive regimen. Therefore, the reluctance to accept alcoholic patients because of the risk of recidivism is no longer relevant.

In conclusion, patients with severe alcoholic cirrhosis benefit from liver transplantation. Most centers recommend a 6-month abstinence for listing the patients. However, this sole criterion is insufficient to predict abstinence after transplantation. Moreover, after transplantation, the recidivism of alcoholism seems to have no effect on the patients' outcome.

REFERENCES

1 Piccinino F, Sagnelli E, Pasquale G *et al.* Complications following liver biopsy: a multicentre retrospective study on 68276 biopsies. *J Hepatol* 1986; **2**: 165–73.

2 Bedossa P, Poynard T, Naveau S *et al.* Observer variation in assessment of liver biopsies of alcoholic patients. *Alc Clin Exp Res* 1988; **12**: 173–8.

3 Torres-Salinas M, Pares A, Caballeria J *et al.* Serum procollagen type III peptide as a marker of hepatic fibrogenesis in alcoholic patients. *Gastroenterology* 1986; **90**: 1241–6.

4 Niemelä O, Ristelli L, Sotaniemi EA *et al.* Aminoterminal propedtide of type III procollagen in serum in alcoholic liver disease. *Gastroenterology* 1983; **85**: 254–9.

5 Annoni G, Colombo M, Cantaluppi MC *et al.* Serum type III procollagen and laminin (Lam-P1) detect alcoholic hepatitis in chronic alcohol abusers. *Hepatology* 1989; **9**: 693–7.

6 Oberti F, Valsesia E, Pilette C *et al.* Noninvasive diagnosis of hepatic fibrosis or cirrhosis. *Gastroenterology* 1997; **113**: 1609–16.

7 Teare JP, Sherman D, Greenfield SM *et al.* Comparison of serum procollagen III peptide concentrations and PGA index for assessment of hepatic fibrosis. *Lancet* 1993; **342**: 895–8.

8 Engström-Laurent A, Loöf L, Nyberg A *et al.* Increased serum levels of hyaluronate in liver disease. *Hepatology* 1985; **5**: 638–42.

9 Nyberg A, Engström-Laurent A, Loöf L. Serum hyaluronate in primary biliary cirrhosis – a biochemical marker for progressive liver damage. *Hepatology* 1988; **8**: 142–6.

10 Plebani M, Giacomini A, Floreani A *et al.* Biochemical markers of hepatic fibrosis in primary biliary cirrhosis. *Ric Clin Lab* 1990; **20**: 269–74.

11 Pilette C, Rousselet MC, Bedossa P *et al.* Histopathological evaluation of liver fibrosis: quantitative image analysis vs semi-quantitative scores. *J Hepatol* 1998; **28**: 439–46.

12 Poynard T, Aubert A, Bedossa P *et al.* A simple biological index for detection of alcoholic liver disease in drinkers. *Gastroenterology* 1991; **100**: 1397–402.

13 Duhamel G, Nalpas B, Goldstein S *et al.* Plama lipoprotein and apolipoprotein profile in alcoholic patients with and without liver disease: on the relative roles of alcohol and liver injury. *Hepatology* 1984; **4**: 577–85.

14 Poynard T, Abella A, Pignon JP *et al.* AI and alcoholic liver disease. *Hepatology* 1986; **6**: 1391–5.

15 Bedossa P, Poynard T, Abella A *et al.* Apolipoprotein AI is a serum and tissue marker of liver fibrosis in alcoholic patients. *Alcohol Clin Exp Res* 1989; **13**: 829–33.

16 Paradis V, Laurent A, Mathurin P *et al.* Role of liver extracellular matrix in transcriptional and post-transcriptional regulation of apolipoprotein A-I by hepatocytes. *Cell Mol Biol* 1996; **42**: 525–34.

17 Paradis V, Mathurin P, Ratziu V *et al.* Binding of apolipoprotein A-I and acetaldehyde-modified apolipoprotein A-I to liver matrix. *Hepatology* 1996; **23**: 1232–8.

18 Mathurin P, Vidaud D, Vidaud M *et al.* Quantification of apolipoprotein A-I and B messenger RNA in heavy drinkers according to liver disease. *Hepatology* 1996; **23**: 44–51.

19 Nalpas B, Boigne JM, Zafrani ES *et al.* Perturbations de dix proteines plasmatiques au cours des hépatopathies alcooliques. *Gastroenterol Clin Biol* 1980; **4**: 646–54.

20 Murrray-Lyon IM, Michin Clarke HG, McPherson K *et al.* Quantitative immuno-electrophoresis of serum proteins in cryptogenic cirrhosis, alcoholic cirrhosis and active chronic hepatitis. *Clin Chim Acta* 1972; **39**: 215–20.

21 Naveau S, Poynard T, Benattar C *et al.* Alpha–2-macroglobulin and hepatic fibrosis. *Dig Dis Sci* 1994; **39**: 2426–32.

22 Bruix J, Barrera JM, Calvet X *et al.* Prevalence of antibodies to hepatitis C virus in Spanish patients with hepatocellular carcinoma and hepatic cirrhosis. *Lancet* 1989; **2**: 1004–6.

23 Di Bisceglie AM, Rustgi VK, Hoofnagle JH *et al.* Hepatocellular carcinoma. *Ann Intern Med* 1988; **108**: 390–401.

24 Poynard T, Aubert A, Lazizi Y *et al.* Independent risk factors for hepatocellular carcinoma in French drinkers. *Hepatology* 1991; **13**: 896–901.

25 Ganne-Carrie N, Chastang C, Chapel F *et al.* Predictive score for the development of hepatocellular carcinoma and additional value of liver large cell dysplasia in western patients with cirrhosis. *Hepatology* 1996; **23**: 1112–18.

26 Anthony PP, Vogel CL, Barker LF. Liver cell dysplasia: a premalignant condition. *J Clin Pathol* 1973; **26**: 217–23.

27 Borzio M, Bruno S, Roncalli M *et al.* Liver cell dysplasia is a major risk factor for hepatocellular carcinoma in cirrhosis: a prospective study. *Gastroenterology* 1996; **108**: 812–17.

28 Pateron D, Ganne N, Trinchet JC *et al.* Prospective study of screening for hepatocellular carcinoma in caucasian patients with cirrhosis. *J Hepatol* 1994; **20**: 65–71.

29 Zoli M, Magalotti D, Bianchi G *et al.* Efficacy of a surveillance program for early detection of hepatocellular carcinoma. *Cancer* 1996; **78**: 977–85.

30 Cottone M, Turri M, Caltagirone M *et al.* Screening for hepatocellular carcinoma in patients with Child's A cirrhosis: an 8-year prospective study by ultrasound and alphafetoprotein. *J Hepatol* 1994; **21**: 1029–34.

31 Mezey E Treatment of alcoholic liver disease. *Semin Liver Dis* 1993; **13**: 210–16.

32 Maddrey WC Alcoholic hepatitis: clinico-pathologic features and therapy. *Semin Liv Dis* 1988; **8**: 91–102.

33 Sacks HS, Berrier J, Reitman D *et al.* Meta-analysis of randomized controlled trials. *N Engl J Med* 1987; **19**: 450–5.

34 Kershenobich D, Vargas F, Garcia-Tsao G *et al.* Colchicine in the treatment of cirrhosis of the liver. *N Engl J Med* 1988; **318**: 1709–13.

35 Akriviadis EA, Steindel H, Pinto PC *et al.* Failure of colchicine to improve short-term survival in patients with alcoholic hepatitis. *Gastroenterology* 1990; **99**: 811–18.

36 Trinchet JC, Beaugrand M, Callard P *et al.* Treatment of alcoholic hepatitis with colchicine. Results of a randomized double blind trial. *Gastroenterol Clin Biol* 1989; **13**: 551–5.

37 Halle P, Pare P, Kaptein K *et al.* Double-blind controlled trial of propylthiouracyl in patients with severe acute alcoholic hepatitis. *Gastroenterology* 1982; **82**: 925–31.

38 Orrego H, Kalant H, Israel Y *et al.* Effect of short-term therapy with propylthiouracil in patients with alcoholic liver disease. *Gastroenterogy* 1978: 105–15.

39 Orrego H, Blake JE, Blendis LM *et al.* Long-term treatment of alcoholic liver disease with propylthiouracil. *N Engl J Med* 1987; **317**: 1421–7.

40 Orrego H, Blake JE, Blendis LM *et al.* Long-term treatment of alcoholic liver disease with propylthiouracil. Part 2: Influence of drop-out rates and of continued alcohol consumption in a clinical trial. *J Hepatol* 1994; **20**(3): 343–9.

41 Bird GL, Prach AT, McMahon AD *et al.* Randomised controlled double-blind trial of the calcium channel antagonist amlodipine in the treatment of acute alcoholic hepatitis. *J Hepatol* 1998; **28**: 194–8.

42 Resnick RH, Boinott J, Iber IL *et al.* Preliminary observations of d-penicillamine therapy in acute alcoholic liver disease. *Digestion* 1974; **11**: 257–365.

43 Pia de la Maza M, Petermann M, Bunout D *et al.* Effects of long-term vitamine E supplementation in alcoholic cirrhosis. *J Am Coll Nutr* 1995; **2**: 192–6.

44 Colman JC, Morgan MY, Sheuer PJ *et al.* Treatment of alcohol-related liver disease with (+)-cyanidanol–3: a randomised double-blind trial. *Gut* 1980; **21**: 965–9.

45 Marshall AW, Graul RS, Morgan MY *et al.* Treatment of alcohol-related liver disease with thioctic acid: a six month randomised double-blind trial. *Gut* 1982; **23**: 1088–93.

46 Multimer D, Brunner H, Berthelot P *et al.* Malotilate in alcoholic hepatitis: lessons from 3 European controlled trials (abstract). *Hepatology* 1988; **8**: 1411.

47 Keiding S, Badsberg JH, Becker U *et al.* The prognosis of patients with alcoholic liver disease. An international randomized, placebo-controlled trial on the effect of malotilate on survival. *J Hepatol* 1994; **20**: 454–60.

48 Ferenci P, Dragsics B, Dittrich H *et al.* Randomized controlled trial of silymarin treatment in patients with cirrhosis of the liver. *J Hepatol* 1989; **9**: 105–13.

49 Parès A, Planas R, Torres M *et al.* Effects of silymarin in alcoholic patients with cirrhosis of the liver: results of a controlled, double-blind, randomized and multicenter trial. *J Hepatol* 1998; **28**: 615–21.

50 Feher J, Cornides A, Romany A *et al.* A prospective multicenter study of insulin and glucagon infusion therapy in acute alcoholic hepatitis. *J Hepatol* 1987; **5**: 224–31.

51 Bird G, Lau JYN, Koskinas J *et al.* Insulin and glucagon infusion in acute alcoholic hepatitis: a randomized controlled trial. *Hepatology* 1991; **14**: 1097–101.

52 Mirouze D, Redeker AG, Reynolds TB *et al.* Traitement de l'hépatite alcoolique aiguë grave par insulin et glucagon: étude controlée sur 26 malades (abstract). *Gastroenterol Clin Biol* 1981; **5**: 1187A–8A.

53 Radvan G, Kanel G, Redeker A. Insulin and glucagon infusion in acute acoholic hepatitis (abstract). *Gastroenterology* 1982; **82**: 1154.

54 Trinchet JC, Balkau B, Poupon RE *et al.* Treatment of severe alcoholic hepatitis by infusion of insulin and glucagon: a multicenter sequential trial. *Hepatology* 1992; **15**: 76–81.

55 Islam N, Islam A. Testosterone propionate in cirrhosis of the liver. A controlled trial. *Br J Clin Pract* 1973; **27**: 125–8.

56 Gluud C, Copenhagen Study Group for Liver Diseases. Testosterone treatment of men with alcoholic cirrhosis: a double-blind study. *Hepatology* 1986; **6**: 807–13.

57 Mendenhall CL, Anderson S, Garcia-Pont P *et al.* Short-term and long-term survival in patients with alcoholic hepatitis treated with oxandrolone and prednisolone. *N Engl J Med* 1984; **311**: 1464–70.

58 Mendenhall CL, Moritz TE, Roselle GA *et al.* A study of oral nutritional support with oxandrolone in malnourished patients with alcoholic hepatitis: results of a Department of Veterans Affairs cooperative study. *Hepatology* 1993; **17**: 564–76.

59 Wells R. Prednisolone and testosterone propionate in cirrhosis of the liver. A controlled trial. *Lancet* 1960; **2**: 1416–19.

60 Blitzer BL, Mutchnick MG, Joshi PH *et al.* Adrenocorticosteroid therapy in alcoholic hepatitis: a prospective, double-blind randomized study. *Am J Dig Dis* 1977; **22**: 477–84.

61 Bories P, Guedj JY, Mirouze D *et al.* Traitement de l'hépatite alcoolique aiguë par la prednisolone. *Presse Med* 1987; **16**: 769–72.

62 Carithers RL Jr, Herlong HF, Diehl AM *et al.* Methylprednisolone therapy in patients with severe alcoholic hepatitis: a randomized multicenter trial. *Ann Intern Med* 1989; **110**: 685–90.

63 Campra JL, Hamlin EM, Kirshbaum RJ *et al.* Prednisone therapy of acute alcoholic hepatitis. *Ann Intern Med* 1973; **79**: 625–31.

64 Depew W, Boyer T, Omata M *et al.* Double-blind controlled trial of prednisolone therapy in patients with severe acute alcoholic hepatitis and spontaneous encephalopathy. *Gastroenterology* 1980; **78**: 524–9.

65 Helman RA, Temko MH, Nye SW *et al.* Natural history and evaluation of prednisolone therapy. *Ann Intern Med* 1971; **74**: 311–21.

66 Lesesne HR, Bozymski EM, Fallon HJ. Treatment of alcoholic hepatitis with encephalopathy. Comparison of prednisolone with caloric supplements. *Gastroenterology* 1978; **74**: 169–73.
67 Maddrey WC, Boitnott JK, Bedine MS *et al.* Corticosteroid therapy of alcoholic hepatitis. *Gastroenterology* 1978; **75**: 193–9.
68 Ramond MJ, Poynard T, Rueff B *et al.* A randomized trial of prednisolone in patients with severe alcoholic hepatitis. *N Engl J Med* 1992; **326**: 507–12.
69 Shumaker JB, Resnick RH, Galambos JT *et al.* A controlled trial of 6-methylprednisolone in acute alcoholic hepatitis. *Am J Gastroenterol* 1978; **69**: 443–9.
70 Theodossi A, Eddleston ALWF, Williams R. Controlled trial of methylprednisolone therapy in severe acute alcoholic hepatitis. *Gut* 1982; **23**: 75–9.
71 Porter HP, Simon FR, Pope CE *et al.* Corticosteroid therapy in severe alcoholic hepatitis. *N Engl J Med* 1971; **284**: 1350–5.
72 Mathurin P, Bernard B, Quichon JP *et al.* L'hémorragie digestive et l'insuffisance rénale: deux facteurs de confusion dans l'analyse de l'efficacité des corticoïdes dans l'hépatite alcoolique aiguë (abstract). *Gastroenterol Clin Biol* 1995; **19**: A162.
73 Imperiale TF, McCullough AJ. Do corticosteroids reduce mortality from alcoholic hepatitis? *Ann Intern Med* 1990; **113**: 299–307.
74 Mathurin P, Duchatelle V, Ramond MJ *et al.* Survival and prognostic factors in patients with severe biopsy-proven alcoholic hepatitis treated by prednisolone: randomized trial, new cohort, and simulation. *Gastroenterology* 1996; **110**: 1847–53.
75 Akriviadis E, Botla R, Birggs W *et al.* Improved short-term survival with pentoxifylline treatment in severe alcoholic hepatitis (abstract). *Hepatology* 1997; **26**: 250A.
76 Mato JM, Camara J, Ortiz P *et al.* S-adenosylmethionine in the treatment of alcoholic cirrhosis: results from a multicentric placebo-controlled, randomized, double-blind clinical trial. *Hepatology* 1997; **26**: 251A.
77 Stefanini GF, Biselli M, Grazi GL *et al.* Orthotopic liver transplantation for alcoholic liver disease: rates of survival, complications and relapse. *Hepatogastroenterology* 1997; **44**: 1356–9.
78 Starzl TE, Van Thiel D, Tzakis AG *et al.* Orthotopic liver transplantation for alcoholic cirrhosis. *JAMA* 1988; **260**: 2542–4.
79 Lucey MR, Merion MR, Henley KS *et al.* Selection for and outcome of liver trasplantation in alcoholic liver disease. *Gastroenterology* 1992; **102**: 1736–41.
80 Poynard T, Barthelemy P, Fratte S *et al.* Evaluation of liver transplantation in alcoholic cirrhosis by a case–control study and simulated controls. *Lancet* 1994; **344**: 502–7.
81 Anand AC, Ferraz-Neto BH, Nightingale P *et al.* Liver transplantation for alcoholic liver disease: evaluation of a selection protocol. *Hepatology* 1997; **25**: 1478–84.
82 Snyder SL, Drooker M, Strain JJ A survey estimate of academic liver transplant teams' selection practices for alcohol-dependent applicants. *Psychosomatics* 1996; **37**: 432–7.
83 Yates WR, Martin M, LaBrecque D *et al.* A model to examine the validity of the 6-month abstinence criterion for liver transplantation *Alcohol Clin Exp Res* 1998; **22**: 513–17.
84 Foster PF, Fabrega F, Karademir S *et al.* Prediction of abstinence from ethanol in alcoholic recipients following liver transplantation. *Hepatology* 1997; **25**: 1469–77.
85 Bird JLA, O'Grady JG, Harvey FAH *et al.* Liver transplantation in patients with alcoholic cirrhosis: selection criteria and rates of survival and relapse. *Br Med J* 1990; **301**: 15–17.
86 Kumar S, Strauber RE, Gavaler JS *et al.* Orthotopic liver transplantation for alcoholic liver disease. *Hepatology* 1990; **11**: 159–64.
87 Osario RW, Ascher NL, Avery M *et al.* Predicting recidivism after orthotopic liver transplantation for alcoholic liver disease. *Hepatology* 1994; **20**: 105–10.
88 Lucey MR, Carr K, Beresford TP *et al.* Alcohol use after liver transplantation in alcoholics: a clinical cohort follow-up study. *Hepatology* 1997; **25**: 1223–7.
89 Shelton W, Balint JA. Fair treatment of alcoholic patients in the context of liver transplantation. *Alcohol Clin Exp Res* 1997; **21**: 93–100.
90 Berlakovich GA, Steininger R, Herbst F *et al.* Efficacy of liver transplantation for alcoholic cirrhosis with respect to recidivism and compliance. *Transplantation* 1994; **58**: 560–5.

Hemochromatosis and Wilson disease: diagnosis and treatment 20

GARY JEFFREY, PAUL C ADAMS

Hemochromatosis is the most common genetic disease in populations of European ancestry. Despite estimates in different countries ranging from 1 in 100 to 1 in 300, hemochromatosis is still considered by many physicians to be a rare disease. The diagnosis can be difficult because of the non-specific nature of the symptoms. The discovery of the hemochromatosis gene in 1996[1] has led to new insights into the pathogenesis of the disease and new diagnostic strategies.[2]

DIAGNOSIS OF HEMOCHROMATOSIS

A paradox of genetic hemochromatosis is the observation that the disease is underdiagnosed in the general population with genetic hemochromatosis, and overdiagnosed in patients with secondary iron overload.

Underdiagnosis of hemochromatosis

Preliminary population studies using genetic testing have demonstrated a prevalence of homozygotes of 1 in 100 in Ireland[3] and 1 in 150 in Australia.[4] The fact that many physicians consider hemochromatosis to be rare implies either a lack of penetrance of the gene (non-expressing homozygote) or a large number of patients that remain undiagnosed in the community. Until larger genetic population studies allow us to estimate the percentage of homozygotes without iron overload, it is likely that both of these factors are contributory.

A major problem in the diagnosis of hemochromatosis is the lack of symptoms and the non-specific nature of symptoms. An elderly patient who presents with joint symptoms and diabetes is not often considered to have genetic hemochromatosis. The presenting features vary depending on age and gender but fatigue is the most common complaint. Women are more likely to have fatigue, arthralgia, and pigmentation than they are to have liver disease and usually present in the post-menopausal period.[5]

Diagnostic tests for hemochromatosis

SERUM IRON

An elevated serum iron is found in most but not all cases. Serum iron can vary throughout the day and it has been estimated that approximately 5–10% of homozygotes have a normal serum iron.[6]

TRANSFERRIN SATURATION

The transferrin saturation is the serum iron/total iron binding capacity. The transferrin saturation has a sensitivity of greater than 90% for hemochromatosis when a phenotypic case definition is used. A fasting value has greater specificity but may not always be practical. The transferrin saturation is elevated even in young adults with hemochromatosis before the development of iron overload and a rising ferritin. The threshold to pursue further diagnostic studies has varied from 45 to 62% in various studies. A lower threshold picks up more patients with hemochromatosis but also leads to more investigations in patients without hemochromatosis. A higher threshold leads to fewer investigations overall with a greater possibility of missing some patients. These concepts are most relevant when considering population screening.[7]

SERUM FERRITIN

The relationship between serum ferritin and total body iron stores has been clearly established by strong correlations with hepatic iron concentration and amount of iron removed by venesection.[8] However, ferritin can be elevated secondary to chronic inflammation and histiocytic neoplasms. A major diagnostic dilemma in the past was whether an elevated serum ferritin value is related to hemochromatosis or to another underlying liver disease such as alcoholic liver disease, chronic viral hepatitis or non-alcoholic steatohepatitis. It is likely that many of these difficult cases will now be resolved by genetic testing.

IRON REMOVED BY VENESECTION

Since hemochromatosis is usually diagnosed when symptoms develop in the fifth or sixth decade, patients have significant iron overload at the time of diagnosis. The removal of 500 ml of blood weekly (0.25 g iron) is well tolerated, often for years, without the development of significant anemia. It used to be felt that if a patient became anemic (hemoglobin <10 g/dl) after only six venesections, it suggested mild iron overload incompatible with the diagnosis of hereditary hemochromatosis. The latter consideration may no longer apply as population and pedigree studies uncover patients in the second and third decade who have far less iron overload.[9] At our center, only 71% of homozygotes would have met the arbitrary criterion that more than 5 g of iron (20 venesections) were removed without anemia.[10] Thus the response to venesection has become a criterion for hemochromatosis which will no longer be relevant in the era of genetic testing.

LIVER BIOPSY

Liver biopsy has been the 'gold standard' diagnostic test for hemochromatosis. Liver biopsy has shifted from a diagnostic tool to a prognostic guide. The need for liver biopsy seems less apparent in the young asymptomatic patient with a low clinical suspicion of cirrhosis based on history, physical examination, and iron studies. Clinical guidelines have been suggested, such as thresholds of serum ferritin of <1000 μg/l or age under 40 to reduce the need for liver biopsy. However, in a study of 304 homozygotes, 20% of patients were cirrhotic with a ferritin <1000 μg/l and 8% of patients aged under 40 had cirrhosis.[11] Clinical judgement and assessment of concomitant risk factors (alcohol, viral hepatitis) would be a better guide for the need for liver biopsy rather than employing an arbitrary threshold. Most non-cirrhotic patients with hemochromatosis have a serum ferritin <1000 μg/l *and* a normal AST.[12]

Patients with cirrhosis due to genetic haemochromatosis have a 5.5-fold relative risk of death compared to the non-cirrhotic hemochromatosis patients.[13,14] Cirrhotic patients are also at risk of hepatocellular carcinoma. The mean age of hepatocellular carcinoma is 68 years in our series, but has been lower in Italian patients with concomitant viral hepatitis.[15] Although early detection has been clearly demonstrated by serial ultrasound and alpha-fetoprotein determination, curative treatment options remain limited. An elderly cirrhotic patient may not withstand a major resection and the residual cirrhotic liver remains a fertile ground for new tumor development. Organ shortages often preclude the possibility of immediate liver transplantation which has shown promising results in solitary tumors <5 cm in diameter. Screening for hepatocellular carcinoma is a time and resource intensive program and in the area of hemochromatosis, resources would be better utilized if directed towards population screening for the disease in the pre-cirrhotic stage to permit early venesection therapy and thus prevent cirrhosis and hepatocellular carcinoma.

HEPATIC IRON CONCENTRATION AND HEPATIC IRON INDEX

The traditional method of assessing iron status by liver biopsy utilizes the semi-quantitative staining method of Perls. However, when moderate iron overload is present, the degree of iron overload can be difficult to interpret. Iron concentration can be measured using atomic absorption spectrophotometry. Since this can be done on paraffin embedded tissue, special preparation is not required at the time of the biopsy. An advantage of cutting the tissue for iron determination from the paraffin block is that it affords greater certainty that the tissue assayed is the same as the tissue examined microscopically. The normal reference range for hepatic iron concentration is 0–35 μmol/g (<2000 μg/g). The hepatic iron concentration (μmol/g) divided by age (years) is the hepatic iron index. This was demonstrated by Bassett *et al* to be a useful test in differentiating the patient with genetic hemochromatosis from the patient with alcoholic siderosis.[16] The index remains a useful test in this clinical setting but has been extrapolated to be a diagnostic criterion for hemochromatosis. A threshold of 1.9 for the hepatic iron index had a 91% sensitivity for hemochromatosis.[17] However, early diagnosis resulting from population screening and from pedigree studies has led to the recognition of many homozygotes with a hepatic iron index <1.9.[18] Moreover, increasing awareness of the concept of moderate iron overload in cirrhosis of any etiology has demonstrated that many patients without hemochromatosis who have a hepatic iron index >1.9.[19] The hepatic iron index will become less useful with the advent of genetic testing. The commentary on liver biopsy reports that the hepatic iron index is greater than 1.9, confirming a diagnosis of genetic hemochromatosis should be strongly discouraged. It may be most useful in the unusual hemochromatosis patient who is negative by conventional genetic testing but clinically seems to have genetic hemochromatosis.

IMAGING STUDIES OF THE LIVER

Magnetic resonance imaging (MRI) can demonstrate moderate to severe iron overload of the liver. The technology is advancing and it is possible that eventually it may be as precise as hepatic iron determination.[20] Proponents of MRI to alleviate the need for liver biopsy emphasized the non-invasive nature of the test for the diagnosis. As previously discussed,

Table 20.1 Prevalence of C282Y homozygotes in hemochromatosis studies

Study	Population[a]	Country	C282Y homozygotes (%)
Adams, 1998[10]	Suspected clinical diagnosis	Canada	122/128 (95)
Feder,1996[1]	Suspected clinical diagnosis	USA	148/178 (83)
Burke, 1998[22]	Suspected clinical diagnosis	USA	121/147 (82)
Jouanolle, 1996[21]	Suspected clinical diagnosis	France	59/65 (93)
Carella, 1997[24]	Suspected clinical diagnosis	Italy	48/75 (64)
UK Consortium, 1997[23]	Suspected clinical diagnosis	United Kingdom	105/115 (91)
Cullen, 1997[4]	Family studies	Australia	112/112 (100)

[a]Suspected clinical diagnosis includes isolated iron loaded probands and probands with discovered relatives.

the role of liver biopsy has now shifted from a diagnostic tool to a prognostic tool. It is likely that the presence of an elevated ferritin with a positive genetic test would satisfy the non-invasive clinician more than an MRI study. The MRI can also demonstrate the clinical features of cirrhosis such as nodularity of the liver, ascites, portal hypertension, and splenomegaly as well as hepatocellular carcinoma. These features can be more readily assessed by abdominal ultrasound at a lower cost. Dual energy CT scanning can also quantitate liver iron concentration but is not widely used. Magnetic susceptibility has been studied using a SQUID machine but the technology is not widely available.

GENETIC TESTING FOR HEMOCHROMATOSIS

A major advance which stems from the discovery of the hemochromatosis gene is the use of a diagnostic genetic test. The original publication reported that 83% of a group of patients with suspected hemochromatosis had the characteristic C282Y mutation of the *HFE* gene. In the original report, the gene was called HLA-H but this name was later changed to *HFE*.[1] The C282Y mutation is also reported as 845A in some laboratories, reflecting the base pair change rather than the amino acid change. Subsequent studies in well defined hemochromatosis pedigrees reported that 90–100% of typical hemochromatosis patients had the C282Y mutation (Table 20.1).[10,17,21–23] The presence of a single mutation in most patients was in marked contrast to other genetic diseases in which multiple mutations were discovered (cystic fibrosis, Wilson disease, α_1-antitrypsin deficiency). A second minor mutation, H63D, was also described in the original report.[1] This mutation does not cause the same intracellular trafficking defect of the *HFE* protein and many homozygotes for H63D have been found without iron overload in the general population. Compound heterozygotes (C282Y/H63D) may resemble homozygotes with mild to moderate iron overload.[25,26]

The interpretation of the test in several settings is shown in Table 20.2. The test may also be done on DNA extracted from paraffin embedded tissue such as liver explants. Studies of explanted livers has demonstrated that many liver transplant patients classified as hemochromatosis patients are negative for the C282Y mutation.[27] This suggests that those patients may have had iron overload secondary to chronic liver disease rather than hemochromatosis. Therefore any interpretation of iron reaccumulation post-liver transplant for hemochromatosis must be viewed with caution.

Genetic discrimination is a concern with the widespread use of genetic testing. A positive genetic test even without iron overload could disqualify a patient for health or life

Table 20.2 Interpretation of C282Y genetic testing for hemochromatosis

Patient/action required	C282Y+/C282Y+	C282Y+/C282Y–	C282Y–/C282–-
Patient found to have elevated transferrin saturation and ferritin without other risk factors	Hemochromatosis homozygote	Hemochromatosis heterozygote	Normal
Action required	Venesection therapy and family investigations	Consider investigations in siblings, consider further genetic testing for H63D	Reconsider HFE negative hemochromatosis or another diagnosis. Venesect if hepatic iron concentration high
Asymptomatic patient with normal transferrin saturation and ferritin	Non-expressing homozygote (incomplete penetrance)	Typical heterozygote	Normal
Action required	Family investigations and repeat iron studies every 2 years	Testing of siblings and spouse to be considered	No further studies
Alcoholic patient, HCV+ with elevated ferritin	Hemochromatosis homozygote	Hemochromatosis heterozygote with secondary iron overload	Most likely secondary iron overload
Action required	Venesection therapy and family investigations	Consider investigations in siblings, consider further genetic testing for H63D	No venesections or family studies

insurance. In the case of hemochromatosis, the advantages of early diagnosis of a treatable disease outweigh the disadvantages of genetic discrimination.

GENOTYPIC–PHENOTYPIC CORRELATION IN HEMOCHROMATOSIS

If we define the presence of homozygosity for the C282Y mutation as the new "gold standard" for hemochromatosis, it provides for the first time a benchmark for the assessment of the phenotypic diagnostic tools that have been used for decades. Transferrin saturation, ferritin, hepatic iron index, and iron removed by venesection were studied in putative homozygotes that had been previously evaluated at this medical center. Patients were homozygous for the C282Y mutation in 122/128 cases (95%). In C282Y homozygotes, the hepatic iron index was >1.9 in 91.3%, transferrin saturation >55% in 90%, serum ferritin >300 μg/l in 96% of men, >200 μg/l in 97% of women, and iron removed >5 g in 70% of men and 73% of women. There were four homozygotes for C282Y with no biochemical evidence of iron overload. The sensitivity of the phenotypic tests in decreasing order was – serum ferritin, hepatic iron index, transferrin saturation, and iron removed by venesection. Although the genetic test is very useful for the diagnosis of hemochromatosis, this study revealed both iron loaded patients without the mutation and homozygous patients without iron overload.[10] C282Y homozygotes have been identified without iron overload but it is important to exclude a false positive genetic test which has been described with a common polymorphism in intron 4 of *HFE*.[28]

NON-EXPRESSSING HOMOZYGOTES

As genetic testing becomes more widespread there is an increasing number of persons found to have the hemochromatosis gene without iron overload. The prevalence of the non-expressing homozygotes is not yet determined from population studies, but this phenomenon may explain the wide discrepancy between the gene frequency and the clinician's perception that this is an uncommon disease. Patients who are homozygous for the C282Y mutation should be considered at risk of developing iron overload. However, if there are no abnormalities in transferrin saturation or ferritin in adulthood, it seems more likely that such patients are non expressing homozygotes rather than patients who will develop iron overload later in life. This needs to be determined in prospective studies.

FAMILY STUDIES IN HEMOCHROMATOSIS

R Grade C

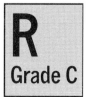

Once the proband case is identified and confirmed with the genetic test for the C282Y mutation, family testing is imperative. Siblings have a 1 in 4 chance of carrying the gene and should be screened with the genetic test, transferrin saturation, and serum ferritin. The risk to a child is dependent on the prevalence of heterozygotes in the community and is probably greater than 1 in 20 and much lower if the spouse is non-caucasian. A cost-effective strategy is now possible with the genetic test is to test the spouse for the C282Y mutation to assess the risk in the children. If the spouse is not a heterozygote or homozygote, the children will be obligate heterozygotes. This assumes paternity and excludes another gene or mutation causing hemochromatosis. This strategy is particularly advantageous where the children are geographically separated or may be under a different physician or health care system.[29] Genetic testing in general raises many perplexing questions which have not yet been tested in hemochromatosis such as pre-marital testing, in utero testing, and paternity issues.

If an isolated heterozygote is detected by genetic testing, it is recommended that siblings be tested. Extended family studies are less revealing than study of a family with an identified homozygote, but are more likely than random population screening to uncover a homozygote.

R Grade C

It is important to remember that there will be patients with a clinical picture indistinguishable from genetic hemochromatosis who will be negative for the C282Y mutation. Most of these patients will be isolated cases, although a few cases of familial iron overload have been reported with negative C282Y testing.[24] In these cases, it may be prudent to do HLA-A typing to facilitate the study of siblings. A negative C282Y test should alert the physician to question the diagnosis of genetic hemochromatosis and reconsider secondary iron overload related to cirrhosis, alcohol, viral hepatitis or iron loading anemias. If no other risk factors are found, the patient should begin venesection treatment similar to any other hemochromatosis patient.

Treatment of hemochromatosis

Patients are initially treated by the weekly removal of 500 ml of blood in an ambulatory care facility. A hemoglobin is done at the time of each venesection. If the hemoglobin decreases to less than 10 g/dl the venesection schedule is modified to 500 ml every other week. Serum ferritin is measured periodically (3-monthly in severe iron overload, monthly in mild iron overload) and weekly venesections are continued until the serum ferritin is approximately 50 μg/l. Transferrin saturation often remains elevated despite therapy. Patients may then begin maintenance venesections three to four times per year.[30] Iron reaccumulation is an inconsistent observation and many patients will remain without treatment without a rise in serum ferritin for many years.[31] Chelation therapy is not used for the treatment of hemochromatosis.

There are no randomized trials comparing venesection therapy to no treatment. Iron depletion before the development of cirrhosis can prevent cirrhosis and the development of hepatocellular carcinoma. Patients with cirrhosis have a 5.5-fold relative risk of death, and non-cirrhotic treated patients have a survival similar to an age- and sex-matched control group.[13,14] Therefore the goal is early detection and treatment before the development of cirrhosis. This concept has led to the introduction of population screening (Table 20.3) for hemochromatosis using a combination of phenotypic and genotypic testing.[32,33] Implementation of population screening is dependent on the willingness of private or government health agencies to pay the initial screening costs to achieve savings many years later.[34]

R
Grade B/C

Table 20.3 Population screening for hemochromatosis

WHO criteria for screening for medical disease	Phenotypic testing (serum iron, transferrin saturation, UIBC, ferritin)	Genotypic testing (C282Y mutation)
Is the disease an important health problem?	Yes (1 in 300)	Yes (1 in 150)
Is there an effective treatment?	Yes	Yes
Are there facilities for diagnosis and treatment?	Yes	Yes
Is there a pre-symptomatic stage?	Yes	Yes
Is the cost of screening reasonable?	Yes	If limited to few mutations
Is continuous case-finding on an ongoing basis feasible?	Yes	Yes
Is there a suitable test?	Yes	Yes
Is the testing acceptable to the population?	Yes	Genetic discrimination?
Is the natural history of disease understood?	Yes	Uncertain in non-expressing homozygotes
Is there agreement on whom to treat?	Yes	Yes

WILSON DISEASE

Clinical features

Wilson disease is an uncommon but important inherited disorder of copper metabolism that is caused by increased copper accumulation in the liver, brain, cornea, kidney, and other tissues. It occurs worldwide with a prevalence of 1 in 30 000 and is inherited as an autosomal recessive disorder.[35] If left untreated the natural history is progressive, with 42% of patients presenting with acute or chronic liver disease, the majority during childhood or early adolescence, although rarely patients may present as late as 58 years. As many as 15% of patients also present with hemolysis in this same young age group. Severe debilitating neurological and psychiatric symptoms are the presenting feature in 44% of patients and these symptoms present somewhat later in adolescence or early adulthood. Prior to the availability of liver transplantation death resulted commonly from the complications of liver failure, although some patients died from progressive neurological dysfunction or hemolysis. Early recognition of Wilson disease allows initiation of treatment that results in the reversal of symptoms and prevents complications and death.

Genetic analysis

The cloning of the Wilson disease gene and the identification of mutations responsible for this disorder has resulted in exciting advances in our understanding of the pathophysiology of this disease.[36–38] The gene encodes for a cation-transporting P-type ATPase that is expressed in the liver and brain. Within the hepatocyte the protein is found diffusely throughout the cytoplasm but is also localized to the golgi.[39] Mutations in the gene result in defective biliary excretion of copper and increased tissue copper levels, however the exact role of the protein in copper excretion remains unknown. The identification of the Wilson disease gene also has implications for the genetic diagnosis of this disorder. However, genotype analysis of the Wilson disease gene has found that no single mutation is responsible for all or even the majority of patients with the disorder and more than 60 different mutations have now been reported. The most common mutation is a His1069Gln substitution, which occurs in between 20 and 60% of patients depending on the population studied. Some studies suggest an association between the His1069Glu mutation and late onset disease and neurological symptoms, however this has not been confirmed by others.[39–41]

Diagnosis

The diagnosis of Wilson disease is made on the basis of clinical and biochemical features with the addition of genotype analysis in family studies (Table 20.4). The diagnostic utility of individual biochemical abnormalities depends on the manner in which a patient presents. In most patients the presence of a serum ceruloplasmin level less than 20 mg/dl and the finding of Kayser–Fleischer rings by slit lamp examination is diagnostic.[42] In those patients with only one of these abnormalities an elevated liver copper level (greater than 250 μg/g dry weight) will confirm the diagnosis. If liver biopsy is contraindicated then an

Table 20.4 Usefulness of diagnostic tests for Wilson disease

Test	Abnormality	Advantage	Disadvantage
Slit lamp examination	Kayser–Fleisher corneal rings	Easily assessed physical finding	Normal in 10–45% of patients, mainly the young
Serum ceruloplasmin	Less than 20 mg/l	Decreased in 73–95% of patients	May be normal, mainly with liver disease
24-hour copper excretion	More than 100 µg/24 hours	Increased in 85% of patients. Useful in acute liver failure	Copper contamination and incomplete sample
Non-ceruloplasmin bound copper	More than 12 µg/dL	Increased when ceruloplasmin levels are normal	Not routinely reported
Liver copper quantitation	More than 250 µg/gram dry weight	Increased in 90% or more of patients	Elevated in chronic cholestasis Sampling errors
Radio-copper scan	Lack of copper binding by ceruloplasmin	Differentiates homozygotes and heterozygotes	Blood samples over 48 hours

elevated 24-hour urinary copper excretion (greater than 100 µg/24 hours), an abnormal radio-copper scan or increased non-ceruloplasmin bound serum copper levels (greater than 12 µg/dl) may be confirmatory.

Screening

Screening the general population for Wilson disease is not cost-effective given the low prevalence of disease and the lack of a single accurate diagnostic test. Screening should be performed in siblings of patients with Wilson disease, as one in four of this group will have homozygous disease. A recent series found that 18% of patients were diagnosed on the basis of family screening and that only one (10%) of these patients was symptomatic at the time of diagnosis.[41] It has been recommended that all psychiatric patients who show signs of liver or neurological disease, or who are refractory to therapy should be screened for Wilson disease. The cost-effectiveness of this strategy has not yet been analyzed. Screening all patients with liver disease with a serum ceruloplasmin estimation found that the positive predictive value of this test was only 5.9%.[42] Screening unselected patients with liver disease was therefore not cost-effective and it was recommended that screening should be restricted to those patients with liver disease of unknown etiology. The cost-effectiveness of this recommendation needs to be further analyzed.

Management

The key to effective drug therapy for Wilson disease is the early detection of disease before the onset of structural neurological abnormalities or cirrhosis. The mainstay of drug

R Grade C

treatment for Wilson disease for the past 40 years has been penicillamine.[40,43] This drug given at a dose of 1.5–2.0 g/day has proven to be an effective copper chelating agent and will reverse or improve the symptoms and signs of Wilson disease. It also prevents the onset of symptoms in asymptomatic patients. Adverse effects occur in 20% of patients within the first month but most of these are due to hypersensitivity and respond to drug cessation and short term prednisolone followed by reintroduction of penicillamine at small doses (250 mg/day). Dose reduction has also been recommended to reduce the adverse effects on skin and elastic tissue. Long term penicillamine therapy needs to be terminated in only 5% of patients. Pyridoxine deficiency may rarely be induced by penicillamine and 25 mg daily supplements are recommended. Unfortunately penicillamine causes significant symptomatic deterioration in 20% of those patients presenting with neurological symptoms and alternative drugs may be required in this situation.

R Grade C

R Grade C

A small number of alternative agents have been shown to be effective in the treatment of Wilson disease. Trientine at a dose of 1–2 g/day is an effective copper chelating agent and may be used in those patients who suffer severe reactions to penicillamine or develop deteriorating neurological symptoms with this drug. Zinc therapy of 75–150 mg/day has been shown to maintain low copper levels in those patients already on maintenance therapy by increasing gastrointestinal copper excretion.[43] It may be useful in those patients unable to tolerate either penicillamine or trientine but is not considered to be the ideal treatment for Wilson disease. Most recently, ammonium thiomolybdate (60–100 mg/day) was shown to effectively bind copper and block intestinal copper absorption, and was able to decrease hepatic copper levels in a limited number of patients.[44] Of 33 patients with neurological symptoms who were initially treated with this drug only, one showed neurological deterioration. Further studies are required to confirm the effectiveness and safety of this agent.

R Grade C

Liver transplantation is required in those patients with acute liver failure or those suffering from complications of cirrhosis. Transplantation cures the hepatic copper excretory abnormality, and survival post-transplantation is similar to patients with other causes of liver disease undergoing this procedure.[45] Transplantation is not recommended for those patients who have only extrahepatic manifestations of Wilson disease.

REFERENCES

1 Feder JN, Gnirke A, Thomas W *et al.* A novel MHC class I-like gene is mutated in patients with hereditary hemochromatosis. *Nature Genet* 1996; **13**: 399–408.

2 Bacon BR, Powell L, Adams PC *et al.* Molecular medicine and hemochromatosis: at the crossroads. *Gastroenterology* 1999; **116**: 193–207.

3 Ryan E, O'Keane C, Crowe J. Hemochromatosis in Ireland and HFE. *Blood Cells Mol Dis* 1998; **24**: 428–32.

4 Cullen LM, Sommerville L, Glassick TCDHG *et al.* Neonatal screening for the hemochromatosis defect. *Blood* 1997; **90**: 4236–7.

5 Moirand R, Adams PC, Bicheler V *et al.* Clinical features of genetic hemochromatosis in women compared to men. *Ann Intern Med* 1997; **127**: 105–10.

6 Adams PC, Valberg LS. Evolving expression of hereditary hemochromatosis. *Semin Liver Dis* 1996; **16**: 47–54.

7 Adams PC. Population screening for hemochromatosis. *Hepatology* 1999; **29**: 1324–7.

8 Brissot P, Bourel M, Herry D *et al.* Assessment of liver iron content in 271 patients: a reevaluation of direct and indirect methods. *Gastroenterology* 1981; **80**: 557–65.

9 Adams PC, Kertesz AE, Valberg LS. Clinical presentation of hemochromatosis: a changing scene. *Am J Med* 1991; **90**: 445–9.

10 Adams PC, Chakrabarti S. Genotypic/phenotypic correlations in genetic hemochromatosis: evolution of diagnostic criteria. *Gastroenterology* 1998; **114**: 319–23.

11 Adams PC, Deugnier Y, Moirand R *et al.* Relationship between age, ferritin, and cirrhosis in genetic hemochromatosis: implications for liver biopsy. [Abstract] *Hepatology* 1997; **26**: 468A.

12 Guyader D, Jacquelinet C, Moirand R *et al.* Non-invasive prediction of fibrosis in C282Y homozygous hemochromatosis. *Gastroenterology* 1998; **115**: 929–36.
13 Adams PC, Speechley M, Kertesz AE. Long-term survival analysis in hereditary hemochromatosis. *Gastroenterology* 1991; **101**: 368–72.
14 Niederau C, Fischer R, Purschel A *et al.* Long-term survival in patients with hereditary hemochromatosis. *Gastroenterology* 1996; **110**: 1107–19.
15 Fargion S, Mandelli C, Piperno A *et al.* Survival and prognostic factors in 212 Italian patients with genetic hemochromatosis. *Hepatology* 1992; **15**: 655–9.
16 Bassett ML, Halliday JW, Powell LW. Value of hepatic iron measurements in early hemochromatosis and determination of the critical iron level associated with fibrosis. *Hepatology* 1986; **6**: 24–9.
17 Adams PC, Bradley C, Henderson AR. Evaluation of the hepatic iron index as a diagnostic criterion in hereditary hemochromatosis. *J Lab Clin Med* 1997; **130**: 509–14.
18 Adams PC, Deugnier Y, Moirand R *et al.* The relationship between iron overload, clinical symptoms and age in 410 patients with genetic hemochromatosis. *Hepatology* 1997; **25**: 162–6.
19 Ludwig J, Hashimoto E, Porayko M *et al.* Hemosiderosis in cirrhosis: a study of 447 native livers. *Gastroenterology* 1997; **112**: 882–8.
20 Guyader D, Gandon Y, Robert JY *et al.* Magnetic resonance imaging and assessment of liver iron content in genetic hemochromatosis. *J Hepatol* 1992; **15**: 304–8.
21 Jouanolle A-M, Gandon G, Jezequel P *et al.* Haemochromatosis and HLA-H. *Nature Genet* 1996; **14**: 251–2.
22 Burke W, Thomson E, Khoury M *et al.* Hereditary hemochromatosis: gene discovery and its implications for population-based screening. *JAMA* 1998; **280**: 172–8.
23 The UK Haemochromatosis Consortium. A simple genetic test identifies 90% of UK patients with haemochromatosis. *Gut* 1997; **41**: 841–5.
24 Carella M, D'Ambrosio L, Totaro A *et al.* Mutation analysis of the HLA-H gene in Italian hemochromatosis patients. *Am J Hum Genet* 1997; **60**: 828–32.
25 Bacon BR, Olynyk J, Brunt E *et al.* HFE genotype in patients with hemochromatosis and other liver diseases. *Ann Intern Med* 1999; **130**: 953–62.
26 Moirand R, Jouanolle A-M, Brissot P *et al.* Phenotypic expression of HFE mutations: a French study of 1110 unrelated iron-overloaded patients and relatives. *Gastroenterology* 1999; **116**: 372–7.
27 Minguillan J, Lee R, Britton R *et al.* Genetic markers for hemochromatosis in patients with cirrhosis and iron overload. [Abstract] *Hepatology* 1997; **26**: 158A.
28 Jeffrey G, Chakrabarti S, Hegele RA *et al.* PC. Polymorphism in intron 4 of HFE may cause overestimation of C282Y homozygote prevalence in haemochromatosis. *Nature Genet* 1999; **22**.
29 Adams PC. Implications of genotyping of spouses to limit investigation of children in genetic hemochromatosis. *Clin Genet* 1998; **53**: 176–8.
30 Adams PC. Factors affecting rate of iron mobilization during venesection therapy for hereditary hemochromatosis. *Am J Hematol* 1998; **58**: 16–19.
31 Adams PC, Kertesz AE, Valberg LS. Rate of iron reaccumulation following iron depletion in hereditary hemochromatosis. Implications for venesection therapy. *J Clin Gastroenterol* 1993; **16**: 207–10.
32 Adams PC, Gregor JC, Kertesz AE *et al.* Screening blood donors for hereditary hemochromatosis: decision analysis model based on a thirty-year database. *Gastroenterology* 1995; **109**: 177–88.
33 Niederau C, Niederau CM, Lange S *et al.* Screening for hemochromatosis and iron deficiency in employees and primary care patients in Western Germany. *Ann Intern Med* 1998; **128**: 337–45.
34 Adams PC, Valberg LS. Screening blood donors for hereditary hemochromatosis: decision analysis model comparing genotyping to phenotyping. *Am J Gastroenterol* 1999; **94**: 1593–600.
35 Bull PC, Thomas GR, Rommens JM *et al.* The Wilson disease gene is a putative copper transporting P-type ATPase similar to the Menkes gene. *Nature Genet* 1993; **5**: 327–37.
36 Tanzi RE, Petrukhin K, Chernov *et al.* The Wilson disease gene is a copper transporting ATPase with homology to the Menkes disease gene. *Nature Genet* 1993; **5**: 344–50.
37 Hung I, Suzuki M, Yamaguchi Y *et al.* Biochemical characterization of the Wilson disease protein and functional expression in the yeast *Saccharomyces cerevisiae*. *J Biol Chem* 1997; **272**: 21461–6.
38 Forbes J, Hsi G, Cox D. Role of the copper-binding domain in the copper transport function of ATP7B, the P-type ATPase defective in Wilson disease. *J Biol Chem* 1999; **274**: 12408–13.
39 Shah A, Chernov I, Zhang H *et al.* Identification and analysis of mutations in the Wilson disease gene (ATP7B): population frequencies, genotype-phenotype correlation, and functional analysis. *Am J Hum Genet* 1997; **61**: 317–28.
40 Thomas G, Forbes J, Roberts E *et al.* The Wilson disease gene: spectrum of mutations and their consequences. *Nature Genet* 1995; **9**: 210–17.
41 Steindl P, Ferenci P, Dienes H *et al.* Wilson's disease in patients presenting with liver disease: a diagnostic challenge. *Gastroenterology* 1997; **113**: 212–18.
42 Cauza E, Dobersberger T, Polli C *et al.* Screening for Wilson's disease in patients with liver disease by

serum ceruloplasmin. *J Hepatol* 1997; **27**: 358–62.
43 Hoogenrad T. Zinc treatment of Wilson's disease. *J Lab Clin Med* 1998; **132**: 240–1.
44 Treatment of Wilson's disease with ammonium tetrathiomolybdate. II. Initial therapy in 33 neurologically affected patients and follow up with zinc therapy. *Arch Neurol* 1996; **53**: 1017–25.
45 Schilsky ML, Scheinberg I, Sternlieb I. Liver transplantation for Wilson's disease: indications and outcome. *Hepatology* 1994; **19**: 583–7.

Primary biliary cirrhosis: diagnosis and treatment

21

Jenny Heathcote

INTRODUCTION

Primary biliary cirrhosis (PBC) is an inflammatory disease of the interlobular and septal bile ducts of the liver thought to be immune-mediated.[1] Granulomatous destruction of these bile ducts leads to ductopenia and hence persistent cholestasis. Progressive fibrosis and eventual cirrhosis develop and liver failure is a terminal event unless intervention with a liver transplant occurs.

This disease predominantly affects middle aged women from all racial groups,[2] but there is considerable geographic variation in its prevalence.[3] It appears to be most common in women of European ancestry, but by no means is this disease confined to caucasians.

DIAGNOSIS OF PBC

When this disease was first described, patients were noted to be jaundiced and to have tuberous xanthoma.[4] It was recognized as a disease of the liver in this century.[5] Once routine biochemical screening at annual check-ups became common practice, patients were diagnosed with primary biliary cirrhosis in the absence of jaundice. In the 1960s, serological tests using immunofluorescence techniques indicated that non-organ and non-species specific mitochondrial antibodies were very specific for patients with primary biliary cirrhosis.[6] At much the same time, the histological characteristics of this disease were first described and "staging" of this disease was introduced later.[7,8] These studies indicated that the early bile duct destruction was often secondary to granulomatous infiltration of the ducts, not dissimilar to that seen in sarcoidosis. In fact, PBC and sarcoidosis have frequently been described as being present at the same time in the same patient.[9] In the 1970s, descriptions of the many autoimmune disorders frequently seen in association with patients with PBC were reported.[10,11]

In the 1980s, it was recognized that the substrates for antimitochondrial antibodies (AMA) were the family of 2-oxo acid dehydrogenase enzymes located on the inner membrane of mitochondria.[12] The isolation of these substrates led to the development of more specific and sensitive testing for AMA using ELISA or immunoblotting, which showed that the AMA test is positive in 95% of patients with PBC. It is extremely rare to find AMA in any other clinical situation apart from otherwise clearcut autoimmune hepatitis, in which this is still very uncommon.[13] AMA are not associated with any other acute or chronic cholestatic condition.

It has now become recognized that sampling error of liver tissue using needle biopsies is common in PBC.[14] It is not unusual to see what are described as early stage I or II lesions in the same sample which, in another area, shows fibrosis and even cirrhosis. It has recently been suggested that in order to accurately diagnose ductopenia in a needle biopsy, 20 portal tracts need to be present for analysis.[15] It is rare for 20 portal tracts to be present in one needle biopsy.

In the early 1970s the natural history of patients with asymptomatic primary biliary cirrhosis was first described.[16] Later it became evident that AMA positive subjects with normal liver biochemistry, often serologically tested because of the presence of another autoimmune disease, may also have the histological lesions of PBC on biopsy.[17] A 10-year follow-up of these patients has shown that the majority develop biochemical cholestasis and many have developed symptomatic disease.[18]

The many presentations of PBC

Primary biliary cirrhosis may be diagnosed in several situations. The classical description of thc paticnt with jaundicc, xanthoma, pruritus, cholestatic liver tests, AMA positive serology, and diagnostic or confirmatory liver biopsy may still present on rare occasions *de novo*. More commonly (60% of the time), PBC is diagnosed in a patient without symptoms but with anicteric cholestatic biochemical tests, with a positive serological test for AMA, and with a diagnostic or confirmatory biopsy. Furthermore, some patients have PBC who are asymptomatic and have normal liver biochemistry, but test positive for AMA and have typical lesions on liver histology. Finally, it has become apparent that some patients may have the clinical, biochemical, and histological features of PBC and also suffer the same associated autoimmune diseases, but test negative for serum AMA.[19–23] These latter patients all test seropositive for antinuclear antibodies (ANA) or smooth muscle antibodies (SMA), generally in high titer. However, the typical histological findings of primary biliary cirrhosis have also been described in a retrospective study of histological tissue and chart review of 200 patients, 12% of whom had no positive serological tests.[24] Until recently, the hallmark for PBC was the presence of AMA ($\geq 1:40$), generally in high titer ($\geq 1:160$), in the serum. Now it appears that the typical histological lesions of PBC may be present in the absence of AMA in serum, and furthermore, even in the absence of abnormal liver tests or symptoms. Thus the diagnosis has become much more diverse. It is unclear whether the same disease process causes the classic histological lesions of PBC or whether there are multiple etiological factors which all cause the same histological response.

NATURAL HISTORY OF PBC

As the diagnosis of primary biliary cirrhosis is made at earlier and earlier stages of the disease, so the natural history appears to have altered. It now seems likely that there is a long preclinical course of this disease when AMA alone are present in the serum. However, the study that described such patients[18] included mostly patients who were well above middle age, ie more than 60 years old. The diagnosis of asymptomatic PBC tends to be made in patients who are 2–10 years older than patients with symptomatic disease.[2] This relationship suggests that asymptomatic disease is not necessarily a precursor to symptomatic disease, but may sometimes be a *form fruste* of symptomatic disease.

However, the natural history of the progression of disease in older patients seems to be no different than that seen in younger patients.

The initial follow-up report of asymptomatic disease suggested that only 50% of asymptomatic patients became symptomatic within 10 years.[16] Another small report indicated that the survival of asymptomatic patients was no different from the age- and gender-matched general population.[25] However, larger studies do indicate that although asymptomatic disease progresses at a much slower rate than symptomatic disease, survival of both symptomatic and asymptomatic patients with PBC is significantly less than that of the general population.[26,27] Mean survival for patients with symptomatic PBC is 8 years whereas that for asymptomatic disease is closer to 16 years.[28] The many randomized controlled trials of therapy in PBC patients conducted over the past 20 years indicate that the course of PBC is not the same for all patients. About one-third of asymptomatic patients develop symptomatic disease within 5 years. The other two-thirds may not develop symptomatic disease for much longer. Once a patient develops biochemical hyperbilirubinemia, the natural history of this disease is much more predictable.

SURROGATE MARKERS OF OUTCOME

Symptoms typical of PBC, such as fatigue, do not correlate with the severity of disease as judged by the height of the serum bilirubin or the Mayo risk score.[29] Pruritus, the next most common symptom in PBC patients, is not a marker of disease severity; in fact pruritus frequently lessens as decompensated disease occurs, just as skin xanthomata diminish with disease progression. Unlike other chronic liver diseases, variceal hemorrhage is not necessarily a sign of progressive liver disease, as the portal hypertension initially is due to presinusoidal causes,[30] ie nodular regenerative hyperplasia, cirrhosis being absent. In this situation, variceal hemorrhage, as long as liver ischemia is avoided, does not necessarily indicate a poor outcome. As PBC is primarily a disease of the biliary system, when signs of failure of hepatocytes develop, such as uncorrectable coagulopathy, these indicate terminal disease. There are no symptoms present in patients with purely compensated disease which correlate with outcome. Some have suggested that the presence of associated autoimmune diseases is associated with a worse prognosis, but the data on which this suggestion was made have recently been refuted.[27,31]

The degree of hyperbilirubinemia has been shown to correlate extremely well with survival.[32] This study was conducted prior to the introduction of liver transplantation for liver failure in PBC and showed that the height of the bilirubin was a valid marker of final outcome, ie death. Standard liver biochemical tests, namely serum levels of alkaline phosphatase and the aminotransferases, have never been shown to correlate with prognosis in patients with PBC. More sophisticated risk scores designed to predict prognosis in patients with primary biliary cirrhosis have been developed by several different authors.[25,33–35] It is noteworthy that serum bilirubin features in each of the scores described. The most widely used composite score, the Mayo risk score,[33] is popular because it does not require any invasive procedures, ie liver biopsy, so is very convenient for everyday use. The components of the Mayo risk score, ie age, serum albumin, coagulation time, and the presence of fluid retention and/or use of diuretics, seem to be sufficient to accurately predict outcome in PBC. However, an earlier study (on a relatively small number of patients) did indicate that patients who have liver fibrosis or cirrhosis on biopsy had a worse survival than those without fibrosis or cirrhosis.[25] On its own, presence or absence of cirrhosis is not a highly predictive surrogate marker for final outcome, ie death, presumably because there are other features which factor into progression of disease. As well, there remains the problem of sampling error.[14]

The recent introduction of ursodeoxycholic acid (UDCA) therapy, which markedly reduces the serum bilirubin concentration, has been shown not to invalidate either the serum bilirubin or the Mayo risk score as a prognostic marker, at least within the first 6 months of therapy.[36] However, it is still unknown whether the serum bilirubin in patients treated with UDCA remains a valid marker of survival in those with endstage disease. The Mayo risk score was first developed and validated for patients who were not treated with a liver transplant for endstage disease. More recently, as liver transplantation has become the alternative endpoint, the Mayo risk score has been re-evaluated along with other factors thought to predict post-transplant survival.[37]

It is only in the context of clinical trials when large numbers of liver biopsy specimens are available that the effect of sampling error is minimized, although it is likely that sampling error will only be truly reduced to an insignificant degree if many hundreds of paired biopsy samples are evaluated. Whereas in the past a composite score for inflammation and fibrosis was developed to stage PBC,[8] it may be more appropriate for the degree of inflammation to be graded separately from the degree of fibrosis, very much like the score that has been developed for the assessment of chronic viral hepatitis. As previously mentioned, the degree of ductopenia can only be adequately assessed in liver tissue specimens with a sufficient number of portal tracts present. Similarly, the degree of inflammation and fibrosis can only be adequately assessed when the tissue specimens are above a minimum size, generally considered to be 0.5–1 cm in length.

There is no evidence that the titer of the AMA in any way correlates with the course of primary biliary cirrhosis.[38] The only biochemical marker with prognostic value is the serum bilirubin concentration. Other factors important in determining outcome have not as yet been validated. These include vascular supply to the liver,[39] or the presence of various inflammatory mediators and markers of tissue fibrosis.[40]

It has now become very difficult to use death as a survival endpoint, since most patients with decompensated PBC, if they have no contraindication, are referred for liver transplantation. The identification of valid surrogate markers is extremely important in evaluating specific therapies in PBC, particularly as the natural history of this disease, even in symptomatic patients, has a long mean survival time (12 years). As more and more asymptomatic patients, whose expected mean survival is even longer, are included in drug trials, trials of very large size and long duration are required in order to effectively evaluate the effect of therapy on survival. Such trials are unwieldly, expensive, and intolerable to patients. Hence the urgent need to establish valid surrogate markers of survival.

TIMING FOR LIVER TRANSPLANTATION

As liver transplantation has become available for patients with PBC in liver failure, the need for this procedure has been used as a final measure of outcome in many therapeutic trials. However, the validity of this surrogate marker can be questioned, since liver transplantation is sometimes performed for intolerable symptoms such as uncontrollable pruritus or severe osteoporosis rather than for liver failure. Even in patients who undergo liver transplanation for decompensated liver disease, timing of the liver transplant will vary considerably between patients simply because of their blood type. Variations will also depend on such external forces as availability of donated organs, health insurance limitations, distance from a major healthcare center, etc. Hence, there are many reasons why time to liver transplantation is a rather variable endpoint and not necessarily as valid as it may appear on the surface.

THERAPEUTIC TRIAL DESIGN: ASSESSMENT OF CREDIBILITY

Randomized controlled trials of therapy in primary biliary cirrhosis have been published for the past 20 years. Over that time, many refinements have been made in trial design in order to enhance accuracy. For instance, the first trial was not double-blind[41] and thus several biases which might have been minimized by blinding were present. In addition, the sample size needed to ensure that the study had adequate power was not calculated, and no "stopping rules" were described.

PBC is a relatively uncommon disease, and as more and more asymptomatic patients are included in order to meet sample size requirements, the frequency of endpoints in the control group over the normal 3–5 year funding period for most trials and the probability of observing an effect of therapy are reduced. Including such low risk patients has resulted in relatively lower event rates than would be observed in trials involving higher risk patients. Therefore the sample size required in the trials has to be very large and generally achievable only in multicenter studies. This has not always been affordable or feasible. The compromise taken has been to perform meta-analyses using data from several published series, or to combine data for analysis in studies where all the raw data are available.

To determine the appropriate sample size for a clinical trial requires not only a large sample of historical data to establish the natural history of the disease in a particular population (event rate in the control group) but also pilot study data, from which an estimate of the expected therapeutic effect can be made. These two conditions have rarely been met in the many trials of therapy reported in PBC.

It is important that a valid primary measure of outcome be established prior to starting a study. This outcome measure needs to be reliable and easy to quantify and should ideally have been validated in both the historical sample and pilot study used to calculate the sample size. The primary measure of outcome in PBC cannot feasibly be death or even need for liver transplantation, in view of the sample size that it would be necessary to recruit (>700 patients).[42] Hence, surrogate markers for outcome are often employed. Unfortunately, some trials have employed surrogate endpoints which have not been shown to correlate with outcome, eg serum alkaline phosphatase concentration. Others have failed to acknowledge the issue of sampling error with liver histology.[14] Recently, "composite failure to respond to treatment" scores have been introduced, but these have not been validated as reliable outcome measures.

The intention to treat principle is vital when performing statistical analysis of outcome in order to avoid as much bias as possible when interpreting the data. This means that all patients who are randomized need to be included in the final analysis, even though they may have been censored at a very early point in the trial because of untimely death, need to withdraw from the study, non-compliance, etc. Using the intention to treat principle allows for only a very conservative analysis of the effectiveness of therapy, but it permits assessment of the "real life" situations, ie assesses the generalizability of the study.

Just as the sample size needs to be adequate to demonstrate an effect of therapy, it also should be adequate to assess the frequency of adverse effects. Whereas this may be obvious with a drug that has a profound systemic effect, ie chlorambucil,[43] it may be less obvious in drugs with fewer adverse effects. As patients with PBC have a quite long natural survival without any therapeutic intervention, it is obviously vital to establish whether adverse effects cause greater morbidity and mortality than if the disease were left untreated. In addition, the effect of any therapy on enhancing the rate of progress of various conditions complicating PBC, such as the effect of prednisolone on osteoporosis, may need to be monitored.[44]

In determining the thoroughness and hence accuracy of any trial report, as much can be learned from what is not written in the methods section as can be gained from the results. The discussion is generally the opinion of the author. For an independent analysis of the validity of the data, a combination of excellent clinical judgement and understanding of the rationale for the intervention, as well as the basic concepts of trial design, need to be considered. Only then can a decision be made whether or not the benefit of an evaluated intervention is generalizable to a specific individual with primary biliary cirrhosis.

RANDOMIZED CONTROLLED TRIALS FOR THE TREATMENT OF PBC

Immunosuppressives

Once it was recognized that PBC was an autoimmune disease, the logical approach to therapy was to employ an immunosuppressive. Because the majority of PBC patients are women and osteoporosis complicates PBC regardless of menopausal status, corticosteroid therapy has for the most part been avoided. Randomized controlled trials of immunosuppressive therapy in PBC have employed azathioprine, cyclosporin, methotrexate, prednisolone, chlorambucil, and more recently, thalidomide.[41,43–52]

Neither of two trials of **azathioprine** showed a beneficial effect of this drug on survival. The first trial was inadequate with respect to sample size,[41] lack of a placebo control group, lack of predetermined stopping rules, and failure to analyse results according to intention to treat. The second azathioprine trial,[45] though much larger (248 patients), did not include a sample size calculation to assure that it had adequate power, and the withdrawal rate was greater than 20% in both the azathioprine and placebo groups. Despite randomization, the two groups were not stratified for factors known to influence survival and were not comparable at baseline. Although employment of the Cox multiple regression analysis to adjust for these baseline differences suggested that there was a benefit of treatment on survival, this procedure does not give as much confidence in the validity of the results as would exist if a stronger design had been employed. The difference between the treatment groups was only measured in months, which may not be clinically important. Patients were followed for as long as 10 years, but the number of patients still being followed at that period was down to nine in the azathioprine and none in the placebo group. It appears that the intention to treat principle was not used in the analysis, since 32 patients were excluded from the analysis because of incomplete data. Thus the small benefit in survival can be further questioned in terms of its validity.

Several small trials and one large trial (349 patients) of **cyclosporin** therapy have been published.[48] This trial ran into the same problems as had been encountered with the large azathioprine trial, ie lack of comparability of the two treatment groups at baseline. Even though there was a similar number of deaths, 30 patients on cyclosporin and 31 in the placebo group, the authors concluded that survival was improved in the cyclosporin treated patients. Renal impairment was observed in 9% and systemic hypertension in 11% of cyclosporin treated patients (1.7% and 1% on placebo). These two serious adverse effects in patients whose disease is relatively slowly progressive precludes the use of this drug in the long term treatment of PBC.

R
Grade A

Methotrexate has been claimed to be of value in pilot studies,[49] while only one randomized controlled trial of therapy has been published in abstract form.[50] Sixty patients were recruited, 30 randomized to low dose therapy (2.5 mg three times per week). At the end of 6 years, the serum bilirubin and Mayo risk score were higher in those receiving methotrexate, suggesting that the drug may be toxic in patients with PBC. However, this report published only in abstract form does not allow for clear definition of methodology, and there may be alternative explanations for these observed findings. A large multicenter trial in the United States comparing ursodeoxycholic acid alone with the same intervention combined with methotrexate is in progress.

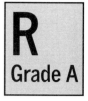

There has been one small, 3-year randomized controlled trial of **prednisolone**.[44] A significant reduction in the serum bilirubin concentration (possibly a valid surrrogate outcome measure) was observed in treated patients, but there was a worsening of osteoporosis in those who received corticosteroids. However, a recent trial of bisphosphonates in PBC patients treated with corticosteroids, indicates that etidronate significantly stabilizes bone mineral density in the vertebrae of PBC patients receiving corticosteroids, compared to corticosteroid treated PBC patients receiving no etidronate.[51] Hence, it is appropriate that corticosteroids are re-evaluated in the therapy of primary biliary cirrhosis now that patients can be given appropriate preventative therapy to avoid the complication of osteoporosis.

R
Grade A

A small study of 13 patients randomized to 0.5–4 mg daily of **chlorambucil** (mean 2 mg daily) compared to placebo has been reported.[43] All treated patients developed some degree of bone marrow suppression and discontinuation of therapy was required in four. A 30% withdrawal rate due to drug toxicity indicates that this drug should not undergo further evaluation in patients with PBC.

A very small and short (6 month) RCT in 18 PBC patients using **thalidomide** has been reported, showing little benefit of this treatment in affected patients. However, this study lacked adequate power to evaluate this form of therapy in any meaningful way. No benefit on serum bilirubin was observed during the 6 months of treatment.[52]

An alternative approach to therapy for PBC has been to use drugs that may not interfere with the primary cause, ie immune mediated duct destruction, but interfere with the progression of the disease, either by **reducing fibrogenesis** or by **reducing cholestasis**.

Two **antifibrotic** drugs have been assessed, colchicine in three small randomized controlled trials and D-penicillamine in many more. The studies of **colchicine** therapy are interesting. Unfortunately, all three trials recruited less than 100 patients each.[53–55] They all used approximately the same dose, so a meta-analysis of these three studies may prove to be worthwhile but has not so far been published. The first study introduced the concept of a multiple criteria "treatment failure" composite index as a measure of outcome. There was no evidence that this composite index had been validated, but similar treatment failure composites indices have been employed in several other clinical trials in PBC. Frequently these indices have included factors not known to be relevant to PBC survival. It was encouraging that two of the colchicine studies suggested that colchicine had a beneficial effect on liver function, ie serum albumin and bilirubin. None of the studies suggested a benefit on symptoms or histology. One study suggested that there was a survival advantage to receiving colchicine, even though only 64 patients were recruited

R
Grade A

R Grade A

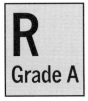

and 10 patients withdrew, eight of whom were randomized to colchicine. The third study also had a high drop-out rate (32%) in those randomized to colchicine. A long term, ie 8-year, follow-up of this latter study indicated that there was no survival advantage in treated patients, although the original sample size was small.[56]

While there were eight randomized controlled trials of **D-penicillamine**, the results were disappointing.[42] Unlike patients with Wilson disease, adverse effects of therapy were common, causing a high withdrawal rate, similar to the experience with rheumatoid arthritis. This drug is no longer recommended for the treatment of PBC.

Reduction of cholestasis

HYDROPHILIC BILE ACIDS

Leuschner, in the early 1980s, reported that administration of ursodeoxycholic acid (UDCA) in patients with gallstones who coincidentally also had chronic hepatitis, led to an improvement of liver biochemistry.[57] A 2-year pilot study in 15 PBC patients conducted by Poupon *et al*[58] indicated that treatment with UDCA in a dose of 13–15 mg/kg daily reduced serum bilirubin concentration in patients who had elevated levels prior to the start of therapy. Many randomized controlled trials of UDCA therapy have been conducted subsequently. The mechanisms of action of UDCA are slowly being identified. The original premise that the introduction of the less toxic hydrophilic dihydroxy bile acid UDCA would reduce the exposure of hepatocyte membranes to the toxic effects of the retained hydrophobic endogenous bile acids has now been proven to be true.[59] In addition, UDCA inhibits the uptake of endogenous bile acids at the terminal ileum,[60] although most of the UDCA is absorbed passively throughout the small bowel in its unconjugated state. There may be other beneficial effects of UDCA in patients with PBC. There is some evidence that it may have an immunoregulatory role[61] and some *in vitro* evidence that it may promote antioxidant activity.[62]

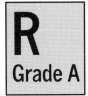

Twelve RCTs evaluating UDCA therapy in PBC have been reported. A meta-analysis[63] of the 11 trials with a follow-up of more than 6 months has recently been accepted for publication, but was not available for critical review during the writing of this chapter. The details of these 12 trials[64–75] are shown in Table 21.1. One trial[75] randomized patients to receive colchicine, UDCA or placebo, and two have been published only as abstracts.[69,74] Unfortunately, few of these randomized UDCA trials are directly comparable. Three were of short duration (6–9 months), and hence did not permit meaningful analysis of survival.[64–66] These trials also used small doses of UDCA (500–600 mg daily). A larger trial, which enrolled 114 patients for a 24-month treatment period, also employed only 500 mg of UDCA.[67] Most trials employed doses between 10 and 15 mg/kg daily.[68–71,73] All trials have demonstrated that treatment with UDCA leads to a marked reduction in elevated total serum bilirubin levels within the first 3 months of introducing therapy. However, a few reports suggest that in those with endstage disease, treatment may cause a sudden rise in bilirubin and hence it is advised that when UDCA is prescribed to patients with decompensated PBC, they should be followed very closely.[76] Such patients are generally on the liver transplant waiting list unless they are unsuitable candidates.

R Grade A

None of the individual studies had adequate power to assess the effect of therapy on survival. Three of the four larger double-blind randomized trials[68,70,71] used the same dose of UDCA (13–15 mg/kg per day), and the results were analyzed according to the intent to treat principle. In two of these a composite "treatment failure" outcome measure was used,

Table 21.1 Baseline patient characteristics in RCT of UDCA vs placebo

Study	No. of patients (UDCA/PL)	Mean age (yr) (UDCA/PL)	Duration of trial (mth)	UDCA dose (mg/kg/d)	Mean baseline bil. (μmol/l)	Histological stage (I/II–III/IV) (UDCA/PL)	Methodological quality score (0–79)
Leuschner, 1989[64]	10/10	ND	9	10	ND	9/1–8/2	27
[a]Hadziyannis, 1989[69]	25/25	ND	24 (19.5)[b]	12–15	ND	ND	18
Poupon, 1991[68]	73/73	54/52	24	13–15	23.2/21.2	36/37–42/31	51
Battezzati, 1993[66]	44/44	54/55	6–9	8.7	31.5/32.5	23/21–22/22[c]	54
Lindor, 1994[70]	89/91	54/52	48 (24)[b]	13–15	32.3/30.6	31/58–26/65	57
Heathcote, 1994[71]	111/111	57.3/55.4	24	14	40/31	50/57–47/60	69
Turner, 1994[72]	22/24	57.5/57.7	24	10	17/17	3/19–5/19	39
Combes, 1995[73]	77/74	49.5/48.9	24	10–12	39.1/34	28/49–22/52	66
Vuoristo 1995[75]	30/31	52/57	24	12–15	22.7/25.5	ND	45
Eriksson, 1997[67]	60/56	57/57	24	7.7	18.9/18.2	ND	48
[a]Pares, 1997[74]	99/93	ND	63.6[b]	15	ND	ND	33

ND, Not determined; PL, placebo.
[a]Abstract only.
[b]Mean.
[c]Stage I/II/III–IV.

and in the third the percentage change in total serum bilirubin over 2 years was used as the primary outcome measure. Detailed sample size calculations and clearcut predetermined definition of study duration were only described for this latter study. Few adverse effects of UDCA were reported and the withdrawal rate was less than 20% in all three studies. A combined analysis of the raw data from these three studies, continued beyond the initial 2 years, has been published.[77] In two of the three trials, some patients initially randomized to placebo were switched to open label UDCA after the first 24 months. However, the results were analyzed according to intention to treat, so that those patients initially randomized to receive placebo and subsequently switched to receive UDCA remained in the placebo group for the purposes of analysis. Intuitively, it seems likely that this procedure would reduce the probability of demonstrating benefit with UDCA in the analysis of the longer term data, should a true benefit exist. Despite this consideration, the combined analysis of survival data from the three trials suggested that UDCA therapy for up to 4 years led to an increase in time free of liver transplantation in treated patients.

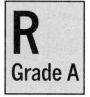

R Grade A

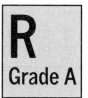

Subgroup analyses did not show any benefit in patients who, at baseline, had a total serum bilirubin of less than 1.4 mg/dl and/or stage I/II liver histology. These subgroup analyses do not prove that UDCA is ineffective in patients with asymptomatic and/or early disease, but they do suggest that clinical trials in such patients would require very large numbers of patients and would be required to be of such long duration to show any benefit of the treatment that they would not be feasible.

R Grade A

The fourth large trial (151 patients) employed a smaller dose (10–12 mg/kg body weight daily) and a different preparation of UDCA. After 2 years of treatment no difference in survival was seen, there being eight deaths in those randomized to UDCA and 12 in those randomized to placebo.[71]

It should be pointed out that the pooled analysis of the three trials is not a systematic review or meta-analysis, but rather was performed by pooling of results from three trials which were of similar design but which had rather dissimilar results. This procedure differs from a systematic review or formal meta-analyis, which includes consideration of all relevant trials, justifies the exclusion of trials from the analysis, and explores heterogeneity between trials and the reasons for variation in results. A formal meta-analysis which demonstrates benefit from an intervention may also include a sensitivity analysis to indicate the number of unpublished or excluded trials of specified size with negative results which would be required to negate the results of the meta-analysis. Meta-analyses may suffer from the opposite weakness cited for the combined analysis of similar trials, ie they may involve pooled analysis of trials which differ sufficiently in their design that they are not truly comparable. Accordingly, caution should be exercised in interpreting both the combined analysis of selected trials[77] on one hand as proof of a beneficial effect of UDCA on mortality in PBC, and the most recent meta-analysis on the other, as evidence that no such effect exists.[63]

Effects of specific therapy on other markers of disease in primary biliary cirrhosis

PORTAL HYPERTENSION

The effect of UDCA on the development of varices and the measurement of intrahepatic sinusoidal portal pressure was evaluated in two of the randomised controlled trials of UDCA therapy. The trial conducted by Lindor *et al.*[78] indicated that esophageal varices were slower to appear in patients randomized to UDCA, but the rate of variceal hemorrhage was not altered. Huet found in a 2-year randomized trial that the increase in intrahepatic portal pressure over baseline was less in UDCA-treated patients than in those receiving placebo.[79] Grade A

OSTEOPOROSIS

R Grade A

No effect of UDCA on bone mineral density (BMD) was demonstrated in the randomized controlled trial of ursodeoxycholic acid in PBC published by Lindor *et al*,[80] although the study may have lacked power. A small study assessing bone mineral density and vertebral fractures in PBC patients randomized to cyclosporin A or placebo suggested that cyclosporin treated patients have less bone loss and better biochemical parameters of bone remodelling.[81]

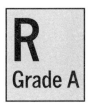

SYMPTOMS OF FATIGUE AND PRURITUS

R Grade C

Although there are very sophisticated methods to measure these symptoms, none of the randomized controlled trials of therapy for PBC employed such instruments to monitor the effect of therapy. There are many anecdotal case reports of marked improvement and marked worsening of both fatigue and pruritus in patients receiving UDCA. Pilot studies of methotrexate have reported dramatic improvement in both fatigue and pruritus, but these uncontrolled studies provide only weak evidence for benefit.

HISTOLOGY

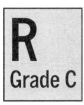

Comments with regard to any therapeutic effect on the histological pattern on primary biliary cirrhosis following specific therapy have been deliberately omitted. Because many patients refuse a second liver biopsy at the end of the trials, hence the number of paired biopsies is often less than anticipated at the beginning of a trial. The problems of adequate amounts of tissue and sampling error have already been addressed. Most of the large studies have employed single observer analysis which reduces inter-observer variation to zero, but there have been no studies of intra-observer error. All these facts, combined with the observation that the degree of fibrosis is not a very valid surrogate outcome measure, lead to the conclusion that the greatest value of liver histology is the assessment of potential drug toxicity.

Assessment of adverse effects in therapeutic trials in PBC

No clearcut hepatotoxic effect of any of the drugs described above has been described, although toxic effects or systemic effects, eg bone marrow suppression with chlorambucil or pulmonary toxicity with methotrexate have been well described. Other drug related adverse effects include the effect of cyclosporin on renal function and systemic blood pressure and a neuropathy thought to be induced by colchicine seen in two the randomized controlled trials of this agent. Certainly the safest and apparently most effective drug to date remains ursodeoxycholic acid.

THE FUTURE FOR PBC

Treatment with UDCA is not curative. It may delay the progression of disease in some patients, but the evidence for this benefit is not clearcut. Several small trials of UDCA in combination with methotrexate,[82–84] colchicine,[85–88] and prednisolone[89,90] have been conducted. The latter two combinations make the most sense, but no study has been large enough to adequately assess the effectiveness of either. The combination of UDCA and methotrexate is accompanied by greater toxicity.[82] Clearly, no randomized controlled trial of liver transplantation is feasible. However, when the assessment of survival following transplantation, compared to the predicted survival using the Mayo risk score at the time transplantation is performed, indicates that liver transplantation leads to a marked survival benefit in patients with primary biliary cirrhosis and currently it remains the only curative therapy for this disease.[91]

REFERENCES

1 Gershwin ME, Mackay IR. Primary biliary cirrhosis: paradigm or paradox for autoimmunity. *Gastroenterology* 1990; **99**: 822–33.

2 Witt-Sullivan H, Heathcote J, Cauch K *et al.* The demography of primary biliary cirrhosis in Ontario, Canada. *Hepatology* 1990; **12**: 98–105.

3 Watson RG, Angus PW, Dewar M *et al.* and the Melbourne Liver Group. Low prevalence of primary biliary cirrhosis in Victoria, Australia. *Gut* 1995; **36**: 927–30.

4 Addison T, Gull W. On a certain affection of the skin, vitiligo idea – plana, tuberosa. *Guy's Hosp Rep* 1851; **7**: 265–76.

5 Ahrens EH, Rayne MA, Kunkle HG *et al.* Primary biliary cirrhosis. *Medicine* 1950; **29**: 299–364.

6 Doniach D, Roitt IM, Walker JG *et al.* Tissue antibodies in primary biliary cirrhosis, active chronic (lupoid) hepatitis, cryptogenic cirrhosis and other liver diseases and their clinical implications. *Clin Exp Immunol* 1966; **1**: 237–62.

7 Scheuer PJ. Primary biliary cirrhosis. *Proc R Soc Med* 1967; **60**: 1257–60.

8 Ludwig J, Dickson ER, Mcdonald GSA. Staging of chronic nonsuppurative destructive cholangitis (syndrome of primary biliary cirrhosis). *Virchows Arch (A)* 1978; **379**: 103–12.

9 Keeffe EB. Sarcoidosis and primary biliary cirrhosis. Literature review and illustrative case. *Am J Med* 1987; **83**: 977–80.

10 Golding PL, Smith M, Williams R. Multisystem involvement in chronic liver disease. *Am J Med* 1973; **55**: 772–82.

11 Culp KS, Fleming CR, Duffy J *et al.* Autoimmune associations in primary biliary cirrhosis. *Mayo Clin Proc* 1982; **57**: 365–70.

12 Fussey S, Guest JR, James O *et al.* Identification and analysis of the major M2 autoantigens in primary biliary cirrhosis. *Proc Natl Acad Sci USA* 1988; **85**: 8654–8.

13 Czaja AJ, Carpenter HA, Manns MP. Antibodies to soluble liver antigen, P455011D6, and mitochondrial complexes in chronic hepatitis. *Gastroenterology* 1993; **105**: 1522–8.

14 Garrido MC, Hubscher SG. Accuracy of staging in primary biliary cirrhosis. *J Clin Pathol* 1996; **49**: 556–9.

15 Tadrous PJ, Goldin RD. How many portal tracts are necessary to make a diagnosis of significant bile duct loss (SBDL)? *J Pathol* 1997; **181**: 11A.

16 Long RG, Scheuer PJ, Sherlock S. Presentation and course of asymptomatic primary biliary cirrhosis. *Gastroenterology* 1977; **72**: 1204–7.

17 Mitchison HC, Bassendine MF, Hendrick A *et al.* Positive antimitochondrial antibody but normal alkaline phosphatase: is this primary biliary cirrhosis? *Hepatology* 1986; **6**: 1279–84.

18 Metcalf JV, Mitchison HC, Palmer JM *et al.* Natural history of early primary biliary cirrhosis. *Lancet* 1996; **348**: 1399–402.

19 Brunner G, Klinge O. Ein der chronisch-destruierenden nicht-eitrigen Cholangitis ähnliches Krankheitsbild mit anti-nukleären Antikörpern (Immunocholangitis)]. *Dtsch Med Wochenschr* 1987; **112**: 1454–8.

20 Ben-Ari Z, Dhillon AP, Sherlock S. Autoimmune cholangiopathy: part of the spectrum of autoimmune chronic active hepatitis. *Hepatology* 1993; **18**: 10–15.

21 Michieletti P, Wanless IR, Katz A *et al.* Antimitochondrial antibody negative primary biliary cirrhosis: a distinct syndrome of autoimmune cholangitis. *Gut* 1994; **35**: 260–5.

22 Taylor SL, Dean PJ, Riely CA. Primary autoimmune cholangitis. An alternative to antimitochondrial antibody-negative primary biliary cirrhosis. *Am J Surg Pathol* 1994; **18**: 91–9.

23 Lacerda MA, Ludwig J, Dickson ER *et al.* Antimitochondrial antibody-negative primary biliary cirrhosis. *Am J Gastroenterol* 1995; **90**: 247–9.

24 Goodman ZD, McNally PR, Davis DR *et al.* Autoimmune cholangitis: a variant of primary biliary cirrhosis. Clinicopathologic and serologic correlations in 200 cases. *Digest Dis Sci* 1995; **40**: 1232–42.

25 Roll J, Boyer JL, Barry D *et al.* The prognostic importance of clinical and histological features in asymptomatic and symptomatic primary biliary cirrhosis. *N Engl J Med* 1983; **308**: 1–7.

26 Balasubramaniam K, Grambsch PM, Wiesner RH *et al.* Diminished survival in asymptomatic primary biliary cirrhosis: a prospective study. *Gastroenterology* 1990; **98**: 1567–71.

27 Springer J, Cauch-Dudek K, O'Rourke K *et al.* Asymptomatic primary biliary cirrhosis: a study of its natural history and progression. *Am J Gastroenterol* 1999; **94**: 47–53.

28 Mahl T, Shockcor W, Boyer JL. Primary biliary cirrhosis: survival of a large cohort of symptomatic and asymptomatic patients followed for 24 years. *J Hepatol* 1994; **20**: 707–13.

29 Cauch-Dudek K, Abbey S, Stewart DE *et al.* Fatigue in primary biliary cirrhosis. *Gut* 1998; **43**: 705–10.

30 Colina F, Pinedo F, Solis JA *et al.* Nodular regenerative hyperplasia of the liver in early histological stages of primary biliary cirrhosis. *Gastroenterology* 1992; **102**: 1319–24.

31 Mitchison HC, Lucey MR, Kelly PJ *et al.* Symptom development and prognosis in primary biliary cirrhosis: a study in two centers. *Gastroenterology* 1990; **99**: 778–84.

32 Shapiro JM, Smith H, Schaffner F. Serum bilirubin: a prognostic factor in primary biliary cirrhosis. *Gut* 1979; **20**: 137–40.

33 Dickson E, Grambsch PM, Fleming TR *et al.* Prognosis in primary biliary cirrhosis: model for decision making. *Hepatology* 1989; **10**: 1–7.

34 Bonsel GJ, Klompmaker IJ, Van 'T Veer F *et al.* Use of prognostic models for assessment of value of liver transplantation in primary biliary cirrhosis. *Lancet* 1990; **335**: 493–7.

35 Hughes MD, Raskino CL, Pocock SJ *et al.* Prediction of short-term survival with an application in primary biliary cirrhosis. *Stat Med* 1992; **11**: 1731–45

36 Kilmurry M, Heathcote EJ, Cauch-Dudek K *et al.* Is the Mayo model for predicting survival useful after the introduction of ursodeoxycholic acid treatment for primary biliary cirrhosis? *Hepatology* 1996; **23**: 1148–53.

37 Ricci P, Therneau TM, Malinchoc M *et al.* A prognostic model for the outcome of liver transplantation in patients with cholestatic liver disease. *Hepatology* 1997; **25**: 672–7.

38 Van Norstrand MD, Malinchoc M, Lindor KD *et al.* Quantitative measurement of autoantibodies to recombinant mitochondrial antigens in patients with primary biliary cirrhosis: relationship of levels of autoantibodies to disease progression. *Hepatology* 1997; **25**: 6–11.

39 Wanless IR, Wong F, Blendis LM *et al.* Hepatic and portal vein thrombosis in cirrhosis: possible role in development of parenchymal extinction and portal hypertension. *Hepatology* 1995; **21**: 1238–47.

40 Poupon RE, Balkau B, Guechot J *et al.* Predictive factors in ursodeoxycholic acid-treated patients with primary biliary cirrhosis: role of serum markers of connective tissue. *Hepatology* 1994; **19**: 635–40.

41 Heathcote J, Ross A, Sherlock S. A prospective controlled trial of azathioprine in primary biliary cirrhosis. *Gastroenterology* 1976; **70**: 656–9.

42 James OFW. D-penicillamine for primary biliary cirrhosis. *Gut* 1985; **26**: 109–13.

43 Hoofnagle JH, Davis GL, Schafer DF *et al.* Randomized trial of chlorambucil for primary biliary cirrhosis. *Gastroenterology* 1986; **91**: 1327–34.

44 Mitchison HC, Palmer JM, Bassendine MF *et al.* A controlled trial of prednisolone treatment in primary biliary cirrhosis. Three-year results. *J Hepatol* 1992; **15**: 336–44.

45 Christensen E, Neuberger J, Crowe J *et al.* Beneficial effect of azathioprine and prediction of prognosis in primary biliary cirrhosis: final results of an international trial. *Gastroenterology* 1985; **89**: 1084–91.

46 Minuk G, Bohme C, Gurgess E *et al.* Pilot study of cyclosporin A in patients with symptomatic primary biliary cirrhosis. *Gastroenterology* 1988; **95**: 1356–63.

47 Wiesner RH, Ludwig J, Lindor K *et al.* A controlled trial of cyclosporine in the treatment of primary biliary cirrhosis. *N Engl J Med* 1990; **322**: 1419–24.

48 Lombard M, Portmann B, Neuberger J. Cyclosporin A treatment in primary biliary cirrhosis: results of a long-term placebo controlled trial. *Gastroenterology* 1993; **104**: 519–26.

49 Kaplan MM, Knox TA. Treatment of primary biliary cirrhosis with low-dose weekly ethotrexate. *Gastroenterology* 1991; **101**: 1332–8.

50 Hendrickse M, Rigney E, Giaffer MH *et al.* Low-dose methotrexate in primary biliary cirrhosis: long-term results of a placebo-controlled trial. *Hepatology* 1997; **26**: 248A.

51 Wolfhagen FHJ, van Buren HR, denOuden JW *et al.* Cyclical etidronate in the prevention of bone loss in corticosteroid-treated primary biliary cirrhosis. A prospective, controlled pilot study. *J Hepatol* 1997; **26**: 325–30.

52 McCormick PA, Scott F, Epstein O *et al.* Thalidomide as therapy for primary biliary cirrhosis: a double-blind placebo controlled pilot study. *J Hepatol* 1994; **21**: 496–9.
53 Kaplan MM, Alling DW, Zimmerman HJ *et al.* A prospective trial of colchicine for primary biliary cirrhosis. *N Engl J Med* 1986; **315**: 1448–54.
54 Warnes TW, Smith A, Lee F *et al.* A controlled trial of colchicine in primary biliary cirrhosis. *Hepatology* 1987; **5**: 1–7.
55 Bodenheimer H, Schaffner F, Pessullo J. Evaluation of colchicine therapy in primary biliary cirrhosis. *Gastroenterology* 1988; **95**: 124–9.
56 Zifroni A, Schaffner F. Long-term follow-up of patients with primary biliary cirrhosis on colchicine therapy. *Hepatology* 1991; **14**: 990–3.
57 Leuschner U, Leuschner M, Sieratzki J *et al.* Gallstone dissolution with ursodeoxycholic acid in patients with chronic active hepatitis and two years follow-up. A pilot study. *Dig Dis Sci* 1985; **30**: 642–9.
58 Poupon R, Poupon RE, Calmus Y *et al.* Is ursodeoxycholic acid an effective treatment for primary biliary cirrhosis? *Lancet* 1987; **i**: 834–6.
59 Setchell KDR, Rodrigues CMP, Clerici C *et al.* Bile acid, concentrations in human and rat liver tissue and in hepatocyte nuclei. *Gastroenterology* 1997; **112**: 226–35.
60 Stiehl A, Raedsch R, Rudolph G. Acute effects of ursodeoxycholic and chenodeoxycholic acid on the small intestinal absorption of bile acids. *Gastroenterology* 1990; **98**: 424–8.
61 Yoshikawa M, Tsujii T, Matsumura K *et al.* Immunomodulatory effects of ursodeoxycholic acid on immune responses. *Hepatology* 1992; **16**: 358–64.
62 Ljubuncic P, Fuhrman B, Oiknine J *et al.* Effect of deoxycholic acid and ursodeoxycholic acid on lipid peroxidation in cultured macrophages. *Gut* 1996; **39**: 475–8.
63 Goulis J, Leandro G, Burroughs AK. No evidence for ursodeoxycholic acid (UDCA) therapy in primary biliary cirrhosis (PBC). *Lancet*, in press.
64 Leuschner U, Fischer H, Kurtz W *et al.* Ursodeoxycholic acid in primary biliary cirrhosis: results of a controlled double-blind trial. *Gastroenterology* 1989; **97**: 1268–74.
65 Oka H, Toda G, Ikeda Y *et al.* A multi-centre double-blind controlled trial of ursodeoxycholic acid for primary biliary cirrhosis. *Gastroenterol Jpn* 1990; **25**: 774–80.
66 Battezati PM, Podda M, Bianchi FB *et al.* Ursodeoxycholic acid for symptomatic primary biliary cirrhosis. Preliminary analysis of a double-blind multicentre trial. *J Hepatol* 1993; **17**: 332–8.
67 Eriksson LS, Olsson R, Glauman H *et al.* Ursodeoxycholic acid treatment in patients with primary biliary cirrhosis. A Swedish multicentre, double-blind, randomized controlled study. *Scand J Gastroenterol* 1997; **32**: 179–86.
68 Poupon RE, Balkau B, Eschwege E *et al.* A multicentre controlled trial of ursodiol for the treatment of primary biliary cirrhosis. *N Engl J Med* 1991; **324**: 1548–554.
69 Hadziyannis SJ, Hadziyannis ES, Makris A. A randomized controlled trial of ursodeoxycholic acid (UDCA) in primary biliary cirrhosis (PBC). *Hepatology* 1989; **10**: 580.
70 Lindor KD, Dickson ER, Baldus WP *et al.* Ursodeoxycholic acid in the treatment of primary biliary cirrhosis. *Gastroenterology* 1994; **106**: 1284–90.
71 Heathcote EJ, Cauch-Dudek K, Walker V *et al.* The Canadian multicentre double-blind randomized controlled trial of ursodeoxycholic acid in primary biliary cirrhosis. *Hepatology* 1994; **19**: 1149–56.
72 Turner IB, Myszor M, Mitchison HC *et al.* A two year controlled trial examining the effectiveness of UDCA in PBC. *J Gastroenterol Hepatol* 1994; **9**: 162–8.
73 Combes B, Carithers RL, Maddrey WC *et al.* A randomized, double-blind, placebo-controlled trial of ursodeoxycholic acid in primary biliary cirrhosis. *Hepatology* 1995; **22**: 759–66.
74 Parés A for the Spanish Association for the Study of the Liver. Long-term treatment of primary biliary cirrhosis with ursodeoxycholic acid: results of a randomized, double-blind, placebo controlled trial. *J Hepatol* 1997; **26** (Suppl 1): 166 (Abstr).
75 Vuoristo M, Farkilla M, Karnonen AL *et al.* A placebo-controlled trial of primary biliary cirrhosis treatment with colchicine and ursodeoxycholic acid. *Gastroenterology* 1995; **108**: 1470–8
76 Poupon R, Poupon RE. Deterioration in primary biliary cirrhosis in a patient on ursodeoxycholic acid. *Lancet* 1988; **ii**: 166.
77 Poupon RE, Lindor KD, Cauch-Dudek K *et al.* Combined analysis of randomized controlled trials of ursodeoxycholic acid in primary biliary cirrhosis. *Gastroenterology* 1997; **113**: 884–90.
78 Lindor KD, Jorgensen RA, Dickson ER. Ursodeoxycholic acid delays the onset of esophageal varices in primary biliary cirrhosis. *Mayo Clin Proc* 1997; **72**: 1137–40.
79 Huet PM, Huet J, Deslauriers J. Portal hypertension in patients with primary biliary cirrhosis. In: Lindor KD, Heathcote EJ, Poupon R (eds), *Primary biliary cirrhosis: from pathogenesis*

to treatment. London: Kluwer Academic, 1998, pp 87–91.
80 Lindor KD, Janes CH, Crippen JS *et al.* Bone disease in primary biliary cirrhosis: does ursodeoxycholic acid make a difference? *Hepatology* 1995; **21**: 389–92.
81 Guanabens N, Pares A, Navasa M *et al.* Cyclosporin A increases the biochemical markers of bone remodeling in primary biliary cirrhosis. *J Hepatol* 1994; **21**: 24–8.
82 Lindor KD, Dickson ER, Jorgenson RA *et al.* The combination of ursodeoxycholic acid and methotrexate for patients with primary biliary cirrhosis: the results of a pilot study. *Hepatology* 1995; **22**: 1158–62.
83 Gonzalez-Koch A, Brahm J, Antezana C *et al.* The combination of ursodeoxycholic acid and methotrexate for primary biliary cirrhosis is not better than ursodeoxycholic acid alone. *J Hepatol* 1997; **27**: 143–9.
84 Buscher HP, Zietzschmann Y, Gerok W. Positive responses to methotrexate and ursodeoxycholic acid in patients with primary biliary cirrhosis responding insufficiently to ursodeoxycholic acid alone. *J Hepatol* 1993; **18**: 9–14.
85 Vuoristo M, Farkkila M, Karvonen A-L *et al.* A placebo-controlled trial of primary biliary cirrhosis treatment with colchicine and ursodeoxycholic acid. *Gastroenterology* 1995; **108**: 1470–8.
86 Shibata J, Fujiyama S, Honda Y *et al.* Combination therapy with ursodeoxycholic acid and colchicine for primary biliary cirrhosis. *J Gastroenterol Hepatol* 1992; **7**: 277–82.
87 Ikeda T, Tozuka S, Noguchi O *et al.* Effects of additional administration of colchicine in ursodeoxycholic acid-treated patients with primary biliary cirrhosis: a prospective randomized study. *J Hepatol* 1996; **24**: 88–94.
88 Poupon RE, Huet PM, Poupon R *et al.* A randomized trial comparing colchicine and ursodeoxycholic acid combination to ursodeoxycholic acid in primary biliary cirrhosis. *Hepatology* 1996; **4**: 1098–103.
89 Leuschner M, Guldutuna S, You T *et al.* Ursodeoxycholic acid and prednisolone versus ursodeoxycholic acid and placebo in the treatment of early stages of primary biliary cirrhosis. *J Hepatol* 1996; **25**: 49–57.
90 Wolfhagen FH, van Buren HR, Schalm SW. Combined treatment with ursodeoxycholic acid and prednisone in primary biliary cirrhosis. *Neth J Med* 1994; **44**: 84–90.
91 Markus BH, Dickson E, Grambsch P *et al.* Efficiency of liver transplantation in patients with primary biliary cirrhosis. *N Engl J Med* 1989; **320**: 1709–13.

22 Autoimmune hepatitis: diagnosis and treatment

Michael Peter Manns, Andreas Schüler

INTRODUCTION

Autoimmune hepatitis (AIH) is a self-perpetuating necroinflammatory disease of unknown etiology, which is characterized by a loss of tolerance towards the patient's own liver tissue. The disease may lead to liver cirrhosis and liver failure. Since the recognition of immunologically based liver disease in the 1950s, efforts have been directed to development of tools for diagnosis, to classification according to serological markers and clinical course, and to distinguishing autoimmune hepatitits from other liver diseases.

In the early years diagnosis of autoimmune hepatitis was hampered by the lack of knowledge about the etiology of most acute and chronic liver diseases. The detection of hepatitis viruses and a better understanding of the etiology of other forms of liver disease allowed the exclusion of patients with these disorders from studies of autoimmune hepatitis and more accurate determination of prognosis and effects of immunosuppressive drugs. The characterization of distinctive autoantibodies and the identification of autoantigens led to a more specific diagnosis of the disease and to the ability to characterize distinct subclasses according to prognosis, treatment response, and outcome.

FEATURES OF AUTOIMMUNE HEPATITIS

Autoimmune hepatitis is a syndrome which is characterized by a set of epidemiological, laboratory, and clinical features: female predominance (female : male ratio 4 : 1), overrepresentation of the HLA alleles DR3 and DR4, hypergammglobulinemia, circulating autoantibodies, response to immunosuppressive therapy, and coexistence of extrahepatic autoimmune diseases.

Epidemiology and genetic predisposition

The incidence of autoimmune hepatitis in Western Europe and ethnically comparable populations is 0.7 cases per 100 000 inhabitants per year.[1] Autoimmune hepatitis is recognized more frequently in geographic areas where the prevalence of viral hepatitis is low.

It is generally accepted that occurrence and probably the severity of autoimmune hepatitis are based on an immunogenetic background. Autoimmune hepatitis is strongly associated with the HLA haplotype A1, B8, DR3 or DR4.[2–5] In caucasian patients autoimmune hepatitis type 1 is strongly associated with the HLA-B8-DR3 haplotype. HLA-B8 is in strong linkage dysequilibrium with HLA-DR3 (94% co-occurrence), which results in a close association between AIH type 1 and B8.[2,5]

HLA-B8 is found in 47%, HLA-A1-B8-DR3 in 37%, HLA-DR3 in 52%, and HLA-DR4 in 42% of patients.[6] Patients with HLA-DR3 have an early onset and a more severe course of the disease. Patients with the HLA-DR4 allele are older, have a more benign disease course, but have extrahepatic autoimmune diseases more frequently. HLA and HLA-B54 are common in Japan where autoimmune hepatitis type 1 is rare.[7]

It is unlikely that a single gene determines susceptibility for autoimmune hepatitis, since HLA-DR3 and DR4 are independent risk factors for the disease and are associated with distinctive clinical syndromes.[3,8]

Prognosis

The mortality rates of untreated autoimmune hepatitis in the placebo control groups of early clinical trials were greater than 50% within 3–5 years of diagnosis.[9–12] However, only cases with severe inflammatory activity or fibrosis were included in these early trials. Although the etiology of the chronic hepatitis was not certain, due to the lack of viral markers, the majority of patients in these trials appear to have been suffering from autoimmune hepatitis. However, it was impossible to exclude hepatitis C infection until the early 1990s.

Verification of these data on naive patients in whom the diagnosis of hepatitis C has been excluded is not possible, since studies including untreated control groups or cohort studies of untreated patients can no longer be justified ethically.

The poor survival observed in the control group in early studies may have been influenced also by the late diagnosis of autoimmune hepatitis, and an over-representation of patients with advanced liver disease. Conversely, the response to newer therapies may also appear to be better today, since more patients are diagnosed at early disease stages without cirrhosis. Nevertheless, it can be concluded that untreated autoimmune hepatitis is associated with a high risk for the development of endstage cirrhosis.

Outcome in untreated autoimmune hepatitis depends on the degree of inflammatory activity and on the stage of fibrosis. In untreated patients more than 10-fold elevation of AST, or more than five-fold elevation of AST together with more than two-fold elevation of gammaglobulins, are associated with an average 50% 3-year and 90% 10-year mortality rate. In contrast, AST elevation less than five-fold together with gammaglobulin elevation less than two-fold are associated with only an average 10% 10-year mortality.[13]

Periportal hepatitis without fibrosis is associated with a 17% incidence of cirrhosis at 5 years, but a normal 5-year survival.[14,15] The presence of bridging necrosis or multilobular necrosis is associated with an incidence of cirrhosis at 5 years as high as 82% and with a 5-year survival of only 55%.[15] Patients with cirrhosis at presentation have a 58% 5-year mortality rate.

Patients in whom remission is achieved have a 10-year life expectancy of 90% which does not differ from that of patients with cirrhosis at the beginning of treatment (89%).[13,16] Thus the presence of cirrhosis before or after therapy does not influence survival.[13,17]

Table 22.1 Extrahepatic autoimmune syndromes in autoimmune hepatitis

Frequent symptoms	Rare symptoms
Arthritis	Mixed connective tissue disease
Vitiligo	Lichen planus
Autoimmune thyroid disease	Ulcerative colitis
Insulin dependent diabetes	
Hirsutism, cushingoid features	

CLINICAL FEATURES

Although autoimmune hepatitis occurs mainly in young women, the disease may develop at any age and in either sex.[17] There appears to be a bimodal distribution to the peak incidence of the disease, with the first peak occurring between ages 10 and 30 and the second over age 40.[17] Data about the distribution of cirrhosis at presentation in these two age groups are not available but differences were not seen when comparing patients with HLA-DR3 which predominates in young patients and DR4.[18] Forty percent of patients present with acute hepatitis.[19] Fulminant liver failure may occur but is rare. In the majority of patients the disease progresses without major symptoms, and the diagnosis is not made until symptoms of severe liver disease are present. Jaundice is present in a large proportion of patients at diagnosis. Patients' complaints include fatigue, anorexia, abdominal pain (10–20%), and fever (20%). Amenorrhea occurs in women with severe hepatic inflammation. Hepatomegaly is common and an enlarged spleen is palpable in 50% of patients. Liver cirrhosis is a presenting feature in 30–80% of patients and 10–20% exhibit signs of decompensated liver disease.

Extrahepatic manifestations

Coexisting extrahepatic autoimmune diseases are frequently found in patients with autoimmune hepatitis. Whereas arthropathies and periarticular swelling both of large and small joints occurs in 6–36% of patients, arthritis with joint erosions is rarely seen. Additional clinical features are listed in Table 22.1.

DIAGNOSIS

Since autoimmune hepatitis is a syndrome of unknown etiology, diagnosis requires the assessment of typical clinical and laboratory features. Histology confirms disease activity and stage but by itself is not sufficient for diagnosis.

Advances in the characterization of autoantibodies and their antigens and the exclusion of etiologically distinct liver diseases facilitate early diagnosis in autoimmune hepatitis. Since treatment of AIH in advanced stages is less effective and is associated with a higher risk of relapse, early treatment improves outcome.

Definitive diagnosis of autoimmune hepatitis requires the presence of circulating autoantibodies at titers of at least 1 : 80 (in children 1 : 20) for most autoantibodies associated with AIH, hypergammaglobulinemia 1 to 1.5 times the upper limit of normal, and periportal or lobular hepatitis on liver biopsy. Other chronic liver diseases must be excluded by a search for the presence of viral markers, the history of parenteral blood exposure, alcoholic liver disease, drug induced liver disease, other forms of autoimmune liver disease including primary biliary cirrhosis, and primary sclerosing cholangitis, and genetically determined diseases like Wilson's disease or hemochromatosis.

The International Autoimmune Hepatitis Group has proposed a scoring system which may help to verify the diagnosis of autoimmune hepatitis[20] and to distinguish it as much as possible from other forms of chronic hepatitis. The system documents clinical, laboratory, and histological findings at presentation as well as response to corticosteroid therapy. The latter response may help to clarify the diagnosis even in patients who lack other typical features (Table 22.2). This scoring system has not yet been validated prospectively, but retrospective validation suggests that it is valuable.[21]

Table 22.2 Scoring system for diagnosis of autoimmune hepatitis

Parameter	Score
Gender	
Female	+2
Male	0
Serum biochemistry	
Alkaline phosphatase-to-AST levels (ratio of elevations above normal)	
>3.0	–2
<3.0	+2
Total serum globulin, gammaglobulin, or IgG (times upper normal limit)	
>2.0	+3
1.5–2.0	+2
1.0–1.5	+1
<l.0	0
Autoantibodies (titers by immunofluorescence on rodent tissues)	
Adults	
ANA, SMA or LKM–1	
>1:80	+3
1:80	+2
1:40	+1
<1:40	0
Children	
ANA or LKM–1	
>1:20	+3
1:10 or 1:20	+2
<1:20	0
SMA	
>1:20	+3
1:20	+2
<1:20	0
Antimitochondrial antibody	
Positive	–2
Negative	0
Viral markers	
IgM anti-HAV, HBsAg or	
IgM anti-HBc positive	–3

Table 22.2 Scoring system for diagnosis of autoimmune hepatitis –*Continued*

Parameter	Score
Anti-HCV positive by ELISA and/or RIBA	–2
HCV positive by PCR for HCV RNA	–3
Positive test indicating active infection with any other virus	–3
Seronegative for all of the above	+3
Other etiological factors	
History of recent hepatotoxic drug usage or parenteral exposure to blood products	
Yes	–2
No	+1
Alcohol (average consumption)	
Male <35 g/day; female <25 g/day	+2
Male 35–50 g/day; female 25–40 g/day	0
Male 50–80 g/day; female 40–60 g/day	–1
Male >80 g/day: female >60 g/day	–2
Genetic factors	
HLA-DR3 or DR4	
Other autoimmune diseases in patient or first degree relatives	+1
Liver histology	
Lobular hepatitis and bridging necrosis	+3
Bridging necrosis	+2
Rosettes	+1
Marked plasma cell infiltrate	+1
Bile duct lesions	–1
Other changes indicating different etiology	–3
Treatment response	
Complete	+2
Partial	0
Treatment failure	0
No response	–2
Relapse	+3
Diagnostic aggregate scores	
Pretreatment	
Definite	>15
Probable	10–15
Post-treatment	
Definite	>17
Probable	12–17

Source: Johnson PJ, McFarlane IG, Alvarez F *et al.* Meeting Report. International Autoimmune Hepatitis Group. *Hepatology* 1993; **18**: 998–1005.

Serologically defined subtypes

Three groups of autoimmune hepatitis can be divided serologically according to the presence of distinct autoantibodies. Although this division into three subgroups is regarded as preliminary and is not conclusively validated, it reflects differences with regard to onset, clinical course, treatment response, and outcome.[22]

AIH TYPE 1

Type is characterized by the presence of antinuclear antibodies (ANA) and/or smooth muscle antibodies (SMA). This group accounts for 80% of AIH patients. Although most patients are young at presentation, the disease may also become manifest in older patients. There is a good response to immunosuppressive therapy in up to 80% of patients.[23] Antinuclear antibodies, and especially the presence of smooth muscle antibodies with anti-actin specificity, are of high diagnostic specificity.[24,25] Seventy percent of patients are women younger than 40 years of age.[23,26] In 17% of patients concurrent autoimmune disease, including immune thyroiditis, Grave's disease, rheumatoid arthritis or ulcerative colitis, are present.[6,26–28] Twenty-five percent of patients with autoimmune hepatitis type 1 are found to have cirrhosis at presentation. Thus the disease may progress without major symptoms, and some patients who present with acute onset may have exacerbation of a longlasting subclinical disease.[16,26,29]

AIH TYPE 2

Type 2 is characterized by liver kidney microsomal (anti-LKM–1) autoantibodies which are targeted against cytochrome P450 IID6, and is predominantly seen in children.[30,31] Anti-LC–1, directed against a cytosolic antigen, is another marker of autoimmune hepatitis type 2.[32] Autoimmune hepatitis type 2 is characterized by a more rapid progression to cirrhosis, a higher relapse rate, and a comparatively poorer response to corticosteroid therapy. The presence of ANA and/or SMA is detected in only 4% of patients in this group.[33]

AIH TYPE 3

Type 3 is characterized by autoantibodies against soluble liver antigen (anti-SLA), which is associated with glutathione S-transferase.[34] The designation of this as a distinct subtype may be premature since clinical course and response to corticosteroid therapy do not differ significantly from AIH type 1. Anti-SLA or anti-LP may indeed be the only markers of autoimmune hepatitis in patients who are negative for ANA, SMA, and LKM–1 autoantibodies.[35] About 13% of patients with autoimmune hepatitis lack classic autoantibodies but present with typical laboratory and clinical features.

Liver histology

Autoimmune hepatitits cannot be diagnosed by liver histology alone, since there are no pathognomonic histological features. Histology can only support the diagnosis and is used to classify disease activity (grading) and the degree of fibrosis (staging). There is a general agreement that bridging necrosis and multilobular necrosis should be regarded as bad prognostic factors.[14,36]

TREATMENT

Corticosteroids should be administered until remission, incomplete response, treatment failure or unacceptable adverse effects occur. Remission is defined by the absence of symptoms, resolution of hepatic inflammation by liver histology, and a normalization of liver enzymes with the exception of AST which may remain up to twice normal.[19]

Conventional corticosteroids

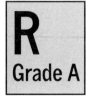

R Grade A

Three controlled trials[10–12] provided evidence that corticosteroid therapy reduces mortality in autoimmune hepatitis (Table 22.3), and this benefit was further substantiated by longer follow-up of the patients in one of these studies[9] (Table 22.4). In these studies steroids also relieved symptoms, improved biochemical abnormalities including transaminases, bilirubin levels, and hypoalbuminemia, and improved liver histology. Each of these early trials enrolled only small numbers of patients. There were also some design flaws, such as lack of blinding, the performance of repeated analyses, and the exclusion from analysis of patients who were withdrawn after randomization because of changes in diagnoses. In one of the trials[10] there were five such examples out of 54 patients who were randomized, and four of these were in the group receiving steroid treatment. However, clinical and biochemical responses to steroid treatment (Figures 22.1–22.3) were sufficiently large, when compared to placebo or azathioprine, that there

Table 22.3 Effect of prednisone on mortality in RCTs in chronic autoimmune hepatitis

Study	Patients	Steroid regimen	Control intervention	Mortality steroid/control		*P*
Cook, 1971[10]	49 patients with CAH, 35 with cirrhosis; no previous steroids; 5 patients (4 in steroid group) excluded from analysis because of change in diagnosis	Prednisone 15 mg (3–72 mth) attempts to withdraw after 1 mth	'No specific treatment'	3/22	15/27	<0.01
Soloway, 1972[11]	35[a] patients with chronic liver disease biochemically and histologically, 16 with cirrhosis	Prednisone 20 mg after 4 wk tapering course from 60 mg (3 mth to 3.5 yr)	Placebo	1/18	7/17	<0.05
Murray-Lyon, 1973[12]	47patients with chronic aggressive hepatitis, 33 with cirrhosis; approximately half had previous steroid or azathioprine	15 mg daily (up to 2 yr); discontinued in 1 mth if no improvement in liver function	Azathioprine 75 mg	1/22	6/25	N/A[b]

[a]Additional patients were randomized to receive prednisone 10 mg plus azathioprine 50 mg (14 patients), or azathioprine 100 mg (14 patients) see text.
[b]N/A, not available. Estimated probability of survival at 2 years: steroid 95%, azathioprine 72%.

Table 22.4 Long term outcome of patients with treated and untreated autoimmune hepatitis (Kirk, 1980[9])

	Control	Prednisolone
Patients treated	22	22
Cirrhosis	15/22	15/21
Alive at 10 yr	6	13
Dead at 10 yr	16[a]	8
Deaths 0–5 yr	14	4
Deaths 6–10 yr	2	4
Lost to follow-up	1	

[a]Two not related to liver disease.

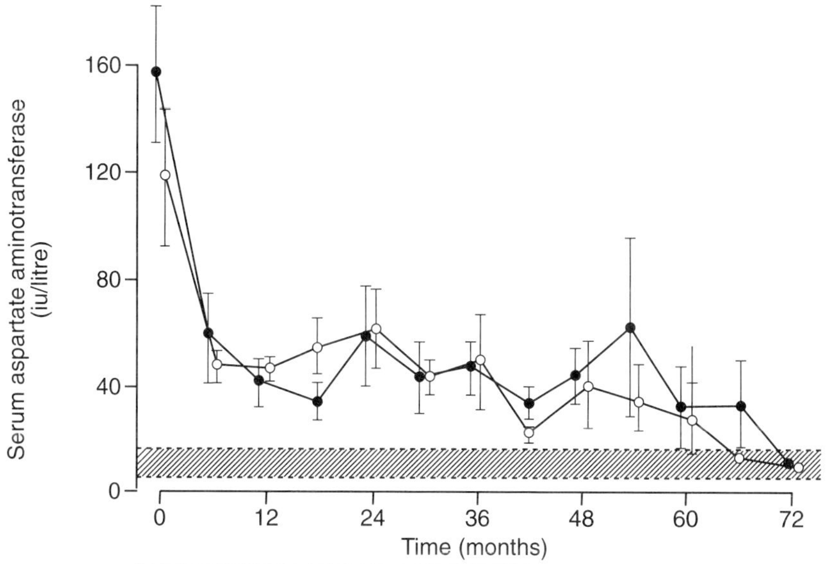

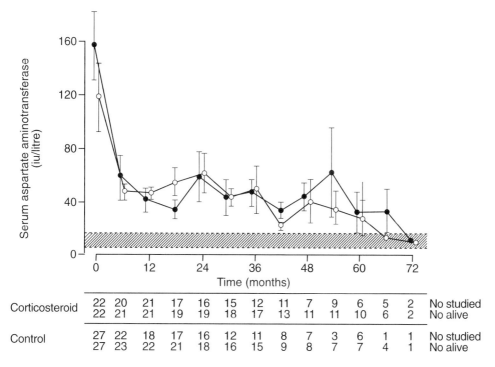

Corticosteroid	22	20	21	17	16	15	12	11	7	9	6	5	2	No studied
	22	21	21	19	19	18	17	13	11	11	10	6	2	No alive
Control	27	22	18	17	16	12	11	8	7	3	6	1	1	No studied
	27	23	22	21	18	16	15	9	8	7	7	4	1	No alive

Figure 22.1 Serum aspartate amniotransferase (Reproduced with permission from Cook GC, Mulligan R, Sherlock S. Controlled prospective trial of corticosteroid therapy in active chronic hepatitis. *Q J Med* 1971; **40**: 159–85)

is a high level of confidence that a significant treatment effect exists. The magnitude of the reduction of mortality produced by steroids can be estimated from the original analysis of Cook's study[10] (control 55%, steroid 14%, ARR 42%, NNT = 3) and from the analysis conducted after 10 years of follow-up of the same patient groups (control 73%, steroid 37%, ARR 36%, NNT = 3).[9]

R
Grade A/C

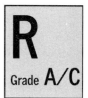

Corticosteroids are now regarded as standard therapy for patients with moderate to severe autoimmune hepatitis. Data from the randomized trials and from uncontrolled studies suggest that the remission rate is approximately 80% with initial therapy within a time frame of 2–4 years.[37] Usually a significant decrease in transaminases is seen within

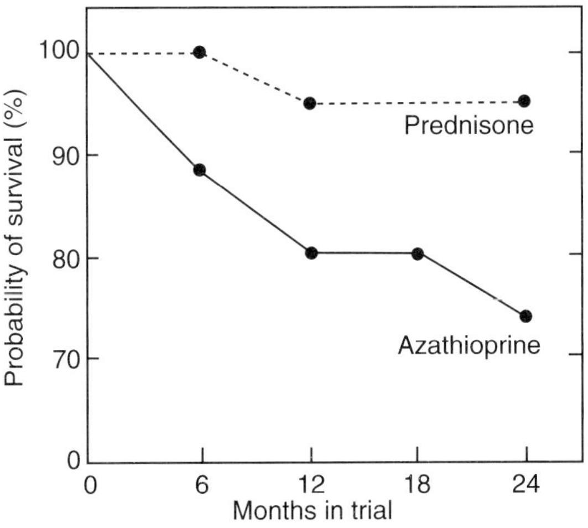

Figure 22.2 The calculated probability of survival in the two groups over the 2 years of treatment (Reproduced with permission from Murray-Lyon IM, Stern RB, Williams R. Controlled trial of prednisone and azathioprine in active chronic hepatitis. *Lancet* 1973; i: 735–7)

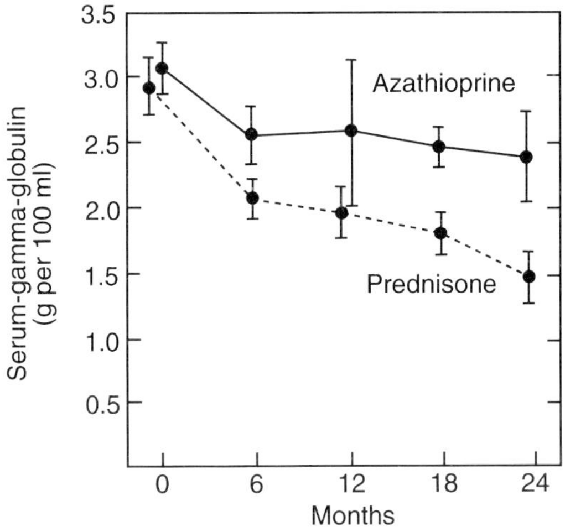

Figure 22.3 Mean values (± SEM) of serum-gamma-globulin in the two treatment groups at 6-month intervals (Reproduced with permission from Murray-Lyon IM, Stern RB, Williams R. Controlled trial of prednisone and azathioprine in active chronic hepatitis. *Lancet* 1973; i: 735–7)

a few months. In the Mayo study of 111 patients treated with daily prednisone alone or prednisone plus azathioprine, 82 (74%) entered remission, 16 (14%) were treatment failures, and 13 patients (12%) neither remitted nor failed therapy. It is important to note that histological remission may lag behind improvement of symptoms and biochemical parameters. In the patients treated in the Mayo study symptoms improved first (87% by 6 months), followed by biochemical resolution (68% by 6 months), while histological resolution was seen in only 8% at 6 months and 29% at 12 months.[38] Complete remission, including histological resolution, was accomplished by 2 years in 61 patients (74%), by 3 years in 73 (89%), and 4 years in 78 (95%).[37] About 10% of patients showed progressive disease in spite of corticosteroid therapy, 13% had an incomplete response after at least 3 years of treatment, and 13% of patients developed severe adverse effects of therapy. Furthermore, the risk of relapse is more than 50% within 6 months and 70% within 3 years after induction therapy or after treatment cessation.[19,39,40] Patients who do not enter remission have a 40% risk of developing cirrhosis within 10 years.[16]

R Grade A/C

The benefits of corticosteroid therapy have been shown only in a subgroup of patients with severe liver disease, symptoms, and markedly elevated transaminases and gammaglobulin levels.[11,38,41,42] For example, the Mayo Clinic studies included patients according to preset criteria,[11,42] which included hepatitis lasting for at least 10 weeks and AST greater than 10 times normal (or AST greater than five times normal together with two-fold elevated gammaglobulins). Disease was verified by liver biopsy in all patients and those with hepatic encephalopathy, malignancy or massive alcohol intake were excluded.

Controlled trials have not been performed in patients with mild asymptomatic AIH. In these patients, who numerically far outnumber patients with severe liver disease, the role for steroid therapy remains unclear.[41]

Since the average duration of treatment until remission is achieved is 22 months (range 6 months to 4 years), treatment withdrawal should not be attempted less than 2 years from the start of therapy to prevent early relapse. Drug withdrawal should be preceded by liver biopsy examination. The relapse rate depends on the degree of continuing inflammation and increases from 20% with complete resolution of hepatic inflammation to 50% with ongoing portal inflammation, and 100% with progression to cirrhosis or persisting periportal hepatitis.[41] The relapse rate after treatment withdrawal is as high as 80%. The remaining 20% of patients have to be regularly assessed by clinical parameters and liver biopsy as the risk of relapse cannot be predicted reliably. Ongoing inflammation may exist without significantly elevated transaminases. Normal liver histology after 2 years of steroid therapy does not exclude relapse following treatment withdrawal.

R Grade C

The proportion of patients who continue without inflammatory activity after treatment withdrawal is low. In some of those patients the initial diagnosis may have been incorrect. Valid data on the long term outcome of this patient group are not available.

Budesonide, a short half-life corticosteroid with 90% hepatic first pass elimination, was shown to improve liver inflammation in an uncontrolled study of patients with acute autoimmune hepatitis.[43] Plasma cortisol levels were suppressed significantly only in cirrhotic patients, possibly due to a reduced capacity of the cirrhotic liver to metabolize steroids. Controlled trials of this drug are not available.

R Grade C

Azathioprine

In one of the trials[11] of prednisone therapy patients were randomized to receive prednisone, azathioprine, a combination of azathioprine and prednisone, or a placebo. No differences in outcomes were observed between the azathioprine and placebo groups, while patients in the combined therapy group appeared to respond in a fashion similar to the prednisone treated patients. In a second study,[12] a direct comparison of steroids and azathioprine was made, and steroids were clearly more effective.

R Grade A

There is no evidence that azathioprine is more effective than placebo for induction of remission, but in uncontrolled studies it was reported to maintain remission induced by combined therapy with azathioprine and corticosteroids for periods of 1–10 years in as many as 83% of patients.[44,45]

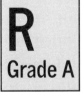

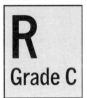

R Grade C

Other immunosuppressive drugs

The impact of novel immunosuppressive drugs like cyclosporin A, FK 506, rapamycin or mycophenolate in the treatment of autoimmune hepatitis has not yet been established and they cannot be recommended for general use in patients with intractable disease.

Liver transplantation

Liver transplantation has resulted in excellent long term survival rates that exceed 90% after five years.[37] Patients who fail to enter remission after 4 years of conventional treatment are regarded as potential candidates for liver transplantation. Autoantibodies and hypergammaglobulinemia disappear within 2 years after transplantation. However, recurrence in the graft may occur. Although the recurrent disease may not respond to adjustments in the immunosuppression regimen, graft function and survival seem not to be decreased in these patients.[46]

REFERENCES

1 Hodges JR, Millward-Sadler GH, Wright R. Chronic active hepatitis: the spectrum of disease. *Lancet* 1982; **i**: 550–2.

2 Mackay IR, Tait BD. HLA associations with autoimmune-type chronic active hepatitis: identification of B8-DRw3 haplotype by family studies. *Gastroenterology* 1980; **79**: 95–8.

3 Donaldson PT, Doherty DG, Hayllar KM *et al.* Susceptibility to autoimmune chronic active hepatitis: human leukocyte antigens DR4 and 4 A1-B8-DR3 are independent risk factors. *Hepatology* 1990; **13**: 701–6.

4 Czaja AJ, Carpenter HA, Santrach PJ *et al.* Significance of HLA DR4 in type 1 autoimmune hepatitis. *Gastroenterology* 1993; **105**: 1502–7.

5 Mackay IR, Morris PJ. Association of autoimmune active chronic hepatitis with HLA-A1,8. *Lancet* 1972; **ii**: 793–5.

6 Czaja AJ, Carpenter HA, Santrach PJ *et al.* Genetic predispositions for the immunological features of chronic active hepatitis. *Hepatology* 1993; **18**: 816–22.

7 Seki T, Kiyosawa K, Inoko H *et al.* Association of autoimmune hepatitis with HLA-Bw54 and DR4 in Japanese patients. *Hepatology* 1990; **12**: 1300–4.

8 Doherty DG, Donaldson PT, Underhill JA *et al.* Allelic sequence variation in the HLA class 11 genes and proteins in patients with autoimmune hepatitis. *Hepatology* 1994; **19**: 609–15.

9 Kirk AP, Jain S, Pocock S *et al.* Late results of the Royal Free Hospital prospective controlled trial of prednisolone therapy in hepatitis B surface antigen negative chronic active hepatitis. *Gut* 1980; **21**: 78–83.

10 Cook GC, Mulligan R, Sherlock S. Controlled prospective trial of corticosteroid therapy in active chronic hepatitis. *Q J Med* 1971; **40**: 159–85.

11 Soloway RD, Summerskill WHJ, Baggenstoss AH *et al.* Clinical, biochemical and histological remission of severe chronic active liver disease: a controlled study of treatments and early prognosis. *Gastroenterology* 1972; **63**: 820–33.

12 Murray-Lyon IM, Stern RB, Williams R. Controlled trial of prednisone and azathioprine in active chronic hepatitis. *Lancet* 1973; **i**: 735–7

13 Roberts SK, Therneau T, Czaja AJ. Prognosis of histologic cirrhosis in type 1 autoimmune hepatitis. *Gastroenterology* 1996; **110**: 848–57.

14 Cooksley WGE, Bradbear RA Robinson W *et al.* The prognosis of chronic active hepatitis without cirrhosis in relation to bridging necrosis. *Hepatology* 1986; **6**: 345–8.

15 Schalm SW, Korman MG, Summerskill WHJ *et al.* Severe chronic active liver disease: prognostic significance of initial morphologic patterns. *Am J Dig Dis* 1977; **22**: 973–80.

16 Davis GL, Czaja AJ, Ludwig J. Development and prognosis of histologic cirrhosis in corticosteroid-treated hepatitis B surface antigen-negative chronic active hepatitis. *Gastroenterology* 1984; **87**: 1222–7.

17 Meyer zum Büschenfelde KH, Hoofnagle J, Manns M. *Immunology and liver*. Dordrecht: Kluwer Academic, 1993; pp 277–83.

18 Czaja AJ, Carpenter HA, Santrach PJ *et al.* Significance of HLA DR4 in Type 1

autoimmune hepatitis. *Gastroenterology* 1993; **105**: 1502–7.
19 Czaja AJ. Diagnosis, prognosis, and treatment of classical autoimmune chronic active hepatitis. In: Krawitt EL, Wiesner RH (eds), *Autoimmune liver diseases*. New York: Raven Press, 1991, pp 143–66.
20 Johnson PJ, McFarlane IG, Alvarez F *et al.* Meeting Report. International Autoimmune Hepatitis Group. *Hepatology* 1993; **18**: 998–1005.
21 Czaja AJ, Carpenter HA. Validation of scoring system for diagnosis of autoimmune hepatitis. *Dig Dis Sci*; **41**: 305–14.
22 Maddrey WC. Subdivisions of idiopathic autoimmune chronic active hepatitis. *Hepatology* 1987; **7**: 1372–5.
23 Czaja AJ. Natural history, clinical features, and treatment of autoimmune hepatitis. *Semin Liver Dis* 1984; **4**: 1–12.
24 Lidman K, Biberfield G, Fagraeus A *et al.* Anti-actin specificity of human smooth muscle antibodies in chronic active hepatitis. *Clin Exp Immunol* 1976; **24**: 266–72.
25 Toh B-H. Smooth muscle autoantibody and autoantigens. *Clin Exp Immunol* 1979; **38**: 621–8.
26 Czaja AJ, Davis GL, Ludwig J *et al.* Autoimmune features as determinants of prognosis in steroid-treated chronic active hepatitis of uncertain etiology. *Gastroenterology* 1983; **85**: 713–17.
27 Perdigoto R, Carpenter HA, Czaja AJ. Frequency and significance of chronic ulcerative colitis in severe corticosteroid-treated autoimmune hepatitis. *J Hepatol* 1992; **14**: 325–31.
28 Czaja AJ, Carpenter HA, Santrach PJ *et al.* Evidence against hepatitis viruses as important causes of severe autoimmune hepatitis in the United States. *J Hepatol* 1993; **18**: 342–52.
29 Nikias GA, Batts KP, Czaja AJ. The nature and prognostic implications of autoimmune hepatitis with an acute presentation. *J Hepatol* 1994; **21**: 866–71.
30 Rizzetto M, Swana G, Doniach D. Microsomal antibodies in active chronic hepatitis and other disorders. *Clin Exp Immunol* 1973; **15**: 331–44.
31 Homberg JC, Abuaf N, Bernard O *et al.* Chronic active hepatitis associated with anti-liver/kidney microsome antibody type I: a second type of "autoimmune hepatitis". *Hepatology* 1987; **197**: 1333–9.
32 Martini E, Abuaf N, Caalli F *et al.* Antibody to liver cytosol (anti-LC1) in patients with autoimmune chronic active hepatitis type 2. *Hepatology* 1988; **8**: 1662–6.
33 Czaja AJ, Manns MP, Homburger HA. Frequency and significance of antibodies to liver/kidney microsome type 1 in adults with chronic active hepatitis. *Gastroenterology* 1992; **103**: 1290–5.
34 Wies I, Brunner S, Henninger J *et al.* Autoimmune hepatitis specific autoantibodies: cloning of the SLA and LP autoantigen. Submitted.
35 Czaja AJ, Manns MP. The validity and importance of subtypes in autoimmune hepatitis: a point of view. *Am J Gastroenterol* 1995; **90**: 1206–11.
36 Combes B. The initial morphologic lesion in chronic hepatitis. Important or unimportant? *Hepatology* 1986; **6**: 518–22.
37 Sanchez-Urdazpal LS, Czaja AJ, van Hoek B *et al.* Prognostic features and role of liver transplantation in severe corticosteroid-treated autoimmune chronic active hepatitis. *Hepatology* 1992; **15**: 215–21.
38 Davis GL, Czaja AJ. Immediate and long term results of corticosteroid therapy for severe idiopathic chronic active hepatitis. In: Czaja AJ, Dickson ER (eds), *Chronic active hepatitis: the Mayo Clinic experience*. New York: Marcel Dekker, 1986, pp 269–83.
39 Hegarty JE, Nouri Aria, KT, Portmann B *et al.* Relapse following treatment withdrawal in patients with autoimmune chronic active hepatitis. *Hepatology* 1993; **3**: 685–9.
40 Czaja AJ, Ammon HV, Summerskill WHJ. Clinical features and prognosis of severe chronic active liver disease (CALD) after corticosteroid-induced remission. *Gastroenterology* 1980; **78**: 518–23.
41 Koretz RL, Lewin KJ, Fagen ND *et al.* Chronic active hepatitis. Who meets treatment criteria? *Dig Dis Sci* 1980; **25**: 695–9.
42 Ammon HV. Assessment of treatment regimens. In: Czaja AF, Dickson ER (eds), *Chronic active hepatitis: the Mayo Clinic experience*. New York: Marcel Dekker, 1986, pp 33–46.
43 Danielsson Å, Prytz H. Oral budesonide for treatment of autoimmune chronic active hepatitis. *Aliment Pharmacol Ther* 1994; **8**: 585–90.
44 Stellon AJ, Keating JJ, Johnson PH *et al.* Maintenance of remission in autoimmune chronic active hepatitis with azathioprine after corticosteroid withdrawal. *Hepatology* 1988; **8**: 781–4.
45 Johnson PJ, McFarlane IG, Williams R. Azathioprine for long-term maintenance of remission in autoimmune hepatitis. *N Engl J Med* 1995; **333**: 958–63.
46 Prados E, Cuervas-Mons V, De la Mata M *et al.* Outcome of autoimmune hepatitis after liver transplantation. *Transplantation* 1998; **66**: 1645–50.

23 Primary sclerosing cholangitis: etiology, diagnosis, prognosis, and treatment

STEPHEN A MITCHELL, ROGER WG CHAPMAN

Primary sclerosing cholangitis (PSC) is a chronic cholestatic liver disease in which a progressive obliterating fibrosis of the intra- and extrahepatic bile ducts leads to biliary cirrhosis, portal hypertension, and eventually hepatic failure. In comparison with some of the conditions discussed in this book, PSC is a rare disease. But the absence of large randomized clinical trials and meta-analyses in PSC does not prevent us from gathering the best evidence with which to attempt an answer to the many questions posed by patients and clinicians about the etiology, diagnosis, prognosis, and management of this disease. Inevitably, where good external evidence is lacking, personal clinical expertise may play a greater role in the decision making process. This integration of clinical expertise and best available clinical evidence from systematic research constitutes the practice of "evidence based gastroenterology".

ETIOLOGY

A number of causative agents have been implicated in the pathogenesis of PSC but no single hypothesis has provided a unifying explanation for all the clinical and pathological features of this disease. PSC is closely associated with inflammatory bowel disease (IBD), the majority (65–86%) of patients with PSC have coexistent ulcerative colitis (UC) and the prevalence of PSC in UC populations is between 2 and 6%.[1–3] In a patient with UC, abnormal liver function tests, particularly an elevated serum alkaline phosphatase, may be the first indication of this insidious condition. Endoscopic retrograde cholangiopancreatography (ERCP) remains the "gold standard" for diagnosis. The close relationship between PSC and UC has inspired a number of hypotheses for the pathogenesis of PSC, involving the enterohepatic circulation of a causative factor. Bacteria and their products,[4] endotoxins,[5] toxic bile acids,[6] and other peptides[7] have all been considered as potential causative agents. It is proposed that the inflamed colonic mucosa becomes "leaky" in UC, permitting bacterial products and toxins to be more rapidly absorbed and to enter the portal circulation. Once in the portal circulation these products may induce liver injury if they are directly hepatotoxic, if they are metabolized within the liver to produce toxic byproducts, or if they activate monocytes or other immune cells to release pro-inflammatory cytokines. The evidence to support these hypotheses has mainly been obtained by collection of samples of portal blood in patients with UC undergoing colectomy. The majority of these studies did not include control samples from patients undergoing abdominal surgery for causes other than UC. These hypotheses also fail to explain the pathogenesis of PSC in the smaller proportion of patients who do not show evidence of underlying IBD.

The detection of portal bacteraemia or endotoxaemia *per se* in severely ill colitics undergoing colectomy does not prove that chronic portal bacteraemia leads to the development of PSC. To provide support for this hypothesis, detection of portal bacteraemia preceding, or at the very least at the onset of the disease, plus some correlation between the degree of bacteraemia and disease severity would be required. Such evidence is unavailable because only a minority of patients with PSC have abdominal surgery or a colectomy, and there is no early marker for the development of PSC. Cohort studies of patients with ulcerative colitis to identify potential etiological factors in PSC have also been considered to be impractical as the disease is rare, may take many years to develop, and requires a relatively invasive procedure for definitive diagnosis. Another approach has been to analyze the incidence and natural history of PSC in different ethnic groups to compare differences in possible risk factors with the incidence PSC. In India[8] and Africa, where perinatal umbilical sepsis and consequent portal bacteraemia is much more common than in the West, the reported incidence of PSC is low. These findings, which seem to argue against the hypothesis that chronic portal sepsis leads to PSC, may reflect differences in access to the appropriate diagnostic tests in developing countries rather than true differences in disease incidence.[9]

In the ultimate experiment to demonstrate that a putative factor leads to development of a PSC the investigator would randomly assign individuals to one of two groups, with one group exposed to the factor and the other not exposed, and compare the outcome. Such an experiment, which exposes a group of patients to a potentially harmful agent would, of course, be unethical. For this reason there is considerable interest in animal models, although many experts question their biological relevance and validity. In the rat model of acetic acid induced colitis a pro-inflammatory bacterial peptide was introduced into the inflamed mucosa, underwent enterohepatic circulation and resulted in hepatic inflammation around the portal areas.[10] The problem is that in this model and many others the histological pattern of damage is more suggestive of acute liver injury than the chronic insidious damage characteristic of PSC. The advent of the technology to "knockout" specific genes in mice and the recognition that this may lead to chronic intestinal inflammation studies has renewed interest in the development of an animal model of PSC. Exposure of knockout colitic mice to potential toxins may provide new insights into the pathogenesis of PSC and potential role of toxins undergoing an enterohepatic circulation.

In the absence of any convincing evidence for the involvement of bacteria, toxic bile acids, toxins or other infective agents in the pathogenesis of PSC, more recent research has concentrated on the possible role of genetic and immune factors. Since the discovery of an association between certain human leukocyte antigens (HLA), HLA B8 and HLA DR3, and PSC in the early 1980s in the United Kingdom[11] and Scandinavia,[12] numerous studies have searched for HLA associations with PSC (see Table 23.1). As susceptibility to a number of autoimmune diseases such as autoimmune hepatitis, insulin dependent diabetes, and myasthenia gravis is associated with HLA B8/DR3, speculation that PSC may also be an autoimmune disease soon arose. By HLA typing a group of patients with PSC, it is possible to show that some HLA alleles occur at higher or lower frequencies in PSC patients than in the general population. The relative risk of developing the disease in individuals who inherit various HLA alleles can then be estimated.

The studies of HLA associations with PSC in various populations are summarized in Table 23.1. The studies agree that there is a close association between PSC and the extended HLA haplotype A1, B8, DR3, DRw52a. Beyond this association apparent differences emerge. The question is whether these differences reflect genuine variation in

Table 23.1 Studies of HLA associations with primary sclerosing cholangitis

Study	No. of PSC patients	Population	Method	Primary associations	Secondary associations	Negative associations	No association
Chapman, 1983[11]	25	UK	S	B8		B12	
Schrumpf, 1982[12]	20	Norway	S	B8			
Prochazka, 1990[13]	29	USA	S	DRw52a			
Donaldson, 1991[14]	81	UK	S	B8, DR3	DR2	B44	DR4
Farrant, 1992[15]	70	UK	G	DRB3*101, DRB5*0101			
Mehal, 1994[16]	83	UK	G	DR52a, Dw2, DR3	DR2	DR4	
Olerup, 1995[17]	75	Sweden	G	DRB1*1301, DQA1*0103 DQB1*0603		DRB1*04	
Underhill, 1995[18]	71	UK	G				DPB1
Moloney, 1996[19]	60	UK	G	DRB1*0301, B8	Cw*0707		
Moloney, 1996[20]	114	UK	G			DR4	
Bittencourt, 1996[21]	18	Brazil	G	DR13.1			
Chen, 1996[22]	n/a	Germany	G	B8, DRB1*0301, DQA1*0103		B12	
Bernal, 1997[23]	120	UK	G	TNFα308A2 TNFβNco1			

S, Serotyping; G, genotyping.

disease susceptibility alleles between ethnic populations or are due to methodological factors. Caution must be exercised in the interpretation of HLA disease associations, as the actual association may be with other alleles that are linked to the "typed allele" and inherited with it. In two studies from King's College Hospital[14,15] DR4 was underrepresented in the PSC group compared to a control group, suggesting that DR4 may offer some protection against developing PSC. In these studies the overrepresentation of the positively associated DR alleles was not considered in the data analysis. No significant difference in the incidence of DR4 was noted in the Oxford[16] and Swedish[17] studies when corrections for the positive DR associations were made. Furthermore, the early studies relied on HLA typing based on serology, a procedure which may not identify the MHC molecules that are truly disease-associated. A single serologically defined allele may actually consist of a family of related HLA alleles that differ slightly from one another in their polymorphic residues. Such differences can only be identified by more detailed molecular studies using restriction fragment length polymorphism, gene amplification, and sequence-specific oligonucleotide probing. For example, Prochazka *et al*[13] reported that 100% of patients with endstage PSC expressed the HLA DRw52a antigen compared to only 35% of controls, suggesting that they had found the prime susceptibility allele for PSC. However, by using serological typing they had overassigned a relatively small number of patients to this allele and were unable to substantiate their earlier finding in a larger group of patients using detailed molecular genotyping.[24]

In addition to HLA A1, B8, DR3 association, Olerup *et al*[17] identified a highly significant association with the allele DRB1*1301 and the DRB1*1301, DQA1*0103 and DQB1*0603 haplotype. This study did not find a significant secondary association between HLA DR2 and PSC as had been reported in the King's and Oxford studies. Although studies of the immunogenetic susceptibility to PSC have concentrated on finding HLA class II associations, recent studies suggest that some HLA class I and class III associations may be at least as strong. In one study[19] the greatest risk of PSC was associated with the Cw*0701-B8-DRB1*0301 haplotype. In another study the association of TNFα-308 A2 allele is far stronger that that for DRB1*0301(DR3) and slightly greater than that for B8.[23] Although the authors suggest that the primary susceptibility allele in PSC may lie closer to the B8 rather than DR3 locus, it is not possible from the current data to identify the prime allele with any certainty.

HLA molecules are intimately involved in the regulation of the immune response and a number of abnormalities in cellular immunity have been detected in PSC, as listed in Table 23.2. Early studies involved the quantification of peripheral blood lymphocyte subsets in PSC patients compared with healthy controls.[44–46] Conflicting results were obtained due to the various methods of lymphocyte quantification (flow cytometry, blood smears, rosetting, and immunofluoresence) and also due to differences in the study populations. Most of these studies also failed to include sufficient numbers of patients with early stage disease and patients with cholestasis from another cause. Although it was initially proposed that there is a reduction in circulating T cells in PSC due to a disproportionate decrease in the $CD8^+$ T cell subset, it is now accepted that in the early stages of PSC the peripheral blood T and B cell populations are normal. As the disease progresses there is a fall in the $CD8^+$ T cell population. Since the biliary epithelium is probably the primary site of inflammation and damage in PSC, the significance of these observations in the periphery is unclear.

Due to the difficulty of obtaining liver tissue, especially in early disease, only a limited number of studies[44,46,47] have attempted to quantify changes in the number of liver infiltrating lymphocytes and their various subsets. All the studies agree that there is a

Table 23.2 Possible pathogenetic mechanisms in primary sclerosing cholangitis

Pathogenetic mechanisms	Evidence	Study
Non-immune mechanisms		
Portal bacteremia		Boden,1959[25]; Warren,1966[4]; Eade,1969[26]
Portal endotoxemia		Jacob,1977[5]
Absorption of colonic toxins		Hobson,1988[10]; Kono,1988[27]
Bile acid toxicity		Carey,1964[6]; Siegel,1977[28]
Copper accumulation and toxicity		Gross,1985[29]; Kowdley,1994[30]
Viral infections	Reovirus type 3	Minuk,1987[31]
	CMV	Mason,1991[32]; Mehal,1992[33]
	Retroviruses	Dowsett,1988[34]; Mason,1998[35]
Ischemic damage		Terblanche,1983[36]
Immune mechanisms		
Humoral immunity	⇑circulating immune complexes	Bodenheimer,1983[37]; Minuk,1985[38]; Garred,1993[39]
	⇑immunoglobulin levels and low titre ANA/SMA	Chapman,1980[40]
	ANCA	Duerr,1991[41]; Lo,1992[42]; Bansi,1996[43]
Cell mediated immunity	⇓circulating peripheral $CD8^+$ T cells	Whiteside,1985[44]; Lindor,1987[45]; Snook,1989[46]
	Portal T cell infiltrate	Whiteside,1985[44]; Snook,1989[46]; Si,1984[47]
	⇑activated and memory T cells	Lindor,1987[48]; Martins,1994[49]
	⇑$\gamma\delta$ T cells	Martins,1996, 1994[50,51]
	Restricted T cell repertoire	Broomé,1997[52]
	Aberrant expression of HLA DR on BECs	Chapman,1988[53]
	Coexpression of CD80 and HLA DR on BECs	Martins,1995[54]
	⇑circulating and tissue bound adhesion molecules	Adams,1991[55]
Immune effector mechanisms	⇑cytokine expression in the liver	Mitchell,1997[56]
Immunogenetic mechanisms	HLA associations	See Table 23.1

BEC, biliary epithelial cells.

portal infiltrate in PSC that is composed predominantly of $CD4^+$ T cells and that B cells are rare. The functional significance of this portal infiltrate is still debated. Immunohistochemical studies have provided evidence of T cell activation, with the portal infiltrate composed mainly of HLA DR^+ and $CD45RO^+$ cells (memory T cells).[48,49,51] The effector phase of the immune response is also enhanced as evidenced by an expanded population of intrahepatic cytokines.[56] Given the close proximity of T cells to the biliary epithelium, which may aberrantly express HLA DR,[53] it has been postulated that the biliary epithelial cells may be capable of presenting antigen to the $CD4^+$ T cells and thus initiating an immune response. Co-stimulatory signals, in addition to the normal T cell receptor and MHC peptide interaction, are needed to determine whether recognition of antigen by T cells leads to activation or T cell anergy. Leon *et al*[57] found that HLA DR^+ biliary epithelial cells when co-cultured with allogeneic lymphocytes did not express the

B7-1 (CD80) or B7-2 (CD86) ligands at either mRNA level or protein level and also failed to induce either lymphoproliferation or IL-2 production. Furthermore, they were not able to induce expression of these ligands on cultured biliary epithelial cells with TNFα, IFNγ or phorbol myrisate acetate. However, none of the biliary epithelial cells in these studies was obtained from PSC patients.[58] Using immunohistochemistry, Martins *et al*[54] detected coexpression of CD80 and HLA DR on 100% of proliferating bile ducts and 25% of interlobular ducts in PSC livers, while there was no expression on proliferating ducts or interlobular ducts in primary biliary cirrhosis. Whether biliary epithelial cells in PSC are capable of acting as antigen presenting cells and activate $CD4^+$ T cells *in vitro* or *vivo* remains controversial.

Although a number of abnormalities in humoral immunity have been described in PSC, many of these findings do not specifically relate to the disease but are secondary to cholestasis or to the development of cirrhosis. Although there were early reports[37] of elevated serum levels of immune complexes in PSC, similar findings have been found in other liver diseases. There is no evidence of complement activation within the liver.[39] Perinuclear anti-neutrophil antibodies (pANCA) have been detected in the serum of 26–85% of patients with PSC with or without coexistent UC.[41,42,59] pANCA may be detected by a variety of techniques including fixed neutrophil ELISA plus immunofluorescence, immunofluorescence alone, or immunoalkaline phosphatase determination. The merits of each technique have been subject to intense debate, but all the techniques detect the antibody with approximately equal sensitivity and specificity.[60] All the studies agree that there is no correlation between the detection of pANCA and clinical or treatment parameters. Therefore this antibody is unlikely to have a role in the pathogenesis of the disease. In one study[61] patients with PSC and UC had higher pANCA titers and increased levels of the IgG3 isotype of ANCA compared to patients with UC alone, hinting at differences in immune regulation. The antigen associated with pANCA in PSC is probably nuclear, but has not yet been identified.

Although there is now a considerable body of evidence that immune mechanisms are involved in the pathogenesis of PSC, we still have little insight into whether these events are triggered by an intrinsic abnormality within the immune system, or by an exogenous agent. As the search for causative agents such as viruses, bacteria, and toxins continues, recently developed animal models of colitis may offer an approach to elucidating pathogenetic mechanisms in PSC.

DIAGNOSIS

Although ERCP remains the gold standard for the diagnosis of PSC, it is an invasive technique which carries a small but significant risk of morbidity and mortality. A non-invasive and inexpensive test could not only be used for diagnosis but also for screening an asymptomatic patient population in order to detect early stage disease. The operating characteristics of such a diagnostic test should be compared with the gold standard and the test should be applied to patients with and without PSC as diagnosed by the gold standard test (ERCP). Although studies of computer assisted tomography (CT),[62,63] magnetic resonance cholangiography (MRC)[64] and pANCA have compared the results of these tests with ERCP findings in a population of PSC patients, only the studies of pANCA have applied the test to patients without PSC. In these studies[61,65] pANCA was measured in patients with UC who did not have PSC and in patients with other liver diseases. Few, if any, of these "controls" underwent ERCP as it would be regarded as unethical to expose patients to the risks of this procedure unless exclusion of biliary obstruction was indicated for clinical diagnosis and management. Even without applying the more rigorous standards that an evidence based approach demands, it is clear that pANCA has limitations as a diagnostic test. At lower titer pANCA can be detected in 50% of patients with autoimmune hepatitis, and even determination of the ANCA titre and IgG subclass does not distinguish between patients with PSC and UC and patients with UC only.[60]

No studies have compared CT or spiral CT and ERCP in a sufficiently large group of PSC patients to determine the specificity and sensitivity of these tests. In comparing CT and ERCP in 20 patients Teefey *et al*[66] found that CT was superior to cholangiography in characterization of the status of the intrahepatic duct system and can provide valuable information about the extent and extrabiliary complications of the disease. Magnetic resonance cholangiography is a new non-invasive technique and minimal data exists on its performance relative to ERCP. In one recent study[64] the ERCP and MRC of 15 patients with a suspected diagnosis of PSC were independently evaluated, and MRC was less sensitive and specific than ERCP, especially in patients with advanced disease and liver cirrhosis. This illustrates the importance of including patients with a wide spectrum of disease stages in these studies. The evidence is that neither CT or MRC can at present be used in place of ERCP to exclude the diagnosis of PSC. However, these tests may provide additional information about the extent of disease and the presence of hepatobiliary malignancy.

PROGNOSIS

Patients frequently ask questions regarding their prognosis. Before we can discuss prognostic factors with them in a meaningful way we must have an understanding of the natural history of the disease. The clinical course of PSC is quite variable; the disease is indolent in some patients and more rapidly progressive in others. The natural history of PSC is described in a number of retrospective studies,with the median survival time from diagnosis to death or transplantation (OLT) reported between 12 and 21 years.[67–69] Differences in survival estimations may reflect the variation in the definition of onset and outcome. As there is no reliable marker of early disease in PSC the onset is difficult to identify clearly. Whether the onset is defined as the occurrence of the first symptoms consistent with PSC, as the time of the first abnormal liver function test, or as the time of diagnosis by ERCP will result in differences in survival estimates. In retrospective studies details of distant events may be sparse and there is likely to be failure to recognize early signs and symptoms. Patients with late stage disease may predominate, while patients who die from rapidly progressive disease may be missed. The ideal study of prognosis is prospective and follows patients from a defined point in the disease process, usually diagnosis. There have been no studies using such an inception cohort in PSC because the disease is rare and its slow progression makes a prospective study impractical. A large retrospective study published by Broomé *et al*[67] did include a high proportion (46%) of patients with early (stage I and II) disease. Forty-four percent of patients were asymptomatic at diagnosis, and these patients exhibited longer survival than symptomatic patients. The estimated median survival for the whole PSC group was 144 months. For patients with symptoms at the time of diagnosis the estimated median survival was significantly less, at 112 months. Over one-fifth of the asymptomatic patients became symptomatic during the median follow-up period of 63 months.

Table 23.3 Studies of prognosis in primary sclerosing cholangitis: multivariate analysis

Study	No. of patients	% asymptomatic	Median survival (yr)	Independent prognostic factors
Helzberg, 1987[70]	53	25	[a]	Hepatomegaly Serum bilirubin >1.5 mg/dl at onset of disease
Wiesner, 1989[68]	174	21	11.9	Age Serum bilirubin Blood hemoglobin conc. Presence of IBD Histological stage
Farrant, 1991[69]	126	16	12.0	Hepatomegaly Splenomegaly Serum alkaline phosphatase Histological stage Age Presence of symptoms not a significant prognostic factor
Broomé, 1996[67]	305	44	12.0	Age Serum bilirubin Histological stage
Kim, 1997[71]	437			Age Serum bilirubin Presence of IBD Splenomegaly Ascites

[a]75% survival = 9 years.

Table 23.4 Studies of prognosis in primary sclerosing cholangitis: univariate analysis

Study	No. of patients	Prognostic indicator	Comments
Craig, 1991[72]	129	Disease assessment by cholangiography	Intrahepatic disease worse than extrahepatic
Mehal, 1994[16]	83	HLA DR4	HLA DR4 associated with poor prognosis
Olsson, 1995[73]	94	Disease assessment by cholangiography	High grade intrahepatic strictures indicate early jaundice and short survival
Moloney, 1996[20]	120	HLA DR4	HLA DR4 not associated with poor prognosis but confers resistance to developing PSC

From these studies a number of prognostic models have been developed, mainly using parameters defined at diagnosis (Tables 23.3, 23.4). Perhaps the most controversial prognostic factor is HLA DR4. Studies from Oxford[16] and the Mayo Clinic[74] suggest that HLA DR4 is associated with poor prognosis, whilst studies from London[20] and Sweden[17] were unable to confirm this association. Although these models successfully predict the natural history of the disease in a cohort of PSC patients, they are less successful when applied to individual patients. The confounding factor is the development of hepatobiliary or colonic cancer.

Cholangiocarcinoma is difficult to diagnose,[75] is associated with poor prognosis,[76] and precludes OLT.[77] In Broomé *et al*'s study cholangiocarcinoma was found in 8% of patients with PSC but occurred in 30% of the 79 patients who died or underwent OLT. In this and other studies none of the investigated clinical or laboratory parameters could identify those patients who would subsequently develop cholangiocarcinoma, although PSC patients with coexistent UC have a three- to four-fold higher risk of developing cholangiocarcinoma. A recent case–control study has suggested that long duration of UC and smoking are independent risk factors associated with the development of hepatobiliary malignancy in PSC.[78]

Patients with UC and PSC are also considered to be at higher risk of developing colonic dysplasia and carcinoma.[79] Studies[80,81] investigating this risk have given conflicting results due to the different methodologies employed, small numbers, design flaws, and different endpoints.[82] A recent study of a retrospectively defined inception cohort[83] has shown that the risk of developing colonic dysplasia or cancer is significantly increased in UC patients with PSC compared with patients with UC alone. A high proportion of right-sided cancers was noted in the PSC patients, consistent with the hypothesis that these cancers arise due to exposure to carcinogenic bile acids. However, the risk of cancer was not lower among the PSC patients treated with ursodeoxycholic acid.[84] PSC patients with UC remain at risk of developing colon cancer or dysplasia even after they have undergone OLT.[85]

The evidence is that physicians can only provide their PSC patients with a tentative survival estimate using the variables derived from prognostic models. The development of cholangiocarcinoma is often insidious and unpredictable. Although a significant impact of screening on mortality is unproven, we recommend that PSC patients with UC should enter a colonoscopic surveillance programme, possibly at an earlier stage than is recommended for UC patients without PSC.

MANAGEMENT

As the disease progresses there is loss of functioning bile ducts until hepatic biliary excretion fails and parenchymal damage, fibrosis, and cirrhosis ensues. The endstage PSC patient with biliary cirrhosis and portal hypertension may suffer from complications which are common to all patients with chronic cholestatic liver disease and cirrhosis. In PSC there is no specific management of these complications (pruritis, malabsorption of fat soluble vitamins, ascites, oesophageal varices, portosystemic encephalopathy). The reader should refer to the relevant chapters in this book for further details.

Over the past 30 years physicians have been searching for a therapeutic agent which delays or reverses disease progression in PSC without causing significant adverse effects. Table 23.5 summarizes results from controlled trials of a number of these agents. Table

Table 23.5 Controlled trials of therapeutic agents in PSC

Study	Agent	No. of patients	Study type	Control	Duration (mth)	Effects of intervention				Adverse effects (%)
						Symptoms	LFTs	Liver histology	Survival	
LaRusso, 1988[86]	Penicillamine oral	70	RCT double blind	Placebo	36	No	No	No	No	21
Knox, 1994[87]	Methotrexate oral	24	RCT double blind	Placebo	24	No	No	No	No	4
Lindor, 1996[88]		19	CCT	UDCA	24	No	No	No	No	26
Lindor, 1991[89]	Corticosteroids oral	12	CCT	Placebo	24	No	No	No	n/a	0
Allison, 1986[90]	Corticosteroids topical	13	RCT	Placebo	0.5	No	No	No	n/a	15
Wiesner, 1991[91]	Cyclosporin oral	34	RCT	Placebo	24	No	No	Yes	No	n/a
Olsson, 1995[92]	Colchicine oral	84	RCT double blind	Placebo	36	No	No	No	No	<5
Lo, 1992[93]	UDCA (<12 mg/kg)	23	RCT double blind	Placebo	24	No	Trend	No	n/a	0
Stiehl, 1994[94]		20	RCT double blind, then open	Placebo	3 (open label up to 48)	No	Yes	Yes	n/a	n/a
Van Thiel, 1992[95]		48	CCT	Placebo	18 (mean)	No	n/a	n/a	n/a	n/a
Beuers, 1992[96]	UDCA (13–15 mg/kg)	14	RCT double blind	Placebo	12	No	Yes	Yes	n/a	14
Lindor, 1997[97]		105	RCT double blind	Placebo	Up to 72 (mean 26)	No	Yes	No	No	0
Mitchell, 1997[98]	UDCA (20 mg/kg)	26	RCT double blind	Placebo	24	No	Yes	Yes	n/a	0

RCT, Randomized controlled trial; CCT, controlled clinical trial (non-randomized); n/a, data not available.

Table 23.6 Uncontrolled trials in PSC

Study	Agent	No. of patients	Duration (mth)	Effects of intervention				
				Symptoms	LFTs	Liver histology	Survival	Adverse effects (%)
Knox, 1991[99]	Methotrexate	10	12	Yes	Yes	Yes	n/a	0
Burgert, 1984[100]	Corticosteroids oral	10	n/a	n/a	Yes	n/a	n/a	n/a
Van Thiel, 1995[101]	FK506 oral	10	12	No	Yes	No	n/a	0
Angulo, 1998[102]	Nicotine oral	8	12	No	No	No	n/a	37.5
Bharucha, 1997[103]	Pentoxifylline oral	20	12	No	No	No	n/a	10
Pockros, 1996[104]	2-Chloro-deoxyadenosine oral	4	12	No	No	Yes	n/a	0
Stiehl, 1989[105]	UDCA (<12 mg/kg)	10	12	n/a	Yes	n/a	n/a	0
O'Brien, 1993[106]	UDCA	14	2–53 (mean 24)	Yes	Yes	n/a	n/a	0

R
Grade A

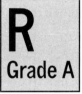

23.6 summarizes studies which lacked controls. Although uncontrolled studies may allow preliminary assessment of an agent, the evidence which they provide is extremely limited and subject to a variety of biases. Many studies of this type report benefit with a new intervention, only to be followed by controlled trials which are "negative". For example, an open pilot study[99] of low dose oral-pulse methotrexate in 10 PSC patients without evidence of portal hypertension produced promising results. The subsequent small randomized placebo controlled trial[87] showed no significant benefit in patients receiving methotrexate, although the relatively small sample size is compatible with a fairly high probability of a type 2 error.

In a majority of the randomized controlled trials which have been performed, surrogate outcomes (liver function tests, liver histology) were used, rather than clinical outcomes such as death or survival free from transplantation. These surrogate outcomes were generally used because the short duration and/or small sample size employed did not encompass a sufficient number of clinically relevant outcomes. The variability in rate of histological progression[107] between disease stages and the incidence of sample variability[108] in PSC patients suggests that even serial liver biopsies may not be reliable as a means of evaluating treatment efficacy.

R
Grade A

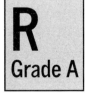

Rather small randomized trials have shown that the cupruretic drug D-penicillamine,[86] the antifibrotic agent colchicine[92] or methotrexate[87] have no beneficial effects on the biochemical tests or liver histology in PSC. While the possibility of a type 2 error exists in these studies, it is unlikely that larger trials will be performed because of the significant toxicity observed. Penicillamine was discontinued in 21% of treated patients due to adverse effects (pancytopenia and proteinuria). Pulmonary complications and alopecia were reported in those treated with methotrexate.[88]

Given the evidence that PSC is immune mediated it is surprising that there have been no RCTs examining the effects of oral corticosteroids in PSC. In a small controlled trial of topical steroids[90] administered via nasobiliary lavage the treatment group experienced no benefits but suffered a high incidence of bacterial cholangitis. Grade A Concerns about the long term adverse effect profile of corticosteroids, especially cortical bone loss, have discouraged larger randomized controlled trials. Cortical bone loss may be accelerated even in male PSC patients, although biphosphonates may reverse this loss. Cyclosporin, the only other immunosuppressant that has been evaluated in a small randomized controlled trial,[91] reduced the symptoms of UC, but had no effect on the course or prognosis of PSC. Grade A

Ursodeoxycholic acid (UDCA) at low (10 mg/kg) to medium (13–15 mg/kg) doses is the only agent that has been shown in a few small controlled trials[95,96] to improve liver biochemical tests, although it has not been demonstrated to have an effect on patients' symptoms. A recent fairly large randomized, placebo controlled trial[97] of medium dose UDCA in PSC found that UDCA significantly improved liver biochemical tests but failed to halt progression in liver histology and had no effect upon survival. Grade A Although the treatment and placebo groups were well matched, a high proportion (45%) of the participants in this trial had advanced disease, which may have precluded any response to medical therapy. In a small RCT[98] high dose UDCA (20 mg/kg) improved liver biochemistry, delayed progression in liver histology as evidenced by unchanged or improved modified histological index scores, but did not improve symptoms. Grade A Although high doses of UDCA were used, no major adverse effects were reported. A further large randomized controlled trial of high dose UDCA using an adequate sample size and study duration is needed to ascertain whether these reported improvements in surrogate outcomes are accompanied by improved clinical outcomes such as survival free of complications.

Dominant strictures particularly, in the extrahepatic biliary tree, may cause rapid deterioration of liver function and hasten progression to biliary cirrhosis. It is often difficult to distinguish dominant strictures from cholangiocarcinoma on cholangiographic appearance alone. Exfoliative brush cytology at ERCP has a high specificity and positive predictive value but low sensitivity and negative predictive value for the diagnosis of cholangiocarcinoma.[109] A combination of serum markers[110] such as Ca 19-9 and CEA may predict the presence of cholangiocarcinoma but ultrasound or CT guided biopsy may more accurately identify a malignant lesion.[111] Dominant strictures may be treated endoscopically by balloon dilation or stent insertion, or surgically.[112,113] Unfortunately there are no randomized trials to prove that endoscopic intervention significantly alters the natural history of strictures. Uncontrolled studies report clinical improvement post dilation, but provide only weak evidence of benefit and there are no trials to indicate which treatment modality offers the most sustained response with lowest risk of complications. Grade C After bilioenteric bypass there is increased risk of ascending cholangitis, and the risk of perioperative mortality at a future OLT may be higher.[114]

For patients with advanced PSC, OLT remains the only therapeutic option. The decision when to transplant a patient with PSC depends on clinical expertise and judgement given the lack of good prognostic models. [115,116] Grade C Advocates of earlier transplantation cite the risk of cholangiocarcinoma and the good 5-year survival rates post-OLT. Against this approach is the accumulation of cholangiographic[117] and histological data[118] from careful follow-up studies showing that PSC recurs in about 20% of grafts within 5 years in the form of non-anastomatic intra- and extrahepatic strictures. Grade C Furthermore, colonic cancer is the most frequent cause of death in PSC patients post-OLT.[119]

CONCLUSION

There is little conclusive evidence from randomized controlled trials concerning the effects of any therapy for PSC. No therapy has been shown to improve survival and halt the progression of the disease, but most reported studies have lacked power to demonstrate modest but clinically significant benefits. In this chronic disease new trials using clinically relevant outcomes should include larger numbers of patients and be of relatively long duration to determine whether proposed interventions do more good than harm.

REFERENCES

1 van Erpecum KJ, Van Berge H. Hepatobiliary abnormalities in inflammatory bowel disease. *Neth J Med* 1989; **35**(Suppl 1): S40–S49.

2 Aitola P, Karvonen AL, Matikainen M. Prevalence of hepatobiliary dysfunction in patients with ulcerative colitis. *Ann Chir Gynaecol* 1994; **83**(4): 275–8.

3 Rasmussen HH, Fallingborg JF, Mortensen PB *et al.* Hepatobiliary dysfunction and primary sclerosing cholangitis in patients with Crohn's disease. *Scand J Gastroenterol* 1997; **32**(6): 604–10.

4 Warren KW, Athanassiades S, Monge JI. Primary sclerosing cholangitis. A study of forty-two cases. *Am J Surg* 1966; **111**(1): 23–38.

5 Jacob AI, Goldberg PK, Bloom N. Endotoxin and bacteria in portal blood. *Gastroenterology* 1977; **72**: 1268–70.

6 Carey JB. Bile acids, cirrhosis and human evolution. *Gastroenterology* 1964; **46**: 490–2.

7 Pereira SP, Rhodes JM, Bain IM *et al.* Biliary lactoferrin concentrations are increased in active inflammatory bowel disease (IBD): a factor in the pathogenesis of primary sclerosing cholangitis? (abstract). *Gut* 1995; **36**(Suppl 1): A56.

8 Acharya SK, Vashisht S, Tandon RK. Primary sclerosing cholangitis in India. *Gastroenterol Jpn* 1989; **24**(1): 75–9.

9 Kochhar R, Goenka MK, Das K *et al.* Primary sclerosing cholangitis: an experience from India. *J Gastroenterol Hepatol* 1996; **11**(5): 429–33.

10 Hobson CH, Butt TJ, Ferry DM *et al.* Enterohepatic circulation of bacterial chemotatic peptide in rats with experimental colitis. *Gastroenterology* 1988; **94**: 1006–13.

11 Chapman RW, Varghese Z, Gaul R *et al.* Association of primary sclerosing cholangitis with HLA-B8. *Gut* 1983; **24**(1): 38–41.

12 Schrumpf E, Fausa O, Forre O *et al.* HLA antigens and immunoregulatory T cells in ulcerative colitis associated with hepatobiliary disease. *Scand J Gastroenterol* 1982; **17**(2): 187–91.

13 Prochazka EJ, Terasaki PI, Park MS *et al.* Association of primary sclerosing cholangitis with HLA-DRw52a. *N Engl J Med* 1990; **322**(26): 1842–4.

14 Donaldson PT, Farrant JM, Wilkinson ML *et al.* Dual association of HLA DR2 and DR3 with primary sclerosing cholangitis. *Hepatology* 1991; **13**(1): 129–33.

15 Farrant JM, Doherty DG, Donaldson PT *et al.* Amino acid substitutions at position 38 of the DR beta polypeptide confer susceptibility to and protection from primary sclerosing cholangitis. *Hepatology* 1992; **16**(2): 390–5.

16 Mehal WZ, Lo YM, Wordsworth BP *et al.* HLA DR4 is a marker for rapid disease progression in primary sclerosing cholangitis. *Gastroenterology* 1994; **106**(1): 160–7.

17 Olerup O, Olsson R, Hultcrantz R *et al.* HLA-DR and HLA-DQ are not markers for rapid disease progression in primary sclerosing cholangitis. *Gastroenterology* 1995; **108**(3): 870–8.

18 Underhill JA, Donaldson PT, Doherty DG *et al.* HLA DPB polymorphism in primary sclerosing cholangitis and primary biliary cirrhosis. *Hepatology* 1995; **21**(4): 959–62.

19 Moloney MM, Thomson LJ, Strettell MDJ *et al.* Human leukocyte antigen-C genes and susceptibility to primary sclerosing cholangitis. *Hepatology* 1998; **28**(3): 660–2.

20 Moloney MM, Donaldson PT, Thomson LJ *et al.* HLA DR4 and DR4 subtypes confer resistance to primary sclerosing cholangitis and are not associated with poor prognosis. *Hepatology* 1996; **24**(4): 169A.

21 Bittencourt PL, Goldberg AC, Cancado EL *et al.* Association of autoimmune hepatitis and primary sclerosing cholangitis with HLA-DR antigens in Brazil (abstract). *Hepatology* 1996; **24**(4): 232A.

22 Chen DF, Tillmann HL, Pastucha L *et al.* HLA polymorphism in German patients with primary sclerosing cholangitis [Abstract]. *Hepatology* 1996; **24**: (4)170A.

23 Bernal W, Moloney M, Underhill J. Does TNF gene polymorphism determine susceptibility to primary sclerosing cholangitis? (abstract) *Hepatology* 1997; **26**: (4)403A.

24 Park MS, Terasaki PI. Inability to attribute susceptibility to primary sclerosing cholangitis to specific amino acid positions of the HLA DRw52 allele (reply to letter). *N Engl J Med* 1991; **325**: 1252.
25 Boden RW, Rankin JG, Goulston SJ *et al.* The liver in ulcerative colitis. The significance of raised alkaline phosphatase. *Lancet* 1959; **2**: 245–8.
26 Eade MN, Brooke BN. Portal bacteraemia in cases of ulcerative colitis submitted to colectomy. *Lancet* 1969; **1**: 1008–9.
27 Kono K, Ohnishi K, Omata M *et al.* Experimental portal fibrosis produced by intraportal injection of killed nonpathogenic *Escherichia coli* in rabbits. *Gastroenterology* 1988; **94**: 787–96.
28 Siegel JH, Barnes S, Morris JS. Bile acids in liver disease associated with inflammatory bowel disease. *Digestion* 1977; **15**: 469–81.
29 Gross JBJ, Ludwig J, Wiesner RH *et al.* Abnormalities in tests of copper metabolism in primary sclerosing cholangitis. *Gastroenterology* 1985; **89**(2): 272–8.
30 Kowdley KV, Knox TA, Kaplan MM. Hepatic copper content is normal in early primary biliary cirrhosis and primary sclerosing cholangitis. *Dig Dis Sci* 1994; **39**(11): 2416–20.
31 Minuk GY, Rascanin N, Paul RW *et al.* Reovirus type 3 infection in patients with primary biliary cirrhosis and primary sclerosing cholangitis. *J Hepatol* 1987; **5**(1): 8–13.
32 Mason AL, Rosen G, White H *et al.* Detection of cytomegalovirus (CMV) DNA in the liver of patients with primary sclerosing cholangitis (PSC) by the polymerase chain reaction. *Hepatology* 1991; **14**: 91A.
33 Mehal WZ, Hattersley AT, Chapman RW *et al.* A survey of cytomegalovirus (CMV) DNA in primary sclerosing cholangitis (PSC) liver tissues using a sensitive polymerase chain reaction (PCR) based assay. *J Hepatol* 1992; **15**(3): 396–9.
34 Dowsett JF, Miller R, Davidson R *et al.* Sclerosing cholangitis in acquired immunodeficiency syndrome. Case reports and review of the literature. *Scand J Gastroenterol* 1988; **23**(10): 1267–74.
35 Mason AL, Xu L, Guo L *et al.* Detection of retroviral antibodies in primary biliary cirrhosis and other idiopathic biliary disorders. *Lancet* 1998; **351**(9116): 1620–4.
36 Terblanche J, Allison HF, Northover JM. An ischemic basis for biliary strictures. *Surgery* 1983; **94**: 52–7.
37 Bodenheimer HCJ, LaRusso NF, Thayer WRJ *et al.* Elevated circulating immune complexes in primary sclerosing cholangitis. *Hepatology* 1983; **3**(2): 150–4.
38 Minuk GY, Angus M, Brickman CM *et al.* Abnormal clearance of immune complexes from the circulation of patients with primary sclerosing cholangitis. *Gastroenterology* 1985; **88**(1 Pt 1): 166–70.
39 Garred P, Lyon H, Christoffersen P *et al.* Deposition of C3, the terminal complement complex and vitronectin in primary biliary cirrhosis and primary sclerosing cholangitis. *Liver* 1993; **13**(6): 305–10.
40 Chapman RW, Arborgh BA, Rhodes JM *et al.* Primary sclerosing cholangitis: a review of its clinical features, cholangiography, and hepatic histology. *Gut* 1980; **21**(10): 870–7.
41 Duerr RH, Targan SR, Landers CJ *et al.* Neutrophil cytoplasmic antibodies: a link between primary sclerosing cholangitis and ulcerative colitis. *Gastroenterology* 1991; **100**(5 Pt 1): 1385–91.
42 Lo SK, Fleming KA, Chapman RW. Prevalence of anti-neutrophil antibody in primary sclerosing cholangitis and ulcerative colitis using an alkaline phosphatase technique. *Gut* 1992; **33**(10): 1370–5.
43 Bansi DS, Fleming KA, Chapman RW. Importance of antineutrophil cytoplasmic antibodies in primary sclerosing cholangitis and ulcerative colitis: prevalence, titre, and IgG subclass. *Gut* 1996; **38**(3): 384–9.
44 Whiteside TL, Lasky S, Si L *et al.* Immunologic analysis of mononuclear cells in liver tissues and blood of patients with primary sclerosing cholangitis. *Hepatology* 1985; **5**(3): 468–74.
45 Lindor KD, Wiesner RH, Katzmann JA *et al.* Lymphocyte subsets in primary sclerosing cholangitis. *Dig Dis Sci* 1987; **32**(7): 720–5.
46 Snook JA, Chapman RW, Sachdev GK *et al.* Peripheral blood and portal tract lymphocyte populations in primary sclerosing cholangitis. *J Hepatol* 1989; **9**(1): 36–41.
47 Si L, Whiteside TL, Schade RR *et al.* T-lymphocyte subsets in liver tissues of patients with primary biliary cirrhosis (PBC), patients with primary sclerosing cholangitis (PSC), and normal controls. *J Clin Immunol* 1984; **4**(4): 262–72.
48 Lindor KD, Wiesner RH, LaRusso NF *et al.* Enhanced autoreactivity of T-lymphocytes in primary sclerosing cholangitis. *Hepatology* 1987; **7**(5): 884–8.
49 Martins EB, Graham AK, Healey CJ *et al.* Activated lymphocytes in the liver of patients with primary sclerosing cholangitis: results of a morphometric study [Abstract]. *Gut* 1994; **35**: S20.
50 Martins EB, Graham AK, Chapman RW *et al.* Elevation of gamma delta T lymphocytes in peripheral blood and livers of patients with primary sclerosing cholangitis and other autoimmune liver diseases. *Hepatology* 1996; **23**(5): 988–93.

51 Martins EB, Healey CJ, Chapman RW *et al.* Increased activation of peripheral blood and liver T-lymphocytes in patients with primary sclerosing cholangitis and autoimmune liver diseases. *Hepatology* 1994; **19**: 98I.
52 Broomé U, Grunewald J, Scheynius A *et al.* Preferential V beta3 usage by hepatic T lymphocytes in patients with primary sclerosing cholangitis. *J Hepatol* 1997; **26**(3): 527–34.
53 Chapman RW, Kelly PM, Heryet A *et al.* Expression of HLA-DR antigens on bile duct epithelium in primary sclerosing cholangitis. *Gut* 1988; **29**(4): 422–7.
54 Martins EB, Chapman RW, Fleming KA. Are bile duct epithelial cells capable of acting as professional antigen presenting cells in primary sclerosing cholangitis? [Abstract]. *Hepatology* 1995; **22**: 109A.
55 Adams DH, Hubscher SG, Shaw J *et al.* Increased expression of intercellular adhesion molecule 1 on bile ducts in primary biliary cirrhosis and primary sclerosing cholangitis. *Hepatology* 1991; **14**(3): 426–31.
56 Mitchell SA, Chapman RW, Fleming KA. Enhanced cytokine mRNA expression in primary sclerosing cholangitis and autoimmune liver disease [Abstract]. *Gastroenterology* 1997; **112**(4): A757.
57 Leon MP, Bassendine MF, Wilson JL *et al.* Immunogenicity of biliary epithelium: investigation of antigen presentation to $CD4^+$ T cells. *Hepatology* 1996; **24**(3): 561–7.
58 Leon MP, Kirby JA, Gibbs P *et al.* Immunogenicity of biliary epithelial cells: study of expression of B7 molecules. *J Hepatol* 1995; **22**: 591–5.
59 Seibold F, Weber P, Klein R *et al.* Clinical significance of antibodies against neutrophils in patients with inflammatory bowel disease and primary sclerosing cholangitis. *Gut* 1992; **33**(5): 657–62.
60 Bansi DS, Bauducci M, Bergqvist A *et al.* Detection of antineutrophil cytoplasmic antibodies in primary sclerosing cholangitis: a comparison of the alkaline phosphatase and immunofluorescent techniques. *Eur J Gastroenterol Hepatol* 1997; **9**(6): 575–80.
61 Bansi DS, Chapman RW, Fleming KA. Prevalence and diagnostic role of antineutrophil cytoplasmic antibodies in inflammatory bowel disease. *Eur J Gastroenterol Hepatol* 1996; **8**(9): 881–5.
62 Teefey SA, Baron RL, Schulte SJ *et al.* Patterns of intrahepatic bile duct dilatation at CT: correlation with obstructive disease processes. *Radiology* 1992; **182**(1): 139–42.
63 Wyatt SH, Fishman EK. Biliary tract obstruction. The role of spiral CT in detection and definition of disease. *Clin Imaging* 1997; **21**(1): 27–34.
64 Scheurlen M, Mork H, Prier S. Comparison of ERCP and magnetic resonance cholangiography (MRC) in primary sclerosing cholangitis. (abstract) *Gastroenterology* 1998; **114**: (4)
65 Seibold F, Slametschka D, Gregor M *et al.* Neutrophil autoantibodies: a genetic marker in primary sclerosing cholangitis and ulcerative colitis. *Gastroenterology* 1994; **107**(2): 532–6.
66 Teefey SA, Baron RL, Rohrmann CA *et al.* Sclerosing cholangitis: CT findings. *Radiology* 1988; **169**(3): 635–9.
67 Broomé U, Olsson R, Lööf L *et al.* Natural history and prognostic factors in 305 Swedish patients with primary sclerosing cholangitis. *Gut* 1996; **38**(4): 610–15.
68 Wiesner RH, Grambsch PM, Dickson ER *et al.* Primary sclerosing cholangitis: natural history, prognostic factors and survival analysis. *Hepatology* 1989; **10**(4): 430–6.
69 Farrant JM, Hayllar KM, Wilkinson ML *et al.* Natural history and prognostic variables in primary sclerosing cholangitis. *Gastroenterology* 1991; **100**(6): 1710–17.
70 Helzberg JH, Petersen JM, Boyer JL. Improved survival with primary sclerosing cholangitis. A review of clinicopathologic features and comparison of symptomatic and asymptomatic patients. *Gastroenterology* 1987; **92**(6): 1869–75.
71 Kim WR, Therneau TM, Wiesner RH. Revised natural history model for primary sclerosing cholangitis obviates the need for liver histology. (abstract) *Hepatology* 1997; **26**: 95A.
72 Craig DA, MacCarty RL, Wiesner RH *et al.* Primary sclerosing cholangitis: value of cholangiography in determining the prognosis. *Am J Roentgenol* 1991; **157**(5): 959–64.
73 Olsson RG, Asztély MS. Prognostic value of cholangiography in primary sclerosing cholangitis. *Eur J Gastroenterol Hepatol* 1995; **7**(3): 251–4.
74 Aguilar HI, Nuako K, Krom RA *et al.* Do primary sclerosing cholangitis (PSC) patients who express HLA-DR4 haplotype have a more rapidly progressive disease? *Hepatology* 1994; **20**: 154A.
75 Miros M, Kerlin P, Walker N *et al.* Predicting cholangiocarcinoma in patients with primary sclerosing cholangitis before transplantation. *Gut* 1991; **32**(11): 1369–73.
76 Kornfeld D, Ekbom A, Ihre T. Survival and risk of cholangiocarcinoma in patients with primary sclerosing cholangitis. A population-based study. *Scand J Gastroenterol* 1997; **32**(10): 1042–5.
77 Herbener T, Zajko AB, Koneru B *et al.* Recurrent cholangiocarcinoma in the biliary tree after liver transplantation. Radiology 1988; **169**(3): 641–2.

78 Bergquist A, Glaumann H, Persson B *et al.* Risk factors and clinical presentation of hepatobiliary carcinoma in patients with primary sclerosing cholangitis: a case-control study. *Hepatology* 1998; **27**(2): 311–16.

79 D'Haens GR, Lashner BA, Hanauer SB. Pericholangitis and sclerosing cholangitis are risk factors for dysplasia and cancer in ulcerative colitis. *Am J Gastroenterol* 1993; **88**(8): 1174–8.

80 Brentnall TA, Haggitt RC, Rabinovitch PS *et al.* Risk and natural history of colonic neoplasia in patients with primary sclerosing cholangitis and ulcerative colitis. *Gastroenterology* 1996; **110**(2): 331–8.

81 Loftus EVJ, Sandborn WJ, Tremaine WJ *et al.* Risk of colorectal neoplasia in patients with primary sclerosing cholangitis. *Gastroenterology* 1996; **110**(2): 432–40.

82 Ahnen DJ. Controlled clinical trials: the controls are the key. *Gastroenterology* 1996; **110**(2): 628–30.

83 Lashner BA, Shetty B, Rybicki L. Risk factors for cancer or dysplasia in ulcerative colitis with primary sclerosing cholangitis. (abstract) *Gastroenterology* 1998; **114**: A1018.

84 Marchesa P, Lashner BA, Lavery IC *et al.* The risk of cancer and dysplasia among ulcerative colitis patients with primary sclerosing cholangitis. *Am J Gastroenterol* 1997; **92**(8): 1285–8.

85 Bleday R, Lee E, Jessurun J *et al.* Increased risk of early colorectal neoplasms after hepatic transplant in patients with inflammatory bowel disease. *Dis Colon Rectum* 1993; **36**(10): 908–12.

86 LaRusso NF, Wiesner RH, Ludwig J *et al.* Prospective trial of penicillamine in primary sclerosing cholangitis. *Gastroenterology* 1988; **95**(4): 1036–42.

87 Knox TA, Kaplan MM. A double-blind controlled trial of oral-pulse methotrexate therapy in the treatment of primary sclerosing cholangitis. *Gastroenterology* 1994; **106**(2): 494–9.

88 Lindor KD, Jorgensen RA, Anderson ML *et al.* Ursodeoxycholic acid and methotrexate for primary sclerosing cholangitis: a pilot study. *Am J Gastroenterol* 1996; **91**(3): 511–15.

89 Lindor KD, Wiesner RH, Colwell LJ *et al.* The combination of prednisone and colchicine in patients with primary sclerosing cholangitis. *Am J Gastroenterol* 1991; **86**(1): 57–61.

90 Allison MC, Burroughs AK, Noone P *et al.* Biliary lavage with corticosteroids in primary sclerosing cholangitis. A clinical, cholangiographic and bacteriological study. *J Hepatol* 1986; **3**(1): 118–22.

91 Wiesner RH, Steiner B, LaRusso NF *et al.* A controlled clinical trial evaluating cyclosporine in the treatment of primary sclerosing cholangitis. (abstract) *Hepatology* 1991; **14**(4): 63A.

92 Olsson R, Broomé U, Danielsson A *et al.* Colchicine treatment of primary sclerosing cholangitis. *Gastroenterology* 1995; **108**(4): 1199–203.

93 Lo SK, Hermann R, Chapman RW *et al.* Ursodeoxycholic acid in primary sclerosing cholangitis: a double-blind placebo controlled trial [Abstract]. *Hepatology* 1992; **16**(92A).

94 Stiehl A. Ursodeoxycholic acid in the treatment of primary sclerosing cholangitis. *Ann Med* 1994; **26**(5): 345–9.

95 Van-Thiel DH, Wright HI, Gavaler JS. Ursodeoxycholic acid therapy for primary sclerosing cholangitis: preliminary report of a randomized controlled trial. (abstract) *Hepatology* 1992; **16**(2 Pt2): 62A.

96 Beuers U, Spengler U, Kruis W *et al.* Ursodeoxycholic acid for treatment of primary sclerosing cholangitis: a placebo-controlled trial. *Hepatology* 1992; **16**(3): 707–14.

97 Lindor KD. Ursodiol for primary sclerosing cholangitis. Mayo Primary Sclerosing Cholangitis-Ursodeoxycholic Acid Study Group. *N Engl J Med* 1997; **336**(10): 691–5.

98 Mitchell SA, Bansi D, Hunt N *et al.* High dose ursodeoxycholic acid (UDCA) in primary sclerosing cholangitis (PSC): results after two years of a randomised double-blind placebo-controlled trial [Abstract]. *Gastroenterology* 1997; **112**((Suppl. 4)): A757.

99 Knox TA, Kaplan MM. Treatment of primary sclerosing cholangitis with oral methotrexate. *Am J Gastroenterol* 1991; **86**(5): 546–52.

100 Burgert SL, Brown BP, Kirkpatrick RB *et al.* Positive corticosteroid response in early primary sclerosing cholangitis. (abstract) *Gastroenterology* 1984; **86**: 1037.

101 Van-Thiel DH, Carroll P, Abu-Elmagd K *et al.* Tacrolimus (FK 506), a treatment for primary sclerosing cholangitis: results of an open-label preliminary trial. *Am J Gastroenterol* 1995; **90**(3): 455–9.

102 Angulo P, Bharucha AE, Jorgensen RA. Oral nicotine in the treatment of primary sclerosing cholangitis: a pilot study. (abstract) *Gastroenterology* 1998; **114**: (4).

103 Bharucha AE, Jorgensen R, Lichtman SN. A pilot study evaluating pentoxifylline in the treatment of primary sclerosing cholangitis. (abstract) *Hepatology* 1998; **26**: (4)402A.

104 Pockros PJ, Younossi ZM, Wilkes LB. An open label pilot study of 2-chlorodeoxyadenosine (2-Cda) in the treatment of early-stage primary sclerosing cholangitis. (abstract) *Hepatology* 1996; **24**: (4)170A.

105 Stiehl A, Raedsch R, Rudolph G *et al.* Treatment of primary sclerosing cholangitis

with ursodexoycholic acid: first results of a controlled study. (abstract) *Hepatology* 1989; **10**(4): A602.

106 O'Brien S, Craig PI, Hatfield AR. The effect of ursodeoxycholic acid treatment in primary sclerosing cholangitis – results of a pilot study. (abstract) *Gastroenterology* 1993; **104**(4): A966.

107 Angulo P, Therneau TM, Larson DR. The time course of histological progression in primary sclerosing cholangitis. (abstract) *Gastroenterology* 1998; **114**: A1204.

108 Olsson R, Hägerstrand I, Broomé U *et al.* Sampling variability of percutaneous liver biopsy in primary sclerosing cholangitis. *J Clin Pathol* 1995; **48**(10): 933–5.

109 Ferrari-Junior AP, Lichtenstein DR, Slivka A *et al.* Brush cytology during ERCP for the diagnosis of biliary and pancreatic malignancies. *Gastrointest Endosc* 1994; **40**(2 Pt 1): 140–5.

110 Ramage JK, Donaghy A, Farrant JM *et al.* Serum tumor markers for the diagnosis of cholangiocarcinoma in primary sclerosing cholangitis. *Gastroenterology* 1995; **108**(3): 865–9.

111 Mirza DF, Davies M, Olliff S *et al.* Preoperative diagnosis of cholangiocarcinoma in primary sclerosing cholangitis in potential liver transplantation candidates. (abstract) *Hepatology* 1994; **20**: 154A.

112 Stiehl A, Benz C, Rudolph G *et al.* Effect of ursodeoxycholic acid and of endoscopic dilation on survival in PSC. Final results of a 8 years prospective study. (abstract) *Gastroenterology* 1996; **110**(4 Suppl.): A1334.

113 Wiesner RH, Porayko MK, Hay JE *et al.* Liver transplantation for primary sclerosing cholangitis: impact of risk factors on outcome. *Liver Transplant Surg* 1996; **2**(5 Suppl 1): 99–108.

114 Ismail T, Angrisani L, Powell JE *et al.* Primary sclerosing cholangitis: surgical options, prognostic variables and outcome. *Br J Surg* 1991; **78**(5): 564–7.

115 Farges O, Malassagne B, Sebagh M *et al.* Primary sclerosing cholangitis: liver transplantation or biliary surgery. *Surgery* 1995; **117**(2): 146–55.

116 Nashan B, Schlitt HJ, Tusch G *et al.* Biliary malignancies in primary sclerosing cholangitis: timing for liver transplantation. *Hepatology* 1996; **23**(5): 1105–11.

117 Sheng R, Zajko AB, Campbell WL *et al.* Biliary strictures in hepatic transplants: prevalence and types in patients with primary sclerosing cholangitis vs those with other liver diseases. *AJR* 1993; **161**(2): 297–300.

118 Harrison RF, Davies MH, Neuberger JM *et al.* Fibrous and obliterative cholangitis in liver allografts: evidence of recurrent primary sclerosing cholangitis? *Hepatology* 1994; **20**(2): 356–61.

119 Narumi S, Roberts JP, Emond JC *et al.* Liver transplantation for sclerosing cholangitis. *Hepatology* 1995; **22**(2): 451–7.

Portal hypertensive bleeding: prevention and treatment

24

JOHN GOULIS, ANDREW K BURROUGHS

INTRODUCTION

Portal hypertension is a major complication of cirrhosis, leading to the development of portosystemic collaterals including gastroesophageal varices. Variceal hemorrhage is associated with a high mortality rate.[1]

During the past decade several new therapeutic approaches have been introduced for the prevention and treatment of variceal bleeding. In addition to sclerotherapy and surgical shunts, interventions for portal hypertensive bleeding include various vasoactive agents, the endoscopic ligation of esophageal varices, and transjugular intrahepatic portosystemic shunts (TIPS).

The number of randomized clinical trials dealing with the treatment of portal hypertension is very large. However, many trials have not used accepted outcomes and lack adequate statistical power. We have evaluated randomized controlled trials for prevention of first bleeding, treatment of acute bleeding, and prevention of recurrent bleeding from esophageal varices, using meta-analysis where applicable. The main clinically relevant outcomes selected for analysis were: (a) first bleeding episode (for primary prevention trials); failure to control bleeding, including very early rebleeding (for trials of acute bleeding) or rebleeding (for trials for prevention of rebleeding); (b) mortality (short term or long term); and (c) incidence of complications. Pooled estimates of efficacy are presented as pooled odds ratio (POR), obtained by the Mantel–Henszel method (fixed effect model) as modified by Robbins,[2] with 95% CI. We used a statistical evaluation of heterogeneity by χ^2 test to assess whether the variation in treatment effect within trials of the same group was greater than might be expected. We considered heterogeneity to be present if $P < 0.05$; in this case the calculation of pooled OR was performed by the Der Simonian and Laird method,[3] which is recommended for meta-analysis of studies with significant heterogeneity.

NATURAL HISTORY – PREDICTION OF THE RISK OF BLEEDING

Development of varices

At the time of diagnosis of cirrhosis, varices are present in about 60% of decompensated and 30% of compensated patients.[1] The minimal portal pressure gradient or its equivalent hepatic venous pressure gradient (HVPG) threshold for the development of varices is 10–12 mmHg.[4] In most patients, esophageal varices enlarge over time, although regression of varices in a minority of patients has also been observed.[5] The presence and size of esophageal varices is associated with the severity of liver disease and with continued alcohol abuse.[6]

Risk of first variceal bleeding

The incidence of variceal bleeding in unselected patients who have never previously bled is low (4.4/100 per year).[7] However, mortality of the first bleeding episode is high (25–50%).[8] The identification of patients with varices who are at risk of bleeding is important in order that effective prophylactic therapy can be offered to those who need it and not to those who do not. Risk factors for the first episode of variceal bleeding are the severity of liver dysfunction, large size of varices, and the presence of endoscopic red color signs. The combination of these three factors is the basis of the NIEC (North Italian Endoscopic Club) index.[9] However only a third of patients that present with variceal hemorrhage have the above risk factors.[10] Hence there is a need to define new predictive factors, such as hemodynamic changes, that could be combined in the NIEC index in order to improve its validity. Variceal bleeding does not occur if HVPG falls below 12 mmHg,[11] and the height of HVPG has been shown to be an independent risk factor for bleeding.[12] Finally, variceal pressure has been also shown, prospectively, to be an independent predictive factor for the first variceal bleeding, and its addition to the NIEC index could result in a significant gain in prognostic accuracy.[13]

RANDOMIZED CONTROLLED TRIALS FOR PREVENTION OF FIRST VARICEAL BLEEDING

Shunt surgery compared with no active treatment

R
Grade A

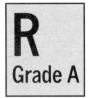

A meta-analysis of the first randomized controlled trials in portal hypertension involving 302 patients in four trials of prophylactic shunt surgery,[14-17] has recently been published.[1] This intervention significantly reduced variceal bleeding (POR 0.31; 95% CI 0.17–0.56) but resulted in decreased survival (POR 1.6; 95% CI 1.02–2.57). The risk of chronic or recurrent encephalopathy was signicantly increased (POR 2.0; 95% CI 1.2–3.1) by the shunt procedure. In view of the mortality data and the serious side effects, prophylactic shunt surgery has been abandoned. The trial reported by Inocuchi *et al* which demonstrated that devascularization procedures or selective shunts[18] significantly reduced bleeding risk and mortality, may be criticized because the method of randomization of patients is unclear. However, this trial is no longer clinically relevant. The advent of liver transplantation removes the rationale for prophylactic surgery of any kind in cirrhotic patients.

Sclerotherapy compared with no active treatment

The success of endoscopic sclerotherapy in the treatment of acute variceal bleeding has led to extensive evaluation of sclerotherapy for the prevention of the first variceal bleed. There are 20 trials,[19-38] of which four were published in abstract form,[34-37] including a total of

1756 patients. The significant heterogeneity (P <0.001) in the direction and size of the treatment effect on bleeding and death, means that meta-analysis is not appropriate. Early trials which reported a reduction in bleeding rate, and in some cases a reduction in overall mortality,[20,26,27] were of poor quality.[39] Subsequently, larger trials did not confirm benefit from this intervention, and some have suggested that prophylactic sclerotherapy is harmful.[31,33] Since prophylactic sclerotherapy is an expensive and invasive intervention, and is associated with potentially serious complications, it would have to be clearly superior to no prophylactic treatment before it could be recommended for widespread use.

R
Grade A

Variceal ligation compared with no active treatment

Variceal ligation has been shown to have fewer adverse effects than sclerotherapy so that it would become the endoscopic treatment of choice.[40] Four studies of prophylactic variceal ligation in patients with high risk esophageal varices,[41,42–44] including 452 patients, have been recently published (two only in abstract form[41,43]). Although variceal ligation significantly reduced the risk of first variceal bleeding (POR 5.6; 95% CI 3.39–9.26) and mortality (POR 3.01; 95% CI 1.94–4.68), the choice of an untreated instead of a beta-blocker control group in these trials is considered by many to be unethical. Thus randomized trials comparing prophylactic variceal ligation and beta-blockers are required. Two studies from which preliminary data are available are inadequate as to sample size and duration of follow-up.[45,46]

Beta-blockers compared with no active treatment

The optimal prophylactic intervention should be effective, easy to administer, and relatively free of adverse effects. Drug therapy potentially fulfils these criteria best. In addition, drug therapy has the potential to protect against gastric mucosal bleeding, which accounts for a sizeable proportion of first bleeding episodes.[47]

Nine trials have studied beta-receptor blockade (seven with propranolol[29,33,36,48,51–53] and two with nadolol[49–50]) as an intervention to prevent bleeding in cirrhotic patients with large varices[29,33,36,48–53] (Table 24.1). One of the two trials[53] published only in abstract form[36,53] reported a very low bleeding rate in non-treated patients. This result caused statistically significant heterogeneity in the meta-analysis which disappeared when this trial was excluded from the analysis. The meta-analysis revealed a statistically significant reduction in bleeding risk with beta-blocker treatment whether this trial was included (POR 0.54; 95% CI 0.39–0.74) or excluded (POR 0.48; 95% CI 0.35–0.66). The NNT, the number of patients that need to be treated with beta-blockers to prevent one bleeding episode, is 11. However, no statistically significant reduction in mortality with this intervention was demonstrated (POR 0.75; 95% CI 0.57–1.06).

R
Grade A

The benefit of beta-blocker therapy was shown to be independent of cause and severity of cirrhosis, presence of ascites, and variceal size in subgroup analysis of individual patient data from four of the above trials.[54] However, bleeding may occur after stopping beta-blocker therapy, suggesting that therapy should be maintained lifelong.[55] Finally, propranolol has been shown to prevent both acute and chronic bleeding from portal hypertensive gastropathy in a single randomized trial.[47] Adverse effects of beta-blockers are usually reversible after discontinuation of the drug, and no fatal complications have been reported.

Table 24.1 Randomized controlled trials of beta-blockers compared to non-active treatment for the prevention of first variceal bleeding

Study	No. of patients C/T	Child C (%)	Bleeding C/T	Death C/T
Pascal, 1987[48]	111/116	46	30/20	40/25
[a]Ideo, 1988[49]	49/30	—	11/1	9/3
[a]Lebrec, 1988[50]	53/53	—	10/7	10/10
IMPPPB (Pasta), 1989[51]	89/85	7	31/18	28/37
Andreani, 1990[29]	41/43	28	13/2	18/13
Conn, 1991[52]	51/51	8	11/2	11/8
PROVA (Bendston), 1991[33]	51/51	8	13/12	14/7
[b]Strauss, 1988[36]	16/20	NR	4/4	7/7
[b]Colman, 1990[53]	25/23	NR	2/8	7/6
POR (95% CI)			0.54 (0.39–0.74)	0.75 (0.57–1.06)

C, control; T, treatment = beta-blockers; NR, not reported; POR, pooled odds ratio.
[a]Nadolol.
[b]Abstract.

There are currently no adequate data to recommend alternatives to non-selective beta-blockers for primary prophylaxis of variceal bleeding. The addition of isosorbide-5-mononitrate to beta-blockade has been evaluated in a single study[56] in which the combination with nadolol was more effective in reducing bleeding, with only a small increase in adverse effects. However, in a direct comparison between propranolol and isosorbide-5-mononitrate for the prevention of variceal bleeding, nitrates were associated with a higher long term mortality.[57]

Conclusion

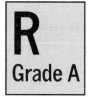

R
Grade A

The data from trials of prophylactic interventions suggest that screening for moderate and large varices in cirrhotics should be part of routine clinical practice, and if these are found, intervention to prevent first variceal bleeding should be offered. Shunt surgery prevents bleeding, but the increase in mortality and the long term risk of encephalopathy make this treatment unacceptable. Prophylactic sclerotherapy should not be used as it is relatively ineffective, costly and potentially dangerous. The intervention of choice is prophylactic beta-blocker therapy. It is cheap, easy to administer, and is effective in preventing the first variceal hemorrhage and bleeding from gastric mucosa. Primary prophylaxis with variceal ligation appears to be safe and may be a reasonable alternative for patients with contraindications to or intolerance of beta-blockers, or who have no hemodynamic response to the drug therapy. However, it is unlikely to be the preferred intervention, as it is much more expensive and less available than beta-blocker therapy and it will not also prevent gastric mucosal bleeding.

OUTCOME OF ACUTE VARICEAL BLEEDING

Acute variceal bleeding is a life-threatening complication in patients with cirrhosis and portal hypertension, with a mortality rate which ranges from 30% to 50%.[1]

Although overall survival may be improving because of new therapeutic approaches, mortality is still closely related to failure to control hemorrhage or early rebleeding which occurs in as many as 50% of patients in the first days to 6 weeks after admission.[58] Severity of liver disease and active bleeding during emergency endoscopy are both risk factors for early rebleeding.[59,60] Increased portal pressure (HVPG >16 mmHg) has been also proposed as a prognostic factor for early rebleeding in an elegant study of continuous portal pressure measurement immediately after the bleeding episode.[61]

There is a strong association between variceal hemorrhage and bacterial infection. Four recent studies have shown that antibiotic therapy (with oral nonabsorbable antibiotics,[62] and more recently with different quinolones or amoxycillin with clavulanic acid[63–65]) prevents bacterial infection in cirrhotic patients with gastrointestinal bleeding.[62–65] Meta-analysis of these four trials shows an absolute risk reduction for infection of 32% (95% CI 19–44) and for mortality of 9.2% (95% CI 2.4–16.0).[66] Bacterial infection, diagnosed on admission, is an independent prognostic factor for failure to control bleeding or early rebleeding.[59] These data may support a role of bacterial infection in the initiation of variceal bleeding.[67]

R Grade A

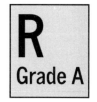

Most clinical trials have focused on esophageal varices. Gastric varices may bleed more initially, and tend to rebleed frequently.[68] The following sections refer to esophageal varices unless specified.

Randomized controlled trials for the treatment of acute variceal bleeding

PHARMACOLOGICAL TREATMENT

Vasoactive drug treatment does not require sophisticated equipment or specialist skills and is available even before the patient is admitted to hospital.[69] Since recent evidence suggests that those patients with high variceal or portal pressure are likely to continue to bleed or rebleed early,[11] prolonged drug therapy that lowers portal pressure over days may be the optimal treatment. The vasoactive drugs that are currently used in the management of acute variceal bleeding are vasopressin, glypressin, somatostatin and octreotide. Vasopressin lowers portal pressure through the induction of smooth muscle contraction, particularly in splanchnic arterioles. However, the drug also causes systemic vasoconstriction which leads to serious adverse effects such as cardiac arrhythmias, myocardial ischemia, mesenteric ischemia and cerebrovascular episodes, resulting in cessation of therapy in up to 25% of cases.[70,71] Terlipressin is a synthetic analogue of vasopressin (triglycyl lysine vasopressin). It has an intrinsic effect as well as being converted *in vivo* into vasopressin. This feature prolongs its biological half-life, so that a continuous intravenous infusion is unnecessary. Somatostatin has been used because of its reported ability to reduce splanchnic blood flow,[72] portal pressure, and azygous blood flow[73] in cirrhotic patients. Bolus injections of somatostatin appear to have greater hemodynamic effects than continuous infusion.[74] Finally octreotide has been reported to cause a reduction in portal pressure[75]and a transient decrease in azygous blood flow,[76] but some studies did not confirm these data, using similar or even greater doses of the drug.[77]

Randomized controlled trials of vasoactive drug treatment of acute variceal bleeding

PLACEBO CONTROLLED TRIALS (TABLE 24.2)

Vasopressin vs placebo

Vasopressin was compared with non-active treatment or placebo in four randomized controlled trials,[70,78–80] which included only 157 patients. In two of these trials the intra-arterial route of administration was used.[70,78] Significant heterogeneity in the effect on control of bleeding was present. No statistically significant differences were shown for control of bleeding or mortality. Complications were reported in up to 64% of patients, which led to discontinuation of treatment in 25% of cases. In order to minimize the

Table 24.2 Randomized controlled trials of drugs compared to placebo for the treatment of the acute bleeding episode

Study	No. of patients	Child C (%)	Event rate D	Event rate C	ARR (95% CI)
Outcome: failure to control bleeding					
Vasopressin vs placebo					
Merigan, 1962[78]	53	NR	13/29	24/24	0.55 (0.37–0.73)
Conn, 1975[70]	33	NR	5/17	12/16	0.46 (0.15–0.76)
Mallory, 1980[79]	38	NR	10/18	17/20	0.29 (0.02–0.57)
Fogel, 1982[80]	33	NR	10/14	12/19	–0.08 (–0.4–0.23)
Total	157		38/78	65/79	0.38 (0.26–0.51)
Terlipressin vs placebo					
Walker, 1986[83]	50	50	5/25	12/25	0.28 (0.03–0.53)
Freeman, 1989[84]	31	29	6/15	10/16	0.22 (–0.11–0.57)
Soderlund, 1990[85]	60	33	5/31	13/29	0.29 (0.06–0.51)
Levacher, 1995[69]	84	81	12/41	23/43	0.24 (0.04–0.45)
Total	225		28/112	58/113	0.26 (0.14–0.38)
Somatostatin vs placebo or inactive treatment					
Flati, 1986[90]	35	40	2/19	9/16	0.46 (0.17–0.74)
Testoni, 1986[91]	29	17	1/15	1/14	0.05 (–0.18–0.18)
Loperfido, 1987[89]	47	19	17/22	21/25	0.07 (–0.16–0.27)
Valenzuela, 1989[86]	84	32	21/48	9/36	–0.19(–0.38–0.01)
Burroughs, 1990[87]	120	41	22/61	35/59	0.23 (0.05–0.1)
Gotzsche, 1995[88]	86	NR	NR	NR	
Total	315		63/165	75/150	0.09 (–0.006–0.18)
Octreotide vs placebo					
[a]Burroughs, 1996[92]	262	40	71/123	85/139	0.03 (–0.08–0.15)
variceal bleeding only	197	40	56/88	75/109	0.05 (–0.08–0.18)
Octreotide vs placebo for early rebleeding					
[b]Primignani, 1995[93]	58	NR	9/26	10/32	–0.04 (–0.28–0.21)
[c]D'Amico, 1998[94]	262	31	31/131	37/131	0.05 (–0.06–0.15)

Table 24.2 Randomized controlled trials of drugs compared to placebo for the treatment of the acute bleeding episode–*Continued*

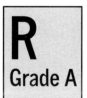

Study	No. of patients	Child C (%)	Event rate D	Event rate C	ARR (95% CI)
Outcome: death					
Vasopressin vs placebo					
Merigan, 1962[78]	53	NR	28/29	23/24	–0.007 (–0.11–0.1)
Conn, 1975[70]	33	NR	9/17	10/16	0.10 (–0.24–0.43)
Mallory, 1980[79]	38	NR	8/18	9/20	0.006 (–031–0.32)
Fogel, 1982[80]	33	NR	7/14	8/19	–0.08 (–0.42–0.26)
Total	157		52/78	50/79	–0004(–0.09–0.09)
Terlipressin vs placebo					
Walker, 1986[83]	50	50	3/25	8/25	0.2 (–0.02–0.4)
Freeman, 1989[84]	31	29	3/15	4/16	0.05 (–0.24–0.34)
Soderlund, 1990[85]	60	33	3/31	11/29	0.28 (0.07–0.49)
Levacher, 1995[69]	84	81	12/41	20/43	0.17 (–0.03–0.38)
Total	225		21/112	43/113	0.19 (0.08–0.3)
Somatostatin vs placebo or inactive treatment					
Flati, 1986[90]	35	40	4/19	7/16	0.23 (–0.08–0.53)
Testoni, 1986[91]	29	17	1/15	0/14	–0.07 (–0.19–0.06)
Loperfido, 1987[89]	47	19	6/22	7/25	0.007 (–0.25–0.26)
Valenzuela, 1989[86]	84	32	15/48	10/36	–0.03 (–0.23–0.16)
Burroughs, 1990[87]	120	41	9/61	7/59	–0.03 (–0.15–0.09)
Gotzsche, 1995[88]	86	NR	16/42	16/44	–0.02 (–0.22–0.19)
Total	401		51/207	47/194	–0.02 (–0.09–0.05)
Octreotide vs placebo					
[a]Burroughs, 1996[92]	262	40	35/71	37/85	–0.02 (–0.13–0.09)
variceal bleeding only	197	40	24/56	32/75	0.02 (–0.1–0.15)
Octreotide vs placebo for early rebleeding					
[c]D'Amico, 1998[94]	262	31	26/131	20/131	–0.05 (–0.14–0.05)

C, controls; D, drugs; NR, not reported.
[a]Der Simonian and Laird method.
[b]Evaluation at 30 days.
[c]Evaluation at 15 days.

systemic complications of vasopressin, nitroglycerin has been added to the regimen. This drug is a powerful venous dilator and reduces the portal vascular resistance and improves myocardial performance. Three randomized controlled trials including 176 patients have compared vasopressin alone with vasopressin plus nitroglycerine (transdermally,[71] sublingually,[81] and intravenously[82]). The combination was more effective for control of bleeding (POR 0.39; 95% CI 0.21–0.72) but no difference in mortality was demonstrated (POR 0.94; 95% CI 0.49–1.79). In two of the trials,[81,82] adverse effects were significantly reduced with the combination treatment. Because of portocollateral shunting nitroglycerine can cause significant systemic effects. Hence this combination therapy must be monitored very closely and is less feasible for immediate therapy.

R
Grade A

Terlipressin vs placebo

The clinical efficacy of terlipressin has been evaluated in four rather small placebo-controlled trials,[69,83–85] which included 225 patients. In one of these trials the drug was given while the patient was being transferred to hospital.[69] Meta-analysis revealed that terlipressin significantly improved control of bleeding (POR 0.33; 95% CI 0.19–0.57) and reduced mortality (POR 0.38; 95% CI 0.22–0.69). However, there is some criticism of these studies. The evidence in the early administration trial[69] of the effect of terlipressin, given only as three doses in the first 8 hours, does not readily explain the apparent beneficial results regarding the mortality rate (only in group C patients) nor the control of bleeding. The benefit of early administration of terlipressin on mortality must be reproduced in other studies.

Somatostatin vs placebo

Three placebo-controlled studies of somatostatin yielded divergent results.[86–88] The trials by Valenzuela *et al*[86] and Gotzsche *et al*[88] suggested that somatostatin was no more effective than placebo. Both studies had a very long recruitment period, suggesting the possibility of patient selection bias. Moreover Gotzsche *et al*[88] did not evaluate outcome of failure to control bleeding, while Valenzuela *et al*[86] reported an extremely high response rate (83%) in the placebo group. Burroughs *et al*[87] reported a statistically significant benefit for somatostatin in controlling variceal bleeding over a 5-day treatment period. These differences in results caused statistically significant heterogeneity (P = 0.006) in the meta-analysis of the six studies that compare somatostatin with placebo[86–88] or no active treatment.[89–91] No statistically significant benefit of somatostatin was demonstrated on bleeding (POR 0.6; 95% CI 0.21–1.65) or mortality (POR 1.02; 95% CI 0.64–1.61).

Octreotide vs placebo

One large randomized trial involving 262 patients[92] compared octreotide, administered as a continuous 5-day infusion of 50 mg/h, with a placebo infusion for the management of acute variceal bleeding. No difference between the treatment groups was demonstrated, whether or not injection sclerotherapy was needed for active bleeding or drug failure. Moreover, two recent studies[93,94] comparing octreotide (100 mg 8-hourly, subcutaneously) with placebo after the control of the initial bleeding episode did not show any difference in early rebleeding or mortality between the two treatment groups.

DRUGS COMPARED TO BALLOON TAMPONADE

There have been six trials comparing vasoactive drugs and balloon tamponade. The drugs used were terlipressin,[95–97] somatostatin,[98,99] and octreotide.[100] Meta-analysis of these six trials showed showed no differences between the treatment groups for failure to control bleeding (POR 1.04; 95% CI 0.63–1.72) or death (POR 0.65; 95% CI 0.36–1.16). Sensitivity analysis showed no effect of type of drug. However, the sample sizes in these trials were small and the outcomes were not very clear, indicating that these results should be interpreted with caution. Tamponade if used properly, provides good control of bleeding. However, the balloons should not be inflated for more than 12 hours and preferably less, and bleeding frequently recurs when the balloons are deflated.

COMPARISONS BETWEEN DRUGS (TABLE 24.3)

Terlipressin vs vasopressin

Terlipressin was compared to vasopressin in five small, unblinded studies,[101–105] involving only 247 patients. In two of these studies, vasopressin was combined with

Table 24.3 Randomized controlled trials of comparisons between drugs for the treatment of the acute bleeding episode

Study	No. of patients	Child C (%)	Event rate D	Event rate C	ARR (95% CI)
Outcome: failure to control bleeding					
Vasopressin vs vasopressin plus nitroglycerin					
Tsai, 1986[81]	39	34	11/20	15/19	0.24 (–0.05–0.5)
Gimson, 1986[82]	72	61	12/38	19/34	0.24 (0.02–0.5)
Bosch, 1989[71]	65	51	8/30	16/35	0.19 (–0.04–0.42)
Total	176		31/88	50/88	0.22 (0.08–0.36)
Terlipressin vs vasopressin					
Freeman, 1982[101]	21	15	3/10	10/11	0.61 (0.28–0.94)
Desaint, 1987[102]	16	43	2/10	1/6	–0.03 (–0.42–0.35)
Lee, 1988[103]	45	27	16/24	17/21	–0.14 (–0.4–0.11)
Chiu, 1988[104]	54	60	13/26	13/28	–0.04 (–0.3–0.23)
D'Amico, 1994[105]	111	9	5/56	13/55	0.15 (0.01–0.28)
Total	247		39/126	54/121	0.1 (0.007–0.2)
Somatostatin vs vasopressin					
Kravetz, 1984[106]	61	41	14/30	13/31	–0.04 (–0.3–0.2)
Jenkins, 1985[107]	22	54	3/10	8/12	0.37 (–0.02–0.8)
Bagarani, 1987[108]	49	69	8/24	17/25	0.35 (0.08–0.6)
Cardona, 1989[109]	38	26	12/20	8/18	–0.16 (–0.47–0.16)
Hsia, 1990[110]	46	65	10/22	15/24	0.17 (–0.1–0.46)
Saari, 1990[111]	54	46	11/32	10/22	0.11 (–0.15–0.38)
Rodriguez-Moreno, 1991[112]	31	30	9/15	6/16	–0.22 (–0.57–0.12)
Total	301		67/153	77/148	0.08 (–0.03–0.19)
Somatostatin vs terlipressin					
Feu, 1996[113]	161	29	13/81	16/80	0.04 (–0.08–0.16)
Walker, 1996[114]	106	12	10/53	5/53	–0.09 (–0.23–0.04)
Octreotide vs vasopressin					
Hwang, 1992[115]	48	44	9/24	13/24	0.17 (–0.11–0.45)
Octreotide vs glypressin					
Silvain, 1993[116]	87	47	10/46	17/41	0.20 (0.05–0.39)
Outcome: death					
Vasopressin vs vasopressin plus nitroglycerin					
Tsai, 1986[81]	39	34	11/19	11/20	0.03 (–0.28–0.34)
Gimson, 1986[82]	72	61	9/34	9/38	0.03 (–0.17–0.23)
Bosch, 1989[71]	65	51	10/35	9/30	–0.01 (–0.24–0.21)
Total	176		30/88	29/78	0.01 (–0.12–0.15)

Table 24.3 Randomized controlled trials of comparisons between drugs for the treatment of the acute bleeding episode–*Continued*

Study	No. of patients	Child C (%)	Event rate D	Event rate C	ARR (95% CI)
Terlipressin vs vasopressin					
Freeman, 1982[101]	21	15	2/10	3/11	0.07 (–0.29–0.43)
Desaint, 1987[102]	16	43	3/10	2/6	0.03 (–0.44–0.5)
Lee, 1988[103]	45	27	10/21	8/24	–0.14 (–0.43–0.14)
Chiu, 1988[104]	54	60	12/26	10/28	–0.10 (–0.37–0.16)
D'Amico, 1994[105]	111	9	14/56	9/55	–0.09 (–0.24–0.06)
Total	247		41/123	32/124	–0.08 (–0.19–0.03)
Somatostatin vs vasopressin					
Kravetz, 1984[106]	61	41	16/30	17/31	0.01 (–0.23–0.26)
Jenkins, 1985[107]	22	54	2/10	4/12	0.13 (–0.23–0.5)
Bagarani, 1987[108]	49	69	6/24	10/25	0.15 (–0.11–0.41)
Cardona, 1989[109]	38	26	6/20	3/18	–0.13 (–0.4–0.13)
Hsia, 1990[110]	46	65	14/22	15/24	–0.01 (–0.29–0.26)
Saari, 1990[111]	54	46	22/32	15/22	–0.57 (–0.26–0.25)
Rodriguez-Moreno, 1991[112]	31	30	3/15	3/16	–0.01 (–0.29–0.27)
Total	301		69/153	67/148	0.01 (–0.09–0.12)
Somatostatin vs terlipressin					
Feu, 1996[113]	161	29	13/81	13/80	0.002 (–0.1–0.12)
Walker, 1996[114]	106	12	11/53	11/53	0.0 (–0.15–0.15)
Octreotide vs vasopressin					
Hwang, 1992[115]	48	44	11/24	12/24	0.04 (–0.24–0.32)
Octreotide vs glypressin					
Silvain, 1993[116]	87	47	10/46	11/41	0.05 (–0.13–0.23)
Outcome: complications					
Somatostatin vs vasopressin					
Kravetz, 1984[106]	61	41	3/30	22/31	0.61 (0.42–0.8)
Jenkins, 1985[107]	22	54	0/10	2/12	0.17 (–0.04–0.38)
Bagarani, 1987[108]	49	69	1/24	3/25	0.08 (–0.07–0.23)
Cardona, 1989[109]	38	26	6/20	15/18	0.53 (0.27–0.8)
Hsia, 1990[110]	46	65	4/22	11/24	0.28 (0.02–0.53)
Saari, 1990[111]	54	46	1/32	11/22	0.47 (0.25–0.69)
Rodriguez-Moreno, 1991[112]	31	30	0/15	11/16	0.69 (0.46–0.91)
Total	301		15/153	75/148	0.36 (0.28–0.43)
Somatostatin vs terlipressin					
Feu, 1996[113]	161	29	19/81	31/80	0.15 (0.01–0.29)
Walker, 1996[114]	106	12	3/53	0/53	–0.06 (–0.12–0.006)
Octreotide vs vasopressin					
Hwang, 1992[115]	48	44	3/24	11/24	0.33 (0.09–0.57)
Octreotide vs glypressin					
Silvain, 1993[116]	87	47	19/46	31/41	–0.05 (–0.21–0.11)

C, controls; D, drugs.

nitroglycerine.[103–105] No statistically significant difference in control of bleeding (POR 0.64; 95% CI 0.36–1.14) or mortality (POR 1.48; 95% CI 0.85–2.57) was demonstrated. The adverse event rate was significantly lower with terlipressin, even when vasopressin was combined with nitroglycerine.

Somatostatin vs vasopressin

Somatostatin was compared with vasopressin in seven studies including 301 patients.[106–112] The meta-analysis did not show a significant difference in the control of bleeding (POR 0.74; 95% CI 0.47–1.16) or mortality (POR 0.93; 95% CI 0.57–1.5) between the two vasoactive agents. However, a statistically significant reduction in complications was observed in the group receiving somatostatin (complication rates: vasopressin 51%, somatostatin 10%; ARR 40%, NNT = 3).

Somatostatin vs terlipressin

Two recent studies involving 267 patients have compared somatostatin with terlipressin.[113,114] These studies did not show a difference with respect to control of variceal bleeding or mortality. In the larger of these studies,[113] a significantly lower incidence of complications in the somatostatin group was reported.

Octreotide vs other drugs

The efficacy of octreotide in comparison to other vasoactive drugs, for acute variceal bleeding, has not been adequately evaluated. Octreotide was not found to be different from vasopressin (n = 48 patients)[115] or terlipressin plus nitoglycerine (n = 87 patients).[116] However, since the sample sizes were small, there is a significant chance of a type 2 error. For this reason, and because the outcomes measures were not very clearly described, these studies should be interpreted with caution.

Randomized controlled trials of emergency sclerotherapy in the management of acute variceal bleeding

Injection sclerotherapy, first introduced in 1939 and "rediscovered" in the late 1970s, has rapidly become the endoscopic treatment of choice for the control of acute variceal bleeding over the past two decades. The best evidence for the value of sclerotherapy in the management of acute variceal bleeding has come from a recently published study by the Veterans Affairs Cooperative Variceal Sclerotherapy Group[117] which compared sclerotherapy, with a sham procedure. The active intervention was effective for control of bleeding (sclerotherapy 91%, sham procedure 60%, P <0.001, ARR 29%, NNT= 3) and reduction in hospital mortality (sclerotherapy 25%, sham procedure 49%, P = 0.04, ARR 24%, NNT = 4).

Sclerotherapy should be performed at the diagnostic endoscopy, which should take place as soon as possible, because early intervention is beneficial.[118,119] No more than two injection sessions should be used to arrest variceal bleeding within a 5-day period.[58] Sclerosing agents in use include polidocanol 1–3%, ethanolamine oleate 5%, sodium tetradecyl sulfate 1–2%, and sodium morrhuate 5%. There is no evidence that any one

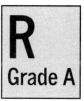

R
Grade A

Table 24.4 Randomized controlled trials of sclerotherapy plus drugs/balloon tamponade vs drugs/balloon tamponade alone for the treatment of the acute bleeding episode

Study	Compared treatment	No. of patients	Child C (%)	Event rate S+D	Event rate D	ARR (95% CI)
Outcome: failure to control bleeding						
Soderlund, 1985[121]	Vasopressin ± tamponade	107	65	3/57	8/50	0.11 (–0.01–0.22)
Larson, 1986[122]	Vasopressin ± tamponade	82	57	5/44	14/38	0.25 (0.07–0.43)
[a]Alexandrino,1990[123]	Vasopressin/nitro glycerin ± tamponade	83	49	12/41	12/42	–0.007(–0.2–0.19)
[a]Novella, 1996[124]	Octreotide	41	NR	3/22	7/19	0.23 (–0.03–0.49)
[a]Ortiz, 1997[125]	Somatostatin	97	26	9/49	21/48	0.25 (0.08–0.43)
Total		410		32/213	62/197	0.15 (0.08–0.23)
Outcome: death						
Soderlund, 1985[121]	Vasopressin ± tamponade	107	65	16/57	18/50	0.08 (–0.1–0.26)
Larson, 1986[122]	Vasopressin ± tamponade	82	57	2/44	5/38	0.09 (–0.04–0.21)
[a]Alexandrino, 1990[123]	Vasopressin/nitro glycerin ± tamponade	83	49	16/41	17/42	0.01 (–0.2–0.23)
[a]Novella, 1996[124]	Octreotide	41	NR	3/22	2/19	–0.03(–0.23–0.17)
[a]Ortiz, 1997[125]	Somatostatin	97	26	NR	NR	
Total		313		37/164	42/149	0.05 (–0.03–0.13)

C, controls; S, sclerotherapy; D, drugs; NR, not reported.
[a]Abstract.

sclerosant is superior. A substantial proportion of intravariceal sclerosant ends up in the paravariceal tissue and *vice versa*, and there is no evidence that one technique is superior. The risk of local and systemic complications of sclerotherapy varies greatly between trials and may be related to the experience of the operator.[120]

SCLEROTHERAPY PLUS CONVENTIONAL THERAPY (DRUGS AND/OR BALLOON TAMPONADE) VS CONVENTIONAL THERAPY

There were five trials comprising 410 patients which compared conventional therapy with vasopressin,[121–123] octreotide,[124] or somatostatin,[125] with or without balloon tamponade, with the addition of sclerotherapy to conventional therapy (Table 24.4). Control of bleeding was evaluated within 24 hours and up to 120 hours. Failure to control bleeding was significantly less common with the regimens that included sclerotherapy (POR 2.59; 95% CI 1.59–4.2), without significant heterogeneity (P = 0.24). The NNT, the number of patients needed to treat with sclerotherapy, in addition to conventional therapy to prevent one rebleeding episode, is 7 (95% CI 4–13). Publication bias assessment showed that 13 null or negative studies would be needed to render the results of this meta-analysis non-significant. There were fewer deaths in the sclerotherapy plus drugs arm than in drugs

Table 24.5 Randomized controlled trials of sclerotherapy compared to drugs for the treatment of the acute bleeding episode

Study	Compared treatment	No. of patients	Child C (%)	Event rate S	Event rate D	ARR (95% CI)
Outcome: failure to control bleeding						
Westaby, 1989[126]	Vasopressin + nitroglycerin	64	34	4/33	11/31	0.23 (0.3–0.44)
[a]Di Febo, 1990[130]	Somatostatin	47	40	2/24	5/23	0.13 (–0.07–0.34)
Shields, 1992[128]	Somatostatin	80	52.5	7/41	9/39	0.06 (–0.12–0.24)
Sung, 1993[131]	Octreotide	98	43	13/49	15/49	0.04 (–0.14–0.22)
Planas, 1994[129]	Somatostatin	70	34	6/35	7/35	0.03 (–0.15–0.21)
[a]Poo, 1996[133]	Octreotide	43	47	2/21	2/22	–0.05 (–0.2–0.1)
[a]Kravetz, 1996[134]	Octreotide	50	NR	7/25	10/25	0.16 (–0.07–0.39)
Jenkins, 1997[132]	Octreotide	150	53	14/77	11/73	–0.03 (–0.15–0.09)
[a]CSFGTBEV, 1997[127]	Terlipressin	219	31	36/114	39/105	0.06 (–0.07–0.18)
[a]El-Jackie, 1998[135]	Octreotide	100	40	3/50	21/50	0.36 (0.21–0.51)
Total		921		94/469	129/452	0.08 (0.03–0.13)
Outcome: death						
Westaby, 1989[126]	Vasopressin + nitroglycerin	64	34	9/33	12/31	0.11 (–0.11–0.34)
[a]Di Febo, 1990[130]	Somatostatin	47	40	5/24	6/23	0.05 (–0.19–0.29)
Shields, 1992[128]	Somatostatin	80	52.5	8/41	12/39	0.11 (–0.07–0.3)
Sung, 1993[131]	Octreotide	98	43	20/49	14/49	–0.12 (–0.31–0.06)
Planas, 1994[129]	Somatostatin	70	34	8/35	10/35	0.06 (–0.15–0.26)
[a]Poo, 1996[133]	Octreotide	43	47	5/21	3/22	–0.1 (–0.33–0.13)
[a]Kravetz, 1996[134]	Octreotide	50	NR	2/25	5/25	0.12 (–0.07–0.31)
Jenkins, 1997[132]	Octreotide	150	53	13/77	22/73	0.13 (–0.002–0.27)
[a]CSFGTBEV, 1997[127]	Terlipressin	219	31	18/114	24/105	0.07 (–0.03–0.18)
[a]El-Jackie, 1998[135]	Octreotide	100	40	NR	NR	
Total		821		88/419	108/402	0.06 (0.006–0.12)
Outcome: complications						
[a]Di Febo, 1990[130]	Somatostatin	47	40	2/24	$\frac{1}{2}$3	–0.04 (–0.18–0.1)
Shields, 1992[128]	Somatostatin	80	52.5	12/41	5/39	–0.16 (–0.34–0.01)
Sung, 1993[131]	Octreotide	98	43	18/49	5/49	–0.27 (–0.42–(–)0.01)
Planas, 1994[129]	Somatostatin	70	34	10/35	5/35	–0.14 (–0.33–0.05)
[a]Poo, 1996[133]	Octreotide	43	47	1/21	1/22	–0.002 (–0.13–0.12)
[a]Kravetz, 1996[134]	Octreotide	50	NR	8/25	9/25	0.04 (–0.22–0.3)
Jenkins, 1997[132]	Octreotide	150	53	15/77	19/73	0.07 (–0.07–0.2)
[a]CSFGTBEV, 1997[127]	Terlipressin	219	31	32/114	33/105	0.03 (–0.09–0.15)
Total		757		98/386	78/371	–0.04 (–0.1–0.009)

C, controls; S, sclerotherapy; D, drugs; NR, not reported.
[a]Abstract.

alone but the difference was not significant (POR 1.33; 95% CI 0.78–2.27). The incidence of complications, when reported, varied considerably between trials, with two of them stating that there were more complications in the sclerotherapy arm and one in the control arm.

SCLEROTHERAPY VS DRUGS

Ten studies including 921 patients compared sclerotherapy with infusion of vasopressin,[126] terlipressin,[127] somatostatin,[128-130] or octreotide[131-135] for 48 to 120 hours (Table 24.5). The outcome measure was control of bleeding at the end of the infusion period. The overall efficacy of sclerotherapy was 85% (range 73–94%) in studies of 12–48 h drug infusion[126,129–133,135] and 74% (68–84%) in studies of 120 h drug infusion.[127,128,134] There was significant heterogeneity (P <0.05) in the evaluation of failure to control bleeding in these studies, which was mainly due to the differences in benefit from sclerotherapy rather than to different outcome measures used in individual studies. Two of the 10 studies[132,133] reported that drugs were better than sclerotherapy but in neither study was this difference statistically significant. Sclerotherapy was significantly more effective than drug therapy (POR 1.68, 95% CI 1.07–2.63; ARR 6%; NNT = 11, 95% CI 6–113). Publication bias assessment showed that nine null or negative studies would be needed to render the results of this meta-analysis non-significant. Sensitivity analyses including only (a) peer-reviewed articles[126,128,129,131,132] (POR 1.3; 95% CI 0.8–2.1), (b) studies using only somatostatin or octreotide,[128–135] (POR 1.65; 95% CI 0.92–2.95), (c) studies with 120 h drug treatment[127,128,134] (POR 1.42; 95% CI 0.9–2.26), (d) studies with cirrhotic patients[126–34] (POR 1.4; 95% CI 0.99–1.9) always showed a strong trend in favor of sclerotherapy.

There was no significant heterogeneity in the evaluation of mortality in these studies: only two studies[131,133] reported a lower mortality in the drug arm which was not statistically significant. Mortality was reduced in the sclerotherapy group (POR 1.43; 95% CI 1.05–1.95; ARR 6%) The NNT to avoid one death is 15 (95% CI 8–69). Publication bias assessment showed that three null or negative studies would be required to render the results of this meta-analysis non-significant.

The type of complications recorded in eight studies[127–134] differed considerably, resulting in a significant heterogeneity (P = 0.04). Four studies reported more complications in the sclerotherapy arm[128–131] while three reported more complications[127,132,134] in the drug arm, and one found equal numbers in both arms.[133] The meta-analysis showed a trend in favor of drug treatment but the result was not statistically significant (Der Simonian and Laird method: POR 0.71; 95% CI 0.41–1.2).

Sclerotherapy plus drugs vs sclerotherapy alone

Table 24.6 summarizes results of five randomized trials[136-140] including 610 patients which have compared sclerotherapy plus somatostatin, octreotide, or terlipressin with sclerotherapy alone. Only three studies were placebo controlled.[136–138] Combination therapy was more effective (POR 0.42; 95% CI 0.29–0.6; failure to control bleeding sclerotherapy + drugs 22%, sclerotherapy alone 38% ARR 16, NNT = 6, 95% CI 4–10). Publication bias assessment showed that 29 null or negative studies would be needed to render the results of this meta-analysis statistically non-significant. No effect on mortality was demonstrated. Only two studies provided data on complications.[136,137] There were no significant differences between the two treatment arms.

SCLEROTHERAPY vs VARICEAL LIGATION

There are only two studies specifically designed to compare sclerotherapy with variceal ligation for the management of the acute bleeding episode.[141;142] Other data come from

Table 24.6 Randomized controlled trials of sclerotherapy plus drugs compared to sclerotherapy alone for the treatment of the acute bleeding episode

Study	Compared treatment	No. of patients	Child C (%)	Event rate S+D	Event rate S	ARR (95% CI)
Outcome: failure to control bleeding						
Besson, 1995[136]	S + octreotide	199	37	11/98	25/101	0.14 (0.03–0.24)
[a]Signorelli, 1996[138]	S + somatostatin	63	NR	6/33	11/30	0.18 (–0.03–0.4)
[a]Brunati, 1996[139]	S + octreotide/ S + terlipressin	55	NR	7/28	11/27	0.16 (–0.09–0.4)
		55	NR	6/28	11/27	0.19(–0.05–0.43)
[a]Signorelli, 1997[140]	S + octreotide	86	NR	7/44	12/42	0.13 (–0.05–0.3)
ABOVE (Avgerinos), 1997[137]	S + somatostatin	152[b]	NR	31/77	48/75	0.24 (0.08–0.39)
Total		610		68/308	118/302	0.16 (0.1–0.23)
Outcome: death						
Besson, 1995[136]	S + octreotide	199	37	12/98	12/101	–0.004 (–0.09–0.09)
[a]Brunati, 1996[139]	S + octreotide/ S + terlipressin	55	NR	4/28	4/27	0.006 (–0.18–0.19)
		55	NR	4/28	4/27	0.006 (–0.18–0.19)
ABOVE (Avgerinos), 1997[137]	S + somatostatin	205[b]	NR	27/101	24/104	–0.04 (–0.15–0.08)
Total		514		47/255	44/259	–0.01 (–0.07–0.05)
Outcome: complications						
Besson 1995[136]	S + octreotide	199	37	34/98	33/101	–0.02 (–0.15–0.11)
ABOVE (Avgerinos), 1997[137]	S + somatostatin	152[b]	NR	37/101	37/104	–0.01 (–0.14–0.12)

C, controls; NR, not reported; S, sclerotherapy; S + D, sclerotherapy plus drugs.
[a]Abstract.
[b]Only patients with variceal bleeding.

10 long term comparisons of sclerotherapy with variceal ligation.[143–152] There was no heterogeneity ($P = 0.21$) in the analysis of failure to control bleeding from the 12 studies,[141–152] which include a total of 419 patients. No difference was demonstrated in the effects of these interventions. Only the two studies specifically designed to compare emergency sclerotherapy with variceal ligation[141,142] reported incidence of complications. Ligation produced significantly fewer complications in one of these[142] and there was a trend in this direction in the other study.[141]

Randomized controlled trials of emergency surgery in the management of acute variceal bleeding

Four randomized trials compared sclerotherapy to emergency staple transection.[153-156] Failure to control bleeding was reported only in two of these studies, with divergent results. Teres *et al*[155] reported that efficacy of transection in their study was only 71%, compared to 83% in the sclerotherapy arm. In the largest study, performed by Burroughs *et al*,[156] a 5-day bleeding-free interval was achieved in 90% of the transected patients (none rebled from varices), compared to 80% in those who had two emergency injection sessions. There was no difference in mortality between the two treatment modalities. Cello *et al* showed that emergency portacaval shunt was more effective than emergency sclerotherapy (followed by elective sclerotherapy) in preventing early rebleeding (19% vs 50%).[157] Hospital and 30-day mortality were not significantly different. Finally Orloff *et al* reported, in a small study,[158] that portacaval shunt, performed in less than 8 hours from admission, was significantly better than medical treatment (vasopressin/balloon tamponade) in the control of acute variceal bleeding. No statistically significant difference in mortality was demonstrated in any of these studies.

Randomized controlled trials of tissue adhesives in the management of acute variceal bleeding

Two types of tissue adhesives – n-butyl-2-cyanoacrylate (Histoacryl) and isobutyl-2-cyanoacrylate (Bucrylate) – harden within seconds upon contact with blood[120] and have been used for the control of variceal bleeding.[159] Two randomized controlled trials compared sclerotherapy alone with the combination of sclerotherapy and Histoacryl for the control of active variceal bleeding.[160,161] The combined treatment was more effective than sclerotherapy alone in both studies. Moreover, in two studies Histoacryl was compared to variceal ligation for the control of bleeding from esophageal[162] or esophagogastric varices.[163] The overall success rate for initial hemostasis was similar for the two interventions in these studies. However, Histoacryl was superior to variceal ligation for the control of fundic variceal bleeding on subgroup analysis, but was less effective for the prevention of rebleeding (67% vs 28%). Finally, in a recent small study,[164] a biological fibrin glue (Tissucol) was more effective than sclerotherapy with polidocanol in the prevention of early rebleeding and had significantly lower incidence of complications. More studies are necessary to confirm these data and examine the potential risks of activation of coagulation, systemic embolism, and transmission of infections with the human plasma derived fibrin glue.

Gastric varices

The reported incidence of bleeding from gastric varices varies between 3% and 30%, but in most series it is less than 10%.[165] Patients with gastric variceal hemorrhage bleed more profusely and require more transfusions than patients with esophageal variceal bleeding.[166] Patients with gastric varices also have a higher risk of rebleeding and decreased survival.[166] The optimal treatment of gastric variceal bleeding is not known. Limited information is available on the role of vasoactive drugs in the control of gastric fundal bleeding and balloon tamponade has been used with little success. Use of standard sclerosants is associated with unacceptable rebleeding, particularly from necrotic ulceration, as gastric mucosa appears to be much more sensitive to this complication than esophageal mucosa.

Because of this, alternative sclerosant agents have been evaluated. The tissue glue isobutyl-2-cyanoacrylate (Bucrylate), mixed with lipiodol to delay premature hardening, was effective in uncontrolled studies.[159,167] Bucrylate has been shown to be superior to ethanolamine, in a non-randomized comparison,[168] achieving hemostasis in 90% of 23 patients, as opposed to 67% of 24 patients, $P < 0.005$. However, reports of cerebral embolism, with the tissue adhesives identified in the cerebral circulation at post mortem, cause concern. Interest has focused on thrombin, which is much easier to administer, and has been shown to provide good early hemostasis.[169] In all of these studies, rebleeding rates have remained high. Hence in patients with rebleeding or uncontrolled bleeding from gastric varices devascularization surgery or portosystemic shunting has been proposed.[170] We have recently described in a case series that "salvage" TIPS is very effective in this situation, with more than 95% success rate for initial hemostasis and an early rebleeding rate of less than 20%.[165]

Uncontrolled variceal bleeding

Uncontrolled variceal bleeding, despite adequate endoscopic and pharmacological therapy, represents a difficult management problem. A recent large consensus conference failed to agree on a suitable definition for this condition.[171] Varices in different locations behave differently, and a variety of interventions is available.

The definition that is commonly used for uncontrolled esophageal variceal bleeding is continued variceal bleeding despite two sessions of emergency endoscopic interventions and vasoactive therapy during a 7-day period, or bleeding past a Sengstaken–Blakemore tube independent of the number of sclerotherapy sessions. Bleeding from gastric varices is said to be uncontrolled when hemorrhage persists despite vasoconstrictor therapy.[165]

There are no randomized controlled trials evaluating different "salvage" therapies in uncontrolled variceal bleeding. However the advent of transjugular intrahepatic portosystemic shunt (TIPS) has offered a valuable option in this condition. TIPS is a radiographically controlled intervention which involves the creation of a communication between hepatic vein and an intrahepatic branch of the portal vein, thus decompressing the portal venous system. Hence TIPS functions in a similar way to surgical shunts. However, the morbidity and mortality due to the procedure is much more favourable. It has been shown in uncontrolled studies that emergency TIPS is highly effective as salvage therapy in patients with uncontrolled esophageal or gastric variceal bleeding.[165,172] This treatment appears to be the best option for patients with poor liver function awaiting liver transplantation.

R
Grade B

Conclusion

The available data suggest that emergency endoscopic treatment with sclerotherapy, at the time of the initial diagnostic endoscopy, should be the standard intervention for the management of the acute variceal bleeding episode. Sclerotherapy is recommended over ligation because it is more feasible in acute situations. A diagnostic endoscopy, with visualization unhindered by the ligation device, should be done first, since varices may not be the source of bleeding. Double intubation (placing ligation device after diagnosis) may increase the risk of complications and lengthens the procedure. Sclerotherapy is significantly better than vasoactive drug treatment alone and there is no need for further studies directly comparing sclerotherapy with currently available drugs. The combination of sclerotherapy with vasoactive drugs has shown promising results and should be tested in randomized controlled trials. The drugs of choice for this combination are terlipressin (as mortality is reduced, albeit in small placebo controlled studies) and somatostatin

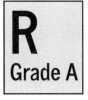

R
Grade A

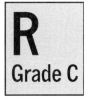

(which has fewer adverse effects and has been successfully tested over five days). Further studies are needed to assess the role of tissue adhesives or fibrin glues in patients unresponsive to vasoactive drugs or sclerotherapy.

R Grade C

The role of emergency TIPS as "salvage therapy" for uncontrolled bleeding from esophageal or gastric varices has been justified, although randomized trials to compare it with emergency surgical shunts or other interventions are still required.

PREVENTION OF RECURRENT VARICEAL BLEEDING

Patients surviving the first episode of variceal bleeding are at very high risk of recurrent bleeding (70% or more) and death (30–50%). There is a consensus that all patients who have previously bled from varices should have secondary therapy to prevent further variceal bleeding.[10] All randomized studies have shown that active intervention is better than observation. Hence the risk indicators for rebleeding are of less clinical value than those for first variceal bleeding. However, severity of liver disease,[7] continued alcohol abuse[6] and variceal size are associated with variceal rebleeding. Hemodynamic indices may identify patients who are more likely to rebleed. Two such indices use the technique of hepatic wedge pressure measurement as an indicator of portal pressure. From the analysis of the Barcelona–Boston–New Haven Primary Prophylaxis trial, it was concluded that variceal bleeding did not occur with an HVPG <12 mmHg, in patients with predominantly sinusoidal portal hypertension.[173]

An alternative hemodynamic index has been recently proposed by Feu *et al*,[174] based on precentage reduction of HVPG, but this approach has not been confirmed[175] and it has not been proven to be more successful than using wedge pressure measurement.

Randomized controlled trials for the prevention of variceal rebleeding

BETA-BLOCKERS COMPARED TO NO TREATMENT

R Grade A

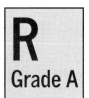

There are 12 trials comprising 769 patients.[53,176–186] A comprehensive meta-analysis of these trials has recently been published.[187] The mean follow-up was 21±5 months. There was significant heterogeneity in the evaluation of rebleeding ($P<0.01$). Treatment with beta-blockers significantly decreased the risk of rebleeding (ARR 21%; 95% CI 10–32; NNT = 5) and death (ARR 5.4%; 95% CI 0–11; NNT = 14). Adverse events occurred in 17% of patients in these randomized controlled trials and were generally mild. No fatal complication has been reported with beta-blockers.

The use of the recently proposed hemodynamic targets to identify patients who are "non-responders" to pharmacological therapy could be a useful tool in the planning of treatment for secondary prevention of variceal bleeding. Patients who fail could be offered alternative interventions. Beta-blockers in association with oral nitrates have been shown to induce a greater drop in portal pressure than beta-blockers alone.[188] Other drugs that may enhance the effect of beta-blockers include molsidomine (an NO donor),[189] serotonin antagonists,[190] and spironolactone [191] but none of these has been evaluated in randomized clinical trials to establish whether they have clinically important benefit.

SCLEROTHERAPY COMPARED TO NO TREATMENT

Meta-analysis of eight trials including 1111 patients[121,183,192–196] demonstrated that sclerotherapy reduced the rebleeding rate (POR 0.63; 95% CI 0.49–0.79) and mortality (POR 0.77; 95% CI 0.61–0.98). However, complications were frequent and did not differ from those of prophylactic or emergency sclerotherapy.

SCLEROTHERAPY COMPARED WITH VASOACTIVE DRUGS

Eleven trials involving 971 patients compared sclerotherapy with propranolol [183,197–205] or nadolol plus isosorbide mononitrate in one,[206] for the prevention of recurrent bleeding (from any source, eg varices, portal hypertensive bleeding, or sclerotherapy ulcers) (Table 24.7). There was a striking heterogeneity in the evaluation of rebleeding (P = 0.004): rebleeding was less frequent in patients randomized to drugs in five studies[183,198,202,203,206] and in patients randomized to sclerotherapy in six,[197,199–201,204,205] and no significant difference in rebleeding or mortality was demonstrated between the two interventions. The number of patients free of adverse events was not significantly different in the two groups (POR 0.85; 95% CI 0.65–1.11).

SCLEROTHERAPY PLUS DRUGS COMPARED TO SCLEROTHERAPY ALONE

There are 12 trials comprising 853 patients which compared sclerotherapy combined with propranolol,[207–214] nadolol[215–217] or isosorbide-5-mononitrate[218] with sclerotherapy alone (Table 24.8). Theoretically, vasoactive drugs might prevent rebleeding before variceal obliteration is achieved. The effect of beta-blockers was evaluated after obliteration[208] of varices in one study, while the drug was stopped at eradication in the others. There was statistically significant heterogeneity caused by differences between studies both in the direction and the size of the treatment effect. Meta-analysis showed that the combined intervention reduced the rebleeding rate (POR 0.54; 95% CI 0.34–0.86; ARR 15; NNT = 7) and mortality (POR 0.65; 95% CI 0.43–0.97; ARR 4; NNT = 22).

SCLEROTHERAPY COMPARED TO VARICEAL LIGATION

Sclerotherapy significantly decreases rebleeding rates and mortality, but it has been associated with serious complications, the most common of which are esophageal stricture and bleeding from treatment-induced ulcers. Variceal ligation was developed with the aim to provide an effective endoscopic intervention with fewer complications. There are 18 studies[141–152,219–224] (n = 1509 patients) comparing sclerotherapy with a variety of sclerosants to variceal ligation, at intervals of 1–3 weeks, for the prevention of recurrent bleeding in patients with cirrhosis,[141–147,219–224] non-cirrhotic portal hypertension,[148–151] or hepatic fibrosis due to schistosomiasis[152] (Table 24.9). Meta-analysis showed that variceal ligation significantly reduced rebleeding (POR 0.54; 95% CI 0.43–0.68; ARR 10; NNT = 10, 95% CI 7–17) and complications (POR 0.3; 95% CI 0.19–0.46). Publication bias assessment showed that there is a need for 99 null or negative studies to render the results of the meta-analysis statistically non-significant. Variceal ligation was also associated with a trend toward lower mortality, but the result did not reach the conventional level of statistical significance (POR 0.78; 95% CI 0.59–1.02;

R
Grade A

Table 24.7 Randomized controlled trials of sclerotherapy compared to beta-blockers for the prevention of rebleeding

Study	No. of patients	Child C (%)	Event rate BB	Event rate S	ARR (95% CI)
Outcome: failure to control bleeding					
Alexandrino, 1988[197]	65	—	25/34	17/31	–0.19 (–0.42–0.04)
Dollet, 1988[198]	55	27	11/27	18/28	0.24 (–0.02–0.49)
Fleig, 1998[199]	115	NR	26/57	26/58	–0.008 (–0.19–0.17)
Westaby, 1990[200]	108	—	29/52	28/56	–0.06 (–0.25–0.13)
Liu, 1990[201]	118	NR	33/58	20/60	–0.24(–0.41–(–)0.06)
Martin, 1991[202]	76	24	18/34	23/42	0.02 (–0.21–0.24)
Rossi, 1991[183]	53	38	13/27	13/26	0.02 (–0.25–0.29)
Andreani, 1991[203]	75	35	12/35	17/40	0.08 (–0.14–0.3)
Dasarathy, 1992[204]	104	34	31/53	19/51	–0.21 (–0.4–(–)0.02)
Teres, 1987[205]	116	14	37/58	26/58	–0.19(–0.37–(–)0.01)
[a]Villanueva, 1996[206]	86	—	11/43	23/43	0.28 (0.08–0.48)
Total	971		246/478	230/493	–0.05 (–0.1–0.01)
Outcome: death					
Alexandrino, 1988[197]	65	—	11/34	9/31	–0.03 (–0.26–0.19)
Dollet, 1988[198]	55	27	12/27	15/28	0.09 (–0.17–0.35)
Fleig, 1988[199]	115	NR	16/57	20/58	0.06 (–0.1–0.23)
Westaby, 1990[200]	108	—	22/52	21/56	–0.05 (–0.23–0.14)
Liu, 1990[201]	118	NR	27/58	17/60	–0.18(–0.35–(–)0.01)
Martin, 1991[202]	76	24	8/34	13/42	0.07 (–0.13–0.27)
Rossi, 1991[183]	53	38	7/27	6/26	–0.03 (–0.26–0.2)
Andreani, 1991[203]	75	35	9/35	17/40	0.1 (–0.04–0.38)
Dasarathy, 1992[204]	104	34	19/53	10/51	–0.16 (–0.33–0.006)
Teres, 1987[205]	116	14	23/58	21/58	–0.03 (–0.21–0.14)
[a]Villanueva, 1996 [206]	86	—	4/43	9/43	0.12 (–0.03–0.27)
Total	971		246/478	230/493	–0.004 (–0.006–0.005)
Outcome: complications					
Alexandrino, 1988[197]	65	—	24/34	28/31	0.2 (0.01–0.38)
Dollet, 1988[198]	55	27	0/27	10/28	0.36 (0.18–0.53)
Westaby, 1990[200]	108	—	4/52	0/56	–0.08 (–0.15–(–)0.004)
Martin, 1991[202]	76	24	0/34	19/42	0.45 (0.3–0.6)
Rossi, 1991[183]	53	38	3/27	8/26	0.2 (–0.02–0.41)
Dasarathy, 1992[204]	104	34	5/53	9/51	0.08 (–0.05–0.21)
Teres, 1987[205]	116	14	10/58	23/58	0.22 (0.06–0.38)
Total	577		46/285	97/292	0.10 (0.05–0.14)

C, controls; BB, beta-blockers; S, sclerotherapy; NR, not reported.
All trials used propranolol except one.
[a]Nadolol plus isosorbide mononitrate.

$P = 0.07$). Variceal ligation reduced the number of treatment sessions needed to achieve variceal obliteration in all the studies (ligation 2.7–4.1 sessions, sclerotherapy 4–6.5 sessions). However, there was no difference in the number of patients with varices

Table 24.8 Randomized controlled trials of sclerotherapy plus drugs compared to sclerotherapy for the prevention of rebleeding

Study	No. of patients	Child C (%)	Event rate S+D	Event rate S	ARR (95% CI)
Outcome: failure to control bleeding					
Westaby, 1986[207]	53	41	7/26	8/27	0.03 (–0.22–0.27)
Jensen, 1989[208]	51	29	3/25	12/26	0.55 (0.26–0.84)
Lundell, 1990[209]	41	51	12/19	11/22	–0.13 (–0.43–0.17)
Bertoni, 1990[215]	28	36	1/14	4/14	0.21 (–0.06–0.49)
Gerunda, 1990[216]	60	NR	6/30	7/30	0.03 (–0.17–0.24)
Vinel, 1992[210]	74	NR	7/39	14/35	0.22 (0.02–0.42)
Avgerinos, 1993[211]	85	7	14/45	21/40	0.21 (0.008–0.42)
Villanueva, 1994[217]	40	NR	12/22	7/18	–0.16 (–0.46–0.15)
Acharya, 1993[213]	114	NR	10/58	12/56	0.04 (–0.1–0.19)
Vickers, 1994[212]	73	34	17/39	14/34	–0.02 (–0.25–0.2)
Bertoni, 1994[218]	76	—	4/39	15/37	0.3 (0.12–0.49)
El-Sayed, 1996[214]	178	—	13/91	34/87	0.25 (0.12–0.37)
Total	853		106/437	159/416	0.15 (0.09–0.2)[a]
Outcome: death					
Westaby, 1986[207]	53	41	9/26	7/27	–0.003 (–0.15–0.14)
Jensen, 1989[208]	51	29	1/25	1 /26	–0.004 (–0.18–0.17)
Lundell, 1990[209]	41	51	NR	NR	0.17 (–0.03–0.38)
Bertoni, 1990[215]	28	36	1/14	3/14	0.14 (–0.11–0.4)
Gerunda, 1990[216]	60	NR	1/30	3/30	0.07 (–0.06–0.19)
Vinel, 1992[210]	74	NR	5/39	5/35	0.01 (–0.14–0.17)
Avgerinos, 1993[211]	85	7	8/45	9/40	0.05 (–0.12–0.22)
Villanueva, 1994[217]	40	NR	2/22	0/18	0.02 (–0.17–0.21)
Acharya, 1993[213]	114	NR	5/58	7/56	0.04 (–0.07–0.15)
Vickers, 1994[212]	73	34	9/39	9/34	0.03 (–0.16–0.23)
Bertoni, 1994[218]	76	—	2/39	9/37	0.19 (0.04–0.35)
El-Sayed, 1996[214]	178	—	11/91	10/87	0.006 (–0.1–0.09)
Total	853		48/437	65/416	0.04 (0.002–0.09)

C, controls; S, sclerotherapy; D, drugs; NR, not reported.
[a]Der Simonian and Laird method.

obliterated, and the recurrence of varices was more frequent in patients treated with ligation (POR 1.48; 95% CI 1.03–2.12). However, rebleeding after initial eradication is unusual if patients are in a regular endoscopic follow-up and varices that recur are re-obliterated.[225]

VARICEAL LIGATION COMPARED TO VARICEAL LIGATION PLUS SCLEROTHERAPY

In an attempt to further improve the results achieved with variceal ligation, it has been suggested that variceal ligation combined with low volume sclerotherapy could lead to more rapid eradication of varices than the use of variceal ligation alone. Meta-analysis of five studies,[226-230] involving 271 patients (Table 24.10) showed no significant differences between the two endoscopic treatments in the number of patients with varices eradicated,

Table 24.9 Randomized controlled trials of sclerotherapy compared to variceal ligation for the prevention of rebleeding

Study	No. of patients	Child C (%)	Event rate VL	Event rate S	ARR (95% CI)
Outcome: failure to control bleeding					
Stiegmann, 1992[143]	129	19	23/64	31/65	0.12 (–0.05–0.29)
Laine, 1993[144]	77	23	10/38	17/39	0.17 (–0.04–0.38)
Gimson, 1993[145]	103	26	16/54	26/49	0.23 (0.05–0.42)
Jensen, 1993[141]	32	NR	6/14	9/18	0.07 (–0.28–0.42)
Mundo, 1993[219]	19	37	2/8	3/11	0.02 (–0.38–0.42)
Young, 1993[220]	23	78	2/10	5/13	0.18 (–0.18–0.55)
Lo, 1995[146]	120	48	20/61	30/59	0.18 (0.007–0.35)
Hou, 1995[147]	134	39	13/67	28/67	0.22 (0.07–0.38)
Jensen, 1995[221]	50	NR	7/24	9/26	0.05 (–0.2–0.31)
Jain, 1996[148]	46	46[a]	9/22	5/24	–0.2 (–0.46–0.06)
Mostafa 1996[149]	158	NR	6/69	9/89	0.01 (–0.08–0.11)
Baroncini, 1997[222]	111	27	9/57	10/54	0.03 (–0.11–0.17)
Lo, 1997[142]	71	60	6/37	10/34	0.17 (–0.04–0.37)
Sarin, 1997[150]	95	14	3/47	10/48	0.14 (0.01–0.28)
Masci, 1997[223]	100	NR	16/50	26/50	0.2 (0.01–0.39)
Avgerinos, 1997[224]	77	8	10/37	19/40	0.2 (–0.006–0.42)
Shiha, 1997[151]	85	NR	6/42	10/43	0.09 (–0.08–0.25)
Fakhry, 1997[152]	84	NR	7/43	6/41	–0.02 (–0.17–0.14)
Total	1509		171/743	263/766	0.1 (0.06–0.14)
Outcome: death					
Stiegmann, 1992[143]	129	19	18/64	29/65	0.16 (0.001–0.33)
Laine, 1993[144]	77	23	4/38	6/39	0.05 (–0.1–0.2)
Gimson, 1993[145]	103	26	21/54	17/49	–0.04 (–0.23–0.14)
Jensen, 1993[141]	32	NR	2/14	3/18	0.02 (–0.23–0.28)
Mundo, 1993[219]	19	37	2/8	4/11	0.11 (–0.3–0.53)
Young, 1993[220]	23	78	2/10	4/13	0.11 (–0.24–0.46)
Lo, 1995[146]	120	48	10/61	19/59	0.16 (0.007–0.31)
Hou, 1995[147]	134	39	14/67	11/67	–0.04 (–0.18–0.09)
Jensen, 1995[221]	50	NR	4/24	9/26	0.18 (–0.06–0.42)
Mostafa, 1996[149]	158	NR	3/69	2/89	–0.02 (–0.08–0.04)
Baroncini, 1997[222]	111	27	12/57	12/54	0.16 (–0.04–0.37)
Lo, 1997[142]	71	60	7/37	12/34	0.01 (–0.14–0.16)
Sarin, 1997[150]	95	14	3/47	3/48	–0.001 (–0.1–0.1)
Masci, 1997[223]	100	NR	12/50	10/50	–0.04 (–0.2–0.12)
Avgerinos, 1997[224]	77	8	8/37	8/40	–0.02 (–0.2–0.17)
Shiha, 1997[151]	85	NR	2/42	2/43	–0.001 (–0.09–0.09)
Total	1384		124/679	151/705	0.01 (–0.02–0.05)
Outcome: variceal obliteration					
Stiegmann, 1992[143]	129	19	27/64	22/65	–0.08 (–0.25–0.08)
Laine, 1993[144]	77	23	22/38	27/39	0.11 (–0.1–0.33)
Gimson, 1993[145]	103	26	32/54	27/49	–0.04 (–0.23–0.15)
Mundo, 1993[219]	19	37	4/8	4/11	–0.14 (–0.58–0.31)
Young, 1993[220]	23	78	9/10	11/13	–0.05 (–0.32–0.22)
Lo, 1995[146]	120	48	45/61	37/59	–0.11 (–0.28–0.05)

Table 24.9 Randomized controlled trials of sclerotherapy compared to variceal ligation for the prevention of rebleeding–*Continued*

Study	No. of patients	Child C (%)	Event rate VL	Event rate S	ARR (95% CI)
Hou, 1995[147]	134	39	58/67	53/67	–0.07 (–0.2–0.05)
Jain, 1996[148]	46	46	20/22	24/24	0.09 (–0.03–0.21)
Mostafa, 1996[149]	158	NR	62/69	82/89	0.008 (–0.08–0.1)
Baroncini, 1997[222]	111	27	53/57	50/54	–0.004 (–0.1–0.09)
Sarin, 1997[150]	95	14	3/47	10/48	0.001 (–0.1–0.1)
Masci, 1997[223]	100	NR	43/50	41/50	–0.04 (–0.18–0.1)
Avgerinos, 1997[224]	77	8	35/37	39/40	0.03 (–0.06–0.12)
Shiha, 1997[151]	85	NR	37/42	37/43	–0.02 (–0.16–0.12)
Fakhry, 1997[152]	84	NR	42/43	40/41	–0.001 (–0.07–0.06)
Total	1509		171/743	263/766	–0.004 (–0.03–0.03)

C, controls; VL, variceal ligation; S, sclerotherapy; NR, not reported.
[a] = Child B and C.

Table 24.10 Randomized controlled trials of variceal ligation compared to variceal ligation plus sclerotherapy for the prevention of rebleeding

Study	No. of patients	Child C (%)	Event rate VL+S	Event rate VL	ARR (95% CI)
Outcome: failure to control bleeding					
Combined					
Laine, 1996[226]	41	44	6/21	6/20	0.01 (–0.26–0.29)
Argonz, 1996[227]	59	NR	5/30	11/29	0.21 (–0.009–0.43)
Saeed, 1997[228]	47	28	8/22	6/25	–0.12 (–0.39–0.14)
Altraif, 1997[229]	60	25	5/29	7/31	0.05 (–0.15–0.25)
El-Khayat, 1997[230]	64	NR	2/34	2/30	0.008 (–0.1–0.13)
Total	171		26/136	32/135	0.03 (–0.06–0.12)
Sequential					
Bhargava, 1997[231]	50	18	5/25	4/25	–0.04 (–0.25–0.17)
Lo, 1998[232]	72	21	3/37	11/35	0.23 (0.06–0.41)
Outcome: death					
Combined					
Laine, 1996[226]	41	44	3/21	3/20	0.007 (–0.21–0.22)
Argonz, 1996[227]	59	NR	4/30	9/29	0.18 (–0.03–0.38)
Saeed, 1997[228]	47	28	8/22	4/25	–0.2 (–0.45–0.04)
Altraif, 1997[229]	60	25	3/29	7/31	0.12 (–0.06–0.31)
El-Khayat, 1997[230]	64	NR	4/34	3/30	–0.02 (–0.17–0.13)
Total	171		22/136	26/135	0.03 (–0.06–0.11)
Sequential					
Lo, 1998[232]	72	21	7/37	10/35	0.09 (–0.11–0.29)

Table 24.10 Randomized controlled trials of variceal ligation compared to variceal ligation plus sclerotherapy for the prevention of rebleeding–*Continued*

Study	No. of patients	Child C (%)	Event rate VL+S	Event rate VL	ARR (95% CI)
Outcome: complications					
Combined					
Laine, 1996[226]	41	44	6/21	2/20	–0.19 (–0.42–0.05)
Argonz, 1996[227]	59	NR	8/30	1/29	–0.23 (–0.4–(–)0.06)
Saeed, 1997[228]	47	28	13/22	5/25	–0.39 (–0.65–(–)0.13)
Altraif, 1997[229]	60	25	6/29	7/31	0.02 (–0.19–0.23)
El-Khayat, 1997[230]	64	NR	6/34	4/30	–0.04 (–0.22–0.13)
Total	171		39/136	19/135	–0.15 (–0.24–(–)0.06)
Sequential					
Bhargava, 1997[231]	50	18	14/25	8/25	–0.24 (–0.51–0.03)
Outcome: variceal eradication					
Combined					
Laine, 1996[226]	41	44	15/21	12/20	–0.11 (–0.4–0.17)
Argonz, 1996[227]	59	NR	24/30	16/29	–0.25 (–0.48–(–)0.02)
Saeed, 1997[228]	47	28	12/22	16/25	0.09 (–0.19–0.38)
Total	147		51/73	44/74	–0.11 (–0.26–0.04)
Sequential					
Bhargava, 1997[231]	50	18	20/25	5/25	–0.6 (–0.38–(–)0.82)

C, controls, VL, variceal ligation; S, sclerotherapy; NR, not reported.

in rebleeding, or mortality. However, complications were significantly more frequent with the combined therapy (ligation + sclerotherapy 29%, ligation alone 14%, ARR 15%, NNT = 7). Moreover, the number of sessions required to achieve eradication was significantly greater in one trial.[226]

Two small studies investigated whether there was an additive effect of sclerotherapy in small varices (inaccessible to variceal ligation) after the completion of repeated variceal ligation treatment,[231,232] with conflicting results. Three trials that compared combined variceal ligation and sclerotherapy with sclerotherapy alone[233,234,235] revealed no difference in rebleeding or mortality. Moreover this comparison is not justified, since sclerotherapy has been replaced by variceal ligation for the secondary prevention of variceal bleeding.

TIPS COMPARED TO SCLEROTHERAPY OR VARICEAL LIGATION

Meta-analysis of 10 trials, involving 719 patients, which compared TIPS with sclerotherapy[236–243] or variceal ligation[244,245] (Table 24.11) revealed that TIPS reduced the rebleeding rate (TIPS 19%, sclerotherapy or ligation 47%, ARR 28%, NNT = 4) with no significant effect on mortality. Hepatic encephalopathy was significantly more common in patients randomized to TIPS (TIPS 35%, sclerotherapy or ligation 19%, ARR 16, NNT =6). These results are similar to results of surgical trials for the secondary prevention of variceal bleeding but are based on shorter follow-up periods. TIPS stenosis occurs in 50–70% of patients within the first year, and this type of shunt requires regular

Table 24.11 Randomized controlled trials of TIPS compared to sclerotherapy/variceal ligation for the prevention of rebleeding

Study	No. of patients	Child C (%)	Event rate TIPS	Event rate S	ARR (95% CI)
Outcome: failure to control bleeding					
GEAIH, 1995[236]	65	100	13/32	20/33	0.2 (–0.04–0.44)
Garcia-Villareal, 1996[237]	37	32	2/18	9/19	0.36 (0.1–0.63)
Cabrera, 1996[238]	63	10	7/31	16/32	0.27 (0.05–0.5)
Sanyal, 1997[239]	80	49	10/41	9/39	–0.01 (–0.2–0.17)
Cello, 1997[240]	49	NR	3/24	12/25	0.35 (0.12–0.59)
Rossle, 1997[241]	126	18	9/61	29/65	0.3 (0.15–0.45)
Sauer, 1997[242]	83	24	6/42	21/41	0.37 (0.18–0.56)
Merli, 1998[243]	81	12	7/38	17/43	0.21 (0.02–0.4)
Jalan, 1997[244]	58	47	3/31	15/27	0.46 (0.24–0.67)
Pomier-Layrargues, 1997[245]	75	NR	10/38	22/37	0.33 (0.12–0.54)
Total	717		70/356	170/361	0.28 (0.21–0.34)
Outcome: death					
GEAIH, 1995[236]	65	100	16/32	14/33	–0.08 (–0.32–0.17)
Garcia-Villareal, 1996[237]	37	32	1/18	8/19	0.37 (0.12–0.61)
Cabrera, 1996[238]	63	10	6/31	5/32	–0.04 (–0.22–0.15)
Sanyal, 1997[239]	80	49	12/41	7/39	–0.11 (–0.3–0.07)
Cello, 1997[240]	49	NR	8/24	8/25	–0.01 (–0.28–0.25)
Rossle, 1997[241]	126	18	8/61	8/65	–0.008 (–0.12–0.11)
Sauer, 1997[242]	83	24	12/42	11/41	–0.02 (–0.21–0.17)
Merli, 1998[243]	81	12	9/38	8/43	–0.05 (–0.23–0.13)
Jalan, 1997[244]	58	47	13/31	10/27	–0.05 (–0.3–0.2)
Pomier-Layrargues, 1997[245]	75	NR	17/38	12/37	–0.12 (–0.34–0.1)
Total	717		102/356	91/361	–0.02 (–0.08–0.04)
Outcome: portal systemic encephalopathy					
Garcia-Villareal, 1996[237]	37	32	4/18	5/19	0.04 (–0.23–0.32)
Cabrera, 1996[238]	63	10	10/31	4/32	–0.2 (–0.4–0.003)
Sanyal, 1997[239]	80	49	12/41	5/39	–0.24 (–0.46–(–)0.002)
Cello, 1997[240]	49	NR	12/24	11/25	–0.06 (–0.34–0.22)
Rossle, 1997[241]	126	18	18/61	9/65	–0.16 (–0.3–(–)0.01)
Sauer, 1997[242]	83	24	14/42	3/41	–0.26 (–0.42–(–)0.01)
Merli, 1998[243]	81	12	21/38	10/43	–0.32 (–0.52–(–)0.12)
Jalan, 1997[244]	58	47	5/31	3/27	–0.05 (–0.23–0.13)
Pomier-Layrargues, 1997[245]	75	NR	13/38	10/37	–0.07 (–0.28–0.14)
Total	636		109/313	60/320	–0.16 (–0.23–(–)0.1)

C, controls; S, sclerotherapy; NR, not reported.

monitoring with doppler/ultrasound and repeat procedures for recanalization.[246] Similarly, a recent trial comparing TIPS to propranolol and isosorbide mononitrate in 91 patients showed that TIPS was effective in reducing rebleeding but did not improve survival, caused hepatic encephalopathy, and had a worse cost–benefit profile than pharmacological treatment.

SURGICAL SHUNTS

The ideal patients for surgical shunting are well compensated cirrhotics who have failed at least one other modality of therapy (drugs or sclerotherapy), have bled from gastric varices despite medical or endoscopic therapy, or live far from suitable medical services. The availability of TIPS has reduced the frequency of surgical shunts. A common indication for a surgical shunt is recurrent symptomatic TIPS stenosis in patients who have had a TIPS without major encephalopathy. These patients have selected themselves as good candidates. Small diameter portacaval H graft or distal splenorenal shunts are the favored surgical options, because they leave the portal vein available should liver transplantation be required.

Selective distal splenorenal shunt (DSRS) was designed to reduce the incidence of hepatic encephalopathy and liver failure following total portacaval shunt (PCS) by partially maintaining portal liver perfusion while decreasing portal blood flow to varices. A meta-analysis[1] of six trials, which included 336 patients,[248–253] showed no significant difference in rebleeding or mortality between the two surgical groups but patients with DSRS had less hepatic encephalopathy (PCS 23%, DSRS 27%, ARR 4%). The calibrated small diameter portacaval H graft shunt (PCHGS) is effective in the control of variceal hemorrhage and has been associated with reduced hepatic encephalopathy when compared to total portacaval shunt.[254] This shunt has been compared to TIPS.[255] Variceal rebleeding, shunt occlusion, shunt revision, and shunt failure occurred significantly more frequently with TIPS.

Table 24.12 Randomized controlled trials of DSRS compared to sclerotherapy for the prevention of rebleeding

Study	No. of patients	Child C (%)	Event rate DSRS	Event rate S	ARR (95% CI)
Outcome: failure to control bleeding					
Henderson, 1990[258]	72	43	1/35	22/37	0.57 (0.4–0.73)
Terés, 1987[257]	93	7.3[a]	6/57	18/55	0.21 (0.05–0.38)
Rikkers, 1987[256]	60	42	5/30	18/30	0.43 (0.21–0.65)
Spina, 1990[259]	66	—	1/34	10/32	0.28 (0.11–0.45)
Total	292		13/142	68/150	0.37 (0.28–0.46)
Outcome: death					
Henderson, 1990[258]	72	43	20/35	12/37	0.08 (–0.09–0.26)
Terés, 1987[257]	93	7.3[a]	9/57	15/55	0.27 (0.02–0.51)
Rikkers, 1987[256]	60	42	12/30	20/30	0.13 (–0.05–0.32)
Spina, 1990[259]	66	—	4/34	8/32	–0.25(–0.47–(–)0.02)
Total	292		45/142	55/150	0.06 (–0.04–0.16)
Outcome: portal systemic encephalopathy					
Henderson, 1990[258]	57	43	5/31	3/26	–0.05 (–0.22–0.13)
Terés, 1987[257]	90	7.3[a]	8/42	3/48	–0.13 (–0.27–0.01)
Rikkers, 1987[256]	58	42	6/29	4/29	–0.07 (–0.26–0.12)
Spina, 1990[259]	59	—	2/30	2/29	0.002 (–0.13–0.13)
Total	264		21/132	12/132	–0.06 (–0.13–0.02)

C, controls; S, sclerotherapy; NR, not reported.
[a]Child score.

A comprehensive meta-analysis[260] of four trials, involving 292 patients,[256–259] in which DSRS was compared to sclerotherapy (Table 24.12) included analysis of individual patient data provided by the principal authors. Rebleeding was statistically significantly reduced by DSRS (ARR = 37, NNT = 3), but no significant difference in mortality or the risk of chronic hepatic encephalopathy was demonstrated. Two trials[261,262] (one published only in abstract form[261]) have compared portacaval shunt with sclerotherapy in the elective treatment of variceal hemorrhage. Rebleeding was significantly less in the portacaval groups. However, the incidence of hepatic encephalopathy was significantly increased with the surgical treatment and there was no difference in survival.

Conclusion

Beta-blocker therapy is a safe and effective long term intervention for the prevention of recurrence of variceal bleeding. Combination of beta-blockers with isosorbide-5-mononitrate needs further testing in randomized controlled trials. The use of hemodynamic targets of HVPG response should be further evaluated during pharmacological therapy for the prevention of rebleeding. If endoscopic treatment is chosen, variceal ligation is the modality of choice. The combination of simultaneous variceal ligation and sclerotherapy does not offer any benefit. However, the use of additional sclerotherapy for the complete eradication of small varices after variceal ligation should be further addressed in future trials. The results of current prospective randomized controlled trials comparing variceal ligation with pharmacological treatment are awaited with great interest. Finally, the use of TIPS for the secondary prevention of variceal bleeding is not recommended on the basis of current data, mainly because of its worse cost–benefit profile compared to other treatments. In contrast there is a limited role for the selective surgical shunts (DSRS or PCHGS) in the modern management of portal hypertension in well compensated cirrhotics who have failed at least one other modality of therapy (drugs or ligation), or have bled from gastric varices despite medical or endoscopic therapy, or who live far from suitable medical services.

R
Grade A

REFERENCES

1 D'Amico G, Pagliaro L, Bosch J. The treatment of portal hypertension. A meta-analytic review. *Hepatology* 1995; **22**: 332–54.
2 Robbins J. Estimators of the Mantel–Haenszel variance consistent in both sparse data and large strata limiting models. *Biometrics* 1986; **42**: 311–23.
3 Der Simonian R, Laird N. Meta-analysis in clinical trials. *Controlled Clin Trials* 1986; **7**: 177–88.
4 Garcia-Tsao G, Groszmann RJ, Fisher RL *et al.* Portal pressure, presence of gastroesophageal varices and variceal bleeding. *Hepatology* 1985; **5**: 419–24.
5 Cales P, Desmorat H, Vinel JP *et al.* Incidence of large esophageal varices in patients with cirrhosis – application to prophylaxis of 1st bleeding. *Gut* 1990; **31**: 1298–302.
6 Vorobioff J, Groszmann RJ, Picabea E *et al.* Prognostic value of hepatic venous pressure gradient measurements in alcoholic cirrhosis: a 10-year prospective study. *Gastroenterology* 1996; **111**: 701–9.
7 Pagliaro L, D'Amico G, Pasta L *et al.* Portal hypertension in cirrhosis: natural history. In: Bosch J, Groszmann R (eds), *Portal hypertension. Pathophysiology and treatment.* Cambridge, MA, Blackwell Scientific, 1994, pp. 72–92.
8 Graham DY, Smith JL. The course of patients after variceal hemorrhage. *Gastroenterology* 1981; **80**: 800–9.
9 Defranchis R. Prediction of the 1st variceal hemorrhage in patients with cirrhosis of the liver and esophageal varices – a prospective multicenter study. *N Engl J Med* 1988; **319**: 983–9.
10 Grace ND, Groszmann RJ, Garcia-Tsao G *et al.* Portal hypertension and variceal bleeding: An

AASLD single topic symposium. *Hepatology* 1998; **28**: 868–80.
11 Armonis A, Patch D, Burroughs AK. Hepatic venous pressure measurement: An old test as new progmostic marker in cirrhosis? *Hepatology* 1997; **25**: 245–8.
12 Merkel C, Gatta A. Can we predict the 1st variceal bleeding in the individual patient with cirrhosis and esophageal varices. *J Hepatol* 1991; **13**: 378.
13 Nevens F, Bustami R, Scheys I *et al.* Variceal pressure is a factor predicting the risk of a first variceal bleeding: a prospective cohort study in cirrhotic patients. *Hepatology* 1998; **27**: 15–19.
14 Conn HO, Lindermuth WW, May CJ *et al.* Prophylactic portacaval anastomosis in cirrhotic patients with esophageal varices. *N Engl J Med* 1965; **272**: 1255–63.
15 Jackson FC, Perrin EB, Smith AG *et al.* A clinical investigation of the portacaval shunt. II. Survival analysis of the prophylactic operation. *Am J Surg* 1968; **115**: 22–42.
16 Resnick RH, Chalmers TC, Ishihara AM *et al.* A controlled study of the prophylactic portacaval shunt. A final report. *Ann Intern Med* 1969; **70**: 675–88.
17 Conn HO, Lindenmuth WW, May CJ *et al.* Prophylactic portacaval anastomosis. *Medicine (Baltimore)* 1972; **51**: 27–40.
18 Inokuchi K. Improved survival after prophylactic portal nondecompression surgery for esophageal varices – a randomized clinical trial. *Hepatology* 1990; **12**: 1–6.
19 Paquet KJ. Prophylactic endoscopic sclerosing treatment of the esophageal wall in varices – a prospective controlled randomized trial. *Endoscopy* 1982; **14**: 4–5.
20 Witzel L, Wolbergs E, Merki H. Prophylactic endoscopic sclerotherapy of esophageal varices – a prospective controlled study. *Lancet* 1985; **1**: 773–5.
21 Koch H, Henning H, Grimm H *et al.* Prophylactic sclerosing of esophageal varices: results of a prospective controlled study. *Endoscopy* 1986; **18**: 40–3.
22 Kobe E, Zipprich B, Schentke KU *et al.* Prophylactic endoscopic sclerotherapy of esophageal varices – a prospective randomized trial. *Endoscopy* 1990; **22**: 245–8.
23 Wordehoff D, Spech HJ. Prophylactic sclerotherapy of esophageal varices – results of a prospective, randomized long term trial over 7 years. *Dtsch Med Wochenschr* 1987; **112**: 947–51.
24 Santangelo WC, Dueno MI, Estes BL *et al.* Prophylactic sclerotherapy of large esophageal varices. *N Engl J Med* 1988; **318**: 814–18.
25 Sauerbruch T, Wotzka R, Kopcke W *et al.* Prophylactic sclerotherapy before the 1st episode of variceal hemorrhage in patients with cirrhosis. *N Engl J Med* 1988; **319**: 8–15.
26 Piai G, Cipolletta L, Claar N *et al.* A prospective controlled randomized study of prophylactic sclerotherapy of esophageal varices prior to 1st hemorrhage. *Ital J Gastroenterol* 1986; **18**: 223
27 Potzi R, Bauer P, Reichel W *et al.* Prophylactic endoscopic sclerotherapy of esophageal varices in liver cirrhosis – a multicenter prospective controlled randomized trial in Vienna. *Gut* 1989; **30**: 873–9.
28 Russo A, Giannone G, Magnano A *et al.* Prophylactic sclerotherapy in nonalcoholic liver cirrhosis – preliminary-results of a prospective controlled randomized trial. *World J Surg* 1989; **13**: 149–53.
29 Andreani T, Poupon RE, Balkau BJ *et al.* Preventive therapy of 1st gastrointestinal bleeding in patients with cirrhosis – results of a controlled trial comparing propranolol, endoscopic sclerotherapy and placebo. *Hepatology* 1990; **12**: 1413–19.
30 Triger DR, Smart HL, Hosking SW *et al.* Prophylactic sclerotherapy for esophageal varices – long term results of a single-center trial. *Hepatology* 1991; **13**: 117–23.
31 Gregory PB. Prophylactic sclerotherapy for esophageal varices in men with alcoholic liver disease – a randomized, single-blind, multicenter clinical trial. *N Engl J Med* 1991; **324**: 1779–84.
32 De Franchis R, Primignani M, Arcidiacono PG *et al.* Prophylactic sclerotherapy (St) in high-risk cirrhotics selected by endoscopic criteria. A multicenter randomized controlled trial. *Gastroenterology* 1989; **101**: 1087–93.
33 Bendsten F, Christensen E, Hardt F *et al.* Prophylaxis of 1st hemorrhage from esophageal varices by sclerotherapy, propranolol or both in cirrhotic-patients – a randomized multicenter trial. *Hepatology* 1991; **14**: 1016–24.
34 Saggioro A, Pallini P, Chiozzini G *et al.* Prophylactic sclerotherapy – a controlled study (abstract). *Dig Dis Sci* 1986; **31**: S504.
35 Fleig WE, Stange EF, Wordehoff D *et al.* Prophylactic (Ps) vs therapeutic sclerotherapy (Ts) in cirrhotic patients with large esophageal varices and no previous hemorrhage – a randomized clinical trial (abstract). *Hepatology* 1988; **8**: 1242.
36 Strauss E, Desa MG, Albano A *et al.* A randomized controlled trial for the prevention of the 1st upper gastrointestinal bleeding due to portal-hypertension in cirrhosis – sclerotherapy or propranolol versus control groups (abstract). *Hepatology* 1988; **8**: 1395.

37 Planas R, Boix J, Dominguez M *et al.* Prophylactic sclerosis of esophageal varices (EV). Prospective trial (abstract). *J Hepatol* 1989; **9**: S73.
38 Paquet KJ, Kalk JF, Klein CP *et al.* Prophylactic sclerotherapy for esophageal varices in high risk cirrhotic patients selected by endoscopic and haemodynamic criteria: a randomized single centre controlled trial. *Endoscopy* 1994; **26**: 733–40.
39 Pagliaro L, D'Amico G, Sorensen TIA *et al.* Prevention of first bleeding in cirrhosis. A meta-analysis of randomized clinical trials of nonsurgical treatment. *Ann Intern Med* 1992; **117**: 59–70.
40 Laine L, Cook D. Endoscopic ligation compared with sclerotherapy for treatment of esophageal variceal bleeding. A meta-analysis [see comments]. *Ann Intern Med* 1995; **123**: 280–7.
41 Lo GH, Hwu JH, Lai KH. Prophylactic banding ligation of high-risk esophageal varices – an interim report (abstract). *Gastroenterology* 1995; **108**: A1112.
42 Sarin SK, Guptan RC, Jain AK *et al.* A randomized controlled trial of endoscopic variceal band ligation for primary prophylaxis of variceal bleeding. *Eur J Gastroenterol Hepatol* 1996; **8**: 337–42.
43 Chen CY, Chang TT. Prophylactic endoscopic variceal ligation (EVL) for esophageal varices (abstract). *Gastroenterology* 1997; **112**: A1240.
44 Lay CS, Tsai YT, Teg CY *et al.* Endoscopic variceal ligation in prophylaxis of first variceal bleeding in cirrhotic patients with high-risk esophageal varices. *Hepatology* 1997; **25**: 1346–50.
45 Sarin SK, Lamba GS, Kumar M *et al.* Randomized trial of propranolol vs. endoscopic variceal ligation (EVL) in the primary prophylaxis of bleeding from high risk varices in cirrhosis: an interim analysis (abstract). *Hepatology* 1997; **26**: 928.
46 Stanley AJ, Forrest EH, Lui HF *et al.* Band ligation versus propranolol or isosorbide mononitrate in the primary prophylaxis of variceal haemorrhage: preliminary results of a randomized controlled trial (abstract). *Gut* 1998; **42**: F74.
47 Perezayuso RM, Pique JM, Bosch J *et al.* Propranolol in prevention of recurrent bleeding from severe portal hypertensive gastropathy in cirrhosis. *Lancet* 1991; **337**: 1431–4.
48 Pascal JP, Cales P. Propranolol in the prevention of first upper gastrointestinal tract haemorrhage in patients with cirrhosis of the liver and esophageal varices. *N Engl J Med* 1987; **317**: 856–61.
49 Ideo G, Bellati G, Fesce E *et al.* Nadolol can prevent the 1st gastrointestinal bleeding in cirrhotics – a prospective, randomized study. *Hepatology* 1988; **8**: 6–9.
50 Lebrec D, Poynard T, Capron JP *et al.* Nadolol for prophylaxis of gastrointestinal bleeding in patients with cirrhosis – a randomized trial. *J Hepatol* 1988; **7**: 118–25.
51 Pasta L. Propranolol prevents 1st gastrointestinal bleeding in non-ascitic cirrhotic-patients – final report of a multicenter randomized trial. *J Hepatol* 1989; **9**: 75–83.
52 Conn HO, Grace ND, Bosch J *et al.* Propranolol in the prevention of the 1st hemorrhage from esophagogastric varices – a multicenter, randomized clinical-trial. *Hepatology* 1991; **13**: 902–12.
53 Colman J, Jones P, Finch C *et al.* Propranolol in the prevention of variceal hemorrhage in alcoholic cirrhotic patients (abstract). *Hepatology* 1990; **8**: 1395A.
54 Poynard T, Cales P, Pasta L *et al.* Beta-adrenergic antagonist drugs in the prevention of gastrointestinal bleeding in patients with cirrhosis and esophageal varices – an analysis of data and prognostic factors in 589 patients from 4 randomized clinical trials. *N Engl J Med* 1991; **324**: 1532–8.
55 Grace ND, Conn HO, Groszmann RJ *et al.* Propranolol for prevention of 1st esophageal variceal hemorrhage (Evh) – a lifetime commitment (abstract). *Hepatology* 1990; **12**: 407.
56 Merkel C, Marin R, Enzo E *et al.* Randomized trial of nadolol alone or with isosorbide mononitrate for primary prophylaxis of variceal bleeding in cirrhosis. Gruppo-Triveneto per l'ipertensione portale (GTIP). *Lancet* 1996; **348**: 1677–81.
57 Angelico M, Carli L, Piat C *et al.* Effects of isosorbide-5-mononitrate compared with propranolol on first bleeding and long term survival in cirrhosis [see comments]. *Gastroenterology* 1997; **113**: 1632–9.
58 Burroughs AK, Mezzanote G, Phillips A *et al.* Cirrhotics with variceal hemorrhage: the importance of the time interval between admission and the start of analysis for survival and rebleeding rates. *Hepatology* 1989; **9**: 801–7.
59 Goulis J, Armonis A, Patch D *et al.* Bacterial infection is independently associated with failure to control bleeding in cirrhotic patients with gastrointestinal hemorrhage. *Hepatology* 1998; **27**: 1207–12.
60 Ben-Ari Z, Cardin F, Wannamethee G *et al.* Prognostic significance of endoscopic active bleeding and early rebleeding from esophageal varices [see comments]. *J Hepatol* 1996; **20**: 92A.
61 Ready JB, Robertson AD, Goff JS *et al.* Assessment of the risk of bleeding from

esophageal varices by continuous monitoring of portal pressure. *Gastroenterology* 1991; **100**: 1403–10.

62 Rimola A, Bory F, Teres J *et al.* Oral, nonabsorbable antibiotics prevent infection in cirrhotics with gastrointestinal hemorrhage. *Hepatology* 1985; **5**: 463–7.

63 Soriano G, Guarner C, Tomas A *et al.* Norfloxacin prevents bacterial infection in cirrhotics with gastrointestinal hemorrhage. *Gastroenterology* 1992; **103**: 1267–72.

64 Blaise M, Pateron D, Trinchet JC *et al.* Systemic antibiotic therapy prevents bacterial infection in cirrhotic patients with gastrointestinal hemorrhage. *Hepatology* 1994; **20**: 34–8.

65 Pauwels A, Mostefa-Kara N, Debenes B *et al.* Systemic antibiotic prophylaxis after gastrointestinal hemorrhage in cirrhotic patients with a high risk of infection. *Hepatology* 1996; **24**: 802–6.

66 Bernard B, Grange JD, Nguyen KE *et al.* Antibiotic prophylaxis (AbP) for the prevention of bacterial infections in cirrhotic patients with gastrointestinal bleeding (GB): a meta-analysis (abstract). *Hepatology* 1996; **24**: 1271.

67 Goulis J, Patch D, Burroughs AK. The role of bacterial infection in the pathogenesis of variceal bleeding. *Lancet* 1999; **353**: 139–42.

68 Sarin SK. Long term follow-up of gastric variceal sclerotherapy: an eleven-year experience. *Gastrointest Endosc* 1997; **46**: 8–14.

69 Levacher S, Letoumelin P, Pateron D *et al.* Early administration of terlipressin plus glyceryl trinitrate to control active upper gastrointestinal bleeding in cirrhotic patients. *Lancet* 1995; **346**: 865–8.

70 Conn HO, Ramsby GR, Storer EH *et al.* Intraarterial vasopressin in the treatment of upper gastrointestinal hemorrhage: a prospective, controlled clinical trial. *Gastroenterology* 1975; **68**: 211–21.

71 Bosch J, Groszmann RJ, Garcia-Pagan JC *et al.* Association of transdermal nitroglycerin to vasopressin infusion in the treatment of variceal hemorrhage: a placebo-controlled clinical trial. *Hepatology* 1989; **10**: 962–8.

72 Sonnenburg GE, Keller U, Perruchud A *et al.* Effect of somatostatin on splanchnic haemodynamics. *Gastroenterology* 1981; **80**: 5226–32.

73 Bosch J, Kravetz D, Rodes J. Effects of somatostatin on hepatic and systemic haemodynamics in patients with cirrhosis of the liver: comparison with vasopressin. *Gastroenterology* 1981; **80**: 518–25.

74 Variceal Bleeding Study Group. A muticenter randomized controlled trial comparing different schedules of somatostatin administration in the treatment of acute variceal bleeding (abstract). *Hepatology* 1998; **28**: 770A.

75 Jenkins SA, Baxter JN, Snowden S. The effects of somatostatin and SMS 201–995 on hepatic haemodynamics inpatients with cirrhosis and portal hypertension. *Fibrinolysis* 1988; **2**: 48–50.

76 McCormick PA, Dick R, Siringo S *et al.* Octreotide reduces azygous blood flow in cirrhotic patients with portal hypertension. *Eur J Gastroenterol Hepatol* 1990; **2**: 489–92.

77 Escorsell A, Bandi JC, Francosis E *et al.* Desensitization to the effects of intravenous octreotide in cirrhotic patients with portal hypertension (abstract). *Hepatology* 1996; **24**: 207A.

78 Merigan TCJ, Poltkin JR, Davidson CS. Effect of intravenously administered posterior pituitary extract on haemorrhage from bleeding esophageal varices. *N Engl J Med* 1962; **266**: 134–5.

79 Mallory A, Schaefer JW, Cohen JR *et al.* Selective intra-arterial vasopressin infusion for upper gastrointestinal tract hemorrhage. A controlled trial. *Arch Surg* 1980; **115**: 30–2.

80 Fogel RM, Knauer CM, Andress LL. Continuous intravenous vasopressin in active upper gastrointestinal bleeding. A placebo controlled trial. *Ann Intern Med* 1982; **96**: 565–9.

81 Tsai YT, Lay CS, Lai KH *et al.* Controlled trial of vasopressin plus nitroglycerin vs. vasopressin alone in the treatment of bleeding esophageal varices. *Hepatology* 1986; **6**: 406–9.

82 Gimson AE, Westaby D, Hegarty J *et al.* A randomized trial of vasopressin and vasopressin plus nitroglycerin in the control of acute variceal hemorrhage. *Hepatology* 1986; **6**: 410–13.

83 Walker S, Stiehl A, Raedsch R *et al.* Terlipressin in bleeding esophageal varices: a placebo-controlled, double-blind study. *Hepatology* 1986; **6**: 112–15.

84 Freeman JG, Cobden MD, Record CO. Placebo-controlled trial of terlipressin (glypressin) in the management of acute variceal bleeding. *J Clin Gastroenterol* 1989; **11**: 58–60.

85 Soderlund C, Magnusson I, Torngren S *et al.* Terlipressin (triglycyl-lysine vasopressin) controls acute bleeding esophageal varices. A double-blind, randomized, placebo-controlled trial. *Scand J Gastroenterol* 1990; **25**: 622–30.

86 Valenzuela JE, Schubert T, Fogel RM *et al.* A multicenter, randomized, double-blind trial of somatostatin in the management of acute hemorrhage from esophageal varices. *Hepatology* 1989; **10**: 958–61.

87 Burroughs AK, McCormick PA, Hughes MD *et al.* Randomized, double-blind, placebo-controlled trial of somatostatin for variceal bleeding. *Gastroenterology* 1990; **99**: 1388–95.

88 Gotzsche PC, Gjorup I, Bonnen H *et al.* Somatostatin v placebo in bleeding esophageal varices – randomized trial and metaanalysis. *Br Med J* 1995; **310**: 1495–8.
89 Loperfido S, Godena F, Tosolini G *et al.* [Somatostatin in the treatment of bleeding esophagogastric varices. Controlled clinical trial in comparison with ranitidine] [Italian]. *Recent Progr Med* 1987; **78**: 82–6.
90 Flati G, Negro P, Flati D *et al.* [Somatostatin. Massive upper digestive hemorrhage in portal hypertension. Results of a controlled study] [Spanish]. *Rev Espanol Enferm Apar Dig* 1986; **70**: 411–14.
91 Testoni PA, Masci E, Passaretti S *et al.* Comparison of somatostatin and cimetidine in the treatment of acute esophageal variceal bleeding. *Curr Ther Res* 1986; **39**: 759–66.
92 Burroughs AK, International Octreotide Varices Study Group. Double blind RCT of 5 day octreotide versus placebo, associated with sclerotherapy for trial failures (abstract). *Hepatology* 1996; **24**: 352A.
93 Primignani M, Andreoni B, Carpinelli L *et al.* Sclerotherapy plus octreotide versus sclerotherapy alone in the prevention of early rebleeding from esophageal varices – a randomized, double-blind, placebo-controlled, multicenter trial. *Hepatology* 1995; **21**: 1322–7.
94 D'Amico G, Politi F, Morabito A *et al.* Octreotide compared with placebo in a treatment strategy for early rebleeding in cirrhosis. A double blind, randomized pragmatic trial. *Hepatology* 1998; **28**: 1206–14.
95 Colin R, Giuli N, Czernichow P *et al.* Prospective comparison of glypressin, tamponade and their association in the treatment of bleeding esophageal varices. In Lebrec D, Blei AT (eds), *Vasopressin analogs and portal hypertension*. Paris, John Libbey Eurotext, 1987, pp 149–53.
96 Fort E, Sauterau D, Silvaine C *et al.* A randomized trial of terlipressin plus nitroglycerin vs balloon tamponade in the control of acute variceal haemorrhage. *Hepatology* 1990; **11**: 678–81.
97 Blanc P, Bories J, Desprez D *et al.* Balloon tamponade with Linton–Michel tube versus terlipressin in the treatment of acute esophageal and gastric variceal bleeding (abstract). *J Hepatol* 1994; **21**: 133S.
98 Jaramillo JL, de la Mata M, Mino G *et al.* Somatostatin versus Sengstaken tube balloon tamponade for primary haemostasis of bleeding esophageal varices.a randomized pilot study. *J Hepatol* 1991; **12**: 100–5.
99 Avgerinos A, Klonis C, Rekoumis G *et al.* A prospective randomized trial comparing somatostatin, baloon tamponade and the combination of both methods in the management of acute variceal haemorrhage. *J Hepatol* 1991; **13**: 78–83.
100 McKee R. A study of octreotide in esophageal varices. *Digestion* 1990; **45** Suppl 1: 60–4.
101 Freeman JG, Cobden MD, Lishaman AH *et al.* Controlled trial of terlipressin ("glypressin") versus vasopressin in the early treatment of esophageal varices. *Lancet* 1989; **2**: 62–8.
102 Desaint B, Florent C, Levy VG. A randomized trial of triglycyl-lysine vasopressin versus lysine vasopressin in active cirrhotic variceal hemorrhage. In Lebrec D, Blei AT (eds), *Vasopressin analogs and portal hypertension*. Paris, John Libbey Eurotext, 1987, pp 155–7.
103 Lee FY, Tsai YT, Lai KH *et al.* A randomized controlled study of triglycyl vasopressin and vasopressin plus nitroglycerin in the control of acute esophageal variceal hemorrhage. *Chin J Gastroenterol* 1988; **5**: 131–8.
104 Chiu WK, Sheen IS, Liaw YF. A controlled study of glypressin versus vasopressin in the control of bleeding from esophageal varices. *J Gastroenterol Hepatol* 1988; **5**: 549–53.
105 D'Amico G, Traina M, Vizzini G *et al.* Terlipressin or vasopressin plus transdermal nitroglycerin in a treatment strategy for digestive bleeding in cirrhosis. A randomized clinical trial. *J Hepatol* 1994; **20**: 206–12.
106 Kravetz D, Bosch J, Teres J *et al.* Comparison of intravenous somatostatin and vasopressin infusion in treatment of acute variceal hemorrhage. *Hepatology* 1984; **4**: 442–6.
107 Jenkins SA, Baxter JN, Corbett W *et al.* A prospective randomized controlled clinical trial comparing somatostatin and vasopressin in controlling acute variceal haemorrhage. *Br Med J* 1985; **290**: 275–8.
108 Bagarani M, Albertini V, Anza M *et al.* Effect of somatostatin in controlling bleeding from esophageal varices. *Ital J Surg Sci* 1987; **17**: 21–6.
109 Cardona C, Vida F, Balanzo J *et al.* Efficacia terapeutica de la somatostatina versus vasopressina mas nitroglycerina en la hemorragia activa por varices esofagogastrica. *Gastroenterol Hepatol* 1989; **12**: 30–4.
110 Hsia HC, Lee FY, Tsai YT *et al.* Comparison of somatostatin and vasopressin in the control of acute esophageal variceal hemorrhage. A randomized,controlled study. *Chin J Gastroenterol* 1990; **7**: 71–8.
111 Saari A, Klvilaasko E, Inberg M *et al.* Comparison of somatostatin and vasopressin in bleeding esophageal varices. *Am J Gastroenterol* 1990; **85**: 804–7.
112 Rodriguez-Moreno F, Santolaria F, Gles-Reimers E *et al.* A randomized trial of somatostatin vs vasopressin plus nitroglycerin in the treatment

of acute variceal bleeding (abstract). *J Hepatol* 1991; **13**: S162.
113 Feu F, DelArbol LR, Banares R *et al.* Double-blind randomized controlled trial comparing terlipressin and somatostatin for acute variceal hemorrhage. *Gastroenterology* 1996; **111**: 1291–9.
114 Walker S, Kreichgauer HP, Bode JC. Terlipressin (glypressin) versus somatostatin in the treatment of bleeding esophageal varices – final report of a placebo-controlled, double-blind study. *Zeitschr Gastroenterol* 1996; **34**: 692–8.
115 Hwang SJ, Lin HC, Chang CF *et al.* A randomized controlled trial comparing octreotide and vasopressin in the control of acute esophageal variceal bleeding. *J Hepatol* 1992; **16**: 320–5.
116 Silvain C, Carpentier S, Sautereau D *et al.* Terlipressin plus transdermal nitroglycerin vs octreotide in the control of acute bleeding from esophageal varices – a multicenter randomized trial. *Hepatology* 1993; **18**: 61–5.
117 Hartigan PM, Gebhard RL, Gregory PB, for the Veterans Cooperative Variceal Sclerotherapy Group. Sclerotherapy for actively bleeding esophageal varices in male alcoholics with cirrhosis. *Gastrointest Endosc* 1997; **46**: 1–7.
118 Prindiville T, Trudeau W. A comparison of immediate versus delayed endoscopic injection sclerosis of bleeding esophageal varices. *Gastrointest Endosc* 1986; **32**: 385–8.
119 Shemesh E, Czerniac A, Klein, E *et al.* A comparison between emergency and delayed endoscopic injection sclerotherapy of bleeding esophageal varices in non-alcoholic portal hypertension. *J Clin Gastroenterol* 1990; **12**: 5–9.
120 De Franchis R, Banares R, Silvain C. Emergency endoscopy strategies for improved outcomes. *Scand J Gastroenterol* 1998; **33** Suppl 226: 25–36.
121 Soderlund C, Ihre T. Endoscopic sclerotherapy v conservative management of bleeding esophageal varices. A 5-year prospective controlled trial of emergency and long term treatment. *Acta Chir Scand* 1985; **151**: 449–56.
122 Larson AW, Cohen H, Zweiban B *et al.* Acute esophageal variceal sclerotherapy. Results of a prospective randomized controlled trial. *JAMA* 1996; **255**: 497–500.
123 Alexandrino P, Alves MM, Fidalgo P *et al.* Is sclerotherapy the first choice treatment for active esophageal variceal bleeding in cirrhotic patients? Final report of a randomized controlled trial (abstract). *J Hepatol* 1990; **11**(Suppl): S1.
124 Novella MT, Villanueva C, Ortiz J *et al.* Octreotide vs sclerotherapy and octreotide for acute variceal bleeding. A pilot study (abstract). *Hepatology* 1996; **24**: 207A.
125 Ortiz J, Villanueva C, Sabat M *et al.* Somatostatin alone or combined with emergency sclerotherapy for acute variceal bleeding (abstract). *Gastrointest Endosc* 1997; **45**: 77A.
126 Westaby D, Hayes P, Gimson AES *et al.* Controlled trial of injection sclerotherapy for active variceal bleeding. *Hepatology* 1989; **9**: 274–7.
127 Cooperative Spanish-French Group for the Treatment of Bleeding Esophageal Varices. Randomized controlled trial comparing terlipressin vs endoscopic injection sclerotherapy in the treatment of acute variceal bleeding and prevention of early rebleeding (abstract). *Hepatology* 1997; **26**: 249A.
128 Shields R, Jenkins SA, Baxter JN *et al.* A prospective randomized controlled trial comparing the efficacy of somatostatin with injection sclerotherapy in the control of bleeding esophageal varices. *J Hepatol* 1992; **16**: 128–37.
129 Planas R, Quer JC, Boix J *et al.* A prospective randomized trial comparing somatostatin and sclerotherapy in the treatment of acute variceal bleeding. *Hepatology* 1994; **20**: 370–5.
130 Di Febo G, Siringo S, Vacirca M *et al.* Somatostatin (SMS) and urgent sclerotherapy (US) in active esophageal variceal bleeding (abstract). *Gastroenterology* 1990; **98**: 583A.
131 Sung JJ, Chung SS, Lai CW *et al.* Octreotide infusion or emergency sclerotherapy for variceal hemorrhage. *Lancet* 1993; **342**: 637–41.
132 Jenkins SA, Shields R, Davies M *et al.* A multicentre randomized trial comparing octreotide and injection sclerotherapy in the management and outcome of acute variceal haemorrhage. *Gut* 1997; **41**: 526–33.
133 Poo JL, Bosques F, Garduno R *et al.* Octreotide versus emergency sclerotherapy in acute variceal hemorrhage in liver cirrhosis (abstract). *Gastroenterology* 1996; **110**: 1297A.
134 Kravetz D, and Group for the Study of Portal Hypertension.Octreotide vs sclerotherapy in the treatment of acute variceal bleeding (abstract). *Hepatology* 1996; **24**: 206A.
135 El-Jackie A, Rowaisha I, Waked I *et al.* Octreotide vs. sclerotherapy in the control of acute variceal bleeding in schistosomal portal hypertension: a randomized trial (abstract). *Hepatology* 1998; **28**: 533A.
136 Besson I, Ingrand P, Person B *et al.* Sclerotherapy with or without octreotide for acute variceal bleeding. *N Engl J Med* 1995; **333**: 555–60.
137 Avgerinos A, Nevens F, Raptis S et al and the ABOVE Study Group. Early administration of somatostatin and efficacy of sclerotherapy in acute esophageal variceal bleeds: the European

Acute Bleeding esophageal Variceal Episodes (ABOVE) randomized trial. *Lancet* 1997; **350**: 1495–9.

138 Signorelli S, Negrini F, Paris B *et al.* Sclerotherapy with or without somatostatin or octreotide in the treatment of acute variceal haemorrhage: our experience (abstract). *Gastroenterology* 1996; **110**: 1326A.

139 Brunati S, Ceriani R, Curioni R *et al.* Sclerotherapy alone vs sclerotherapy plus terlipressin vs sclerotherapy plus octreotide in the treatment of acute variceal haemorrhage (abstract). *Hepatology* 1996; **24**: 207A.

140 Signorelli S, Paris B, Negrini F *et al.* Esophageal varices bleeding: comparison between treatment with sclerotherapy alone vs sclerotherapy plus octreotide (abstract). *Hepatology* 1997; **26**: 137A.

141 Jensen DM, Kovacs TOG, Randall GM *et al.* Initial results of a randomized prospective study of emergency banding vs sclerotherapy for bleeding gastric or esophageal varices (abstract). *Gastrointest Endosc* 1993; **39**: 128A.

142 Lo GH, Lai KH, Cheng JS *et al.* Emergency banding ligation versus sclerotherapy for the control of active bleeding from esophageal varices. *Hepatology* 1997; **25**: 1101–4.

143 Stiegmann GV, Goff JS, Michaletz-Onody PA *et al.* Endoscopic sclerotherapy as compared with endoscopic ligation for bleeding esophageal varices. *N Engl J Med* 1992; **326**: 1527–32.

144 Laine L, El-Newihi HM, Migikovsky B *et al.* Endoscopic ligation compared with sclerotherapy for the treatment of bleeding esophageal varices. *Ann Intern Med* 1993; **119**: 1–7.

145 Gimson AES, Ramage JK, Panos MZ *et al.* Randomized trial of variceal banding ligation versus injection sclerotherapy forbleeding esophageal varices. *Lancet* 1993; **342**: 391–4.

146 Lo GH, Lai KH, Cheng JS *et al.* A prospective, randomized trial of sclerotherapy versus ligation in the management of bleeding esophageal varices. *Hepatology* 1995; **22**: 466–71.

147 Hou MC, Lin HC, Kuo BIT *et al.* Comparison of endoscopic variceal injection sclerotherapy and ligation for the treatment of esophageal variceal hemorrhage: a prospective randomized trial. *Hepatology* 1995; **21**: 1517–22.

148 Jain AK, Ray RP, Gupta JP. Management of acute variceal bleed: randomized trial of variceal ligation and sclerotherapy (abstract). *Hepatology* 1996; **23**: 138P.

149 Mostafa I, Omar MM, Fakhry S *et al.* Prospective randomized comparative study of injection sclerotherapy and band ligation for bleeding esophageal varices (abstract). *Hepatology* 1996; **23**: 185P.

150 Sarin SK, Govil A, Jain AK *et al.* Prospective randomized trial of endoscopic sclerotherapy versus variceal band ligation for esophageal varices: influence on gastropathy, gastric varices and variceal recurrence. *J Hepatol* 1997; **26**: 826–32.

151 Shiha GE, Farag FM. Endoscopic variceal ligation versus endoscopic sclerotherapy for the management of bleeding varices: A prospective randomized trial (abstract). *Hepatology* 1997; **26**: 136A.

152 Fakhry S, Omar MM, Mustafa I *et al.* Endoscopic sclerotherapy versus endoscopic variceal ligation in the management of bleeding esophageal varices: a final report of a prospective randomized study in schistisomal hepatic fibrosis (abstract). *Hepatology* 1997; **26**: 137A.

153 Cello JP, Crass RA, Trunkey DD. Endoscopic sclerotherapy versus esophageal transection in Child's class C patients with variceal hemorrhage. Comparison with results of portacaval shunt. Preliminary report. *Surgery* 1982; **91**: 333–8.

154 Huizinga WKJ, Angorn PA, Baker WW. Oesophageal transection versus injection sclerotherapy in the management of bleeding esophageal varices in patients at high risk. *Surg Gynecol Obstet* 1985; **160**: 539–46.

155 Teres J, Baroni R, Bordas JM *et al.* Randomized trial of portacaval-shunt, stapling transection and endoscopic sclerotherapy in uncontrolled variceal bleeding. *J Hepatol* 1987; **4**: 159–67.

156 Burroughs AK, Hamilton G, Phillips A *et al.* A comparison of sclerotherapy with staple transection of the esophagus for the emergency control of bleeding from esophageal varices. *N Engl J Med* 1989; **321**: 857–62.

157 Cello JP, Grendell JH, Crass RA *et al.* Endoscopic sclerotherapy versus portacaval-shunt in patients with severe cirrhosis and acute variceal hemorrhage – long term follow-up. *N Engl J Med* 1987; **316**: 11–15.

158 Orloff MJ, Bell RH, Orloff MS *et al.* Prospective randomized trial of emergency portacaval-shunt and emergency medical therapy in unselected cirrhotic-patients with bleeding varices. *Hepatology* 1994; **20**: 863–72.

159 Soehendra N, Grimm H, Nam VC *et al.* N-butyl-2-cyanoacrylate: a supplement to endoscopic sclerotherapy. *Endoscopy* 1987; **19**: 221–4.

160 Feretis C, Dimopoulos C, Benakis P *et al.* N-butyl-cyanoacrylate (Histoacryl) Plus sclerotherapy alone in the treatment of bleeding esophageal varices: a randomized prospective study. *Endoscopy* 1995; **27**: 355–7.

161 Thakeb F, Salama Z, Salama H *et al.* The value of combined use of N-butyl-2-cyanoacrylate and ethanolamine oleate in the management of bleeding esophagogastric varices. *Endoscopy* 1995; **27**: 358–64.
162 Sung JY, Lee YT, Suen R *et al.* Banding is superior to cyanoacrylate for the treatment of esophageal variceal bleeding. A prospective randomized study (abstract). *Gastrointest Endosc* 1998; **47**: 210.
163 Duvall GA, Haber G, Kortan P *et al.* A prospective randomized trial of cyanoacrylate (CYA) vs endoscopic variceal ligation (EVL) for acute esophagogastric variceal hemorrhage (abstract). *Gastrointest Endosc* 1997; **45**: 172.
164 Zimmer T, Rucktaschel F, Stolzel U *et al.* Endoscopic sclerotherapy with fibrin glue as compared with polidocanol to prevent early esophageal variceal rebleeding. *J Hepatol* 1998; **28**: 292–7.
165 Chau TN, Patch D, Chan YW *et al.* "Salvage" transjugular intrahepatic portosystemic shunts: gastric fundal compared with esophageal variceal bleeding. *Gastroenterology* 1998; **114**: 981–7.
166 Sarin SK, Lahoti D, Saxena SP *et al.* Prevalence, classification and natural-history of gastric varices – a long term follow-up study in 568 portal-hypertension patients. *Hepatology* 1992; **16**: 1343–9.
167 Ramond MJ, Valla D, Mosnier JF *et al.* Successful endoscopic obturation of gastric varices with butyl cyanoacrylate. *Hepatology* 1989; **10**: 488–93.
168 Oho K, Iwao T, Sumino M *et al.* Ethanolamine oleate versus butyl cyanoacrylate for bleeding gastric varices – a nonrandomized study. *Endoscopy* 1995; **27**: 349–54.
169 Williams SGJ, Peters RA, Westaby D. Thrombin – an effective treatment for gastric variceal hemorrhage. *Gut* 1994; **35**: 1287–9.
170 Merican I, Burroughs AK. Gastric varices. *Eur J Gastroenterol Hepatol* 1992; **4**: 511–20.
171 De Franchis R. Developing consensus in portal hypertension. *J Hepatol* 1996; **25**: 390–4.
172 Sanyal AJ, Freedman AM, Luketic VA *et al.* Transjugular intrahepatic portosystemic shunts for patients with active variceal hemorrhage unresponsive to sclerotherapy. *Gastroenterology* 1996; **111**: 138–46.
173 Groszmann RJ, Bosch J, Grace ND *et al.* Hemodynamic events in a prospective randomized trial of propranolol versus placebo in the prevention of a 1st variceal hemorrhage. *Gastroenterology* 1990; **99**: 1401–7.
174 Feu F, Garcia-Pagan JC, Bosch J *et al.* Relation between portal pressure response to pharmacotherapy and risk of recurrent variceal haemorrhage in patients with cirrhosis [see comments]. *Lancet* 1995; **346**: 1056–9.
175 McCormick PA, Patch D, Greenslade L *et al.* Clinical vs haemodynamic response to drugs in portal hypertension. *J Hepatol* 1998; **28**: 1015–19.
176 Lebrec D, Poynard T, Bernuau J *et al.* A randomized controlled-study of propranolol for prevention of recurrent gastrointestinal bleeding in patients with cirrhosis – a final report. *Hepatology* 1984; **4**: 355–8.
177 Burroughs AK, Jenkins WJ, Sherlock S *et al.* Controlled trial of propranolol for the prevention of recurrent variceal hemorrhage in patients with cirrhosis. *N Engl J Med* 1983; **309**: 1539–42.
178 Villeneuve JP, PomierLayrargues G, Infanterivard C *et al.* Propranolol for the prevention of recurrent variceal hemorrhage – a controlled trial. *Hepatology* 1986; **6**: 1239–43.
179 Cerbelaud P, Lavignolle A, Perrin D *et al.* Propranolol et prevention des recidives de rupture de varice esophagienne du cirrhotique (abstract). *Gastroenterol Clin Biol* 1986; **18**: A10.
180 Queuniet AM, Czernichow P, Lerebours E *et al.* Controlled trial of propranolol for the prevention of recurrent gastrointestinal-bleeding in patients with cirrhosis. *Gastroenterol Clin Biol* 1987; **11**: 41–7.
181 Sheen IS, Chen TY, Liaw YF. Randomized controlled-study of propranolol for prevention of recurrent esophageal varices bleeding in patients with cirrhosis. *Liver* 1989; **9**: 1–5.
182 Garden OJ, Mills PR, Birnie GG *et al.* Propranolol in the prevention of recurrent variceal hemorrhage in cirrhotic-patients – a controlled trial. *Gastroenterology* 1990; **98**: 185–90.
183 Rossi V, Cales P, Burtin P *et al.* Prevention of recurrent variceal bleeding in alcoholic cirrhotic patients – prospective controlled trial of propranolol and sclerotherapy. *J Hepatol* 1991; **12**: 283–9.
184 Gatta A, Merkel C, Sacerdoti D *et al.* Nadolol for prevention of variceal rebleeding in cirrhosis – a controlled clinical-trial. *Digestion* 1987; **37**: 22–8.
185 Kobe E, Schentke KU. Unsichere rezidivprophylaxe von osophagusvarizen-blutungen durch Propranolol bei Leberzirrhotikern: eine prospektive kontrollierte studie. *Zeitschr Klin Med-Zkm* 1987; **42**: 507–10.
186 Colombo M, Defranchis R, Tommasini M *et al.* Beta-blockade prevents recurrent gastrointestinal bleeding in well compensated patients with alcoholic cirrhosis – a multicenter randomized controlled trial. *Hepatology* 1989; **9**: 433–8.

187 Bernard B, Lebrec D, Mathurin P *et al.* Beta-adrenergic antagonists in the prevention of gastrointestinal rebleeding in patients with cirrhosis: a meta-analysis. *Hepatology* 1997; **25**: 63–70.
188 Garciapagan JC, Feu F, Bosch J *et al.* Propranolol compared with propranolol plus isosorbide-5-mononitrate for portal-hypertension in cirrhosis – a randomized controlled study. *Ann Intern Med* 1991; **114**: 869–73.
189 Vinel JP, Monnin JL, Combis JM *et al.* Hemodynamic evaluation of molsidomine – a vasodilator with antianginal properties in patients with alcoholic cirrhosis. *Hepatology* 1990; **11**: 239–42.
190 Vorobioff J, Garciatsao G, Groszmann R *et al.* Long term hemodynamic effects of ketanserin, a 5-hydroxytryptamine blocker, in portal hypertensive patients. *Hepatology* 1989; **9**: 88–91.
191 Nevens F, Lijnen P, VanBilloen H *et al.* The effect of long term treatment with spironolactone on variceal pressure in patients with portal hypertension without ascites. *Hepatology* 1996; **23**: 1047–52.
192 Terblanche J, Kahn D, Campbell JH *et al.* Failure of repeated injection sclerotherapy to improve long term survival after esophageal variceal bleeding – a 5-year prospective controlled clinical-trial. *Lancet* 1983; **2**: 1328–32.
193 The Copenhagen Esophageal Varices Sclerotherapy Project. Sclerotherapy after first variceal hemorrhage in cirrhosis. A randomized multicenter trial. *N Engl J Med* 1984; **311**: 1594–600.
194 Westaby D, Macdougall BD, Williams R. Improved survival following injection sclerotherapy for esophageal varices – final analysis of a controlled trial. *Hepatology* 1985; **5**: 827–30.
195 Korula J, Balart LA, Radvan G *et al.* A prospective, randomized controlled trial of chronic esophageal variceal sclerotherapy. *Hepatology* 1985; **5**: 584–9.
196 Burroughs AK, McCormick PA, Siringo S *et al.* Prospective randomized trial of long term sclerotherapy for variceal rebleeding, using the same protocol to treat rebleeding in all patients. Final report (abstract). *J Hepatol* 1989; **9**: S12.
197 Alexandrino PT, Alves MM, Correia JP. Propranolol or endoscopic sclerotherapy in the prevention of recurrence of variceal bleeding – a prospective, randomized controlled trial. *J Hepatol* 1988; **7**: 175–85.
198 Dollet JM, Champigneulle B, Patris A *et al.* Endoscopic sclerotherapy versus oral propranolol after variceal hemorrhage in cirrhosis – results of a 4-year prospective randomized trial. *Gastroenterol Clin Biol* 1988; **12**: 234–9.
199 Fleig WE, Stange EF, Schonborn W *et al.* Final analysis of a randomized trial of propranolol (P) vs sclerotherapy (Eps) for the prevention of recurrent variceal hemorrhage in cirrhosis (abstract). *Hepatology* 1988; **8**: 1220.
200 Westaby D, Polson RJ, Gimson AS *et al.* A controlled trial of oral propranolol compared with injection sclerotherapy for the long term management of variceal bleeding. *Hepatology* 1990; **11**: 353–9.
201 Liu JD, Jeng YS, Chen PH *et al.* Endoscopic injection sclerotherapy and propranolol in the prevention of recurrent variceal bleeding (abstract). *1990 Gastroenterology World Congress abstract book* 1990; FP 1181.
202 Martin T, Taupignon A, Lavignolle A *et al.* Prevention of recurrent bleeding in patients with cirrhosis – results of a controlled trial of propranolol versus endoscopic sclerotherapy. *Gastroenterol Clin Biol* 1991; **15**: 833–7.
203 Andreani T, Poupon RE, Balkau BJ *et al.* Efficacite comparée du propranolol et des scleroses endoscopiques du varices esophagiennes dans la prevention des recidives d'hemorragies digestives au cours des cirrhoces. Etude controlée (abstract). *Gastroenterol Clin Biol* 1991; **15** (Suppl 2): A215.
204 Dasarathy S, Dwivedi M, Bhargava DK *et al.* A prospective randomized trial comparing repeated endoscopic sclerotherapy and propranolol in decompensated (Child class B and class C) cirrhotic patients. *Hepatology* 1992; **16**: 89–94.
205 Teres J, Bosch J, Bordas JM *et al.* Endoscopic sclerotherapy (Es) vs propranolol (Pr) in the elective treatment of variceal bleeding – preliminary-results of a randomized controlled clinical-trial (abstract). *J Hepatol* 1987; **5**: S210.
206 Villanueva C, Balanzo J, Novella MT *et al.* Nadolol plus isosorbide mononitrate compared with sclerotherapy for the prevention of variceal rebleeding [see comments]. *N Engl J Med* 1996; **334**: 1624–9.
207 Westaby D, Melia W, Hegarty J *et al.* Use of propranolol to reduce the rebleeding rate during injection sclerotherapy prior to variceal obliteration. *Hepatology* 1986; **6**: 673–5.
208 Jensen LS, Krarup N. Propranolol in prevention of rebleeding from esophageal varices during the course of endoscopic sclerotherapy. *Scand J Gastroenterol* 1989; **24**: 339–45.
209 Lundell L, Leth R, Lind T *et al.* Evaluation of propranolol for prevention of recurrent bleeding from esophageal varices between sclerotherapy sessions. *Acta Chir Scand* 1990; **156**: 711–15.

210 Vinel JP, Lamouliatte H, Cales P *et al.* Propranolol reduces the rebleeding rate during endoscopic sclerotherapy before variceal obliteration. *Gastroenterology* 1992; **102**: 1760–3.
211 Avgerinos A, Rekoumis G, Klonis C *et al.* Propranolol in the prevention of recurrent upper gastrointestinal bleeding in patients with cirrhosis undergoing endoscopic sclerotherapy – a randomized controlled trial. *J Hepatol* 1993; **19**: 301–11.
212 Vickers C, Rhodes J, Chesner I *et al.* Prevention of rebleeding from esophageal varices – 2-year follow-up of a prospective controlled trial of propranolol in addition to sclerotherapy. *J Hepatol* 1994; **21**: 81–7.
213 Acharya SK, Dasarathy S, Saksena S *et al.* A prospective randomized study to evaluate propranolol in patients undergoing long term endoscopic sclerotherapy. *J Hepatol* 1993; **19**: 291–300.
214 Elsayed SS, Shiha G, Hamid M *et al.* Sclerotherapy versus sclerotherapy and propranolol in the prevention of rebleeding from esophageal varices: a randomized study. *Gut* 1996; **38**: 770–4.
215 Bertoni G, Fornaciari G, Beltrami M *et al.* Nadolol for prevention of variceal rebleeding during the course of endoscopic injection sclerotherapy – a randomized pilot study. *J Clin Gastroenterol* 1990; **12**: 364–5.
216 Gerunda GE, Neri D, Zangrandi F *et al.* Nadolol does not reduce early rebleeding in cirrhotics undergoing endoscopic variceal sclerotherapy (Evs) – A multicenter randomized controlled trial (abstract). *Hepatology* 1990; **12**: 988.
217 Villanueva C, Martinez FJ, Torras X *et al.* [Nadolol as an adjuvant to sclerotherapy of esophageal varices for prevention of recurrent hemorrhaging] [Spanish]. *Rev Espan Enferm Dig* 1994; **86**: 499–504.
218 Bertoni G, Sassatelli R, Fornaciari G *et al.* Oral isosorbide-5-mononitrate reduces the re-bleeding rate during the course of injection sclerotherapy for esophageal varices. *Scand J Gastroenterol* 1994; **29**: 363–70.
219 Mundo F, Mitrani C, Rodriguez G *et al.* Endoscopic variceal treatment, is band ligation taking over sclerotherapy? (abstract). *Am J Gastroenterol* 1993; **88**: 1493A.
220 Young HS, Sanowski RA, Rasche R. Comparison and characterization of ulcerations induced by endoscopic ligation of esophageal varices versus endoscopic sclerotherapy. *Gastrointest Endosc* 1993; **39**: 119–22.
221 Jensen DM, Kovacs TOG, Jutabha R *et al.* Randomized, blinded prospective study of banding vs. sclerotherapy for preventing recurrent variceal hemorrhage for patients without active bleeding at endoscopy (abstract). *Gastrointest Endosc* 1995; **41**: 351A.
222 Baroncini D, Milandri GL, Borioni D *et al.* A prospective randomized trial of sclerotherapy versus ligation in the elective treatment of bleeding esophageal varices. *Endoscopy* 1997; **29**: 235–40.
223 Masci E, Norberto L, D'Imperio N *et al.* Prospective multicentric randomized trial comparing banding ligation with sclerotherapy of esophageal varices (abstract). *Gastrointest Endosc* 1997; **45**: 874A.
224 Avgerinos A, Armonis A, Manolakopoulos S *et al.* Endoscopic sclerotherapy versus variceal ligation in the long term management of patients with cirrhosis after variceal bleeding. A prospective randomized study. *J Hepatol* 1997; **26**: 1034–41.
225 delaPena J, Rivero M, Hernandez ES *et al.* Variceal recurrence after ligation and endoscopic sclerotherapy (abstract). *Hepatology* 1998; **28**: 1173.
226 Laine L, Stein C, Sharma V. Randomized comparison of ligation versus ligation plus sclerotherapy in patients with bleeding esophageal varices. *Gastroenterology* 1996; **110**: 529–33.
227 Argonz J, Kravetz D, Suarez A *et al.* Banding plus sclerotherapy is more effective than banding alone in preventing variceal rebleeding (abstract). *Hepatology* 1996; **24**: 327A.
228 Saeed ZA, Stiegmann GV, Ramirez FC *et al.* Endoscopic variceal ligation is superior to combined ligation and sclerotherapy for esophageal varices: a muticenter, prospective, randomized trial. *Hepatology* 1997; **25**: 71–4.
229 Altraif I, Sbeih F, Al-Johani M *et al.* Randomized trial of ligation vs combined ligation and sclerotherapy (ST) for bleeding esophageal varices (abstract). *Hepatology* 1997; **26**: 1372A.
230 El-Khayat HR, Omar MM, Moustafa I. Comparative evaluation of combined endoscopic variceal ligation together with low volume sclerotherapy versus ligation alone for bleeding esophageal varices (abstract). *Hepatology* 1997; **26**: 38.
231 Bhargava DK, Pokharna R. Endoscopic variceal ligation versus endoscopic variceal ligation and endoscopic sclerotherapy: a prospective randomized study [see comments]. *Am J Gastroenterol* 1997; **92**: 950–3.
232 Lo GH, Lai KH, Cheng JS *et al.* The additive effect of sclerotherapy to patients receiving repeated endoscopic variceal ligation: a prospective, randomized trial. *Hepatology* 1998; **28**: 391–5.
233 Jensen DM, Jutabha R, Kovacs TOG *et al.* Final results of a randomized prospective study of combination banding and sclerotherapy versus

sclerotherapy alone for hemostasis of bleeding esophageal varices (abstract). *Gastrointest Endosc* 1998; **47**: 184A.

234 El-Khayat HR, Khamis AA. Comparative evaluation of combined endoscopic variceal ligation (EVL) together with low volume endoscopic sclerotherapy (ES) versus sclerotherapy or band ligation alone for bleeding esophageal varices (abstract). *Gastroenterology* 1995; **108**: A1061.

235 Koutsomanis D. Endoscopic variceal ligation combined with sclerotherapy versus sclerotherapy alone: 5-years follow-up (abstract). *Gastroenterology* 1997; **112**: 1308A.

236 Groupe d'Etude des Anastomoses Intrahepatiques. Tips vs sclerotherapy plus propranolol in the prevention of variceal rebleeding – preliminary-results of a multicenter randomized trial (abstract). *Hepatology* 1995; **22**: 761.

237 GarciaVillarreal L, MartinezLagares F, Sierra A *et al.* Tips vs sclerotherapy (SCL) for the prevention of variceal rebleeding. Preliminary results of a randomized study (abstract). *Hepatology* 1996; **24**: 326.

238 Cabrera J, Maynar M, Granados R *et al.* Transjugular intrahepatic portosystemic shunt versus sclerotherapy in the elective treatment of variceal hemorrhage. *Gastroenterology* 1996; **110**: 832–9.

239 Sanyal AJ, Freedman AM, Luketic VA *et al.* Transjugular intrahepatic portosystemic shunts compared with endoscopic sclerotherapy for the prevention of recurrent variceal hemorrhage. A randomized, controlled trial [see comments]. *Ann Intern Med* 1997; **126**: 849–57.

240 Cello JP, Ring EJ, Olcott EW *et al.* Endoscopic sclerotherapy compared with percutaneous transjugular intrahepatic portosystemic shunt after initial sclerotherapy in patients with acute variceal hemorrhage. A randomized, controlled trial [see comments]. *Ann Intern Med* 1997; **126**: 858–65.

241 Rossle M, Deibert P, Haag K *et al.* Randomized trial of transjugular-intrahepatic portosystemic shunt versus endoscopy plus propranolol for prevention of variceal rebleeding. *Lancet* 1997; **349**: 1043–9.

242 Sauer P, Theilmann L, Stremmel W *et al.* Transjugular intrahepatic portosystemic stent shunt versus sclerotherapy plus propranolol for variceal rebleeding. *Gastroenterology* 1997; **113**: 1623–31.

243 Merli M, Salerno F, Riggio O *et al.* Transjugular intrahepatic portosystemic shunt versus endoscopic sclerotherapy for the prevention of variceal bleeding in cirrhosis. a randomized multicenter trial. Gruppo Italiano Studio TIPS (G.I.S.T.). *Hepatology* 1998; **27**: 48–53.

244 Jalan R, Forrest EH, Stanley AJ *et al.* A randomized trial comparing transjugular intrahepatic portosystemic stent-shunt with variceal band ligation in the prevention of rebleeding from esophageal varices. *Hepatology* 1997; **26**: 1115–22.

245 PomierLayrargues G, Dufresne MP, Bui B *et al.* TIPS versus endoscopic variceal ligation in the prevention of variceal rebleeding in cirrhotic patients: a comparative randomized clinical trial (interim analysis) (abstract). *Hepatology* 1997; **26**: 35.

246 Casado M, Bosch J, Garcia-Pagan JC *et al.* Clinical events after transjugular intrahepatic portosystemic shunt. Correlation with hemodynamic findings. *Gastroenterology* 1998; **114**: 1296–303.

247 Escorsell A, Banares R, Gilabert R *et al.* Transjugular intrahepatic portosystemic shunt (TIPS) vs propranolol + isosorbide-mononitrate (P+I) for the prevention of variceal rebleeding in patients with cirrhosis: results of a randomized controlled trial (abstract). *Hepatology* 1998; **28**: 770A.

248 Reichle FA, Fahmy WF, Golsorkhi M. Prospective comparative clinical trial with distal splenorenal and mesocaval shunts. *Am J Surg* 1979; **137**: 13–21.

249 Fischer JE, Bower RH, Atamian S *et al.* Comparison of distal and proximal splenorenal shunts – a randomized prospective trial. *Ann Surg* 1981; **194**: 531–44.

250 Langer B, Taylor BR, Mackenzie DR *et al.* Further report of a prospective randomized trial comparing distal splenorenal shunt with end-to-side portacaval-shunt – an analysis of encephalopathy, survival, and quality of life. *Gastroenterology* 1985; **88**: 424–9.

251 Millikan WJ, Warren WD, Henderson JM *et al.* The Emory prospective randomized trial – selective versus nonselective shunt to control variceal bleeding – 10-year follow-up. *Ann Surg* 1985; **201**: 712–22.

252 Harley HJ, Morgan T, Redeker AG *et al.* Results of a randomized trial of end-to-side portacaval shunt and distal splenorenal shunt in alcoholic liver disease and variceal bleeding. *Gastroenterology* 1986; **91**: 802–9.

253 Grace ND, Conn HO, Resnick RH *et al.* Distal splenorenal vs portal systemic shunts after hemorrhage from varices – a randomized controlled trial. *Hepatology* 1988; **8**: 1475–81.

254 Sarfeh IJ, Rypins EB. Partial versus total portacaval-shunt in alcoholic cirrhosis – results of a prospective, randomized clinical-trial. *Ann Surg* 1994; **219**: 353–61.

255 Rosemurgy AS, Goode SE, Zwiebel B *et al.* A prospective trial of TIPS vs small diameter prosthetic H-graft portacaval shunt in the

treatment of bleeding varices. *Ann Surg* 1996; **224**: 378–84.

256 Rikkers LF, Burnett DA, Volentine GD *et al.* Shunt surgery versus endoscopic sclerotherapy for long term treatment of variceal bleeding – early results of a randomized trial. *Ann Surg* 1987; **206**: 261–71.

257 Teres J, Bordas JM, Bravo D *et al.* Sclerotherapy vs distal splenorenal shunt in the elective treatment of variceal hemorrhage – a randomized controlled trial. *Hepatology* 1987; **7**: 430–6.

258 Henderson JM, Kutner MH, Millikan WJ *et al.* Endoscopic variceal sclerosis compared with distal splenorenal shunt to prevent recurrent variceal bleeding in cirrhosis – a prospective, randomized trial. *Ann Intern Med* 1990; **112**: 262–9.

259 Spina GP, Santambrogio R, Opocher E *et al.* Distal splenorenal shunt versus endoscopic sclerotherapy in the prevention of variceal rebleeding. First stage of a randomized, controlled trial. *Ann Surg* 1990; **211**: 178–86.

260 Spina GP, Henderson JM, Rikkers LF *et al.* Distal splenorenal shunt versus endoscopic sclerotherapy in the prevention of variceal rebleeding – a metaanalysis of 4 randomized clinical trials. *J Hepatol* 1992; **16**: 338–45.

261 Korula J, Yellin A, Yamada S *et al.* A prospective randomized controlled comparison of chronic endoscopic variceal sclerotherapy and portasystemic shunt for variceal hemorrhage in Child's class-A cirrhotics (abstract). *Hepatology* 1988; **8**: 1242.

262 Planas R, Boix J, Broggi M *et al.* Portacaval-shunt versus endoscopic sclerotherapy in the elective treatment of variceal hemorrhage. *Gastroenterology* 1991; **100**: 1078–86.

Ascites, hepatorenal syndrome, and spontaneous bacterial peritonitis: prevention and treatment

25

PERE GINÈS, VICENTE ARROYO, JUAN RODÉS

Patients with cirrhosis frequently develop a disturbance in body fluid regulation, which results in increased extracellular fluid volume that is accumulated in the peritoneal cavity as ascites and the interstitial tissue as edema.[1,2] Although the pathogenesis of ascites is incompletely understood, most available evidence indicates that fluid retention is the consequence of the homeostatic activation of vasoconstrictor and sodium-retaining systems triggered by a marked arterial vasodilatation located mainly in the splanchnic vascular bed. The existence of marked abnormalities in the splanchnic microcirculation due to portal hypertension facilitates the accumulation of the retained fluid in the peritoneal cavity. Ascites is frequently complicated by abnormalities of renal function such as an impaired ability to eliminate water and a vasoconstriction of the renal circulation, which may lead to development of dilutional hyponatremia and hepatorenal syndrome, respectively.[1,3] Finally, the coexistence of ascites and abnormalities in the host defense mechanisms against infection, which occur frequently in patients with advanced cirrhosis, account for the spontaneous infection of ascitic fluid, a condition known as spontaneous bacterial peritonitis.[4,5]

The aim of the current chapter is to review, on the basis of available evidence, the efficacy of therapeutic methods used in the management of ascites, hepatorenal syndrome and spontaneous bacterial peritonitis in cirrhosis. The pathogenesis of these complications is briefly discussed to provide the reader with an understanding of the pathophysiological basis of the different therapeutic approaches. A comprehensive review of the pathophysiology of these disorders may be found elsewhere.[1,6]

THERAPY OF ASCITES

As previously mentioned, a large body of evidence indicates that in cirrhosis sodium retention, with subsequent ascites and edema formation, results from the action of neurohumoral factors on the kidney, which are activated as a homeostatic response to a disturbed systemic circulation (Figure 25.1).[1,2,6,7] The initial abnormality would be sinusoidal portal hypertension causing marked arterial vasodilatation located mainly in the splanchnic circulation. The mechanism of this vasodilatation is not known, but may involve the increased synthesis/release of vasodilating substances, including nitric oxide and/or vasodilator peptides.[2,6,8] Arterial vasodilatation would then result in an abnormal distribution of blood volume with reduced effective arterial blood volume, ie the blood

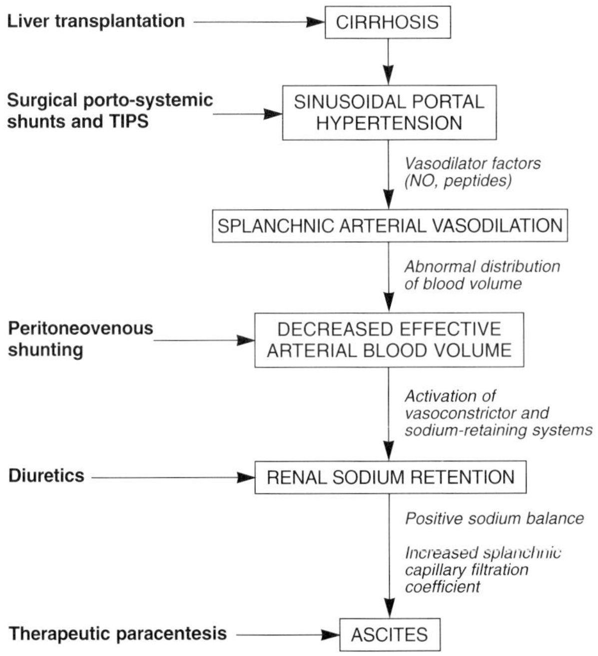

Figure 25.1 Proposed pathogenesis of ascites formation in cirrhosis according to the arterial vasodilatation hypothesis and available therapeutic interventions (in bold)

volume in the heart, lungs and central arterial tree that is sensed by arterial receptors, and subsequent renal sodium retention due to the activation of vasoconstrictor and sodium-retaining factors.

Sodium restriction

In all diseases associated with generalized edema (cirrhosis, heart failure, renal failure), the amount of exogenous fluid retained depends on the balance between sodium intake and the renal excretion of sodium. Because sodium is retained iso-osmotically in the kidney, 1 liter of extracellular fluid is gained for every 130–140 mmol of sodium retained. If sodium excretion remains constant, the gain of extracellular fluid volume (and the consequent increase in weight) depends exclusively on sodium intake and increases proportionally to the amount of sodium taken with the diet. Nevertheless, because sodium excretion may be increased pharmacologically by the administration of diuretics, the sodium balance depends not only on sodium intake but also on the natriuretic response achieved by diuretics.

On this background, it seems reasonable that a reduction in sodium intake (low salt diet) will favor a negative sodium balance and facilitate the disappearance of ascites and edema. This contention, was demonstrated in earlier studies[9,10] and is supported by the common clinical observation that the management of ascites is more difficult in patients who are not compliant with a low sodium diet. Non-compliant patients usually require higher doses of diuretics to achieve resolution of ascites and are readmitted more frequently to hospital for recurrence of ascites. Surprisingly, however, several randomized comparative studies have not demonstrated an advantage of low sodium diet as compared with an unrestricted sodium diet in the management of ascites.[11–13] Nevertheless, it should be pointed out that in these studies most patients had mild sodium retention (urine sodium in the absence of diuretic therapy was close to sodium intake) and showed an excellent response to diuretic therapy (only less than 5% of patients did not respond to diuretics).

Therefore, on the basis of available data, it can be concluded that in patients with mild sodium retention a restriction of dietary sodium is probably not necessary because the hypothetical benefit of low salt diet in the achievement of a negative sodium balance is overridden by the marked natriuretic effect of diuretics. By contrast, in patients with marked sodium retention, who usually have a less intense natriuretic response to diuretics compared with patients with moderate sodium retention, dietary sodium restriction (40–60 mmol of sodium per day) may facilitate the elimination of ascites and delay the reaccumulation of fluid after ascites has been removed. A more severe restriction of sodium (<40 mmol/day) is not recommended because it is poorly accepted by patients and may impair their nutritional status.

R Grade C

Therapeutic paracentesis

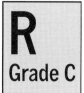

During the current decade, therapeutic paracentesis has progressively replaced diuretics as the treatment of choice in the management of patients with cirrhosis and large ascites in many centers.[14,15] This change in treatment strategy is based on the results of several randomized controlled trials comparing paracentesis (either removal of all ascitic fluid in a single tap or repeated taps of 4–6 liters/day) associated with plasma volume expansion vs diuretics.[16–20] Because paracentesis does not modify renal sodium retention, patients should receive diuretics after paracentesis to avoid reaccumulation of ascites.[21]

Two aspects concerning the use of therapeutic paracentesis in patients with cirrhosis and ascites deserve specific discussion: (1) the population of patients with cirrhosis in whom therapeutic paracentesis should be used; and (2) the use of plasma expanders to prevent disturbances in circulatory function after paracentesis. While most physicians consider that therapeutic paracentesis is the treatment of choice for all patients with large ascites,[14,15] others believe that therapeutic paracentesis should be used only in those patients with large ascites who show a poor or no response to diuretics.[22] Results obtained in randomized trials indicate that therapeutic paracentesis is faster and in several trials was associated with lower incidence of adverse effects compared with diuretics (Table 25.1).[16–20] Moreover, therapeutic paracentesis may have a better cost-effectiveness profile compared with diuretic treatment, which may result in prolonged hospital admissions. Therefore, on the basis of available data, it seems clear that the use of therapeutic paracentesis should not be restricted to patients failing to respond to diuretics and should be considered the treatment of choice for all patients with large ascites (Table 25.2).

R Grade A

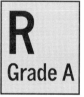

The removal of large volumes of ascitic fluid is associated with circulatory dysfunction characterized by a reduction of effective blood volume.[23–29] Several lines of evidence indicate that this circulatory dysfunction and/or the mechanisms activated to maintain circulatory homeostasis have detrimental effects in cirrhotic patients. First, circulatory dysfunction is associated with rapid reaccumulation of ascites.[29] Second, approximately 20% of these patients develop irreversible renal failure and/or water retention leading to dilutional hyponatremia.[23] Third, portal pressure increases in patients developing circulatory dysfunction after paracentesis, probably owing to an increased intrahepatic resistance due to the action of vasoconstrictor systems on the hepatic vascular bed.[27] Finally, the development of circulatory dysfunction is associated with a shortened survival.[29]

Table 25.1 Adverse effects in randomized studies comparing the efficacy and safety of diuretics vs therapeutic paracentesis and plasma volume expansion in patients with cirrhosis and large ascites[a]

Study	Diuretics	Paracentesis and plasma volume expansion	*P* values	Type of plasma expander
Renal impairment				
Ginès *et al*[16]	16/59[b] (27%)	3/58 (5%)	0.003	Albumin
Salerno *et al*[17]	1/21(5%)	1/20 (5%)	NS	Albumin
Hagège *et al*[18]	1/27 (4%)	1/26 (4%)	NS	Albumin
Acharya *et al*[19]	1/20 (5%)	0/20 (0%)	NS	Dextran-40
Solà *et al*[20]	5/40 (12%)	1/40 (2%)	NS	Dextran-40
Hyponatremia				
Ginès *et al*[16]	18/59 (30%)	3/58(5%)	0.0009	Albumin
Salerno *et al*[17]	–	–	—	Albumin
Hagège *et al*[18]	8/27 (30%)	2/26 (8%)	0.07	Albumin
Acharya *et al*[19]	1/20 (5%)	3/20 (5%)	NS	Dextran-40
Solà *et al*[20]	8/40 (20%)	5/40 (12%)	NS	Dextran-40
Encephalopathy				
Ginès *et al*[16]	17/59 (29%)	6/58 (10%)	0.02	Albumin
Salerno *et al*[17]	3/21 (14%)	2/20 (10%)	NS	Albumin
Hagège *et al*[18]	4/27 (15%)	1/26 (4%)	NS	Albumin
Acharya *et al*[19]	1/20 (5%)	0/20 (0%)	NS	Dextran-40
Solà *et al*[20]	12/40 (22%)	1/40 (2%)	0.0015	Dextran-40

[a]Differences in the rate of adverse effects among the studies may be due, at least in part, to differences in the populations of patients included.
[b]Figures represent the number of patients developing the adverse effects compared with the total number of patients in each treatment group.

Table 25.2 Recommendations for the management of patients with cirrhosis and large ascites

1 Total paracentesis plus intravenous albumin[a] (8 g/l of ascites removed). Patients can be treated as outpatients. Hospitalization is recommended in patients with associated complications (ie encephalopathy, bacterial infection, gastrointestinal bleeding)
2 After removal of ascitic fluid, start with moderate sodium restriction (40–60 mmol/day) and diuretics, either aldosterone antagonists alone (ie spironolactone 50–400 mg/day) or in combination with loop diuretics (ie frusemide 20–160 mg/day). If patients were on diuretics before the development of large ascites, check compliance with sodium diet and diuretic therapy. Compliant patients should be given doses of diuretics higher than those received before paracentesis
3 Consider liver transplantation

[a]Although a survival benefit of albumin over other plasma expanders has not been demonstrated, albumin is more effective than other plasma expanders in the prevention of paracentesis-induced circulatory dysfunction when more than 5 liters of ascitic fluid are removed.

Table 25.3 Complications in randomized studies assessing the efficacy and safety of therapeutic paracentesis without plasma volume expansion or with different plasma volume expanders in patients with cirrhosis and large ascites

Study	No plasma expander	Polygeline	Dextran-70	Albumin	*P* values
Renal impairment					
Ginès *et al*[23]	6/53[a](11%)	–	–	0/52(0%)	0.03
Ginès *et al*[29]	–	10/100 (10%)	8/93 (9%)	7/97 (7%)	NS
Planas *et al*[30]	–	–	1/42 (2%)	1/43 (2%)	NS
Salerno *et al*[31]	–	1/27 (4%)	–	1/27 (4%)	NS
Fassio *et al*[32]	–	–	1/20 (5%)	1/21 (5%)	NS
Hyponatremia					
Ginès *et al*[23]	9/53 (17%)	–	–	1/52 (2%)	0.02
Ginès *et al*[29]	–	19/100 (19%)	23/93 (25%)	14/97 (14%)	NS
Planas *et al*[30]	–	–	4/45 (9%)	3/43 (7%)	NS
Salerno *et al*[31]	–	5/27 (18%)	–	4/27 (15%)	NS
Fassio *et al*[32]	–	–	3/20 (15%)	4/21 (19%)	NS

[a]Figures represent the number of patients developing the complication compared with the total number of patients in each treatment group.

At present, the only effective method to prevent circulatory dysfunction is the administration of plasma expanders. A randomized trial has shown that albumin is more effective than other plasma expanders (dextran-70, polygeline), at preventing circulatory dysfunction as estimated by plasma renin activity, probably owing to its longer persistence in the intravascular compartment.[29] When less than 5 liters of ascites are removed, dextran-70 or polygeline show efficacy similar to that of albumin. However, albumin is more effective than these two artificial plasma expanders when more than 5 liters of ascites are removed.[29] Despite this greater efficacy, randomized trials have not shown differences in survival of patients treated with albumin compared with those treated with other plasma expanders.[29–32] Larger trials would be required to demonstrate a benefit of albumin on survival as well as on circulatory function, should one exist. Table 25.3 shows the incidence of adverse effects observed in randomized trials comparing therapeutic paracentesis without plasma volume expansion or with three different plasma expanders in patients with cirrhosis and large ascites.

Conclusive results from a randomized trial with adequate power to demonstrate a benefit on mortality are not available. However, the currently available data indicate that circulatory dysfunction after therapeutic paracentesis is potentially harmful to patients with cirrhosis. Albumin appears to be the plasma expander of choice when more than 5 liters of ascites are removed.

R
Grade A

Diuretics

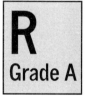

Diuretics eliminate the excess of extracellular fluid present as ascites and edema by increasing renal sodium excretion, thus achieving a negative sodium balance.[33] The diuretics most frequently used in patients with cirrhosis and ascites are aldosterone antagonists, mainly spironolactone and potassium canrenoate, drugs that antagonize selectively the sodium-retaining effects of aldosterone in the renal collecting tubules, and loop diuretics, especially ferosomide, that inhibit the Na^+-K^+-$2Cl^-$ cotransporter in the loop of Henle.[33,34]

R
Grade A

Despite the use of diuretics in clinical practice for more than 30 years, few randomized trials have been reported comparing the efficacy of different diuretic agents in the treatment of ascites.[34–36] In patients without renal failure, aldosterone antagonist spironolactone in a dose of 150 mg/day (increased to 300 mg/day if there was no response) was shown in one small randomized trial to be more effective than the loop diuretic ferosomide (furosemide) in a dose of 80 mg/day (increased to 160 mg/day if there was no response.[35] This increased efficacy of aldosterone antagonists has also been suggested by several physiological studies and case series.[13,37–40] Based on these findings, aldosterone antagonists are considered the diuretics of choice in the management of cirrhotic ascites.

In clinical practice, aldosterone antagonists are frequently given in combination with loop diuretics. Theoretical advantages of this combination include greater natriuretic potency, earlier onset of diuresis, and less tendency to induce hyperkalemia. Two different schedules of combined administration have been proposed. In the first, the dose of aldosterone antagonists is increased progressively (usually up to to 400 mg/day of spironolactone) and loop diuretics (ferosomide up to 160 mg/day) are added only if no response is achieved with the highest dose of aldosterone antagonists. In the second, both drugs are given in combination from the start of therapy. Whether one of these two combined schedules has advantages over the other has not been assessed.

Diuretic therapy is effective in the elimination of ascites in 80–90% of all patients with ascites, a percentage that may increase up to 95% when only patients without renal failure are considered.[13,16–20,35–40] The remaining patients either do not respond to diuretic therapy or develop diuretic-induced complications that prevent the use of high doses of these drugs. This condition is known as refractory ascites.[41] Complications of diuretic therapy in patients with cirrhosis include hepatic encephalopathy, hyponatremia, renal impairment, potassium disturbances, gynecomastia, and muscle cramps.[34,42] The incidence of renal and electrolyte disorders and encephalopathty varies depending on the population of patients studied, being higher in patients with marked sodium retention and renal failure (who require higher doses of diuretics) and lower in patients with moderate sodium retention and without renal failure. Although some of these complications may be unrelated to diuretic therapy and due to the existence of advanced liver disease,[43] there is no doubt that diuretics are a major cause of these complications because their frequency is markedly lower if ascites is removed by therapeutic paracentesis (see Table 25.1).

Because therapeutic paracentesis has replaced diuretics as the treatment of choice for hospitalized cirrhotic patients with large ascites in most centers,[14,15] at present the main indications for use of diuretics in cirrhosis are as follows:

1 treatment of patients with mild or moderate ascites or those with large ascites in whom paracentesis is not effective because of compartmentalization of ascitic fluid due to peritoneal adhesions;
2 treatment of patients with edema without ascites;
3 prevention of ascites recurrence after therapeutic paracentesis.

Peritoneovenous shunt

Peritoneovenous shunting causes the passage of ascitic fluid from the peritoneal cavity to the systemic circulation, which results in the improvement of effective arterial blood volume with subsequent reduction in the activity of vasoconstrictor and antinatriuretic systems.[44] These favorable hemodynamic effects result in an increase in sodium excretion and, to a lesser extent, renal blood flow and glomerular filtration rate which facilitate the management of ascites in most patients.[45] Randomized trials of peritoneovenous shunting and therapeutic paracentesis plus iv albumin in patients with refractory ascites have not shown differences in survival or in number of hospital admissions. However, the probability of readmission to hospital for ascites as well as the number of readmissions for ascites recurrence are markedly lower in patients treated by peritoneovenous shunting compared with those treated by therapeutic paracentesis.[46,47] Unfortunately, the use of the shunt is associated with a number of important adverse effects, including coagulopathy, bacterial infections, peritoneal fibrosis or shunt obstruction, which limit its clinical applicability.[48,49] Obstruction is the most common complication and may be located either within the valve or due to thrombosis of the superior vena cava. Obstruction is associated with recurrence of ascites and requires surgical intervention with replacement of the clotted shunt.[50] Although peritoneovenous shunting is an effective therapy for refractory ascites, the high incidence of adverse effects and the existence of an alternative therapy (eg therapeutic paracentesis) has resulted in a marked decline in its use in most centers.

Portosystemic shunts

The reduction in portal pressure by surgical portosystemic shunts, especially side-to-side portacaval shunts, is associated with increased sodium excretion, suppression of antinatriuretic systems and elimination of ascites in patients with cirrhosis and refractory ascites.[51,52] Furthermore, cirrhotic patients with variceal bleeding treated with surgical portosystemic shunts show a markedly lower probability of ascites occurrence during the course of their disease compared with patients treated with procedures that do not reduce portal pressure, such as sclerotherapy or esophageal transection.[53] Nevertheless, despite these benefits, surgical portosystemic shunts have not become a standard intervention for management of refractory ascites because of a high operative mortality and an exceedingly high risk of chronic encephalopathy.

The usefulness of portosystemic shunting in the management of ascites is currently being reevaluated due to the introduction of TIPS (transjugular intrahepatic portosystemic shunts), a non-surgical method of portal decom-pression that acts as a side-to-side portacaval shunt and has the advantage over surgical shunts of an extremely low operative mortality.[54] The most frequent complications of TIPS are hepatic encephalopathy and obstruction of the stent. The available information regarding the use of TIPS in patients with ascites is derived from several uncontrolled studies and only one randomized controlled trial which included only a small number of patients.[55–60] In the randomized trial, patients with decompensated liver disease graded as Pughs grade C, had a significantly worse survival.[60] As with surgical portosystemic shunts, TIPS can be associated with favorable effects on renal function, including an increase in sodium excretion and reduction in the activity of antinatriuretic systems, which results in the elimination of ascites in some patients and decrease ßof diuretic requirements in others. Controlled trials of adequate power are needed before the role of TIPS in the management of refractory ascites in cirrhosis can be clearly defined.[61]

Liver transplantation

Liver transplantation has become a frequent intervention for patients with advanced cirrhosis. Although randomized trials comparing liver transplantation with conventional medical therapy in patients with ascites are not available for obvious reasons, the 70–80% 5-year probability of survival obtained in adult cirrhotic patients treated with liver transplantation in most centers is markedly greater than the expected 20% in non-transplanted patients with cirrhosis and ascites.[62]

Earlier recommendations suggested that ascites *per se* was not an indication for liver transplantation, and patients had to be considered for transplantation only when ascites was refractory to diuretic therapy or was associated with severe complications, such as spontaneous bacterial peritonitis (SBP) or hepatorenal syndrome. However, with these guidelines a large proportion of these patients die while registered on the transplantation waiting list. This is because of the short survival associated with these conditions. The median survival time is less than 1year for patients with refractory ascites and those recovering from SBP and is even shorter in patients with HRS, particularly in those with the progressive form of this syndrome – type I – who have a median survival time of less than 1 month.[46,47,63,64]

With the growing knowledge of the natural history of ascites in cirrhosis, it is now known that a number of factors predictive of survival can be used to identify candidates for liver transplantation.[65,66] The most useful predictive factors are related to abnormalities in renal function and systemic hemodynamics and include:

- an impaired ability to excrete a water load (urine volume <8 ml/min after a water load of 5% dextrose 20 ml/kg iv);
- dilutional hyponatremia (serum sodium <130 mmol/l in the absence of diuretic therapy);
- arterial hypotension (mean arterial pressure <80 mmHg in the absence of diuretic therapy);
- reduced glomerular filtration rate (even moderate reductions, as indicated by serum creatinine >1.2 mg/dl in the absence of diuretic therapy);
- marked sodium retention (urine sodium <10 mmol/day under a moderate sodium-restricted diet and in the absence of diuretic therapy).

R
Grade B

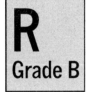

Interestingly, in patients with ascites these parameters are better than liver function tests as predictors of prognosis.[65] Therefore, patients with one or more of these predictive factors have a poor survival expectancy and should be considered for liver transplantation.

THERAPY OF HEPATORENAL SYNDROME

Hepatorenal syndrome (HRS) is the worst end of the clinical spectrum of abnormalities of renal function in patients with cirrhosis and ascites.[3,6,41,67] HRS may occur in two different clinical patterns.[41]

1 Type 1 HRS is characterized by rapid and progressive impairment of renal function as defined by a 100% increase of the initial serum creatinine to a level greater than 2.5 mg/dl or a 50% reduction of the initial 24-hour creatinine clearance to a level

Table 25.4 Diagnostic criteria of hepatorenal syndrome

Major criteria
1 Low glomerular filtration rate, as indicated by serum creatinine greater than 1.5 mg/dl or 24-hour creatinine clearance lower than 40 ml/min
2 Absence of shock, ongoing bacterial infection, fluid losses and current treatment with nephrotoxic drugs
3 No sustained improvement in renal function (decrease in serum creatinine to 1.5 mg/dl or less or increase in creatinine clearance to 40 ml/min or more) following diuretic withdrawal and expansion of plasma volume with 1.5 l of a plasma expander
4 Proteinuria lower than 500 mg/day and no ultrasonographic evidence of obstructive uropathy or parenchymal renal disease

Additional criteria
1 Urine volume lower than 500 ml/day
2 Urine sodium lower than 10 mmol/l
3 Urine osmolality greater than plasma osmolality
4 Urine red blood cells less than 50 per high power field
5 Serum sodium concentration lower than 130 mmol/l

[a]All major criteria must be present for the diagnosis of hepatorenal syndrome. Additional criteria are not necessary for the diagnosis, but provide supportive evidence.
Reproduced from Arroyo V *et al.* Definition and diagnostic criteria of refractory ascites and hepatorenal syndrome in cirrhosis. *Hepatology* 1996;**23**:164.

lower than 20 ml/min in less than 2 weeks; in some patients, this type of HRS develops spontaneously without any identifiable precipitating factor, while in others it occurs in close chronological relationship with some complications, particularly after the resolution of spontaneous bacterial peritonitis.[68]

2 Type 2 HRS is characterized by a less severe and non-progressive reduction of glomerular filtration rate (at least in the short term); the main clinical consequence of this type of HRS is refractory ascites.

Because of the lack of specific diagnostic tests, the diagnosis of HRS is currently made according to several criteria, as proposed by the International Ascites Club, which are based on demonstration of a marked reduction in glomerular filtration rate (serum creatinine >1.5 mg/dl in the absence of diuretic therapy) and the exclusion of other causes of renal failure that may occur in patients with cirrhosis[41] (Table 25.4).

Although a variety of therapeutic modalities have been used in patients with HRS, the only effective methods, besides liver transplantation, are those that improve effective arterial blood volume or decrease portal pressure.[69] A recent uncontrolled study in a small series of patients showed that the administration of ornipressin, a vasopressin analogue with a potent vasoconstrictor action on the splanchnic circulation but with a weak antidiuretic action, combined with plasma expansion with albumin for a prolonged period of time (up to 2 weeks), reverses HRS.[70] However, this treatment is associated with a significant incidence of ischemic complications that may limit its applicability in clinical practice. Another vasopressin analogue, terlipressin, which probably has a better safety profile than ornipressin, also appears to be effective, but more information on its potential benefit is required.[71,72] On the other hand, several studies, albeit also with small numbers of patients, have demonstrated that TIPS improves renal function in patients with HRS.[59,73] However, as previously mentioned, TIPS has the risk of hepatic encephalopathy and may also impair liver function. Therefore, the role that these two new approaches may have in clinical practice should be evaluated in prospective controlled investigations. The treatment of choice for HRS in selected candidates is liver transplantation.[74] Grade B However, as discussed previously, liver transplantation should be performed, whenever possible, before the development of HRS. Factors predictive of poor survival in patients with cirrhosis and ascites are also predictive for the development of HRS.[64,66]

THERAPY AND PROPHYLAXIS OF SPONTANEOUS BACTERIAL PERITONITIS

Spontaneous bacterial peritonitis (SBP) is a common and severe complication of cirrhotic patients with ascites characterized by infection of ascitic fluid with no apparent intra-abdominal source of infection.[4,5] Most episodes of SBP are caused by Gram-negative bacteria from the intestinal flora, especially *Escherichia coli*. The diagnosis of SBP is based on the demonstration of an absolute number of polymorphonuclear cells in ascitic fluid greater than 250/mm^3. The clinical spectrum of SBP is very variable and ranges from complete absence of symptoms to a classical clinical picture of peritonitis. For this reason and because of the high prevalence of SBP among patients with ascites, ascitic fluid polymorphonuclear count should be checked routinely in all patients with cirrhosis admitted to hospital with ascites and in those hospitalized patients who develop signs and/or symptoms suggestive of peritoneal or systemic infection (ie abdominal pain, rebound tenderness, ileus, fever, leukocytosis, shock), hepatic encephalopathy or impairment in renal function. Cirrhotic patients with hydrothorax may also develop a spontaneous infection of pleural fluid that is pathogenically akin to SBP and should be managed similarly.[75]

Therapy

Antibiotic therapy should be started whenever the polymorphonuclear count in ascitic fluid is greater than 250/mm^3 and before obtaining microbiological culture results.[4,5] Grade B Third generation cephalosporins are the antibiotics of choice as initial empirical treatment for patients with SBP, because of their broad antibacterial spectrum, high efficacy, and safety.[76–79] Grade A Cefotaxime (2 g/8–12 h) has been the drug most commonly used in randomized trials, but other third generation cephalosporins can be used .[80] Cefotaxime has been shown to be more effective than other antibiotics, such as aztre-onam or the combination of aminoglycosides plus ampicillin.[76,81] Amoxicillin-clavulanic acid is also effective,[82] but randomized trials comparing this agent with third generation cephalosporins have not been reported. Ofloxacin (400 mg/12 h, orally), a quinolone rapidly absorbed with high diffusion into the ascitic fluid and very active against Gram-negative and Gram-positive bacteria, is as effective as cefotaxime in terms of resolution of infection and survival.[83] Grade A Because of simplicity and lower cost, oral ofloxacin appears to be an excellent alternative to third generation cephalosporins in the treatment of SBP. Nevertheless, in patients who are severely ill (ie septic shock, severe renal failure) or with complications that may impair the absorption of the drug (gastrointestinal hemorrhage or ileus), iv third generation cephalosporins should be the treatment of choice. Antibiotic therapy is maintained until the complete disappearance of all signs of infection and decrease of polymorphonuclear count in ascitic fluid below the threshold value of 250/mm^3. In most patients, resolution of SBP is achieved in a short period of time, usually less than 6 days. Recommendations for the management of SBP are summarized in Table 25.5.

Table 25.5 Recommendations for the management of spontaneous bacterial peritonitis

1	After diagnosis of peritonitis has been made (>250 polymorphonuclear cells/mm^3 in ascitic fluid), start with third generation cephalosporins (ie cefotaxime 2 g/8–12 h iv). In non-severely ill patients,[a] oral ofloxacin 400 mg/12 h may be used. In patients on antibiotic prophylaxis, third generation cephalosporins are the treatment of choice
2	Give albumin 1.5 g/kg iv at the diagnosis of the infection and 1 g/kg 48 h later
3	Maintain antibiotic therapy until disappearance of signs of infection and reduction of polymorphonuclear cells in ascitic fluid below 250/mm^3
4	After resolution of infection, start long term norfloxacin 400 mg/day po

[a]Absence of shock, severe renal failure (serum creatinine >3 mg/dl), gastrointestinal hemorrhage or ileus.

Resolution of SBP is obtained in up to 90% of patients, but hospital mortality remains very high, around 30% in most series.[4,5,77–80] Advanced liver failure and associated complications (ie gastrointestinal hemorrhage, renal failure) probably account for this high mortality rate. The most important predictor of survival in patients with SBP is the development of renal failure during the infection.[68] Recent data indicate that the development of renal failure in the setting of SBP can be effectively prevented by the administration of albumin together with the antibiotic therapy.[83a] The incidence of renal failure is markedly lower in patients receiving albumin compared with that of patients not receiving albumin. Most importantly, albumin administration also improves survival in these patients. The beneficial effect of albumin is probably related to its capacity to prevent the impairment in the effective arterial blood volume and subsequent activation of vasoconstrictor systems that occurs during the infection. As previously discussed, long term prognosis of patients who have recovered from an episode of SBP is poor, and patients should be evaluated for liver transplantation. Recurrent SBP is very common in these patients and constitutes a major cause of death.[63]

Prophylaxis

The identification of subsets of patients with an increased risk of developing SBP has stimulated the search for prophylactic methods to prevent the development of this complication. Conditions associated with an increased risk of SBP include: gastrointestinal bleeding, low protein concentration in ascitic fluid, advanced liver failure (high serum bilirubin and/or markedly prolonged prothrombin time), and past history of SBP.[4,5] Because most episodes of SBP are caused by Gram-negative bacteria present in the normal intestinal flora, the rationale for the prophylaxis of SBP has been based mainly on the administration of antibiotics that produce a selective decontamination of the gastrointestinal tract, with elimination of aerobic Gram-negative bacteria without affecting aerobic Gram-positive bacteria and anaerobes.

The efficacy of this approach has been demonstrated in patients with gastrointestinal hemorrhage[84–87] and patients who have recovered from the first SBP episode (Table 25.6).[88] In patients with gastrointestinal hemorrhage, the short term administration of norfloxacin reduces markedly the incidence of SBP or bacteremia as compared with patients not receiving prophylactic antibiotics.[85] Other effective approaches consist of the administration of parenteral antibiotics, such as ofloxacin or the combination of ciprofloxacin and amoxicillin-clavulanic acid.[86,87] The absolute risk reduction in four trials of antibiotic prophylaxis in patients with gastrointestinal hemorrhage ranges from

R
Grade A

Table 25.6 Incidence of spontaneous bacterial peritonitis in randomized studies assessing the efficacy of antibiotic prophylaxis in cirrhosis[a]

	Antibiotic prophylaxis	*P* values	Control	Antibiotic used
Primary prophylaxis[b]				
Gastrointestinal hemorrhage				
Rimola *et al*[84]	Non-absorbable antibiotics[c] po	0.05	15/72 (21%)	6/68(%)
Soriano *et al*[85]	Norfloxacin 400 bid po	0.02	10/59 (17%)	2/60 (3%)
Blaise *et al*[86]	Ofloxacin 400 mg/day iv	NS	7/45 (16%)	3/46 (7%)
Pauwels *et al*[87]	Ciprofloxacin 200 mg iv + amoxicillin and clavulanic acid 1 g/200 mg po tid	0.05	7/34 (21%)	1/30 (3%)
Ascites				
Soriano *et al*[92]	Norfloxacin 400 mg/day po	0.005	7/31 (23%)	0/32 (0%)
Rolanchon *et al*[93]	Ciprofloxacin 750 mg weekly po	0.05	7/32 (22%)	1/28 (4%)
Singh *et al*[94]	Trimethoprim-sulfamethoxazole 160 mg/800 mg 5 days a week po	0.03	8/30 (27%)	1/30 (3%)
Novella *et al*[95]	Norfloxacin 400 mg/day po	0.007	9/53 (17%)[d]	1/56 (2%)
Grange *et al*[96]	Norfloxacin 400 mg/day po	NS	4/54 (7%)	0/53 (0%)
Secondary prophylaxis				
Ginès *et al*[88]	Norfloxacin 400 mg/day po	0.03	14/40 (35%)	5/40 (12%)

[a]Figures represent the number of patients developing spontaneous bacterial peritonitis during follow-up compared with the total number of patients in each treatment group.
[b]Refers to the antibiotic prophylaxis given to prevent the first episode of spontaneous bacterial peritonitis.
[c]Combination of gentamicin, vancomycin and nystatin or neomycin, colistin, and nystatin.
[d]The control group received norfloxacin only during hospitalizations.

9 to 23% (NNT 4–11). The results of a recent meta-analysis, published so far only in abstract form, indicate that antibiotic prophylaxis in patients with gastrointestinal bleeding not only prevents infection but also improves survival.[89]

R Grade A

Long term norfloxacin administration is very effective in the prevention of SBP recurrence (Table 25.6).[88] Patients under long term norfloxacin therapy demonstrate a reduction of Gram-negative bacteria from fecal flora, with no significant changes in Gram-positive cocci or anaerobic bacteria counts.[88] Gram-negative bacteria resistant to norfloxacin have been isolated from fecal flora of patients under chronic norfloxacin therapy,[90] but the occurrence of episodes of SBP caused by resistant organisms is extremely uncommon.[91] Therefore, antibiotic prophylaxis should be given to all patients after resolution of SBP.

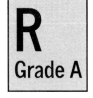

Antibiotic prophylaxis (norfloxacin, ciprofloxacin, or trimethoprim-sulfamethoxazole) also appears to be effective in the prevention of the first SBP episode (primary prophylaxis) in patients with low ascitic fluid protein (<10–15 g/l), who have a relatively high risk of developing the first episode of SBP (Table 25.6).[92–96] However, the published studies summarized in Table 25.6 have included only small numbers of patients and were of short duration or were not placebo controlled. Additional studies involving larger numbers of patients with longer periods of follow-up are needed before antibiotic prophylaxis can be recommended routinely for this patient population.[97]

REFERENCES

1 Arroyo V, Ginès P, Planas R *et al.* Pathogenesis, diagnosis and treatment of ascites in cirrhosis. In: McIntyre N, Benhamou JP, Bircher J (eds), *Oxford textbook of clinical hepatology*, 2nd edn,1999, pp 697–732.

2 Ginès P, Fernández-Esparrach G, Arroyo V *et al.* Pathogenesis of ascites in cirrhosis. *Semin Liver Dis* 1997; **17**: 175–91.

3 Ginès P, Rodés J. Clinical disorders of renal function in cirrhosis with ascites. In: Arroyo V, Ginès P, Rodés J *et al* (eds), *Ascites and renal dysfunction in liver disease. Pathogenesis, diagnosis and treatment*. Malden, Blackwell Science, 1999, pp 36–62.

4 Rimola A, Navasa M. Infections in liver diseases. In: McIntyre N, Benhamou JP, Bircher J *et al* (eds), *Oxford textbook of clinical hepatology*, 2nd edn, Oxford, Oxford University Press, 1999, pp 1861–76.

5 Guarner C, Soriano G. Spontaneous bacterial peritonitis. *Semin Liver Dis* 1997; **17**: 203–18.

6 Arroyo V, Ginès P, Jiménez W *et al.* Renal dysfunction in cirrhosis. In: McIntyre N, Benhamou JP, Bircher J *et al* (eds), *Oxford textbook of clinical hepatology*, 2nd edn, 1999, pp 733–64.

7 Schrier RW, Arroyo V, Bernardi M *et al.* Peripheral arterial vasodilation hypothesis: a proposal for the initiation of renal sodium and water retention in cirrhosis. *Hepatology* 1988; **8**: 1151–7.

8 Martin PY, Ginès P, Schrier RW. Role of nitric oxide as mediator of hemodynamic abnormalities and sodium and water retention in cirrhosis. *N Engl J Med* 1998; **339**: 533–41.

9 Farnsworth EB, Krakusin JS. Electrolyte partition in patients with edema of various origins. *J Lab Clin Med* 1948; **33**: 1545–54.

10 Eisenmenger WJ, Blondheim SH, Bongiovanni AM *et al.* Electrolyte studies on patients with cirrhosis of the liver. *J Clin Invest* 1950; **29**: 1491–9.

11 Reynolds TB, Lieberman FL, Goodman AR. Advantages of treatment of ascites without sodium restriction and without complete removal of excess fluid. *Gut* 1978; **19**: 549–53.

12 Gauthier A, Levy VG, Quinton A *et al.* Salt or no salt in the treatment of cirrhotic ascites: a randomised study. *Gut* 1986; **27**: 705–9.

13 Bernardi M, Laffi G, Salvagnini M *et al.* Efficacy and safety of the stepped care medical treatment of ascites in liver cirrhosis: a randomized controlled clinical trial comparing two diets with different sodium content. *Liver* 1993; **13**: 156–62.

14 Ascione A, Burroughs AK. Paracentesis for ascites in cirrhotic patients. *Gastroenterol Int* 1990; **3**: 120–3.

15 Arroyo V, Ginès A, Saló J. A European survey on the treatment of ascites in cirrhosis. *J Hepatol* 1994; **21**: 667–72.

16 Ginès P, Arroyo V, Quintero E *et al.* Comparison of paracentesis and diuretics in the treatment of cirrhotics with tense ascites. Results of a randomized study. *Gastroenterology* 1987; **93**: 234–41.

17 Salerno F, Badalamenti S, Incerti P *et al.* Repeated paracentesis and iv albumin infusion to treat "tense" ascites in cirrhotic patients: A safe alternative therapy. *J Hepatol* 1987; **5**: 102–8.

18 Hagège H, Ink O, Ducreux M *et al.* Traitement de l'ascite chez les malades atteints de cirrhose sans hyponatrémie ni insuffisance rénale. Résultats d'une étude randomisée comparant les diurétiques et les ponctions compensées par l'albumine. *Gastroenterol Clin Biol* 1992; **16**: 751–5.

19 Acharya SK, Balwinder S, Padhee AK *et al.* Large-volume paracentesis and intravenous dextran to treat tense ascites. *J Clin Gastroenterol* 1992; **14**: 31–5.

20 Solà R, Vila MC, Andreu M *et al.* Total paracentesis with dextran 40 vs diuretics in the treatment of ascites in cirrhosis: a randomized controlled study. *J Hepatol* 1994; **20**: 282–8.

21 Fernández-Esparrach G, Guevara M, Sort P *et al.* Diuretic requirements after therapeutic paracentesis in non-azotemic patients with cirrhosis. A randomized double-blind trial of spironolactone versus placebo. *J Hepatol* 1997; **26**: 614–20.

22 Runyon BA. Treatment of patients with cirrhosis and ascites. *Semin Liver Dis* 1997; **17**: 249–60.

23 Ginès P, Titó Ll, Arroyo V *et al.* Randomized comparative study of therapeutic paracentesis with and without intravenous albumin in cirrhosis. *Gastroenterology* 1988; **94**: 1493–502.

24 Pozzi M, Osculati G, Boari G *et al.* Time course of circulatory and humoral effects of rapid total paracentesis in cirrhotic patients with tense, refractory ascites. *Gastroenterology* 1994; **106**: 709–19.

25 Luca A, Garcia-Pagan JC, Bosch J *et al.* Beneficial effects of intravenous albumin infusion on the hemodynamic and humoral changes after total paracentesis. *Hepatology* 1995; **22**: 753–8.

26 Saló J, Ginès A, Ginès P *et al.* Effect of therapeutic paracentesis on plasma volume and transvascular escape rate of albumin in patients with cirrhosis. *J Hepatol* 1997; **27**: 645–53.

27 Ruiz del Arbol L, Monescillo A, Jiménez W *et al.* Paracentesis-induced circulatory dysfunction: mechanism and effect on hepatic hemodynamics in cirrhosis. *Gastroenterology* 1997; **113**: 579–86.

28 Vila MC, Solà R, Molina L *et al*. Hemodynamic changes in patients developing effective hypovolemia after total paracentesis. *J Hepatol* 1998; **28**: 639–45.
29 Ginès A, Fernández-Esparrach G, Monescillo A *et al*. Randomized trial comparing albumin, dextran-70 and polygelin in cirrhotic patients with ascites treated by paracentesis. *Gastroenterology* 1996; **111**: 1002–10.
30 Planas R, Ginès P, Arroyo V *et al*. Dextran 70 vs albumin as plasma expanders in cirrhotic patients with tense ascites treated with total paracentesis. Results of a randomized study. *Gastroenterology* 1990; **99**: 1736–44.
31 Salerno F, Badalamenti S, Lorenzano E *et al*. Randomized comparative study of Hemaccel vs albumin infusion after total paracentesis in cirrhotic patients with refractory ascites. *Hepatology* 1991; **13**: 707–13.
32 Fassio E, Terg R, Landeira G *et al*. Paracentesis with dextran 70 vs paracentesis with albumin in cirrhosis with tense ascites: results of a randomized study. *J Hepatol* 1992; **14**: 310–16.
33 Bataller R, Ginès P, Arroyo V. Practical recommendations for the treatment of ascites and its complications. *Drugs* 1997; **54**: 571–80.
34 Angeli P, Gatta A. Medical treatment of ascites in cirrhosis. In Arroyo V, Ginès P, Rodés J *et al* (eds), *Ascites and renal dysfunction in liver disease. Pathogenesis, diagnosis and treatment*. Malden, Blackwell Science, 1999, pp 442–63.
35 Pérez-Ayuso RM, Arroyo V, Planas R *et al*. Randomized comparative study of efficacy of furosemide versus spironolactone in nonazotemic cirrhosis with ascites. Relationship between the diuretic response and the activity of the renin-aldosterone system. *Gastroenterology* 1983; **84**: 961–8.
36 Angeli P, Pria MD, De Bei E *et al*. Randomized clinical study of the efficacy of amiloride and potassium canreonate in nonazotemic cirrhotic patients with ascites. *Hepatology* 1994; **19**: 72–9.
37 Campra JL, Reynolds TB. Effectiveness of high-dose spironolactone therapy in patients with chronic liver disease and relatively refractory ascites. *Dig Dis Sci* 1978; **23**: 1025–30.
38 Eggert RC. Spironolactone diuresis in patients with cirrhosis and ascites. *Br Med J* 1970; **4**: 401–3.
39 Strauss E, De SaMF, Lacet CM *et al*. Standardization of a therapeutic approach for ascites due to chronic liver disease. A prospective study of 100 patients. *Gastrointest Endosc Digest* 1985; **4**: 79–86.
40 Gatta A, Angeli P, Caregaro L *et al*. A pathophysiological interpretation of unresponsiveness to spironolactone in a stepped care approach to the diuretic treatment of ascites in nonazotemic cirrhotic patients. *Hepatology* 1991; **14**: 231–6.
41 Arroyo V, Ginès P, Gerbes A *et al*. Definition and diagnostic criteria of refractory ascites and hepatorenal syndrome in cirrhosis. *Hepatology* 1996; **23**: 164–76.
42 Angeli P, Albino G, Carraro P *et al*. Cirrhosis and muscle cramps: evidence of a causal relationship. *Hepatology* 1996; **23**: 264–73.
43 Gregory PB, Broekelschen PH, Hill MD *et al*. Complications of diuresis in the alcoholic patient with ascites: a controlled trial. *Gastroenterology* 1977; **73**: 534–8.
44 Blendis LM, Greig PD, Langer B *et al*. Renal and hemodynamic effect of the peritoneovenous shunt for intractable hepatic ascites. *Gastroenterology* 1979; **77**: 250–7.
45 Greig PD, Blendis LM, Langer B *et al*. Renal and hemodynamic effect of the peritoneovenous shunt. II. Long-term effect. *Gastroenterology* 1981; **80**: 119–25.
46 Ginès P, Arroyo V, Vargas V *et al*. Paracentesis with intravenous infusion of albumin as compared with peritoneovenous shunting in cirrhosis with refractory ascites. *N Engl J Med* 1991; **325**: 829–35.
47 Ginès A, Planas R, Angeli P *et al*. Treatment of patients with cirrhosis and refractory ascites by LeVeen shunt with titanium tip. Comparison with therapeutic paracentesis. *Hepatology* 1995; **22**: 124–31.
48 Epstein M. Peritoneovenous shunt in the management of ascites and hepatorenal syndrome. In Epstein M (ed), *The kidney in liver disease*, 4th edn. Philadelphia, Hanley and Belfus, 1996, pp 491–506.
49 Ring-Larsen H. Treatment of refractory ascites. In Arroyo V, Ginès P, Rodés J, Schrier RW (eds) *Ascites and renal dysfunction in liver disease. Pathogenesis, diagnosis and treatment*. Malden, Blackwell Science, 1999, pp 480–91.
50 LeVeen HH, Vujic I, D'Ovidio N *et al*. Peritoneovenous shunt occlusion. Etiology, diagnosis, therapy. *Ann Surg* 1984; **200**: 212–23.
51 Orloff MJ. Pathogenesis and surgical treatment of intractable ascites associated with alcoholic cirrhosis. *Ann NY Acad Sci* 1970; **170**: 213–38.
52 Franco D, Vons C, Traynor C *et al*. Should portosystemic shunt be reconsidered in the treatment of intractable ascites in cirrhosis? *Arch Surg* 1988; **123**: 987–91.
53 Castells A, Saló J, Planas R *et al*. Impact of shunt surgery for variceal bleeding in the natural history of ascites in cirrhosis: a retrospective study. *Hepatology* 1994; **20**: 584–91.
54 Shiffman ML, Jeffers L, Hoofnagle JH *et al*. The role of transjugular intrahepatic portosystemic shunt for treatment of portal hypertension and its complications: a conference sponsored by the

National Digestive Disease advisory board. *Hepatology* 1995; **25**: 1591–7.

55 Ferral H, Bjarnason H, Wegryn SA *et al.* Refractory ascites: early experience in treatment with transjugular intrahepatic portosystemic shunt. *Radiology* 1993; **189**: 7905–801.

56 Somberg KA, Lake JR, Tomlanovich SJ *et al.* Transjugular intrahepatic portosystemic shunt for refractory ascites: assessment of clinical and humoral response and renal function. *Hepatology* 1995; **21**: 709–16.

57 Quiroga J, Sangro B, Nuñez M *et al.* Transjugular intrahepatic portal-systemic shunt in the management of refractory ascites: effect on clinical, renal, humoral and hemodynamic parameters. *Hepatology* 1995; **21**: 986–994.

58 Wong F, Sniderman K, Liu P *et al.* Transjugular intrahepatic portosystemic stent shunt: effects on hemodynamics and sodium homeostasis in cirrhosis and refractory ascites. *Ann Intern Med* 1995; **122**: 816–22.

59 Ochs A, Rössle M, Haag K *et al.* The transjugular intrahepatic portosystemic stent shunt procedure for refractory ascites. *N Engl J Med* 1995; **332**: 1192–7.

60 Lebrec D, Giuily N, Hadengue A *et al.* Transjugular intrahepatic portosystemic shunts: comparison with paracentesis in patients with cirrhosis and refractory ascites: a randomized trial. *J Hepatol* 1996; **25**: 135–44.

61 Arroyo V, Ginès P. TIPS and refractory ascites. Lessons from recent history of ascites therapy. *J Hepatol* 1996; **25**: 221–3.

62 Rimola A, Navasa M, Grande L. Liver transplantation in cirrhotic patients with ascites. In Arroyo V, Ginès P, Rodés J *et al* (eds), *Ascites and renal dysfunction in liver disease. Pathogenesis, diagnosis and treatment.* Malden, Blackwell Science, 1999, pp 522–537.

63 Tító L, Rimola A, Ginès P *et al.* Recurrence of spontaneous bacterial peritonitis in cirrhosis. Frequency and predictive factors. *Hepatology* 1988; **8**: 27–31.

64 Ginès A, Escorsell A, Ginès P *et al.* Incidence, predictive factors, and prognosis of the hepatorenal syndrome in cirrhosis with ascites. *Gastroenterology* 1993; **105**: 229–36.

65 Llach J, Ginès P, Arroyo V *et al.* Prognostic value of arterial pressure, endogenous vasoactive systems, and renal function in cirrhotic patients admitted to the hospital for the treatment of ascites. *Gastroenterology* 1988; **94**: 482–7.

66 Ginès P, Fernández-Esparrach G. Prognosis of cirrhosis with ascites. In Arroyo V, Ginès P, Rodés J *et al* (eds), *Ascites and renal dysfunction in liver disease. Pathogenesis, diagnosis and treatment.* Malden, Blackwell Science, 1999; 431–42.

67 Schrier RW, Niederbeger M, Weigert A *et al.* Peripheral arterial vasodilation: determinant of functional spectrum of cirrhosis. *Semin Liver Dis* 1994; **14**: 14–22.

68 Follo A, Llovet JM, Navasa M *et al.* Renal impairment after spontaneous bacterial peritonitis in cirrhosis: incidence, clinical course, predictive factors and prognosis. *Hepatology* 1994; **20**: 495–501.

69 Arroyo V, Bataller R, Guevara M. Treatment of hepatorenal syndrome in cirrhosis. In Arroyo V, Ginès P, Rodés J *et al* (eds), *Ascites and renal dysfunction in liver disease. Pathogenesis, diagnosis and treatment.* Malden, Blackwell Science, 1999, pp 492–510.

70 Guevara M, Ginès P, Fernández-Esparrach G *et al.* Reversibility of hepatorenal syndrome by prolonged administration of ornipressin and plasma volume expansion. *Hepatology* 1998; **27**: 35–41.

71 Ganne–Carrié N, Hadengue A, Mathurin P *et al.* Hepatorenal syndrome. Long-term treatment with terlipressin as a bridge to liver transplantation. *Dig Dis Sci* 1996; **41**: 1054–6.

72 Hadengue A, Gadano A, Moreau R *et al.* Beneficial effects of the 2-day administration of terlipressin in patients with cirrhosis and hepatorenal syndrome. *J Hepatol* 1998; **29**: 565–70.

73 Guevara M, Ginès P, Bandi JC *et al.* Transjugular intrahepatic portosystemic shunt in hepatorenal syndrome. Effects on renal function and vasoactive systems. *Hepatology* 1998; **28**: 416–22.

74 Gonwa TA, Morris CA, Goldstein RM *et al.* Long-term survival and renal function following liver transplantation in patients with and without hepatorenal syndrome – experience in 300 patients. *Transplantation* 1991; **51**: 428–30.

75 Castellví JM, Guardiola J, Sesé E *et al.* Spontaneous bacterial empyema of cirrhotic patients: a prospective study. *Hepatology* 1996; **23**: 719–24.

76 Felisart J, Rimola A, Arroyo V *et al.* Cefotaxime is more effective than is ampicillin-tobramycin in cirrhotics with severe infections. *Hepatology* 1985;**5**:457–62.

77 Toledo C, Salmerón JM, Rimola A *et al.* Spontaneous bacterial peritonitis in cirrhosis: predictive factors of infection resolution and survival in patients treated with cefotaxime. *Hepatology* 1993; **17**: 251–7.

78 Rimola A, Salmerón JM, Clemente G *et al.* Two different dosages of cefotaxime in the treatment of spontaneous bacterial peritonitis in cirrhosis: results of a prospective, randomized, multicenter study. *Hepatology* 1995; **21**: 674–9.

79 Runyon BA, McHutchinson JG, Antillon MR. Short-course versus long-course antibiotic treatment of spontaneous bacterial peritonitis: a

randomized, controlled study of 100 patients. *Gastroenterology* 1991; **100**: 1737–42.

80 Gómez-Jiménez J, Ribera E, Gasser I *et al.* Randomized trial comparing ceftriaxone with cefonicid for treatment of spontaneous bacterial peritonitis in cirrhotic patients. *Antimicrob Agents Chemother* 1993; **37**: 1587–92.

81 Ariza J, Xiol X, Esteve M *et al.* Aztreonam vs Cefotaxime in the treatment of gram-negative spontaneous peritonitis in cirrhotic patients. *Hepatology* 1991; **14**: 91–8.

82 Grange JD, Amiot X, Grange V *et al.* Amoxicillin-clavulanic acid therapy of spontaneous bacterial peritonitis: a prospective study of twenty-seven cases in cirrhotic patients. *Hepatology* 1990; **11**: 360–4.

83 Navasa M, Follo A, Llovet JM *et al.* Randomized, comparative study of oral ofloxacin versus intravenous cefotaxime in spontaneous bacterial peritonitis. *Gastroenterology* 1996; **111**: 1011–7.

83a Sort P, Navasa M, Arroyo V *et al.* Effect of plasma volume expansion on renal impairment and mortality in patients with cirrhosis and spontaneous bacterial peritonitis. *N Engl J Med* 1999, in press.

84 Rimola A, Bory F, Terés J *et al.* Oral non-absorbable antibiotics prevent infection in cirrhosis with gastrointestinal hemorrhage. *Hepatology* 1985; **5**: 463–7.

85 Soriano G, Guarner C, Tomás A *et al.* Norfloxacin prevents bacterial infection in cirrhotics with gastrointestinal hemorrhage. *Gastroenterology* 1992; **103**: 1267–72.

86 Blaise M, Pateron D, Trinchet JC *et al.* Systemic antibiotic therapy prevents bacterial infections in cirrhotic patients with gastrointestinal hemorrhage. *Hepatology* 1994; **20**: 34–8.

87 Pauwels A, Mostefa-Kara N, Debenes B *et al.* Systemic antibiotic prophylaxis after gastrointestinal hemorrhage in cirrhotic patients with a high risk of infection. *Hepatology* 1996; **24**: 802–6.

88 Ginès P, Rimola A, Planas R *et al.* Norfloxacin prevents spontaneous bacterial peritonitis recurrence in cirrhosis: results of a double blind, placebo-controlled trial. *Hepatology* 1990; **12**: 716–24.

89 Bernard B, Grangé JD, Khac NE *et al.* Antibiotic prophylaxis for the prevention of bacterial infections in cirrhotic patients with gastrointestinal bleeding: a meta-analysis. *Hepatology* 1999; **29**: 1655–61.

90 Dupeyron C, Mangeney N, Sedrati L *et al.* Rapid emergence of quinolone resistance in cirrhotic patients treated with norfloxacin to prevent spontaneous bacterial peritonitis. *Antimicrob Agents Chemother* 1994; **38**: 340–4.

91 Llovet J, Rodríguez-Iglesias P, Moitinho E *et al.* Spontaneous bacterial peritonitis in patients with cirrhosis undergoing selective intestinal decontamination. A retrospective study of 229 spontaneous bacterial peritonititis episodes. *J Hepatol* 1997; **26**: 88–95.

92 Soriano G, Guarner C, Teixidó M *et al.* Selective intestinal decontamination prevents spontaneous bacterial peritonitis. *Gastroenterology* 1991; **100**: 77–81.

93 Rolanchon A, Cordier L, Bacq Y *et al.* Ciprofloxacin and long-term prevention of spontaneous bacterial peritonitis: results of a prospective controlled trial. *Hepatology* 1995; **22**: 1171–4.

94 Singh N, Gayowski T, Yu VL *et al.* Trimethoprim-sulfamethoxazole for the prevention of spontaneous bacterial peritonitis in cirrhosis: a randomized trial. *Ann Intern Med* 1995; **122**: 595–8.

95 Novella M, Solá R, Soriano G *et al.* Continuous versus inpatient prophylaxis of the first spontaneous bacterial peritonitis with norfloxacin. *Hepatology* 1997; **25**: 532–6.

96 Grange JD, Roulot D, Pelletier G *et al.* Norfloxacin primary prophylaxis of bacterial infections in cirrhotic patients with ascites: a double-blind randomized trial. *J Hepatol* 1998; **29**: 430–6.

97 Ginès P, Navasa M. Antibiotic prophylaxis for spontaneous bacterial peritonitis: how and whom? *J Hepatol* 1998; **29**: 490–4.

Hepatic encephalopathy: treatment

26

PETER FERENCI, CHRISTIAN MÜLLER

Because the pathogenesis of hepatic encephalopathy (HE) is unknown,[1] no truly "specific" treatment exists. Nevertheless, a variety of compounds have been introduced for treatment of HE (Table 26.1). Some of these treatments are based on clinical observations, some on extrapolation of experimental data obtained in animal models of HE.

Table 26.1 Treatments for hepatic encephalopathy

	Controlled studies	
	vs lactulose	vs placebo
Decrease of ammoniagenic substrates		
Enemas with lactulose		+
Reduction of dietary protein		?
Inhibition of ammonia production		
Antibiotics		
Neomycin	=	=
Rifaximin	=	vs neomycin =
Vancomycin	= / +	nd
Disaccharides		
Lactulose		? =
Lactitol	=	nd
Lactose in lactase deficiency		+
Modification of colonic flora		
Lactobacillus SF 68	=	nd
Metabolic ammonia removal		
Ornithine aspartate iv		+
Benzoate	=	nd
BCAA supplementation		
Modified AA solutions ("FO80" type)	=	±
Dietary BCAA supplementation		+
Neuroactive drugs		
Flumazenil iv		+
L-Dopa, bromocriptine		=

+ Superior to control treatment; = equal to control treatment; ± conflicting results; nd, not done.

DESIGN OF CLINICAL TRIALS IN HEPATIC ENCEPHALOPATHY

A large spectrum of clinical conditions is summarized under the term "HE" and includes a variety of neuropsychiatric symptoms, ranging from minor, not readily discernible signs of altered brain function, overt psychiatric and/or neurological symptoms to deep coma. Accordingly, the methods to quantitate treatment effects and treatment endpoints are highly variable. Another variable is the treatment of control groups. Most studies compare a new drug to "standard treatment" (which by itself may be highly effective) such as oral lactulose, for which efficacy has not been demonstrated in a randomized placebo controlled trial for ethical reasons. However, in view of the natural history of HE, the inclusion of a placebo group in trials of new agents is highly desirable. In studies comparing a new drug with effective "standard treatment" demonstration of effectiveness of the new drug will require a very large sample size. Table 26.2 summarizes the appropriate study endpoints in various patient groups.

Natural history of HE

The natural history of HE is not well studied. However, examination of the outcomes in the placebo treatment groups in nine randomized controlled trials (Table 26.3) reveals that patients with grade III and IV HE may have recovery rates from 22% to greater than 90%. Therefore, in studies of new agents which lack controls, high response rates may be anticipated, and trials of new agents may require quite large numbers of patients to demonstrate benefits. Short term mortality of patients with HE appears to be low if unstable patients are excluded. The course of patients with *subclinical* HE is unknown, and it is by definition impossible to detect clinical improvement in such cases. Studies of new agents with subclinical illness should focus on progression to more severe levels of HE. The grade of encephalopathy of patients selected for clinical trials may be expected to have a substantial influence on results.

Table 26.2 Methods to assess treatment in various groups of patients with hepatic encephalopathy

Study group	Treatment endpoint	Assessment of treatment effects	Natural history	Problems
Overt hepatic encephalopathy	Clinical improvement	Clinical grading, EEG, SEP	Well documented	High mortality, precipitating factors
Chronic PSE	Clinical improvement	Clinical grading, PSE index[a]	Well documented	
Patients recovered from hepatic coma	Recurrence	PSE index, MDF	Variable	Compliance
TIPS or portocaval shunts (surgical)	Prevention of HE	PSE index, psychometry, MDF,	Well documented	
Subclinical HE	Psychometry EEG	Psychometry, MDF, P300	Unknown	Clinical meaning of certain tests

[a] PSE index according to Conn *et al.*[2]
SEP, somatosensory evoked potentials; MDF, mean dominant frequency; P300, event related acoustic evoked responses.

Methods to quantify

CLINICAL ASSESSMENT

The simplest assessment of HE is a description of the mental state according to Conn,[2] which grades HE in stages I–IV based on changes in consciousness, intellectual function and behavior. It does not include neurological changes or asterixis. The Glasgow Coma scale is useful in stages III and IV.

THE PSE (PORTAL–SYSTEMIC ENCEPHALOPATHY) INDEX

In 1977 the "PSE index"[3] was introduced in a trial comparing neomycin with lactulose and has been subsequently used by other investigators. The main problem with this index is the inclusion of arterial ammonia estimations. Hyperammonemia is possibly a cause, but not a symptom or effect of HE. Measurements of arterial ammonia concentrations require serial arterial punctures. The scoring of actual arterial ammonia concentrations is arbitrary and not based on a sound statistical analysis. Furthermore, the other parameters of the PSE index – mental state, EEG, and number connection tests (NCT) – are also graded by arbitrary units. No age-dependent normal values are used for NCT.[13] Finally, the PSE index does not discriminate between overt, mild or subclinical HE and has not been validated prospectively. In clinically overt HE the PSE index does not appear to be superior to simple clinical grading.

Table 26.3 Survival rates and improvement of hepatic encephalopathy in placebo treated patients in randomized controlled trials

Study	Test drug	HE grade	No. of patients	Observation time	Exclusion criteria	Survival % (on placebo)	HE better % (on placebo)
[a]Barbaro, 1998[4]	Flumazenil	III IV	265 262	6 days	HR, RF, acidosis	97.3 91.3	>90 >90
Kircheis, 1997[5]	Ornithine-aspartate	SHE I II	27 19 27	7 days	GI bleed, HR, RF	100 100 100	0 22 44
Stauch, 1998[6]	Ornithine-asparate	SHE I + II	 20	14 days	Unstable patients	100 100	0 40
Marchesini, 1990[7]	BCAA oral	I	34	3 mth	Unstable patients	100	38
Michel, 1980[8]	L-Dopa	I–III	38	7 days	None	61	37
Michel, 1984[9]	BCAA iv	I–III	24	5 days	Unstable patients	74	26
Wahren, 1983[10]	BCAA iv	II–IV	25	5 days	None	80	48
Blanc, 1994[11]	Neomycin + lactulose	II–IV	40	5 days	?	85	70
Strauss, 1992[12]	Neomycin	II–IV	19	5 days	MOF	89.5	89.5

[a] All patients were on neomycin!
HR, hepatorenal syndrome; RF, respiratory failure; MOF, multiorgan failure; BCAA, branched chain amino acids; SHE, subclinical hepatic encephalopathy.

PSYCHOMETRIC TESTS

Grading of HE does not allow the documentation of subtle changes. To quantify the impairment of mental function in mild stages of HE several psychometric tests have been evaluated.[14–16] Detailed psychometric testing is more sensitive in the detection of minor deficits of mental function than either conventional clinical assessment or the EEG.[17] However, the tests are cumbersome, and when applied repeatedly the reliability of most of them is adversely affected by the learning effect. Few are useful in routine practice. The most frequently applied test is the number connection test.[16] This test is easily administered and the results can be quickly quantified. One important consequence of the application of psychometric tests in cirrhotic patients was the finding that even patients with apparently normal mental status have a measurable deficit in their intellectual performance.[14] These patients are usually referred to as suffering from "subclinical HE" or "stage 0 HE". However, psychometric tests may overdiagnose subclinical HE, because scores are usually not corrected for age.[13,17] Furthermore, it is unknown whether abnormalities of test results correlate with impaired quality of life or performance in daily life.[18] On the contrary, the driving ability of patients with test results classifying them as "unable to drive a car"[14] was not different from that of healthy controls.[19] A quality-of-life questionnaire (sickness impact profile – SIP) detects the extent and frequency of deficits in daily functioning in patients without clinically apparent HE. From the 136 statements, five were selected as predictive of subclinical HE.[18]

ELECTROPHYSIOLOGICAL TESTS

The simplest EEG assessment of HE is to grade the degree of abnormality of the conventional EEG trace. A more refined assessment by computer assisted techniques allow variables in the EEG such as the mean dominant EEG frequency and the power of a particular EEG rhythm to be quantified. Evoked responses (by visual, somatosensory, or acoustic stimuli) or event related responses, like the P300 peak after auditory stimuli, are sensitive to detect subtle changes of brain function and can be used for diagnosis of subclinical HE.[20]

EVIDENCE BASED MEDICINE AND HEPATIC ENCEPHALOPATHY

Evidence based medicine is a process of systematically finding, appraising, and using research findings as the basis for clinical decisions[21] based on the formulation of relevant questions concerning a patient's problem.

The answer to the question "Does treatment with specific drugs, compared to placebo, improve HE?" should be addressed separately for overt and subclinical HE. In the following sections we have identified the studies that attempt to answer this question and we have critically appraised the evidence for the most important treatment regimens. The magnitude of the treatment effect of various interventions has been assessed. This assessment is difficult in HE because of the use of different methods which are not readily comparable for quantifying the severity of this disease. The question of the clinical applicability and generalizability of the findings of randomized controlled studies in HE must be addressed in the context of the treatment and the grade of encephalopathy studied.

Table 26.4A Medline Search, 1966–1999

Search parameter	No. of articles
Hepatic encephalopathy (HE)	6178
Treatment of HE	1320
Placebo and HE	66
Randomized and HE	128
Double-blind and HE	54
Randomized controlled trial (RCT) and HE	19
HE/all subheadings (MESH term)	5499
HE and publication type (PT) = RCT	125
Randomized studies with the endpoint "improvement of HE" and more than 10 patients per study group	34

Table 26.4B Randomized trials with endpoint "improvement of HE"

	Control				
Test drug	Placebo	Standard therapy[a]	Lactulose	Neomycin	Total
Flumazenil	6				6
BCAA iv	4	2			6
BCAA oral	2				2
Lactulose	2			3	5
Lactitol			3		3
Neomycin	1				1
Lactulose + neomycin	1				1
Lactulose/lactose enemas	1			1	2
Zinc		2			2
Benzoate			1		1
L-Dopa	1				1
Rifaximine			1	2	3
SF-68			1		1
Total	18	4	6	6	34

[a]Usually includes lactulose or neomycin.

Data base

To identify all randomized controlled trials in HE, a Medline search was conducted using several terms (Table 26.4A). A total of 1320 papers dealt with treatment of HE, less than a hundred represent some form of controlled trials. In this group, 34 randomized trials had the endpoint "improvement of HE" and included more than 10 patients per study group (Table 26.4B). In addition, two meta-analyses have been published.[22,23]

TREATMENT OF HEPATIC ENCEPHALOPATHY

Clinically overt HE (grade I–IV) in patients with cirrhosis

SUPPORTIVE CARE AND TREATMENT OF PRECIPITATING CAUSES OF HE

It is important to recognize that HE, acute and chronic, is reversible and that a precipitating cause rather than worsening of hepatocellular function can be identified in the majority of patients.[1,2] These causes include gastrointestinal bleeding, increased protein intake, hypokalemic alkalosis, infection, and constipation (all of which increase arterial ammonia levels), hypoxia, and the use of sedatives and tranquilizers. Patients with advanced cirrhosis may be particularly sensitive to benzodiazepines.

R Grade C

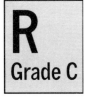

Treatment of these precipitating events is typically associated with a prompt and permanent improvement of HE. As a result, every attempt should be made to identify and to treat such precipitating events. This approach has never been tested formally but is based on common clinical experience. As judged from the outcomes observed in placebo groups of controlled studies (see Table 26.3) standard medical care is highly effective.

ENEMAS

R Grade A

Cleansing of the colon by enemas is a rapid and effective procedure to remove ammoniagenic substrates. The efficacy of enemas of 1–3 liters of 20% lactulose or lactitol solutions was proven in randomized controlled trials; a favorable response was noted in 78–86% of patients (ARR 0.4%, NNT = 2.5).[24,25] Interestingly, enemas with tap water were ineffective, raising the possibility that colonic acidification rather than bowel cleansing was the effective therapeutic mechanism.

NUTRITION

Patients with grade III–IV HE usually do not receive oral nutrition. In general, there is no need for parenteral nutritional, if patients improve within 2 days.

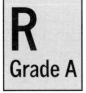

R Grade A

Based on the "false neurotransmitter hypothesis", total parenteral nutrition with specific amino acid solutions has been proposed. A number of randomized controlled studies have evaluated the use of solutions with a high content of branched chain amino acids (BCAA) and a low content of aromatic amino acids (AAA). These studies differ with respect to the amino acid solutions used, the study protocols, patient selection, and the duration of treatment, and are difficult to compare. The results have been conflicting, but most studies did not find any improvement in HE or any reduction in mortality in patients treated with BCAA.[26,27] Although a meta-analysis revealed a significant trend toward improvement in these outcomes, it was concluded that further randomized controlled trials are needed.[22] At present, infusions of modified amino acid solutions should not be used in the standard treatment of patients with HE.

There is no proven need for a specific diet for patients with HE. Although mentioned in all textbooks, the recommendation of a low protein diet in patients with advanced liver disease is not supported by good clinical or experimental evidence. On the contrary, in patients with alcoholic hepatitis, low protein intake is associated with worsening HE while a higher protein intake correlates with improvement in HE.[28] The recommendations of the European Society of Parenteral and Enteral Nutrition (ESPEN) are that oral protein intake should not exceed 70 g/day in a patient with a history of HE; a level below 70 g/day is rarely necessary and minimum intake should not be lower than 40 g/day to avoid negative nitrogen balance.[29]

R
Grade B

Pharmacotherapy

FLUMAZENIL

Based upon the GABA-benzodiazepine hypothesis of the pathogenesis of HE, the benzodiazepine receptor antagonist flumazenil has been tested for treatment of HE in five randomized placebo controlled trials involving over 600 patients. Four were crossover trials, and one used a parallel group design. Flumazenil was superior to placebo in four of these studies (Table 26.5). In the only large double-blind, placebo controlled crossover trial 537 cirrhotic patients with grade III (265 patients) or IVa (262 patients) hepatic encephalopathy were randomised to receive intravenous flumazenil or a placebo over a 3–5 minute period. Patients subsequently received the other study medication if they were still in grade III or IVa encephalopathy after the first study period. Treatment was begun within 15 minutes of randomisation. Outcome measures included both a neurological score and a grading derived from continuous EEG recordings. Table 26.5 shows the results obtained by combining the scores from the initial and crossover period. Improvement of the neurological score was documented in 46 of grade III and in 39 of grade IVa patients

Table 26.5 Randomized controlled trials of flumazenil for hepatic encephalopathy

						Number improved/Number of treatment periods(%)			
						Flumazenil		Placebo	
	Study design	No. of patients	Dose (mg)	Outcome measure	HE grade	clinical	EEG	clinical	EEG
Barbaro, 1998[3]	Crossover RCT	527	1	EEG and neurological score	3	46/262* (17.6)	73/262* (27.9)	10/262 (3.8)	13/262 (5)
					4	39/265* (14.7)	57/265* (21.5)	3/265 (1.1)	9/265 (3.4)
Gyr, 1996[30]	RCT	49[a]	1/hr×3hr	PSE score dependent on neuro symptoms	2–4	5/14* (35) (28)[b]*		0/11 (0) (0)	
Pomier-Layrargues, 1994[31]	Crossover RCT	21	2	HE grade EEG	2–4	6/13* (46)	4/12 (33)	0/15 (0)	2/13 (15)
Cadranel, 1995[32]	Crossover RCT	14[c]	1	HE grade EEG	2–4	d	12/18* (67)		0/8 (17)
van der Rijt, 1995[33]	Crossover RCT	18	0.25 mg/hr × 3 days	HE grade EEG	0–4	6/18** (35)	0/18	2/18 (12)	0/18

[a] 24 patients excluded from analysis (see text)
[b] intent to treat analysis
[c] 18 episodes of HE in 14 patients
[d] "modest improvement"
*$P < 0.05$
**$P = 0.06$

during the combined flumazenil treatment periods and in 10 (Grade III) and 3 (Grade IVa) of the patients during placebo treatment periods. Improvement of the EEG score occurred in 73 (Grade III) and 57 (Grade IVa) patients during flumazenil treatment and 13 (Grade III) and 9 (Grade IVa) patients during placebo treatment. The effects of flumazenil were statistically significant ($P<0.01$). In the second study,[30] 24 of 49 randomized patients were excluded from the final analysis, mainly due to inadequate benzodiazepine screening. However, flumazenil was superior to placebo even when the data were evaluated by intention to treat analysis; among the 25 patients who were not excluded, clinically relevant improvement was seen in 35% compared to 0% in patients given placebo. In the Canadian trial,[31] very strict exclusion criteria resulted in the rejection of 56 of 77 potential patients. Improvement in neurological symptoms was observed in 6 of 11 flumazenil treatment periods compared to zero of 10 placebo periods; a few patients showed improvement in the EEG during both treatments. The beneficial effect of flumazenil was not related to the presence of identifiable benzodiazepines in the blood. In the fourth positive study,[32] drug effects were evaluated on continuous EEG recordings obtained before, during, and 10 minutes after a bolus dose of the drug. No patient improved on placebo; on flumazenil the EEG recording improved in 12 out of 18 cases (66%) and was associated with a shortlasting modest clinical improvement. In the fifth study the response rate with flumazenil was greater than that observed with placebo, but the result was not statistically significant.[33]

Taken together, these studies suggest that some patients with severe HE will experience clinical improvement when flumazenil is added to standard treatment.

ANTIBIOTICS

R Grade A

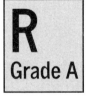

Neomycin has been used as standard treatment of HE for almost 40 years. Surprisingly, there is no evidence that neomycin is effective. The only randomized placebo controlled study found no benefit of neomycin compared to standard treatment alone.[12] Based on this negative study and the potential for serious adverse effects of this drug, neomycin should not be prescribed for this condition. The combination of neomycin with lactulose was not superior to placebo.[23] Other antibiotics including paromomycin, metronidazole, vancomycin[34] and rifaximine[35] are better tolerated, but there is no evidence supporting their efficacy.

DISACCHARIDES

Synthetic disaccharides (lactulose, lactitol, lactose in lactase deficiency) are currently the mainstay of therapy of HE. The dose of lactulose (45–90 g/day) should be titrated in every patient to achieve two to three soft stools with a pH below 6 per day. Lactitol has been evaluated in a number of clinical trials. It appears to be as effective as lactulose, is more palatable, and may have fewer adverse effects.[23,36] In patients with lactase deficiency, lactose has most of the same effects as the synthetic disaccharides in the colon.[37]

R Grade C

Although a properly conducted placebo controlled trial has not been performed, the efficacy of these disaccharides is considered to be beyond doubt.[2,36] Approximately 70–80% of patients with HE improve on lactulose treatment, a response rate comparable to that observed in patients treated with neomycin.[3,38] Treatment is usually well tolerated, and the principal toxicity is abdominal cramping, diarrhea, and flatulence. Nevertheless, in view of the questionable efficacy of neomycin, the efficacy of oral lactulose or lactitol for treatment of clinically overt HE has to be questioned. Since most new treatment are considered to be effective if improvement rates are not different from a group treated with lactulose, a randomized, placebo controlled study of lactulose for treatment of overt HE would be desirable. The only placebo controlled trial (with a crossover design) involved just seven patients, of whom[39] only two had clinical symptoms. One patient improved on lactulose. This result is clearly not significant, and the trial lacked adequate power. In contrast to oral lactulose administration, the efficacy of lactulose or lactose enemas is beyond any doubt (see above).

ORNITHINE ASPARTATE

Ornithine and aspartate increase ammonia removal. In cirrhotics, ornithine aspartate infusions prevented hyperammonemia after an oral protein load in a dose-dependent fashion.[40] In a randomized, placebo controlled trial of patients with HE, ornithine aspartate (20 g/day given intravenously over 4 hours for 7 days) improved fasting and postprandial blood ammonia levels compared to placebo treated patients.[5] There was also symptomatic improvement (assessed by psychometric tests and the PSE index) in patients with grade I or II HE, but no effect was observed in those with subclinical HE. The results of this study are encouraging, and a confirmatory trial is needed.

BENZOATE

A different approach to elimination of ammonia is the use of benzoate. Benzoate reacts with glycine to form hippurate. For each mole of benzoate, one mole of waste nitrogen is excreted into the urine. In a prospective, randomized double-blind study of 74 patients with acute HE, sodium benzoate (5 g bid) was compared with lactulose.[41] Treatment effects were evaluated using the PSE index, visual, auditory, and somatosensory evoked potentials, and a battery of psychometric tests. The improvement in encephalopathy parameters and the incidence of adverse effects were similar in the two treatment groups. In view of the unknown efficacy of lactulose, a confirmatory placebo controlled trial is needed.

Chronic (overt) HE

Patients with chronic HE that is refractory to standard therapy are rare. Most have surgical shunts or a large diameter transjugular intrahepatic portosystemic shunt (TIPS). Due to the small number of such patients, there are no controlled studies. Case reports on individual patients describe successful approaches by narrowing or closure of the shunt, protein restriction together with BCAA supplementation, supplementation of zinc and thiamin, and the use of bromocriptin and oral flumazenil. The only controlled study was performed in 37 hospitalized patients with documented severe protein intolerance.[42] Addition of BCAA to the diet enabled the daily protein intake to be increased to up to 80 g without worsening of cerebral function. Many control patients who received casein as a protein source deteriorated after increasing dietary protein intake. No benefit of BCAA-supplementation was observed in protein-tolerant patients.

In protein-intolerant patients vegetable proteins appear to be better tolerated than proteins derived from fish, milk or meat. In three controlled studies a vegetable diet was better tolerated then a diet which also included meat.[43,44] Other studies did not show these favorable effects.[45] The beneficial effects of a vegetable diet on the protein tolerance of patients with HE cannot be explained by the amino acid compositions of the proteins alone.[46]

Subclinical HE

Although the number of patients with subclinical HE is large, good clinical studies are rare. Even among experts, there is no agreement on how to define subclinical HE or whether subclinical HE even exists. Efficacy of treatment is judged by the improvement of psychometric tests or of electrophysiological measurements. The clinical relevance of these outcomes is uncertain. Substances that improved responses in psychometric tests in randomized trials include lactulose[47,48] modification of colonic flora to increase lactobacilli,[49] ornithin aspartate,[5] and oral BCAA.[6,50,51]

Prevention of HE

The occurrence of HE is a problem after TIPS insertion.[52] Although most clinicians administer prophylactic treatments after TIPS placement, the frequency of episodes of overt HE was about 10% per month. The manifestation of HE before TIPS and/or reduced liver function were identified as independent risk factors.

SUMMARY OF RECOMMENDED TREATMENT OF HEPATIC ENCEPHALOPATHY IN CLINICAL PRACTICE

Treatment of acute HE

Treatment of acute HE in cirrhotics involves two steps. The first is to identify and to correct precipitating causes:

- gastrointestinal bleeding
- sedatives or tranquilizers
- infections
- hypovolemia, hypoxia, electrolyte imbalance, hypoglycemia.

R
Grade C

The second step is initiation of measures to lower blood ammonia concentrations using:

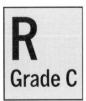

- lactulose enemas
- ornithine aspartate iv
- parenteral or enteral nutrition, if patient is unable to eat
- flumazenil if the patient has been given benzodiazepines.

Chronic therapy

Chronic management of the patient with recurrent HE requires individual adjustment of treatment. The titration of protein tolerance after an episode of acute HE should permit the design of an individual diet for each patient. Limitation of protein intake is reasonable in some patients, but protein restriction should be avoided if possible, since it will lead to negative nitrogen balance. In protein-intolerant patients, vegetable proteins are better tolerated than proteins derived from fish, milk, or meat. The supplementation of a low protein diet with branched chain amino acids should be considered. Additionally, patients may benefit from zinc and thiamin supplementation. The long term benefit of all other treatments (including lactulose and neomycin) is uncertain. The need for treatment of subclinical HE is not established and unproven therapy should be administered in the context of randomized controlled clinical trials.

REFERENCES

1 Ferenci P, Püspök A, Steindl P. Current concepts in the pathophysiology of hepatic encephalopathy. *Eur J Clin Invest* 1992; **22**: 573–81.

2 Conn HO, Lieberthal MM. *The hepatic coma syndromes and lactulose*. Baltimore, MD: Williams & Wilkins, 1979.

3 Conn HO, Leevy CM, Vlahcevic ZR *et al.* Comparison of lactulose and neomycin in the treatment of chronic portal-systemic encephalopathy. *Gastroenterology* 1977; **72**: 573–83.

4 Barbaro G, Di Lorenzo G, Soldini M *et al.* Flumazenil for hepatic encephalopathy grade III and IVa in patients with cirrhosis: an Italian multicenter double-blind, placebo-controlled, cross-over study. *Hepatology* 1998; **28**: 374–8.

5 Kircheis G, Nilius R, Held C *et al.* Therapeutic efficacy of L-ornithine-L-aspartate infusions in patients with cirrhosis and hepatic encephalopathy: results of a placebo-controlled, double-blind study. *Hepatology* 1997; **25**: 1351–60.

6 Stauch S, Kircheis G, Adler G *et al.* Oral L-ornithine-L-aspartate therapy of chronic hepatic encephalopathy: results of a placebo-controlled double-blind study. *J Hepatol* 1998; **28**: 856–64.

7 Marchesini G, Dioguardi FS, Bianchi GP *et al.* Long-term oral branched-chain amino acid treatment in chronic hepatic encephalopathy. A randomized double-blind casein-controlled trial. The Italian Multicenter Study Group. *J Hepatol* 1990; **11**: 92–101.

8 Michel H, Solere M, Granier P *et al.* Treatment of cirrhotic hepatic encephalopathy with L-dopa. A controlled trial. *Gastroenterology* 1980; **79**: 207–11.

9 Michel H, Pomier-Layrargues G, Aubin JP *et al.* Treatment of hepatic encephalopathy by infusion of a modified amino acid solution: results of a study in 47 cirrhotic patients. In: Capocaccia L, Fischer JE, Rossi-Fanelli F (eds) *Hepatic encephalopathy and chronic liver failure* New York/London: Plenum Press, 1984, pp 301–10.

10 Wahren J, Denis J, Desurmont P *et al.* Is intravenous administration of branched chain amino acids effective in the treatment of hepatic encephalopathy? A multicenter study. *Hepatology* 1983; **3**: 475–80.

11 Blanc P, Daures JP, Liautard J *et al.* Lactulose-neomycin combination versus placebo in the treatment of acute hepatic encephalopathy. Results of a randomized controlled trial. *Gastroenterol Clin Biol* 1994; **18**: 1063–8.

12 Strauss E, Tramote R, Silva EP *et al.* Double-blind randomized clinical trial comparing neomycin and placebo in the treatment of exogenous hepatic encephalopathy. *Hepatogastroenterology* 1992; **39**: 542–5.

13 Weissenborn K, Ruckert N, Hecker H *et al.* The number connection tests A and B: interindividual variability and use for the assessment of early hepatic encephalopathy. *J Hepatol* 1998; **28**: 646–53.

14 Schomerus H, Hamster W, Blunck H *et al.* Latent portosystemic encephalopathy I. Nature of cerebral functional defects and fitness to drive. *Dig Dis Sci* 1981; **26**: 622–30.

15 Rikkers L, Jenko P, Rudman D *et al.* Subclinical hepatic encephalopathy: detection, prevalence and relationship to nitrogen metabolism. *Gastroenterology* 1978; **75**: 462–9.

16 Conn HO. Trailmaking and number connection tests in the assessment of mental state in portal systemic encephalopathy. *Am J Dig Dis* 1977; **22**: 541–50.

17 JC Quero, IJ Hartmann, J Meulstee *et al.* The diagnosis of subclinical hepatic encephalopathy in patients with cirrhosis using neuropsychological tests and automated electroencephalogram analysis. *Hepatology* 1996; **24**: 556–60.

18 Groeneweg M, Quero JC, De Bruijn I *et al.* Subclinical hepatic encephalopathy impairs daily functioning. *Hepatology* 1998; **28**: 45–9.

19 Srivastava A, Mehta R, Rothke SP *et al*. Fitness to drive in patients with cirrhosis and portal systemic shunting: a pilot study evaluating driving performance. *J Hepatol* 1994; **21**: 1023–8.
20 Kullmann F, Hollerbach S, Holstege A *et al*. Subclinical hepatic encephalopathy: the diagnostic value of evoked potentials. *J Hepatol* 1995; **22**: 101–10.
21 Rosenberg W, Donald A. Evidence based medicine: an approach to clinical problem-solving. *Br Med J* 1995; **310**: 1122–6.
22 Naylor CD, O'Rourkee K, Detsky AS *et al*. Parenteral nutrition with branched-chain amino acids in hepatic encephalopathy. A meta-analysis. *Gastroenterology* 1989; **97**: 1033–42.
23 Blanc P, Daures JP, Rouillon JM *et al*. Lactitol or lactulose in the treatment of chronic hepatic encephalopathy: results of a meta-analysis. *Hepatology* 1992; **15**: 222–8.
24 Uribe M, Berthier J, Lewis H, *et al*. Lactose enemas plus placebo tablets vs. neomycin tablets plus starch enemas in acute portal systemic encephalopathy. A double-blind randomized controlled study. *Gastroenterology* 1981; **81**: 101–6.
25 Uribe M, Campollo O, Vargas-F *et al*. Acidifying enemas (lactitol and lactose) vs. nonacidifying enemas (tap water) to treat acute portal-systemic encephalopathy: a double-blind, randomized clinical trial. *Hepatology* 1987; **7**: 639–43.
26 Ferenci, P. Critical evaluation of the role of branched chain amino acids in liver disease. In: Thomas JC, Jones EA (eds), *Recent advances in hepatology* 2. New York: Churchill Livingstone, 1986, pp. 137–54.
27 Fabbri A, Magrini N, Bianchi G *et al*. Overview of randomized clinical trials of oral branched-chain amino acid treatment in chronic hepatic encephalopathy. *J Parent Ent Nutr* 1996; **20**: 159–64.
28 Morgan TR, Moritz TE, Mendenhall CL *et al*. Protein consumption and hepatic encephalopathy in alcoholic hepatitis. VA Cooperative Study Group #275. *J Am Coll Nutr* 1995; **14**: 152–8.
29 Plauth M, Merli M, Kondrup J *et al*. ESPEN Guidelines for nutrition in liver disease and transplantation. *Clin Nutr* 1997; **16**: 43–55.
30 Gyr K, Meier R, Haussler J *et al*. Evaluation of the efficacy and safety of flumazenil in the treatment of portal systemic encephalopathy: a double blind, randomized, placebo controlled multicenter study. *Gut* 1996; **39**: 319–25.
31 Pomier-Layrargues G, Giguere JF, Lavoie J *et al*. Flumazenil in cirrhotic patients in hepatic coma: a randomized double-blind placebo-controlled crossover trial. *Hepatology* 1994; **19**: 32–7.
32 Cadranel JF, el Younsi M, Pidoux B *et al*. Flumazenil therapy for hepatic encephalopathy in cirrhotic patients: a double-blind pragmatic randomized, placebo study. *Eur J Gastroenterol Hepatol* 1995; **7**: 325–9.
33 Van der Rijt CC, Schalm SW, Meulstee J *et al*. Flumazenil therapy for hepatic encephalopathy. A double-blind cross over study. *Gastroenterol Clin Biol* 1995; **19**: 572–80.
34 Tarao K, Ikeda T, Hayashi K *et al*. Successful use of vancomycin hydrochloride in the treatment of lactulose resistant chronic hepatic encephalopathy. *Gut* 1990; **31**: 702–6.
35 Bucci L, Palmieri GC. Double-blind, double-dummy comparison between treatment with rifaximin and lactulose in patients with medium to severe degree hepatic encephalopathy. *Curr Med Res Opin* 1993; **13**: 109–18.
36 Morgan MY, Hawley KE. Lactitol vs lactulose in the treatment of acute hepatic encephalopathy in cirrhotic patients: a double blind, randomized trial. *Hepatology* 1987; **7**: 1278–84.
37 Uribe-Esquivel M, Moran S, Poo JL *et al*. In vitro and in vivo lactose and lactulose effects on colonic fermentation and portal-systemic encephalopathy parameters. *Scand J Gastroenterol* 1997; 222 (Suppl):49.
38 Orlandi F, Freddara U, Candelaresi MT *et al*. Comparison between neomycin and lactulose in 173 patients with hepatic encephalopathy: a randomized clinical study. *Dig Dis Sci* 1981; **26**: 408–506.
39 Elkington SG, Floch MH, Conn HO. Lactulose in the treatment of chronic portal-systemic encephalopathy. A double-blind clinical trial. *N Engl J Med* 1969; **281**: 498–12.
40 Staedt U, Leweling H, Gladisch R *et al*. Effects of ornithine aspartate on plasma ammonia and plasma amino acids in patients with cirrhosis. A double-blind, randomized study using a four-fold crossover design. *J Hepatol* 1993; **19**: 424–30.
41 Sushma S, Dasarathy S, Tandon RK *et al*. Sodium benzoate in the treatment of acute hepatic encephalopathy: a double-blind randomized trial. *Hepatology* 1992; **16**: 138-44.
42 Horst D, Grace ND, Conn HO *et al*. Comparison of dietary protein with an oral, branched chain-enriched amino acid supplement in chronic portal-systemic encephalopathy: a randomized controlled trial. *Hepatology* 1984; **4**: 279–87.
43 Uribe M, Marquez MA, Ramos GG *et al*. Treatment of chronic portal-systemic encephalopathy with vegetable and animal protein diets. *Dig Dis Sci* 1982; **27**: 1109–16.
44 Bianchi GP, Marchesini G, Fabbri A *et al*. Vegetable versus animal protein diet in cirrhotic patients with chronic encephalopathy. A randomized cross-over comparison. *J Intern Med* 1993; **233**: 385–92.

45 Greenberger NJ, Carley J, Schenker S *et al.* Effect of vegetable and animal protein diets in chronic hepatic encephalopathy. *Dig Dis* 1977; **22**: 845–55.
46 Keshavarzian A, Meek J, Sutton C *et al.* Dietary protein supplementation from vegetable sources in the management of chronic portal systemic encephalopathy. *Am J Gastroenterol* 1984; **79**: 945–9.
47 Watanabe A, Sakai T, Sato S *et al.* Clinical efficacy of lactulose in cirrhotic patients with and without subclinical hepatic encephalopathy. *Hepatology* 1997; **26**: 1410–4.
48 Horsmans Y, Solbreux PM, Daenens C *et al.* Lactulose improves psychometric testing in cirrhotic patients with subclinical encephalopathy. *Aliment Pharmacol Ther* 1997; **11**: 165–70.
49 Loguercio C, Abbiati R, Rinaldi M *et al.* Long-term effects of *Enterococcus faecium* SF68 versus lactulose in the treatment of patients with cirrhosis and grade 1–2 hepatic encephalopathy *J Hepatol* 1995; **23**: 39–46.
50 Egberts EH, Schomerus H, Hamster W *et al.* Branched chain amino acids in the treatment of latent portosystemic encephalopathy. A double-blind placebo-controlled crossover study. *Gastroenterology* 1985; **88**: 887–95.
51 Plauth M, Egberts EH, Hamster W *et al.* Long-term treatment of latent portosystemic encephalopathy with branched-chain amino acids. A double-blind placebo-controlled crossover study. *J Hepatol* 1993; **17**: 308–14.
52 Nolte W, Wiltfang J, Schindler C *et al.* Portosystemic hepatic encephalopathy after transjugular intrahepatic portosystemic shunt in patients with cirrhosis: clinical, laboratory, psychometric, and electroencephalographic investigations. *Hepatology* 1998; **28**: 1215–25.

27 Hepatocellular carcinoma: screening and treatment

Massimo Colombo

Since the widespread adoption of ultrasound (US) scan for screening high risk patients, the number of patients identified with a small, potentially treatable hepatocellular carcinoma (HCC) has more than doubled.[1,2] However, due to the lack of randomized controlled studies, it is not clear whether the mortality rate for HCC has been reduced in parallel. Such features of the natural history of HCC as the long lasting subclinical incubation period of HCC that have been observed in many patients, as well as the large number of tumors which grow as a solitary mass to a size at which they can be detected by US, seem to favor screening programs. Conversely, in many patients such aspects of HCC as multinodal onset of the tumor and great variations in the growth rates of single nodes, with doubling volume times from 1 to 20 months, may hinder the effectiveness of screening.[3]

TARGET POPULATION

HCC is linked to environmental, dietary and lifestyle factors. Not surprisingly, therefore, epidemiological surveys were instrumental in identifying groups of individuals who are at risk for HCC. In two Consensus Conferences, held in Anchorage (Alaska, USA)[4] and in Milan (Italy),[5] patients with cirrhosis, chronic carriers of HBsAg, and patients with rare metabolic liver diseases were identified as populations at risk for HCC. The cost-effectiveness of screening would certainly be improved if we could assess an individual's cancer risk. However, this assessment is difficult because of individual variations in the metabolism of carcinogens, DNA repair capacities, genomic stability, and inherited cancer predisposition.

Patients with cirrhosis

Three to four percent of all patients with cirrhosis due to chronic viral hepatitis or alcohol abuse develop HCC each year.[6–8] HCC develops also in patients with chronic viral hepatitis without histological evidence of cirrhosis, but at lower incidence rates (1%).[9] HCC risk is particularly high in patients with cirrhosis and histological markers of increased liver cell proliferation. In a cohort study of 307 Italian patients with viral cirrhosis followed up for 4 years, HCC developed in 60% of 27 patients with liver cell dysplasia compared to 18% of 40 patients without it.[10] HCC risk was also high in cirrhotic patients with either fluctuating or persistently elevated serum levels of α-fetoprotein (AFP)[7,11] as well as in cirrhotic patients presenting with more than one risk factor for liver cell damage and regeneration (eg hepatitis B and C).[12] Liver cell regeneration is thought to be the crucial oncogenic event promoting selection and clonal expansion of committed hepatocytes after damage caused by genotoxic agents.

Chronic carriers of HBsAg

More than 250 million persons worldwide are persistently infected with HBV.[13] Epidemiological, clinical and experimental studies have established a strong link between chronic infection with this virus and HCC. HBV is responsible for both genotoxic lesions of the liver cells and tumor promotion through increased liver cell proliferation associated with persisting hepatitis. HBV does not necessarily require the step to cirrhosis to be oncogenic.[14] In a prospective cohort study in Taiwan, the risk of HCC in 3454 HBsAg carriers was 102 times greater than in 19 253 non-carriers.[15] However, the carriers at especially high risk for developing HCC were those with actively replicating HBV ($HBeAg^+$/$HBV\text{-}DNA^+$) and those with cirrhosis. Healthy carriers may develop HCC, but are at substantially lower risk.[16] Often, distinguishing between clinical subsets of HBsAg carriers may be difficult, unless the patients are periodically assessed with laboratory or histological investigations. The strong link between HBV and HCC has been further confirmed by the decrease of HCC that has been observed among Taiwanese children since the start of mass vaccination of all newborns against HBV.[17]

Patients with rare metabolic diseases

Patients with porphyria cutanea tarda, genetic hemochromatosis, alpha-1-antitrypsin deficiency, tyrosinemia, and hypercitrullinemia are also at high risk for HCC. Patients with glycogenosis type I and III, Wilson disease and hereditary fructose intolerance may also develop HCC, but are at substantially lower risk.[3] HCC has developed also in patients with primary biliary cirrhosis, probably reflecting treatment related improvement in patients' survival. HCC was also found in 64% of 160 Japanese patients and in 48% of 101 South African Blacks with Budd–Chiari syndrome.[18,19] However, in these studies the possible role of other unidentified carcinogens could not be excluded.

SCREENING TESTS

Serum AFP

AFP is a normal serum protein synthesized by fetal liver cells and by yolk sac cells. The normal range for serum AFP is 0–20 ng/ml for the healthy adults. Serum levels of 400 ng/ml are very suggestive of HCC. However, two-thirds of patients with small HCCs have less than 200 ng/ml and more than 30% of patients with HCC do not have abnormal circulating levels of AFP, even in advanced stages.[6–8,20] Moreover, in the range of 20–200 ng/ml, patients with chronic liver disease and false positive results due to hepatitis flares outnumber those with HCC.

In patients with borderline elevations of serum AFP, the microheterogeneity of the sugar component of AFP can be assessed by lectin affinity electrophoresis coupled with antibody affinity blotting. Serum AFP in patients with HCC has greater proportions of this atypical AFP than serum AFP of patients with cirrhosis. In a prospective study of 361 cirrhotics, 33 showed elevated atypical AFP 3–18 months before HCC was detected by imaging techniques.[11]

Abdominal ultrasound

To minimize the false results of AFP determinations, cirrhotics are undergoing surveillance by means of real-time US. As a general rule, a lesion seen as a discrete node in the liver should be presumed to be a preneoplastic lesion or HCC, and should be investigated accordingly. Most HCCs can be detected as a hypodysechoic mass.[21] Tumors may escape detection when located in the upper and posterior portion of the right lobe, an area that is technically difficult to assess by US, or because HCC nodes are present as isoechoic masses or are too small to be detected. One major problem in US screening of cirrhotics are false diagnoses due to regenerative macronodules smaller than 2 cm and small hyperechoic hemangiomas. In a 12-year prospective cohort study of 447 cirrhotics, we found that 83 patients had had an initial diagnosis of benign node that later turned out to be HCC in 7 (8%).

SCREENING STRATEGIES

In population based studies, most individuals are asymptomatic, and therefore the screening intervals can be easily standardized. Serum AFP is the screening method of choice for such studies because they include thousands of healthy persons and relatively few patients with liver disease who are at risk of false positive results with AFP. Between 1982 and 1992, 18 299 AFP determinations were performed on 2230 symptomless Alaskan natives who were HBsAg carriers.[22] At least one AFP determination was elevated (>25 ng/ml) for 371 persons, including 292 pregnant women, 24 patients with hepatitis related events, and 16 patients with HCC. Because of the high risk of false results, AFP is not appropriate for screening cirrhotics. Abdominal US is the screening and surveillance method of choice. In fact, in 25–60% of the cirrhotics studied by US, HCC would have gone undetected if the patients had been screened by AFP only (Table 27.1).[7,8,11] In a prospective cohort study of 447 cirrhotics in Milan, the negative predictive value of US was 92% and the positive predictive value was 66%. At the Milan Conference,[5] it was recommended that patients with cirrhosis or with certain congenital conditions known to

Table 27.1 Prospective cohort studies of patients with compensated cirrhosis undergoing surveillance by ultrasound examination

Study	Screening interval (mth)	Patients with cirrhosis (no.)	Hepatocellular carcinoma No.	Annual rate (%)	Single node (%)	<3 cm (%)	AFP(-) (%)
Sato, 1993[11]	3	361	33	3.0	88	64	41
Cottone, 1994[8]	6	157	30	4.4	87	53	60
[a]Colombo, 1998[7]	12	417	88	3.1	56	27	33

[a]Unpublished data.

be risk factors for HCC should be screened by US and AFP twice a year, whereas HBsAg carriers should be screened for HCC by determinations of serum AFP levels once a year.

R
Grade B/C

TREATMENT

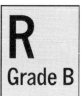

Treatment options have been selected according to the presence or absence of cirrhosis, number and size of tumors, and degree of hepatic deterioration. Staging is a crucial variable in treatment outcome, since many therapeutic failures have resulted from incorrect patient selection. When patients are scanned by biphasic spiral computed tomography (CT) during the arterial phase (about 20 seconds after the start of injection), highly vascularized tumors appear against a background of relatively unenhanced liver that is primarily enhanced during the late portal vein phase.[23] However, most tumors smaller than 2 cm are hypovascular and therefore escape detection with such gold standard staging techniques as biphasic spiral CT.[24] For staging clinical status, the Child–Pugh scoring system provides accurate estimates of patient survival. The 3-year survival of untreated patients with a small tumor and well compensated cirrhosis was approximately 25%.[25]

A review of treatments offered for this disease encounters a number of difficulties. First, few controlled trials comparing the efficacy of the available surgical or loco-regional ablative treatments have been performed. Second, there is substantial heterogeneity of survival between control groups in various trials, making it even riskier than usual to compare the results of small individual trials. Some trials have not been analyzed on the basis of intention to treat and probably yield exaggerated estimates of treatment effects.

PATIENTS WITH NORMAL LIVERS

Hepatic resection is the primary option for the few patients with HCC who present with normal livers and well preserved hepatic function. In two case series,[26,27] the cumulative 5-year survival for 128 such patients treated in two centers with hepatic resection was approximately 45%, compared to 12–26% for the 51 treated with orthotopic liver transplantation (OLT). The good results with hepatic resection probably depended on the absence of cirrhosis, which allowed for extensive resection of the liver without affecting survival. The poor results with OLT probably reflected bias in selection of patients, for example transplantation may have been performed in patients with advanced HCC who were judged to be unsuitable candidates for resection.

R
Grade B

PATIENTS WITH CIRRHOSIS AND A SMALL TUMOR

The functional capacity of the liver not involved by HCC is the major factor in these patients' prognosis. Thus, starting in 1950, surgical resection of the tumor was frequently performed in China and Japan for treating HCC in cirrhotic livers, with substantial benefit for patients with small tumors and well preserved hepatic function. More recently, in the wake of substantial improvements in transplantation technology and better understanding of the natural history of HCC, liver transplantation has gained more popularity as curative treatment for patients with HCC and cirrhosis.

Table 27.2 Five-year survival of patients with HCC treated by transplantation in 82 European centers between 1988 and June 1994

Indication for transplantation	No. of patients	% alive	
HCC with cirrhosis	361	46	
HCC without cirrhosis	446	34	
Cirrhosis with HCC	176	54	$P = 0.0004$

Source: European Transplantation Register, 1995

Orthotopic liver transplantation

Transplants eliminate both detectable and undetectable tumor nodes and all the preneoplastic lesions in the cirrhotic liver. Removal of the diseased liver also reduces the risk of morbidity and mortality from portal hypertension. Opposing these "pros" for OLT are several important "cons" for example, shortage of donated organs, high costs of the procedure, the need for stringent criteria for selection of patients, high risk of early tumor recurrence due to faulty staging of the disease and immunosuppression, and recurrence of hepatitis.

Overall survival after OLT has improved markedly since the introduction of cyclosporin and more accurate criteria for patient selection. One major obstacle to the interpretation of OLT results is the large differences between transplantation centers in terms of time lag between candidacy and operation. The best long term survivors (90% at 5 years) were patients for whom HCC was not the primary indication for OLT but was discovered by chance as a minute nodule during examination of the explanted liver.[27] Between January 1988 and June 1994, the 5-year survival of 834 patients with HCC (7% of total) who were given transplants in 82 European Centers was 39%. This included the 54.5% survival of 176 patients in whom cirrhosis was the primary indication for OLT and 45.5% of 361 cirrhotics in whom HCC was the primary indication (Table 27.2). In Milan, 48 consecutive patients with viral cirrhosis and a single <5 cm tumor or fewer than three <3 cm nodes were treated by OLT.[28] The 4-year actuarial survival was 92% for the 35 patients who were confirmed at the operation as having met the selection criteria, compared to 60% for the 13 patients who did not, because they were found to have ancillary nodes.

Although survival of transplanted patients seems to be largely influenced by tumor size and number, there is no general agreement on the ideal tumor size that entails the least risk of recurrence, mostly because small tumor volume does not mean an early biological stage for all cases. Indeed, vascular invasion by the tumor and perihepatic lymph nodes can occur even in patients with small HCCs.[26,27] Unfortunately, vascular invasion can be assessed only during the operation and lymph nodes can be precisely assessed only during laparoscopy or laparotomy. The most common cause of early death, within 3 months of OLT, was graft failure. In all studies, the most common cause of late death, from 3 months after OLT, was recurrence of the original tumor. The outcome of OLT may be influenced by recurrence of viral hepatitis, since infection of the graft may facilitate rejection and re-establish the oncogenic potential of the liver. The efficacy of interferon and the nucleoside analogue ribavirin against hepatitis C is under evaluation. For hepatitis B, hyperimmune gamma-globulins and the nucleoside analogue Lamivudine are protective but costly.[29,30]

Hepatic resection

Liver transplantation cannot be offered to all patients with cirrhosis who are found to harbor a small HCC. Thus, in many countries, hepatic resection remains the primary therapeutic option for these patients. Since the functional capacity of the remaining liver is a major factor affecting prognosis for patients undergoing hepatic resection, limited hepatic resections (segmentectomy and subsegmentectomy) are the technical procedures of choice. Since 1983 the widespread adoption of intraoperative US has changed the outlook of this treatment. The best results in terms of both short term and long term survival were for patients with single tumors less than 2 cm in diameter and well preserved hepatic function. In 347 Japanese patients, the 5-year survival rate was as high as 60.5%,[31] with very low mortality rates (0–5%). Considering all patients in Japan treated with hepatic resection, the most powerful predictor of survival was a combination of the three factors AFP, tumor size, and number of tumors.[32] Portal invasion by the tumor and metachronous multifocal tumorigenesis are the mechanisms by which HCC may recur after resection. In a series of 102 patients with tumors smaller than 3 cm, without portal vein invasion or intrahepatic metastases, recurrence 5 years after resection was recorded as 68%,[33] with the highest recurrence rates being observed in patients with more compromised hepatic function, for example high ALT and low albumin values. In fact, survival of patients undergoing hepatic resection is influenced not only by the tumor size and invasiveness, but also by the functional status of the liver expressed as the Child–Pugh score. The 3-year cumulative survival was 50% for 78 Japanese patients with single tumors and Child's A status, 35% for 26 with Child's B status and 0 for three with Child's C status.[34] For 72 European patients, these figures were 51% for Child's A patients and 12% for Child's B–C (Table 27.3).[35] In patients with Child–Pugh A cirrhosis, portal hypertension is the most reliable predictor of survival after resection. None of the 14 operated patients with less than 10 mmHg hepatic venous pressure gradient had had unresolved hepatic decompensation, compared to 11 of the 15 patients with higher gradients.[36] Thus, resection is definitely contraindicated for patients with deteriorated cirrhosis or severe portal hypertension in view of the high operative risk and short life expectancy. There are no controlled data demonstrating that chemotherapy improves the survival of resected patients by eradicating occult nests of tumor cells.[37] Also, there are no controlled studies comparing OLT and resection. In Paris[38] the policy for dealing with small tumors in cirrhotic patients is resection when it is feasible and transplantation when it is not. These procedures yielded similar medium term results: 50% (resection) and 47% (transplantation) survival at 3 years. However, the survival rates without recurrence were better after OLT than after resection (46% vs 27%). In patients with small single or

R
Grade B

R
Grade B

R
Grade B

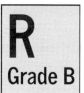

Table 27.3 Three-year survival of patients with a small HCC treated by hepatic resection, according to the degree of hepatic impairment (Child–Pugh class)

Liver stage	Nagasue, 1989[34]		Franco, 1990[35]	
(Child–Pugh)	No. treated	% alive	No. treated	% alive
A	78	50	54	57
B	26	35	14	
			+ }	12
C	3	0	4	

binodular tumors (<3 cm), transplantation had much better outcomes than resection (83% vs 13%).

PATIENTS WITH CIRRHOSIS NOT ELIGIBLE FOR SURGERY

Patients could be refused surgery because of advanced age, deteriorated liver function, large tumors, tumors localized in strategic positions or associated clinical conditions that contraindicate surgery.

Percutaneous interstitial treatments

R Grade B

R Grade B

Ultrasound guided interstitial treatments include tumor injection with absolute ethanol, 50% acetic acid or hot saline, or tumor thermoablation with radiofrequency, microwaves or laser. Most treatments were carried out with intratumor ethanol injection (PEI), which causes extensive coagulative necrosis of the tumor cells, and thrombosis of the tumor vessels, and is well tolerated. Up to 73% of the lesions treated with PEI underwent complete coagulative necrosis. Once more, survival was largely influenced by liver function, size, and number of tumors. The 5-year survival of 293 Italian patients with Child's A cirrhosis was 47%, compared to 29% for 149 with Child's B cirrhosis (Table 27.4).[39] Life expectancy of Child's A patients with a small tumor treated by PEI appeared to be as good as that of similar patients treated with hepatic resection, and associated with a low risk of severe complications (1.7%) and mortality (0.1%). In the multicenter study of PEI performed in Italy, the 5-year survival of 28 patients with larger than 5 cm HCC was 30% compared to 47% for the 392 patients with smaller than 5 cm tumors and compensated cirrhosis. The 5-year survival of 121 patients with two or three tumor nodes and compensated cirrhosis was 36%. PEI is thought to be successful for small HCCs because these tumors are often hypovascular, and therefore trap the injected ethanol better. In fact, patients with smaller than 2 cm tumors that were hypovascular by US–CO_2 scan survived longer than similar patients with hypervascular tumors (5-year survival rate: 86% vs 37%, $P = 0.02$).[24]

Tumor disease recurred in virtually all treated patients, more often in those with high levels of serum AFP and those without peritumoral capsule or with cirrhosis.[40,41] Up to 26% of the patients had loco-regional metastases of HCC; in the remaining cases, recurrence was due to development of second primary HCCs.[26,42] In 60 randomly selected patients with tumors smaller than 3 cm and compensated cirrhosis, injection with 50%

Table 27.4 Five-year survival of patients with cirrhosis and tumors smaller than 5 cm treated by percutaneous ethanol injection

Liver stage (Child–Pugh)	No. of patients	% alive
A	293	47
B	149	29
C	20	0

Source: Livraghi *et al.*, 1995[39]

acetic acid was superior to ethanol in terms of 2-year cancer-free survival (acetic acid 92%, alcohol 63%, $P = 0.02$, NNT = 3). The benefits of acetic acid injection appeared to be most marked in patients with hypervascular tumors.[43] However, this study may have a problem of patient selection, since the 3-year survival of patients treated with PEI was half that reported in previous studies in patients who appeared to be comparable with respect to tumor size and liver function. Retreatment of patients with tumor recurrence is thought to prolong patient survival.

R
Grade A

Radiofrequency thermoablation is safe and convenient in patients with compensated cirrhosis and a small HCC. An 8-minute course of thermoablation results in complete necrosis of a 3 cm tumor. However, radiofrequency may cause complications in patients with strategically located tumors and usually requires general anesthesia.[44] In a randomized trial of 86 patients with compensated cirrhosis and small HCC, radiofrequency was superior to PEI in terms of complete tumor necrosis (90% vs 80%), and numbers of treatments (1.2 vs 4.8), but it caused more complications (9.5% vs 0).[45]

R
Grade A

There are no guidelines on how to prevent tumor recurrence after percutaneous interstitial therapy. In a single randomized trial, the risk of second primary tumors in 44 patients who were successfully treated with hepatic resection or PEI was reduced by 12 months administration of polyprenoic acid.[46] The incidence of recurrent or new hepatomas at 38 months of follow-up was 49% in the placebo group and 22% in the treatment group ($P = 0.04$, NNT = 5).

R
Grade A

Transcatheter arterial chemo-embolization

Transcatheter arterial chemo-embolization (TACE) of HCC is possible because the liver has a dual blood supply, while HCC is supplied virtually only from the hepatic artery. TACE through the femoral artery leads to ischemic necrosis of the tumor and makes hepatic arterial injection of antitumor agents possible, giving higher local concentrations of drugs with fewer systemic adverse effects. TACE of the proximal hepatic artery (conventional TACE) has been widely employed in Eastern and Western countries as an alternative to hepatic resection and has now been improved, as segmental or subsegmental TACE. The procedure is contraindicated for patients with venous tumor supply (hypovascular tumors), advanced liver deterioration, complete thrombosis of the portal vein trunk, renal failure or extrahepatic metastases. In the past decade, three randomized controlled trials of TACE and one randomized controlled trial of transarterial embolization (TAE, without chemotherapy) treatment of patients with unresectable HCC have been conducted (Table

Table 27.5 Randomized controlled studies of transarterial embolization therapy in patients with advanced HCC

			1-yr survival		*P*-value
Study	Treatment	No. of patients	Treated (%)	Controls (%)	
Pelletier, 1990[47]	TACE	42	24	31	ns
Groupe d'Etude … (Trinchet), 1995[48]	TACE	96	62	44	ns
Pelletier, 1998[49]	TACE	73	51	55	ns
Bruix, 1998[50]	TAE[a]	80	70	80	ns

[a]Transarterial embolization without chemotherapy.

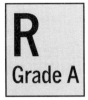

R Grade A

R Grade B

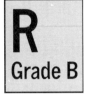

27.5).[47–50] One trial[48] showed a significant reduction of tumor growth in the treated patients. The substantial heterogeneity of survival between control groups suggests that the four studies included patients with different degrees of liver failure and tumor progression. Thus, we have chosen not to perform a meta-analysis of the results from the individual trials. However, no trial showed improved survival and TACE is not recommended for cirrhotic patients with a multifocal or large HCC. Conversely, non-controlled studies of segmental TACE in 63 Japanese patients with Child–Pugh A cirrhosis and small HCC reported 4-year survivals comparable to those for similar patients treated with resection or PEI.[51] Thus, TACE should be compared with these interventions in a randomized trial in patients with compensated cirrhosis and a small vascularized HCC.

Other treatments

R Grade A

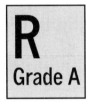

R Grade A

Systemic chemotherapy has been widely used to treat inoperable HCC, but the response rate is very low (20%). In the only randomized controlled trial[52] doxorubicin not only failed to prolong survival of 60 patients with inoperable HCC but also caused fatal complications in 15 (25%) due to cardiotoxicity. The possible sex hormone dependence of HCC and the presence of tumor hormone receptors have suggested a potential for hormonal manipulation of tumor growth, particularly using anti-estrogens. Initially, three small randomized controlled trials in patients considered to be unsuitable for any treatment because of advanced tumors or impaired hepatic function showed improved survival.[53–55] However, in two large randomized trials of 120 and 477 patients with inoperable HCC, but less deteriorated liver functions, treatment with the anti-estrogen tamoxifen did not improve survival or the quality of life, compared to controls.[56,57] Differences in patient selection reflected in large differences in survival between control groups may explain the contrasting results. The 1-year survival of control groups in the two studies which showed a benefit with tamoxifen was 5% and 9% compared to 43% and 56% for the two studies with negative results. A meta-analysis[57] of the five randomized studies comparing tamoxifen alone versus no active treatment yielded a pooled odds ratio of being alive at 1 year of 1.19 (95% CI 0.88–1.61).

Perhaps hormonal treatment of patients with inoperable HCC could be refined on the basis of the type of estrogen receptor expressed by tumor cells as indicated by the high response rate in patients with the wild-type estrogen receptor.[58] In a randomized trial of 58 patients with advanced HCC, treatment with subcutaneous octreotide 250 μg twice daily increased survival from 13% to 56% at 12 months.[59]

The conventional method of external irradiation is not effective against HCC. Using three-dimensional radiation planning (conformal radiotherapy) the beam scatter can be minimized to deliver the therapeutic dose, making selective irradiation of the liver possible. Local radiation was performed safely in patients with Child A cirrhosis and smaller than 8 cm tumor, with a partial response rate of 64%.[60] With proton radiation therapy, a large amount of radiation is focused only on the lesion, and the exposure of surrounding non-tumoral liver can be limited. Of 83 patients so treated only 19% had a complete response without any appreciable effect on survival.[61]

Acknowledgement

This work was supported by a grant from Fondazione Italiana Ricerca Cancro.

REFERENCES

1 Collier J, Sherman M. Screening for hepatocellular carcinoma. *Hepatology* 1998; **27**: 273–8.

2 Sallie R. Screening for hepatocellular carcinoma in patients with chronic viral hepatitis: can the result justify the effort? *Viral Hep Rev* 1995; **1**: 77–95.

3 Colombo M. Hepatocellular carcinoma in cirrhotics. *Semin Liv Dis* 1993; **13**: 374–83.

4 McMahon BJ, London T. Workshop on screening for hepatocellular carcinoma. *J Natl Cancer Inst* 1991; **83**: 916–19.

5 Colombo M. Early diagnosis of hepatocellular carcinoma in Italy. A summary of a Consensus Development Conference held in Milan, 16 November 1990 by the Italian Association for the Study of the Liver (AISF). *J Hepatol* 1992; **14**: 401–3.

6 Oka H, Kurioka N, Kim K *et al.* Prospective study of early detection of hepatocellular carcinoma in patients with cirrhosis. *Hepatology* 1990; **12**: 680–7.

7 Colombo M, de Franchis R, Del Ninno E *et al.* Hepatocellular carcinoma in Italian patients with cirrhosis. *N Engl J Med* 1991; **325**: 675–80.

8 Cottone M, Turri M, Caltagirone M *et al.* Screening for hepatocellular carcinoma in patients with Child's A cirrhosis: a 8 year prospective study by ultrasound and alphafetoprotein. *J Hepatol* 1994; **21**: 1029–34.

9 Tsukuma H, Hiyama T, Tanaka S *et al.* Risk factors for hepatocellular carcinoma among patients with chronic liver disease. *N Engl J Med* 1993; **328**: 1797–1801.

10 Borzio M, Bruno S, Roncalli M *et al.* Liver cell dysplasia is a major risk factor for hepatocellular carcinoma in cirrhosis: a prospective study. *Gastroenterology* 1995; **108**: 812–17.

11 Sato Y, Nakata K, Kato Y *et al.* Early recognition of hepatocellular carcinoma based on altered profiles of alpha-fetoprotein. *N Engl J Med* 1993; **328**: 1802–6.

12 Donato F, Boffetta P, Puoti M. A meta-analysis of epidemiological studies on the combined effect of hepatitis B and C virus infections in causing hepatocellular carcinoma. *Int J Cancer* 1998; **30**: 347–54.

13 Maynard JE. Hepatitis B: global importance and need for control. *Vaccine* 1990; **8**: S18–20.

14 Rogler CE. Cellular and molecular mechanisms of hepatocarcinogenesis associated with hepadnavirus infection. In: Mason WS, Seager C (eds), *Hepadnavirus molecular biology and pathogenesis.* Berlin: Springer-Verlag, 1991, pp 102–40.

15 Beasley RP. Hepatitis B virus. The major etiology of hepatocellular carcinoma. *Cancer* 1988; **61**: 1842–56.

16 de Franchis R, Meucci G, Vecchi M *et al.* The natural history of asymptomatic hepatitis B surface antigen carriers. *Ann Intern Med* 1993; **118**: 191–4.

17 Chang MH, Chen CJ, Lai MS *et al.* Universal hepatitis B vaccination in Taiwan and the incidence of hepatocellular carcinoma in children. *N Engl J Med* 1997; **336**: 1855–9.

18 Nakamura T, Nakamura S, Aikawa T *et al.* Obstruction of the inferior vena cava in the hepatic portion and the hepatic vein: report of eight cases and review of the Japanese literature. *Angiology* 1968; **19**: 479–98.

19 Kew MC, McKnight A, Hodkingson H *et al.* The role of membranous obstruction of the inferior vena cava in the etiology of hepatocellular carcinoma in Southern African Blacks. *Hepatology* 1989; **9**: 121–5.

20 Okuda K. Early recognition of hepatocellular carcinoma. *Hepatology* 1986; **6**: 729–38.

21 Okuda K. Hepatocellular carcinoma: recent progress. *Hepatology* 1992; **5**: 948–63.

22 McMahon BJ, Alberts SR, Wainwright RB *et al.* Hepatitis B sequelae: prospective study in 1400 hepatitis B surface antigen-positive Alaska Native carriers. *Arch Intern Med* 1990; **150**: 1051–4.

23 Ros PR, Davis GL. The incidental focal liver lesion: photon, proton or needle? *Hepatology* 1998; **27**: 1183–90.

24 Toyoda H, Kumuda T, Nakano S *et al.* The significance of tumor vascularity as a predictor of long-term prognosis in patients with small hepatocellular carcinoma treated by percutaneous ethanol injection. *J Hepatol* 1997; **26**: 1055–62.

25 Livraghi T, Bolondi L, Buscarini L *et al.* No treatment, resection and ethanol injection in hepatocellular carcinoma: a retrospective analysis of survival in 391 patients with cirrhosis. *J Hepatol* 1995; **22**: 522–6.

26 Ringe B, Pichlmayr R, Wittekind C *et al* Surgical treatment of hepatocellular carcinoma: experience with liver resection and transplantation in 198 patients. *World J Surg* 1991; **15**: 270–85.

27 Iwatsuki S, Starzl TE, Sheahan DG *et al.* Hepatic resection versus transplantation for hepatocellular carcinoma. *Ann Surg* 1991; **214**: 221–9.

28 Mazzaferro V, Regalia E, Doci R *et al.* Liver transplantation for the treatment of small hepatocellular carcinomas in patients with cirrhosis. *N Engl J Med* 1996; **334**: 693–9.

29 Samuel D, Muller R, Alexander G *et al.* Liver transplantation in European patients with the hepatitis B surface antigen. *N Engl J Med* 1993; **329**: 1842–7.

30 Bain VG, Kneteman NM, Ma MM *et al*. Efficacy of Lamivudine in chronic hepatitis B patients with active viral replication and decompensated cirrhosis undergoing liver transplantation. *Transplantation* 1996; **62**: 1456–62.
31 Tobe T, Arii S. Improving survival after resection of hepatocellular carcinoma: characteristics and current status of surgical treatment of primary liver cancer in Japan. In: Tobe T, Kameda H, Okudaira M *et al*. *Primary liver cancer in Japan*. Tokyo/Berlin: Springer, 1992, pp 215–20.
32 The Liver Cancer Study Group of Japan. Predictive factors for long term prognosis after partial hepatectomy for patients with hepatocellular carcinoma in Japan. *Cancer* 1994; **74**: 2772–80.
33 Adachi E, Maeda T, Matsumata T *et al*. Risk factors for intrahepatic recurrence in human small hepatocellular carcinoma. *Gastroenterology* 1995; **108**: 768–75.
34 Nagasue N, Yukaya H. Liver resection for hepatocellular carcinoma: results from 150 consecutive patients. *Cancer Chemother Pharmacol* 1989; **23**: S78–S82.
35 Franco D, Capussotti L, Smadja C *et al*. Resection of hepatocellular carcinomas. Results in 72 European patients with cirrhosis. *Gastroenterology* 1990; **98**: 733–8.
36 Bruix J, Castells A, Bosch J *et al*. Surgical resection of hepatocellular carcinoma in cirrhotic patients: prognostic value of preoperative portal pressure. *Gastroenterology* 1996; **111**: 1018–23.
37 Harada T, Shigemura T, Kodama S *et al*. Hepatic resection is not enough for hepatocellular carcinoma. A follow-up study of 92 patients. *Am J Gastroenterol* 1992; **14**: 245–50.
38 Bismuth H, Chiche L, Adam R *et al*. Liver resection versus transplantation for hepatocellular carcinoma in cirrhotic patients. *Ann Surg* 1993; **218**: 145–51.
39 Livraghi T, Giorgio T, Marin G *et al*. Hepatocellular carcinoma in cirrhosis in 746 patients: long-term results of percutaneous ethanol injection. *Radiology* 1995; **197**: 101–8.
40 Castellano L, Calandra M, Del Vecchio Blanco *et al*. Predictive factors of survival and intrahepatic recurrence of hepatocellular carcinoma in cirrhosis after percutaneous ethanol injection: analysis of 71 patients. *J Hepatol* 1997; **27**: 862–70.
41 Pompili M, Rapaccini GL, de Luca F *et al*. Risk factors for intrahepatic recurrence of hepatocellular carcinoma in cirrhotic patients treated by percutaneous ethanol injection. *Cancer* 1997; **79**: 1501–8.
42 Ebara M, Otho M, Sugiura N *et al*. Percutaneous ethanol injection for the treatment of small hepatocellular carcinoma. Study of 95 patients. *J Gastroenterol Hepatol* 1990; **5**: 616–26.
43 Ohnishi K, Yoshioka H, Ito S *et al*. Prospective randomized controlled trial comparing percutaneous acetic acid injection and percutaneous ethanol injection for small hepatocellular carcinoma. *Hepatology* 1998; **27**: 67–72.
44 Nagata Y, Abe M, Hiroada M *et al*. Radiofrequency hyperthermia and radiotherapy for hepatocellular carcinoma. In: Tobe T, Kameda H, Okudaira M *et al* (eds), *Primary liver cancer in Japan*. Tokyo/Berlin: Springer, 1992, pp 315–25.
45 Livraghi T, Goldberg SN, Lazzaroni S *et al*. Small hepatocellular carcinoma treatment with radio-frequency ablation versus ethanol injection. *Radiology* 1999; **210**(3): 655–61.
46 Muto Y, Moriwaki H, Ninomiya M *et al*. Prevention of second primary tumors by an acyclic retinoid, polyprenoic acid, in patients with hepatocellular carcinoma. *N Engl J Med* 1996; **334**: 1561–7.
47 Pelletier G, Roche A, Ink O *et al*. A randomized trial of hepatic arterial chemoembolization in patients with unresectable hepatocellular carcinoma. *J Hepatol* 1990; **11**: 181–4.
48 Groupe d'Etude et de Traitement du Carcinome Hépatocellulaire. A comparison of Lipiodol chemoembolization and conservative treatment for unresectable hepatocellular carcinoma. *N Engl J Med* 1995; **332**: 1256–61.
49 Pelletier G, Ducreux M, Gay F *et al*. Treatment of unresectable hepatocellular carcinoma with lipiodol chemoembolization: a multicenter randomized trial. *J Hepatol* 1998; **28**: 129–34.
50 Bruix J, Llovet JM, Castells A *et al*. Transarterial embolization versus symptomatic treatment in patients with advanced hepatocellular carcinoma: results of a randomized controlled trial in a single institution. *Hepatology* 1998; **27**: 1578–83.
51 Matsui O, Kodoya M, Yoshikawa J *et al*. Small hepatocellular carcinoma: treatment with subsegmental transcatheter arterial embolization. *Radiology* 1993; **188**: 79–83.
52 Lai CL, Wu PC, Chan GCB *et al*. Doxorubicin versus no antitumor therapy in inoperable hepatocellular carcinoma. A prospective randomized trial. *Cancer* 1988; **62**: 479–83.
53 Farinati F, Salvagnini M, De Maria N *et al*. Unresectable hepatocellular carcinoma: a prospective controlled trial with tamoxifen. *J Hepatol* 1990; **11**: 297–301.
54 Martinez Cerezo FJ, Tomas A, Donoso L *et al*. Controlled trial of tamoxifen in patients with advanced hepatocellular carcinoma. *J Hepatol* 1994; **20**: 702–6.
55 Elba S, Giannuzzi V, Misciagna G *et al*. Randomized controlled trial of tamoxifen versus placebo in inoperable hepatocellular carcinoma. *Ital J Gatroenterology* 1994; **26**: 66–8.

56 Castells A, Bruix J, Bru C *et al.* Treatment of hepatocellular carcinoma with tamoxifen: a double-blind placebo-controlled trial in 120 patients. *Gastroenterology* 1995; **109**: 917–22.

57 CLIP Group. Tamoxifen in treatment of hepatocellular carcinoma: a randomised controlled trial. *Lancet* 1998; **352**: 17–20.

58 Villa E, Camellini L, Dugani A *et al.* Variant estrogen receptor messenger RNA species detected in human primary hepatocellular carcinoma. *Cancer Res* 1995; **55**: 498–500.

59 Kouroumalis E, Skordilis P, Thermos K *et al.* Treatment of hepatocellular carcinoma with octreotide: a randomised controlled study. *Gut* 1998; **42**: 442–7.

60 Lawrence TS, Tesser RJ, Tam Haken RK. An application of dose volume histograms to the treatment of intrahepatic malignancies with radiation therapy. *Int J Radiat Oncol Biol Phys* 1991; **20**: 555–61.

61 Matsuzaki Y, Osuga T, Saito Y *et al.* A new, effective and safe therapeutic option using proton irradiation for hepatocellular carcinoma. *Gastroenterology* 1994; **106**: 1032–41.

28 Fulminant hepatic failure: treatment

Nick Murphy, Julia Wendon

INTRODUCTION

Intensive care medicine has developed over the past 40 years in response to the need to support failing organ systems in critically ill patients. The majority of methods used have been introduced without the prior benefit of controlled clinical trials.

The small numbers of patients and their heterogeneity within general intensive care units have hampered the search for proven remedies. This lack of evidence of benefit in intensive care medicine is also present in the treatment of patients with fulminant hepatic failure who require the full spectrum of organ support in the ICU.

The management of fulminant hepatic failure can be split into two main headings: (1) general supportive care and (2) therapies aimed at managing the failing liver and its complications.

Definition

In 1970 Trey and Davidson[1] introduced the term fulminant hepatic failure (FHF) to describe a syndrome of rapidly progressing liver failure in which encephalopathy follows

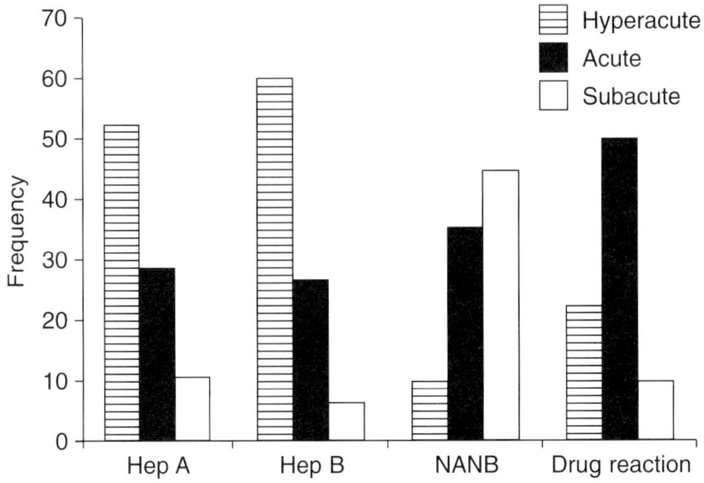

Figure 28.1 Speed of onset according to etiology. (Note that the majority of paracetamol poisoning would appear in the hyperacute group[4])

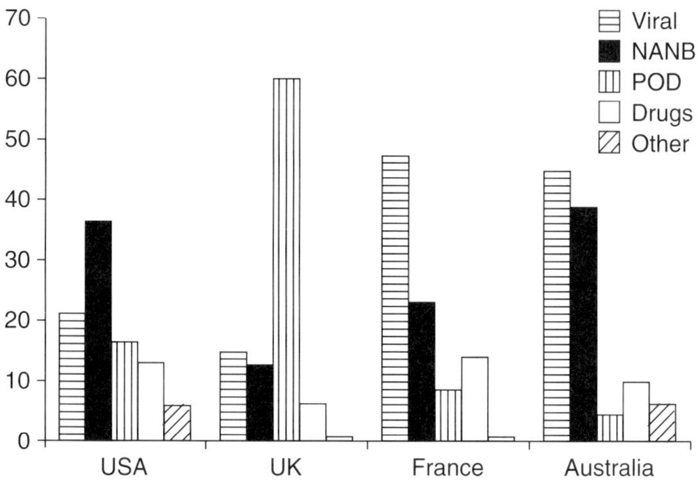

Figure 28.2 Etiology of FHF in some developed countries. POD, paracetamol overdose.

the onset of symptoms within 8 weeks in someone without previous liver disease. This definition is still used today; however, it has become clear that this definition is too broad and that subgroups exist. Both etiology and speed of progression to encephalopathy from the onset of jaundice can be used to define subgroups. This is important, as both factors have been shown to be independent predictors of prognosis[2] (Figure 28.1). Interestingly, it is the hyperacute group that have the best chance for spontaneous recovery, although it also carries the highest risk of cerebral oedema.[2,3]

Etiology

FHF has many causes (see Figure 28.2). World wide, viral hepatitis is by far the most common cause. Within the UK, paracetamol (acetaminophen) self-poisoning is the most frequent cause of FHF.

Pathogenesis

FHF is not a disease but a syndrome whose severity is proportional to the degree of hepatic necrosis. FHF causes profound physiological derangement characterized by encephalopathy, vasoparesis,[5] and coagulopathy. As the syndrome progresses, cerebral oedema[6] and renal failure are prominent and there is impaired immunity with increased susceptibility to infection.[7]

The rate of progression of FHF can be unpredictable in the hyperacute group. The syndrome typically evolves over several days, but deep coma can occur within hours. The mainstay of treatment in FHF is supportive while the decision to proceed to hepatic transplantation is being considered.

The cause of death in FHF can be split into two main groups: those with cerebral oedema who die of brain ischemia or brain stem compression, and those who succumb to sepsis and multiple organ failure.[8]

Intensive care management versus ward management

There have been no controlled clinical trials comparing intensive care with ward management, but considering the almost 100% mortality before the adoption of modern intensive care units[9] it seems likely that intensive care management improves mortality. Patients with grade III and IV encephalopathy should be intubated, ventilated, and managed within an intensive care unit. The use of high dependency areas for patients with liver failure and lower levels of coma is to be encouraged.[10]

Management in a liver unit

R
Grade C

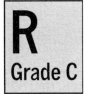

Again management of FHF in a liver unit has not been subjected to a controlled clinical trial but the access to a liver transplant program has obvious advantages. Survival rates for FHF with medical therapy alone in cases that progress to grade III or IV encephalopathy are poor, varying between 10 and 40%. With the introduction of orthotopic liver transplantation (OLT) as a therapeutic option for patients with FHF, survival rates have increased to 60–80%[11] (see Figure 28.3).

Criteria have been developed to help advise peripheral hospitals when patients should be transferred to a liver unit (see Box 28.1).[12] These criteria are based on clinical judgement and have not been subjected to a controlled clinical trial.

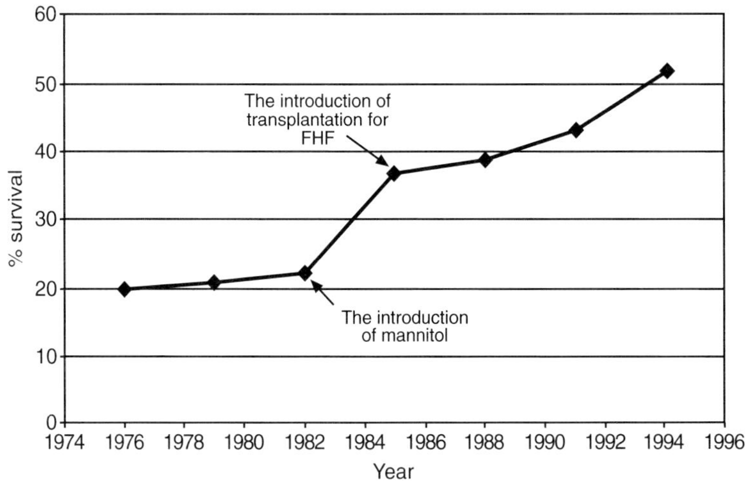

Figure 28.3 Improving survival in FHF

Box 28.1 Transfer criteria

INR >3.0
Prothrombin time in seconds greater than the time in hours since the overdose. (For paracetamol poisoning)
Any evidence of encephalopathy
Hypotension following fluid resuscitation
Evidence of a metabolic acidosis

GENERAL SUPPORTIVE MANAGEMENT

Fluid resuscitation and circulatory management

Patients with FHF develop marked hemodynamic changes. Vasodilatation can be profound and is invariably accompanied by a compensatory increase in cardiac output.[13] This distributive shock, with relative hypovolemia, causes hypotension despite the increased cardiac output. Prognostic criteria such as acidosis and renal function should only be assessed following adequate resuscitation, as there can be marked improvement in these following fluid replacement. There have not been any controlled clinical trials comparing fluid regimens in FHF. Recent systematic reviews comparing the use of crystalloids and colloids[14] and the use of human albumin solutions[15] in the critically ill found an excess mortality associated with colloid (4%) and albumin (6%) use. Both of these systematic reviews have been criticized within the medical literature,[16] mainly due to the limitations associated with the individual trials. The reviews used mortality as an outcome, which had not been used as an outcome measure in any of the individual studies. Widely different patient populations, from neonates to adults with severe burns, were included. The wide range of different fluids used in the colloid group again makes interpretation difficult.[17] Practice has not changed since the publication of these reviews and the reality is that albumin use has declined over the past: 10 years in response to the introduction of larger molecular weight and cheaper colloids. Properly conducted controlled clinical trials are needed, the results of which could be used as the basis for a change in current practice.

It is not known what endpoints for resuscitation should be used, and which vasopressors are most appropriate. A normal blood pressure cannot often be achieved with fluid infusion alone. While an adequate perfusion pressure is required, there are no firm data to define what is adequate. However, some assessment of tissue perfusion is needed. Central venous pressure (CVP) and pulmonary artery occlusion pressure (PAOP) are often used to assess preload and the adequacy of resuscitation, but the correlation between CVP, PAOP, and blood volume is poor.[18] The use of trends and the response to a series of fluid challenges improve their usefulness. Despite the limitations of using intravascular pressures to assess the adequacy of preload to the heart, PAOP is used as a marker for left ventricular end diastolic volume because of the lack of an available alternative. In practice it is used alongside clinical examination, together with assessment of adequate oxygen delivery.

The observational study by Connors *et al*[2] demonstrated an increased mortality associated with the use of the pulmonary artery catheter in critically ill patients during the first 24 hours of intensive care compared with case-matched control individuals.[2] However, the calls for a moratorium on the use of PA catheters following publication of this paper have not stopped their use. The results of prospective trials into the therapeutic use of PA catheter directed therapy are eagerly awaited.

R
Grade C

Pulmonary artery flotation catheterization has been used as both a diagnostic aid and a tool to assess the achievement of treatment targets (PAOP, oxygen delivery ($\dot{D}o_2$), consumption ($\dot{V}o_2$), and oxygen extraction ratio). There is no clear evidence whether PA catheters can be used to provide adequate endpoints for resuscitation or what targets should be aimed for. However, there is evidence that failure to achieve normal or greater than normal oxygen delivery in critical illness is associated with a poor outcome.[19]

Oxygen delivery or oxygen flux ($\dot{D}o_2$) is the amount of oxygen transported to the tissues of the body per unit time and is a product of cardiac output and blood oxygen content. In health $\dot{D}o_2$ far outstrips oxygen consumption until a critical level is reached below which consumption becomes dependent on delivery.

During the early 1970s it was first suggested that a pathological supply–dependency line is seen in critical illness.[20] This was proposed because markedly increased resting oxygen consumption was noted in critical illness associated with systemic inflammation. Oxygen delivery increases to meet the demand. It was noted that survivors had higher oxygen transport parameters than non-survivors and that if oxygen delivery was increased by fluid resuscitation and/or inotropic drugs, oxygen consumption also increased. This suggested that covert tissue hypoxia exists and that this could be the cause of multiple organ failure.

Work by Bihari and Gimson suggested the presence of a pathological supply–dependency for oxygen in patients with FHF. The patients with FHF who failed to survive had both a lower baseline $\dot{V}O_2$ than survivors and greater increases in $\dot{V}o_2$ following infusion of epoprosternol, suggesting a greater oxygen debt.[21] Whether improvements in mortality can be achieved by targeting survivor parameters in terms of oxygen in all critically ill patients or patients with FHF is unknown.

R Grade A

An early study in high risk surgical patients suggested an improvement in mortality.[22] This study has been criticized due to combination of two different pools of data using different randomization schemes to achieve the statistically significant result.[23] More recent randomized controlled trials investigating the augmentation of oxygen delivery have not shown any advantage when applied indiscriminately to all patients. In fact an increase in mortality was shown in a group of patients achieving supranormal goals with the aid of inotropes.[24] A European consensus conference concluded that the continued aggressive attempts to increase oxygen transport in all critically ill patients is unwarranted, although timely resuscitation and achievement of normal hemodynamics is essential.[25]

The whole premise of this debate, that there exists a pathological oxygen supply dependency in critical illness, has been questioned because of the inevitable increase in calculated oxygen consumption when delivery is increased due to mathematical coupling.[23] Studies are awaited in which changes in $\dot{V}o_2$ are measured directly via expired gas.

R Grade C

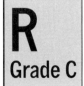

If the global increase in $\dot{D}o_2$ has not proved to be beneficial in critically ill patients, improvements in regional oxygenation and the prevention of regional ischemia may be a target for therapy. At present gastrointestinal intramucosal pH (pHi) is the only available method in clinical practice and it has been shown to be of greater value in monitoring trauma patients rather than monitoring oxygen transport parameters.[26] Therapy aimed at protecting the gut via selective splanchnic vasodilation may have a role in the prevention of multiple organ failure.[27] Dopamine probably enhances renal perfusion in the setting of low flow shock accompanying left ventricular dysfunction. However, in high output hypotension, such as sepsis and FHF, recent studies suggest that low dose dopamine does not increase renal perfusion (although it may increase urine volume by its natriuretic effects) and may actually divert blood flow away from the gastric mucosa.[28] Thus, at the present time low dose dopamine cannot be recommended in FHF. Experimental studies have shown that dopexamine can improve splanchnic oxygenation, and clinical studies also support an effect of dopexamine on splanchnic blood flow. However, the effects of dopexamine on pHi are inconclusive. Dobutamine has been shown both experimentally and clinically to consistently improve splanchnic blood flow and increase pHi.[27] Epinephrinee and norepinephrinee are effective agents and are frequently employed to improve MAP in FHF, commencing at 0.1 μg/kg per minute. Both of these agents have been shown to improve MAP. Significantly, the addition of epoprostenol (a microcirculatory vasodilator) to norepinephrinee increases oxygen delivery while maintaining MAP.[29] Epoprosternol has been shown in animal models to selectively increase splanchnic blood flow and to increase pHi in patients with septic shock.[27] The effects of norepinephrine and epinephrine on splanchnic perfusion are inconsistent.[27] α_1-adrenergic agonists such as norepinephrinee, and to a lesser extent dobutamine,[30] have also been shown to produce structural liver damage in a septic porcine model, as have β_2 antagonists.[30,31] Combinations of vasoactive drugs may prove to be more useful than any individual in the protection of the gut mucosa.

Blood pressure is important in maintaining flow to essential organs. The optimal target blood pressure in FHF is unknown. However, cerebral autoregulation is disturbed in FHF, making cerebral blood flow directly proportional to cerebral perfusion pressure.[32] This implies that hypotension will result in cerebral ischemia, which may be a factor precipitating brain swelling in FHF,[33] and that hypertension will result in cerebral hyperemia and increased ICP.

Mechanical ventilation

Intubation of the trachea and mechanical ventilation is indicated for several reasons in FHF but not usually for hypoxemia.[13] As patients progress from grade II to grade III encephalopathy, decreasing consciousness can lead to airway compromise with the risk of aspiration. Grade III encephalopathy is often characterized by agitation and aggressive behaviour. Sedation in these patients is required to allow appropriate monitoring and treatment but requires intubation and ventilation.

As opposed to other causes of systemic inflammatory response syndrome, the lungs are relatively spared early in the course of FHF. However, a proportion of patients progress to multiple organ dysfunction in which lung disease is prominent.[34]

The normal lung can tolerate "conventional" ventilation with physiological tidal volumes and low levels of positive end expiratory pressure (PEEP) for extended periods without apparent harm. The situation is different for damaged lungs and particularly so in patients with acute respiratory distress syndrome (ARDS). There is increasing evidence that mechanical ventilation in the setting of ARDS can increase lung injury and negatively impinge on outcome. Ventilator induced lung injury (VILI) encompasses a wide spectrum of damage, consisting of conventional barotrauma, pneumothorax, pneumomediastinum, and alveolar damage increasing pulmonary edema.[35] Recent controlled clinical trials have shown improvements in mortality with a protective ventilatory strategy[36] and a recent consensus conference has recommended certain steps to minimize damage to the lungs during mechanical ventilation.[37]

R Grade A

- Minimize the inspired oxygen level and take aggressive steps to do this if the inspired fraction is greater than 0.65.
- Recruit alveoli by increasing PEEP. The amount of PEEP necessary to prevent cyclic opening and closure of alveoli is approximately 10–15 cmH_2O.
- Minimize high airway pressures. Transalveolar pressures should not exceed 25–30 cmH_2O. This corresponds to an end inspiratory static (plateau) pressure of 30–40 cmH_2O.
- Prevent atelectasis by employing larger breaths periodically to re-expand collapsed units during tidal ventilation with small tidal volumes.

Sedation and paralysis

Patients with acute hepatic failure requiring mechanical ventilation are deeply encephalopathic. The need for sedation varies between patients and should be tailored individually. Sedation scoring with, for example, the 6-point Ramsay scale[38] has not been validated in FHF and is difficult to interpret in the setting of hepatic encephalopathy. Mechanical ventilation is usually tolerated with minimum amounts of opiate and little if any hypnotic agent. Deep sedation is unnecessary and will only add to cardiovascular depression and prolong recovery in patients with impaired liver function. These considerations, however, have to be balanced with the need to prevent surges in intracranial pressure during routine nursing care. Supplemental sedation or small doses of non-depolarizing neuromuscular blocker may be useful during suctioning of the patient's trachea. The issue of paralysis in FHF should be considered. It had been common practice to paralyse all ventilated patients with FHF while they are at risk from cerebral oedema. However, there have not been any controlled clinical trials of paralysis in FHF, or in other critically ill patients. A recent retrospective review of 1030 patients with acute traumatic brain injury showed that ICU stay and infectious complications were higher in patients who received routine paralysis.[39] Many anecdotal reports have also suggested an association between long term paralysis and a necrotizing myopathy that may prolong ICU stay and impinge adversely on outcome.[40,41] Thus, there is no indication for routine paralysis in FHF.

R
Grade C

Nutrition in FHF, enteral versus parenteral nutrition

It seems obvious that nutrition is of benefit in critically ill patients but this has not been proven in controlled clinical trials. Data from the hunger strikes in Northern Ireland and from Nazi Germany confirm that death is inevitable within 60–80 days without nutrition, providing that fluids and electrolytes are given.

In common with other forms of critical illness, FHF is associated with increased catabolism. Depending on the severity of the injury and the duration of the disease, weight loss associated with the loss of body fat and skeletal muscle mass may vary from being relatively insignificant to being life-threatening, primarily through the development of immunosuppression and reduced or delayed wound healing and tissue repair.[42,43] The loss of body protein cannot be prevented by nutrition but the rate of loss can be slowed. It is the treatment of the underlying problem that eventually reverses the catabolic phase of the illness and it is at that time that anabolism can be promoted by nutrition.[44]

R
Grade C

The route used in supplying nutrition is more easily compared. Where possible, enteral nutrition is the preferred method. Intestinal stimulation from enteral nutrition helps to maintain the gastrointestinal integrity and results in reduced infection rates when compared to total parenteral nutrition.[45] Recent interest has been shown in the supplementation of both enteral nutrition and TPN. Immuno-enhanced enteral feeds containing arginine, purine nucleotides, and omega-3 fatty acids have been compared with standard enteral nutrition in intensive care units. There appears to be a reduction in the number of infectious complications and other adverse events, including length of hospital stay and the number of days on ventilation.[46] However, this reduction in morbidity has not yet translated into a decrease in mortality.[46,47]

R
Grade A

TPN when given to well nourished elective surgical patients preoperatively actually results in an increase in postoperative infectious complications.[48] The risk of coagulase-negative staphylococcal bacteremia in neonates is increased six times by the administration of lipid emulsions.[49] The Veterans Affairs group found that a group of severely malnourished patients benefited from 10 days perioperative TPN.[48] However, TPN has not been shown to benefit patients with FHF, or other critically ill patients.

Glutamine is a non-essential amino acid in health. During critical illness, because of its central role in protein metabolism, glutamine deficiency is common. Original TPN formulations did not contain glutamine because of problems with its stability in solution and standard enteral feed contains minimal amounts. There is evidence that glutamine-enriched TPN can reduce gut atrophy, infectious complications, and 6-month mortality in critically ill patients.[50] A recent randomized trial supports the view that glutamine-enhanced nutrition is of benefit in critical illness.[51]

R Grade A

Stress ulcer prophylaxis

Many small randomized controlled clinical trials over the past 20 years have looked at the prevention of stress ulceration. While the incidence of stress ulcer has fallen over this period, the cause of this decline is unclear. It is probably the result of both improved resuscitation and the widespread use of stress ulcer prophylaxis.

H_2-blockers are effective in the prevention of stress ulceration in FHF. Macdougall *et al*[52] investigated the effects of H_2-blockers and antacid solutions in two small controlled trials. They found a significant decrease in the incidence of stress ulceration and blood transfusions with the use of H_2-blockers, but not with antacids. There was a trend toward an improved survival in the treated patients but this was not statistically significant.[52]

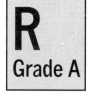

R Grade A

Stress ulceration is probably the result of ischemic injury to the gastric mucosa, and adequate resuscitation is the single most important factor in its prevention. Apart from good general ICU care there have been two broad approaches to reducing the incidence of stress ulceration: decreasing the acidity of the stomach with the use of antacids, H_2-blockers, or proton pump inhibitors, and the use of sucralfate, a cytoprotective agent. The role of acid suppression in encouraging an increase in bacterial overgrowth, and the ensuing microaspiration of colonized pharyngeal fluid thus promoting the development of hospital acquired pneumonia, has led to the comparison of the ulcer, pneumonia, and mortality rates between the two methods.

Recently several meta-analyses have attempted to resolve the uncertainty regarding efficacy on one hand and adverse effects of the drugs on the other.[53] After combining their efforts, the two main groups of investigators published a meta-analysis which included all relevant published and unpublished randomized clinical trials.[54] The meta-analysis demonstrated similar efficacy for H_2-blockers and sucralfate for the outcome of reduction in stress ulceration bleeding, but an increase in the incidence of pneumonia and an excess mortality in the H_2-blocker group.[54] A more recent trial conducted by some of the same authors suggests a significantly higher rate of stress ulceration with sucralfate compared to ranitidine without any difference in pneumonia or mortality rates.[55]

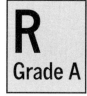

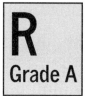

R Grade A

R Grade A

FHF was excluded in most of the trials comparing sucralfate to pH-altering drugs and was not included in the meta-analysis. It is therefore difficult to make firm conclusions. Patients with FHF tend to fall into the high risk group by virtue of both being ventilated and having a coagulopathy. The balance of evidence suggests that pH-altering drugs such as H_2-blockers or proton pump inhibitors provide the best defence against stress ulceration, but that this may be offset by an increased incidence of pneumonia.

Prophylactic antibiotics and selective decontamination of the digestive tract

Patients with acute liver failure (ALF) have increased susceptibility to infections, principally as a result of impaired phagocytic function, reduced complement levels, and the need for invasive procedures[56] Bacteriologically proven infection is recorded in up to 80% of patients with FHF, and fungal infection (predominantly candidiasis) in 32%. Clinical signs such as fever and elevated WBC are absent in 30% of the cases. Pneumonia accounts for 50% of infective episodes.[7] Risk factors for infection that have been identified are a high maximum INR, grade III or IV encephalopathy, and intubation of the trachea.[56,57]

Because of the high incidence of infection the use of prophylactic antimicrobial agents has been investigated. Both parenteral antibiotics and the use of selective decontamination of the digestive tract (SDD), in combination and individually, have been studied.

Intravenous antibiotics if given prophylactically will reduce the incidence of infection in patients with FHF to approximately 20%.[56,57] Grade A However, the use of prophylactic antibiotics has not been shown to improve outcome or reduce the length of stay in patients with FHF.[56] The role of SDD is less clear and has not been evaluated in controlled trials compared with placebo or intravenous antibiotics alone in FHF. Rolando reported that SDD used in combination with intravenous antibiotics provided no additional benefit.[56–58] Grade A

The most recent systematic review of randomized controlled trials of antibiotic prophylaxis in intensive care units was published in the Cochrane database of systematic reviews.[59] This systematic review evaluated 32 RCTs, which included 5639 unselected general ICU patients. Selected groups, eg patients with FHF, were excluded from the review. Pooled estimates of the 16 RCTs testing the effect of the SDD and systemic antibiotic combination indicate a significant reduction of both respiratory tract infections (OR 0.35, 95% CI 0.29–0.41) and total mortality (OR 0.80, 95% CI 0.68–0.93) (Figure 28.4). The number needed to treat to prevent one infection is 5, and the NNT to prevent one death is 23. When the data on the effect of SDD alone compared to control were pooled from the 16 available trials a marked reduction in respiratory tract infections was demonstrated (OR 0.56, 95% CI 0.46–0.68) but no corresponding effect on overall mortality (OR 1.01, 95% CI 0.84–1.22) was found (Figure 28.5).

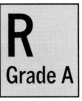

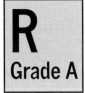

R Grade A

R Grade A

Although prophylactic intravenous antibiotics have been shown to reduce the number of proven infections in FHF, improvements in outcome have not been demonstrated. SDD on its own has not been shown to reduce infection or improve outcome in FHF. There is also a risk of promoting the emergence of multiply resistant organisms within intensive care units by the blanket use of broad spectrum antimicrobials. SDD selects for an increase in Gram-positive organisms, especially methicillin resistant staphylococcus (MRSA) and vancomycin resistant enterococcus (VRE). Future research should be aimed at determining the cost-effectiveness of SDD, with inclusion of estimates of the effects of the emergence of resistant microorganisms. However, for the individual patient the evidence in favor of the use of prophylactic antimicrobials is compelling.

MANAGEMENT OF CEREBRAL EDEMA

The etiology of cerebral edema in acute liver failure is an area of active research. The link with increasing grade of encephalopathy, the relative absence of cerebral edema in

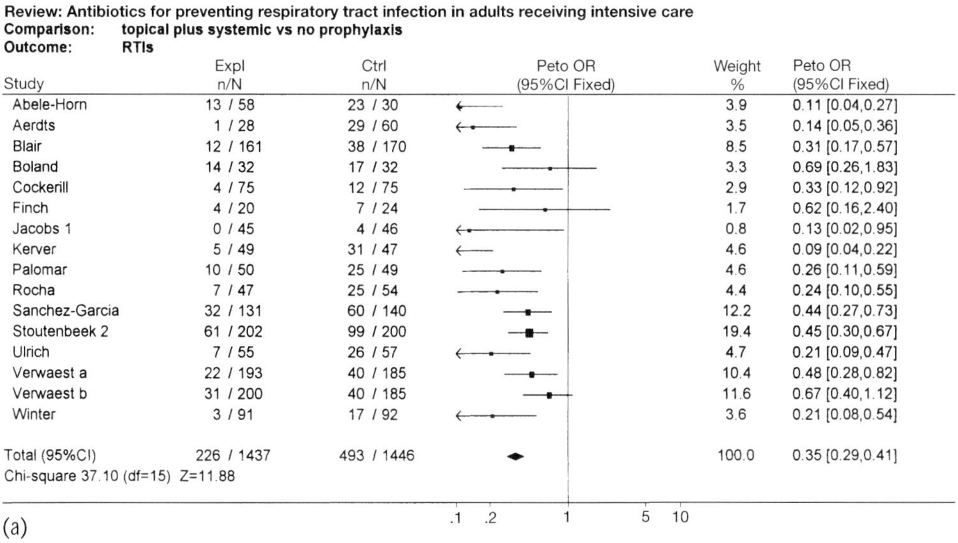

Review: Antibiotics for preventing respiratory tract infection in adults receiving intensive care
Comparison: topical plus systemic vs no prophylaxis
Outcome: RTIs

Study	Expl n/N	Ctrl n/N	Weight %	Peto OR (95%CI Fixed)
Abele-Horn	13 / 58	23 / 30	3.9	0.11 [0.04,0.27]
Aerdts	1 / 28	29 / 60	3.5	0.14 [0.05,0.36]
Blair	12 / 161	38 / 170	8.5	0.31 [0.17,0.57]
Boland	14 / 32	17 / 32	3.3	0.69 [0.26,1.83]
Cockerill	4 / 75	12 / 75	2.9	0.33 [0.12,0.92]
Finch	4 / 20	7 / 24	1.7	0.62 [0.16,2.40]
Jacobs 1	0 / 45	4 / 46	0.8	0.13 [0.02,0.95]
Kerver	5 / 49	31 / 47	4.6	0.09 [0.04,0.22]
Palomar	10 / 50	25 / 49	4.6	0.26 [0.11,0.59]
Rocha	7 / 47	25 / 54	4.4	0.24 [0.10,0.55]
Sanchez-Garcia	32 / 131	60 / 140	12.2	0.44 [0.27,0.73]
Stoutenbeek 2	61 / 202	99 / 200	19.4	0.45 [0.30,0.67]
Ulrich	7 / 55	26 / 57	4.7	0.21 [0.09,0.47]
Verwaest a	22 / 193	40 / 185	10.4	0.48 [0.28,0.82]
Verwaest b	31 / 200	40 / 185	11.6	0.67 [0.40,1.12]
Winter	3 / 91	17 / 92	3.6	0.21 [0.08,0.54]
Total (95%CI)	226 / 1437	493 / 1446	100.0	0.35 [0.29,0.41]
Chi-square 37.10 (df=15) Z=11.88				

(a)

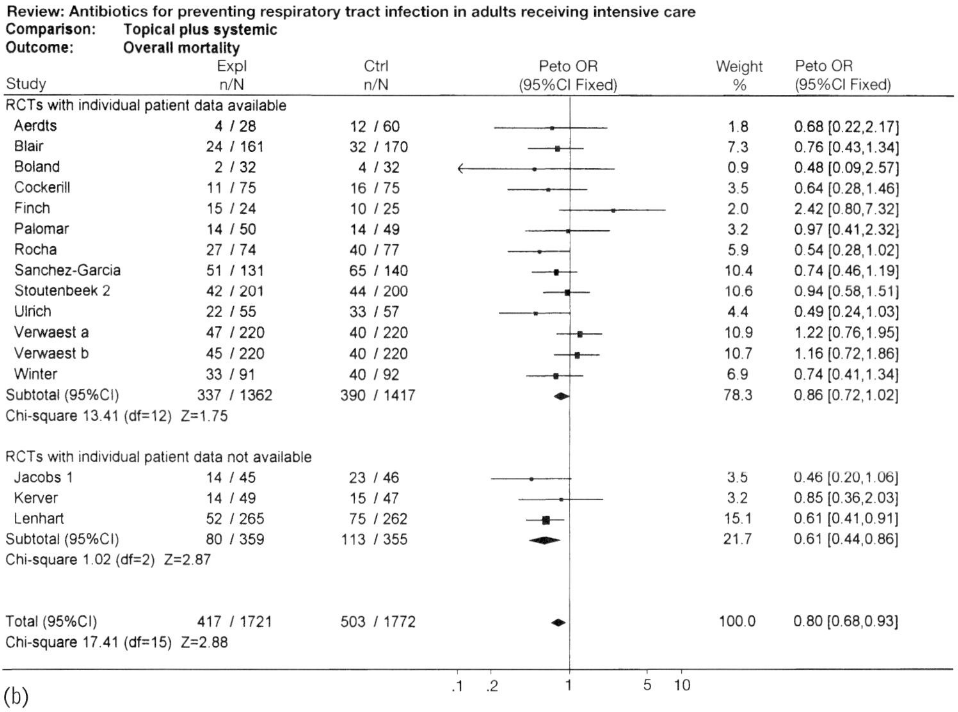

Review: Antibiotics for preventing respiratory tract infection in adults receiving intensive care
Comparison: Topical plus systemic
Outcome: Overall mortality

Study	Expl n/N	Ctrl n/N	Weight %	Peto OR (95%CI Fixed)
RCTs with individual patient data available				
Aerdts	4 / 28	12 / 60	1.8	0.68 [0.22,2.17]
Blair	24 / 161	32 / 170	7.3	0.76 [0.43,1.34]
Boland	2 / 32	4 / 32	0.9	0.48 [0.09,2.57]
Cockerill	11 / 75	16 / 75	3.5	0.64 [0.28,1.46]
Finch	15 / 24	10 / 25	2.0	2.42 [0.80,7.32]
Palomar	14 / 50	14 / 49	3.2	0.97 [0.41,2.32]
Rocha	27 / 74	40 / 77	5.9	0.54 [0.28,1.02]
Sanchez-Garcia	51 / 131	65 / 140	10.4	0.74 [0.46,1.19]
Stoutenbeek 2	42 / 201	44 / 200	10.6	0.94 [0.58,1.51]
Ulrich	22 / 55	33 / 57	4.4	0.49 [0.24,1.03]
Verwaest a	47 / 220	40 / 220	10.9	1.22 [0.76,1.95]
Verwaest b	45 / 220	40 / 220	10.7	1.16 [0.72,1.86]
Winter	33 / 91	40 / 92	6.9	0.74 [0.41,1.34]
Subtotal (95%CI)	337 / 1362	390 / 1417	78.3	0.86 [0.72,1.02]
Chi-square 13.41 (df=12) Z=1.75				
RCTs with individual patient data not available				
Jacobs 1	14 / 45	23 / 46	3.5	0.46 [0.20,1.06]
Kerver	14 / 49	15 / 47	3.2	0.85 [0.36,2.03]
Lenhart	52 / 265	75 / 262	15.1	0.61 [0.41,0.91]
Subtotal (95%CI)	80 / 359	113 / 355	21.7	0.61 [0.44,0.86]
Chi-square 1.02 (df=2) Z=2.87				
Total (95%CI)	417 / 1721	503 / 1772	100.0	0.80 [0.68,0.93]
Chi-square 17.41 (df=15) Z=2.88				

(b)

Figure 28.4 (a) and (b) (Source: Antibiotics for preventing respiratory tract infections (Cochrane Review). In: *The Cochrane Library*, issue 2, 1999. Oxford: Update Software)

encephalopathic patients with chronic liver disease and the increased incidence in those with hyperacute FHF, continue to be debated.

Both cytotoxic and to a lesser extent vasogenic mechanisms seem to play a role in the etiology of brain swelling during FHF. Accumulation of glutamine within astrocytes may be a cause of increased osmolar activity. The increase in glutamine due to combination of ammonia with glutamate, via the action of glutamine synthetase, a reaction localized to

Review: Antibiotics for preventing respiratory tract infection in adults receiving intensive care
Comparison: topical vs control
Outcome: RTIs

Study	Expl n/N	Ctrl n/N	Weight %	Peto OR (95%CI Fixed)
topical plus systemic vs systemic				
Ferrer	7 / 51	11 / 50	3.8	0.57 [0.21,1.58]
Hammond	25 / 162	30 / 160	11.7	0.79 [0.44,1.41]
Laggner	1 / 33	4 / 34	1.2	0.29 [0.05,1.76]
Lingnau a	38 / 90	71 / 177	14.8	1.09 [0.65,1.83]
Lingnau b	34 / 90	71 / 177	14.7	0.91 [0.54,1.52]
Stoutenbeek 1	2 / 49	8 / 42	2.3	0.22 [0.06,0.82]
Subtotal (95%CI)	107 / 475	195 / 640	48.5	0.81 [0.61,1.08]
Chi-square 6.98 (df=5) Z=1.42				
topical vs no prophylaxis				
Brun-Buisson	3 / 65	6 / 68	2.2	0.52 [0.13,1.99]
Gastinne	26 / 220	33 / 225	13.1	0.78 [0.45,1.35]
Georges	4 / 31	15 / 33	3.5	0.22 [0.07,0.62]
Jacobs 2	3 / 35	4 / 35	1.6	0.73 [0.16,3.45]
Korinek	20 / 96	37 / 95	10.3	0.42 [0.23,0.78]
Pugin	4 / 38	24 / 41	4.7	0.13 [0.05,0.32]
Quinio	19 / 76	38 / 73	9.1	0.32 [0.17,0.62]
Rodriguez-Roldan	1 / 14	11 / 17	1.9	0.10 [0.02,0.40]
Unertl	1 / 19	9 / 20	2.0	0.13 [0.03,0.54]
Wiener	8 / 30	8 / 31	3.1	1.04 [0.34,3.24]
Subtotal (95%CI)	89 / 624	185 / 638	51.5	0.39 [0.30,0.52]
Chi-square 23.31 (df=9) Z=6.58				
Total (95%CI)	196 / 1099	380 / 1278	100.0	0.56 [0.46,0.68]
Chi-square 43.02 (df=15) Z=5.71				

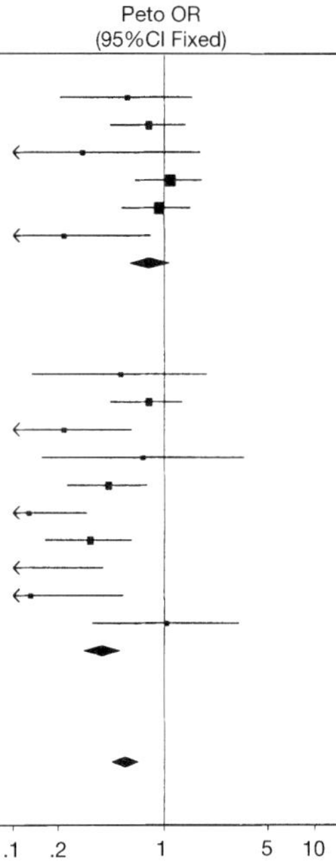

(a)

Review: Antibiotics for preventing respiratory tract infection in adults receiving intensive care
Comparison: topical vs control
Outcome: overall mortality

Study	Expl n/N	Ctrl n/N	Weight %	Peto OR (95%CI Fixed)
topical plus systemic vs systemic				
Ferrer	15 / 51	14 / 50	4.8	1.07 [0.45,2.52]
Gaussorgues	29 / 59	29 / 59	6.9	1.00 [0.49,2.05]
Hammond	34 / 162	31 / 160	12.0	1.10 [0.64,1.90]
Laggner	9 / 33	14 / 34	3.5	0.54 [0.20,1.48]
Lingnau a	9 / 90	17 / 177	4.9	1.05 [0.45,2.46]
Lingnau b	13 / 90	17 / 177	5.5	1.62 [0.73,3.62]
Stoutenbeek 1	2 / 49	8 / 42	2.1	0.22 [0.06,0.82]
Subtotal (95%CI)	111 / 534	130 / 699	39.6	0.98 [0.73,1.32]
Chi-square 8.08 (df=6) Z=0.14				
topical vs no prophylaxis				
Brun-Buisson	14 / 65	15 / 68	5.3	0.97 [0.43,2.20]
Cerra	13 / 25	10 / 23	2.8	1.40 [0.46,4.29]
Gastinne	88 / 220	82 / 225	24.3	1.16 [0.79,1.70]
Georges	3 / 31	5 / 33	1.6	0.61 [0.14,2.66]
Jacobs 2	15 / 35	19 / 35	4.1	0.64 [0.25,1.62]
Korinek	22 / 96	17 / 95	7.2	1.36 [0.67,2.74]
Pugin	10 / 38	11 / 41	3.6	0.97 [0.36,2.63]
Quinio	12 / 76	10 / 73	4.4	1.18 [0.48,2.91]
Rodriguez-Roldan	5 / 14	7 / 17	1.7	0.80 [0.19,3.34]
Unertl	5 / 19	6 / 20	1.9	0.84 [0.21,3.32]
Wiener	11 / 30	15 / 31	3.5	0.62 [0.23,1.71]
Subtotal (95%CI)	198 / 649	197 / 661	60.4	1.04 [0.81,1.32]
Chi-square 4.05 (df=10) Z=0.30				
Total (95%CI)	309 / 1183	327 / 1360	100.0	1.01 [0.84,1.22]
Chi-square 12.22 (df=17) Z=0.14				

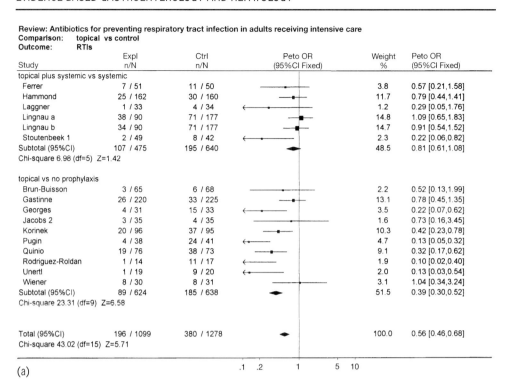

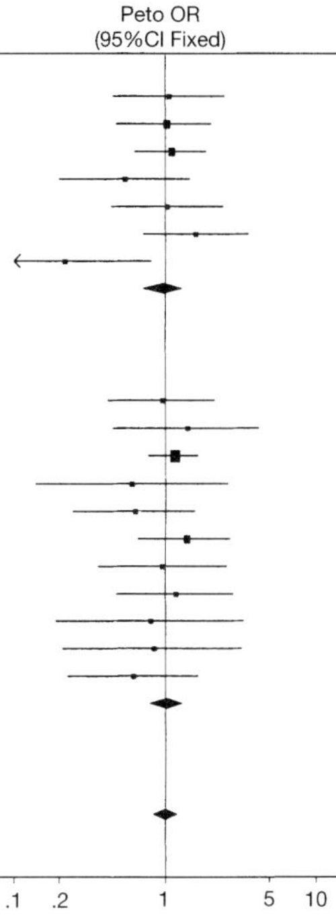

(b)

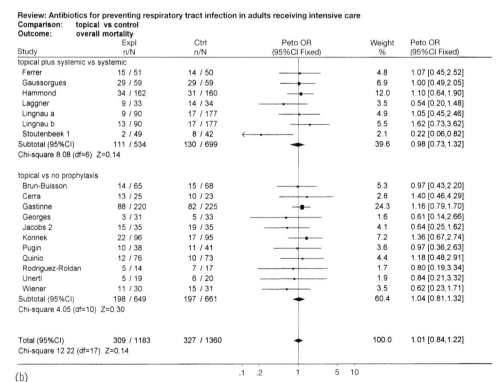

Figure 28.5 (a) and (b) (Source: Antibiotics for preventing respiratory tract infections (Cochrane Review) *The Cochrane Library*, issue 2, 1999. Oxford: Update Software)

astrocytes, is in direct response to the ammonia load in liver failure. In subacute hepatic failure loss of organic osmolytes from the brain may help to offset this rise in osmolality and prevent edema formation. Inhibition of the membrane bound Na^+/K^+ ATPase within astrocytes via a circulating factor has been proposed as a cause of astrocyte swelling.[60]

A partial breakdown of the blood–brain barrier has been shown in experimental animals although it has never been proven in humans. As osmotherapy plays a large part in the treatment of intracranial hypertension in FHF it appears that the blood–brain barrier is not damaged to a great extent, at least in the initial stages of brain swelling.

There are three components within the cranial vault that make up the volume – the brain tissue itself, cerebrospinal fluid, and blood. Any one of these components, if increased in volume, could be responsible for the rise in pressure seen in FHF. The evidence suggests that an increase in the brain tissue itself, cerebral edema, is the main factor. CSF volume probably decreases in FHF as it is displaced from the intracranial compartment. Blood volume appears to be variable and maneuvers to decrease blood volume may be useful in the control of intracranial hypertension during the latter stages, when small changes in volume have profound effects on the pressure within the skull. Until recently, it was assumed that arterial blood volume within the skull was always increased because of hyperemia, and that blood flow may well be in excess of metabolic needs, which are often very low in FHF. However, evidence suggests that blood flow may be inadequate for the metabolic needs of the brain in the early stages of the disease and that cerebral ischemia may be one of the causes of a cytotoxic cerebral edema.[33] The situation is further complicated by the fact that autoregulation of blood flow appears to be lost in FHF.[32] Increases in mean arterial pressure are accompanied by a parallel increase in intracranial pressures as arterial blood volume increases within the brain. The arterial response to CO_2 appears to remain intact in FHF but concerns about exacerbating cerebral ischemia have led to a decrease in the use of routine hyperventilation in patients with FHF. Venous blood volume within the skull is less amenable to manipulation than is the arterial volume. However, raising the head of the bed 20 degrees improves venous drainage and optimizes cerebral perfusion pressure, reducing intracranial pressure.[61]

Intracranial pressure monitoring

The use of intracranial pressure (ICP) monitors in FHF has not been subjected to a randomized controlled trial. As with any monitor used in critical illness, finding a positive outcome related to their use is difficult. At best, studies have suggested they may help with the management of patients with raised ICP. One study using historical controls suggested greater interventions associated with their use, and assuming the interventions were appropriate, this may be of benefit. The duration of survival from the onset of grade IV encephalopathy was significantly greater in the ICP monitored group (median 60 vs 10 hours, $P < 0.01$), although overall survival was unchanged.[62] Blei *et al* performed a postal survey of complications in 262 patients from liver transplant centers across the USA.[63] Epidural transducers were the most commonly used devices and had the lowest complication rate (3.8%); subdural bolts and parenchymal monitors (fiberoptic pressure transducers in direct contact with brain parenchyma and intraventricular catheters) were associated with complication rates of 20% and 22%, respectively. Fatal hemorrhage occurred in 1% of patients undergoing epidural ICP monitoring, whereas subdural and intraparenchymal devices had fatal hemorrhage rates of 5% and 4%. They concluded that epidural transducers were the safest form of monitoring even if not the most accurate.[63]

R
Grade C

R
Grade C

Their use may help in the decision as whether to list a patient for transplantation or not. A cerebral perfusion pressure (mean arterial pressure minus intracranial pressure) of less than 50 mmHg has in the past been considered a contraindication for OLT.[64] This was because of concern regarding cerebral ischemia resulting in poor neurological outcome. Recent reports of patients with CPPs of less than 50 mmHg in which full neurological recovery has taken place have called this practice into question. Davies[65] reported four patients with fulminant hepatic failure who developed prolonged intracranial hypertension (>35 mmHg for 24–38 hours) that was refractory to standard therapy and associated with impaired cerebral perfusion pressure (<50 mmHg for 2–72 h). All survived with complete neurological recovery.

CT scanning

CT scanning, since its introduction into routine clinical practice, has become a standard investigation in any patient with suspected intracranial pathology. In FHF correlation between ICP measurements and pressures predicted by CT imaging have been generally poor.[66] As little information is gained in relation to the difficulty associated with transporting these very sick patients to the CT scanner, a decision regarding the need for a CT must be carefully considered. CT may be of help if there is any diagnostic difficulty as to the cause of the coma or if a complication of ICP bolt insertion is suspected.

Jugular venous saturation

The insertion of a catheter into the jugular vein (JV) in a retrograde fashion until its tip lies in the jugular bulb is a relatively easy technique associated with little morbidity, and venous oxygen saturation and lactate can be sampled.

Jugular venous saturation of less than 55% indicates an ischemic brain in which there is pathologically increased oxygen extraction from the arterial blood. If this is present, steps can be taken to improve the blood flow to the brain, either by increasing blood flow, decreasing ICP or reducing the metabolic demands of the brain. A high JV saturation (>85%) may represent a hyperemic brain and measures can be taken to reduce cerebral blood volume if ICP is raised. Very high JV saturations are often seen as a terminal event and may represent a complete loss of oxygen extraction by the brain. Recently jugular venous catheters with thermistors have been used to measure cerebral blood flow. The technique has been validated at the bedside in comatose patients compared to the Kety–Schmidt method.[67]

All these techniques are relatively new, and controlled trials showing improvement in outcome are needed. However, together with ICP monitoring they give more information about the state of cerebral oxygenation and provide measurable parameters which can be manipulated in the hope of improving outcome.

R
Grade A

Treatment of intracranial hypertension

Osmotherapy initially with urea and then mannitol has been used for many years to treat cerebral edema associated with traumatic brain injury. Canalese *et al*[68] showed that 1 g/kg of mannitol was an effective treatment for established intracranial hypertension in FHF and that dexamethasone was ineffective for prevention. Since then, the same workers have shown that 0.5 g/kg of mannitol is as effective.[69] They suggest that boluses should be delivered rapidly to achieve maximum effect.

Hypertonic saline was the original experimental agent used as an osmolar load to treat intracranial hypertension during the early part of this century. However, it was not used clinically. Over the past 10 years there has been increased interest in hypertonic saline as osmotherapy in traumatic brain injury.[70] In health, the blood–brain barrier is relatively impermeable to sodium ions and sodium is actively pumped out of astrocytes via a Na^+/K^+ ATPase. As discussed above, the etiology of the cerebral edema in FHF appears to be mainly associated with astrocyte swelling, but the blood–brain barrier remains relatively intact.[71]

Hyperventilation decreases ICP by inducing cerebrovascular vasoconstriction – this reduces cerebral blood volume. It has not been shown to be any advantage in the long term in controlling ICP in FHF.[72] A short term period of hyperventilation in patients with raised ICP unresponsive to osmotherapy may be tried, while monitoring jugular venous saturation to assess cerebral oxygenation.

R Grade C

Barbiturates decrease cerebral metabolic rate via their anesthetic action and cause cerebral vasoconstriction. They have been used as agents to prevent secondary brain damage in traumatic brain injury. However, myocardial depression and hypotension with a possible compromise in cerebral perfusion pressure have limited the enthusiasm for routine use. There have not been any randomized controlled clinical trials evaluating barbiturate infusions in FHF. Forbes *et al*[73] investigated the role of thiopentone infusions in 13 patients with FHF in an uncontrolled study. The overall survival rate of five out of 13 was claimed to be better than expected, but it is difficult to come to any conclusions from these data.[73] Prolonged recovery and hypotension limit the use of thiopentone in FHF, although it may be tried when all else fails. A recent study in traumatic brain injury found barbiturate infusion to be of no additional benefit to acute hyperventilation.[74]

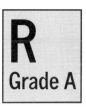

R Grade A

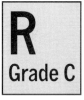

N-acetylcysteine (NAC) has been shown to reduce clinical signs of intracranial hypertension in patients with FHF following paracetamol hepatotoxicity.[75] NAC treated patients had a lower incidence of cerebral oedema (10/25, 40%) than was observed in control patients (17/25, 68%; $P = 0.047$, 95% CI for difference in incidence 2–54).[75]

Anticonvulsant therapy

There is no evidence that prophylactic anticonvulsant therapy improves outcome in FHF.

RENAL FAILURE

The incidence of acute renal failure associated with FHF is high; up to 70% of all patients develop renal failure (defined as urine output of less than 300 ml/24 hours and a serum creatinine of greater than 300 mmol/l in the presence of adequate intravascular filling).[6] The etiology of renal failure in FHF is multifactorial with both pre-renal and renal components. Relative hypovolemia and hypotension contribute to pre-renal causes. Disordered renal vascular autoregulation, present in sepsis, may also exist in the hyperdynamic circulatory failure of FHF, making renal blood flow directly dependent on blood pressure. Direct renal toxicity in patients with FHF secondary to paracetamol poisoning contributes to the very high incidence of renal failure in this group of patients.[6] The contribution of the hepatorenal syndrome, or functional renal failure in the presence of FHF, is difficult to quantify and it probably represents one end of a continuum of disordered renal function from the hepatorenal syndrome to acute tubular necrosis.[76]

Renal protection

There is no proven protective strategy or treatment of renal dysfunction in FHF. Various strategies have been tried with little success.

Dopamine has agonist activity at all adrenergic receptors depending on concentration. Dopamine increases urine output because of its naturitic effect on the proximal tubule and it increases cardiac output and renal blood flow in cardiogenic shock. In FHF and other forms of distributive circulatory failure it has been difficult to demonstrate an increase in renal blood flow.[77] It has been suggested that dopamine may exacerbate renal dysfunction by delivering a sodium load to an already ischemic renal medulla.[78] The use of "low dose" dopamine has been questioned because of the wide variation in plasma concentration in critically ill patients,[79] and because of concern about the long term effect of "low dose" dopamine on anterior pituitary function.[80] Other strategies include infusion of low dose frusemide and aminophylline. Atrial natriuretic peptide, while showing promise in animal models, to date has not been shown to be useful in the clinical setting.[81]

Renal replacement therapy

While the incidence of renal failure in FHF remains high and attempts to prevent or treat it remain poor, renal replacement therapy has become a major part of the routine management. Proving that renal replacement therapy improves outcome is difficult, as no randomized controlled trials have been performed, but it can be assumed that it has contributed in part to the improvement in survival over the past 30 years.

The type of replacement has been investigated in critically ill patients. It has been shown that intermittent forms of therapy cause more hemodynamic compromise than continuous forms of therapy. This has been examined in FHF. Davenport *et al*[82] investigated the effect of various modes of renal replacement therapy in 30 consecutive patients referred with both fulminant hepatic and acute renal failure. Continuous forms of therapy were associated with more hemodynamic stability during the first hour of treatment. Intracranial pressure remained stable during the continuous modes but increased significantly during intermittent machine hemofiltration.[82]

SPECIFIC THERAPIES

N-acetylcysteine (NAC) in paracetamol poisoning and other etiologies

Paracetamol poisoning is the single largest cause of FHF in the UK, accounting for between 50 and 60% of cases seen.[83] NAC can prevent hepatic damage following paracetamol poisoning. Smilkstein *et al*[84] evaluated the time interval from poisoning to treatment with NAC in relation to the incidence of hepatic damage as defined by increased transaminase values. NAC was found to be most effective when given during the first 8 hours following ingestion.[84] More recent data suggest that NAC is effective when given up to 72 hours after ingestion with a decrease in the occurrence of grade III/IV encephalopathy, cerebral edema, hypotension requiring inotropic support, and mortality when compared to untreated controls.[75,85]

R
Grade A/C

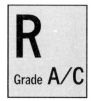

The mechanism of action of NAC in patients with established hepatic necrosis is unclear. Improvements in oxygen transport parameters have been shown with its use in patients with FHF due to paracetamol poisoning and FHF due to other etiology.[86] Although NAC has not been shown to reduce mortality with FHF due to causes other than paracetamol, a hemodynamic effect of this agent is seen when it is used in conjunction with epoprostenol. The beneficial effects may be attributable to a repletion of glutathione status and/or the antioxidant properties of NAC. NAC is also a sulphydryl donor and this may be beneficial in patients in whom sulphydryl groups may be oxidized, impairing microcirculatory function. Infusion of NAC has been shown to increase serum cGMP with no change in atrial natriuretic peptide, suggesting it may indeed have a role in the nitric oxide pathway in patients with acute liver failure.[87]

Blood purification: dialysis, plasmapheresis, hemofiltration, sorbant hemoperfusion, and artificial hepatic support

To effectively support the acutely failing liver requires a thorough understanding of the functional role of the liver in homeostasis. In the past the main focus was the hepatocyte as the only functional unit of the liver with little consideration to the functions of the Kupffer cells and endothelial cells which comprise up to a third of the liver mass. These cells and others are important in many aspects of hepatic function, including the immunological activity of the liver.

There have been two main theories as to the pathophysiology of FHF. The first is the metabolic mass theory, which states that there is a critical mass of functioning hepatocytes and if this is reduced end organ dysfunction will occur, leading to the manifestations of FHF and ultimately death. The second is the toxic liver hypothesis which states that it is the toxins produced by the failing liver itself which cause the syndrome of FHF. The truth probably lies somewhere in between, and any extracorporeal system should clear the serum of any toxins produced by the failing liver and also clear toxins and bacteria produced in the gut and not filtered by the liver. It should also provide enough metabolic support for the other organs of the body. The systemic inflammatory response syndrome produced by other pathological mechanisms such as trauma and pancreatitis is also produced by FHF. It is probable that there is a cascade of events, including the systemic release of cytokines and immune cell activation triggered by FHF, which can ultimately lead to multiple organ failure and death. Purification of the blood will not reverse this process once end organ damage is severe.

Experience with extracorporeal systems designed to clear the blood through physiochemical means alone consist of dialysis, sorbant hemoperfusion, hemofiltration, and plasmapheresis, and combinations of these interventions. Early work with hemodialysis showed improved coma scores in patients with chronic liver disease. With increasing pore size and improving biocompatibility with polyacrylonitrile (PAN) membranes, the hope was to improve middle-molecule clearance. No improvement in mortality in FHF was shown.[88] Hemoperfusion involves the adsorbtion of lipophilic chemicals onto activated charcoal or synthetic resins. Again, early studies suggested an

R Grade A

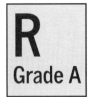

improvement in coma scores,[89] but controlled studies failed to show an improved outcome with this intervention.[6] Plasmapheresis or the exchange of plasma by fresh frozen plasma (FFP) has theoretical advantages over other forms of blood cleansing regimens in that it removes both low molecular weight molecules and the higher molecular weight middle molecules, both bound and unbound. The Copenhagen group have been studying high volume plasmapharesis with exchanges of 1 liter/hour for three consecutive days.[81] Their studies suggest an improvement in hemodynamics and improved CPP but no reduction in ICP. They also noted a decrease in Glasgow coma score, decreased INR, and reduced serum bilirubin.[90] Improvement in mortality has not been shown with the technique. Grade C

R Grade A

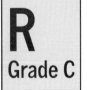

Bioreactors containing hepatocytes have been the basis for biological extracorporeal support systems. These remain experimental and confined to clinical trials. Experience with the systems so far suggest few problems with biocompatibility but there are few data to suggest an improvement in clearance or synthesis by the artificial liver. The systems at the present time are divided into those utilizing porcine hepatocytes or immortalized hepatoblastoma cell lines. The ELAD system comprises a continuous system using a hepatoblastoma cell line. A randomized study utilizing this system, assessing biocompatibility, showed an improvement in galactose clearance at 6 hours but no other measured variables were significantly different between the treatment and control groups. [91] The system of Demetriou utilizes plasma separation and passage of the plasma over charcoal and thence over pig hepatocytes on a daily basis for 6 hours. The system has not yet been subjected to a randomized controlled trial but has been reported to demonstrate improved level of consciousness and improvements in mean arterial pressure, intracranial pressure, and cerebral perfusion pressure.[93] Grade C

Temporizing hepatectomy

R Grade C

The toxic liver theory of FHF has led to the introduction of temporizing hepatectomy in an attempt to regain hemodynamic control or a reduction in ICP in patients on the super-urgent transplant list. There have been several published case reports of successful liver transplantation following a prolonged anhepatic state. Ringe *et al*[93] presented the results of 30 patients who underwent hepatectomy (and temporary portacaval shunting to provide an outflow of the transected portal vein) between 1986 and 1993. Improvement in hemodynamic parameters was seen in 17 of the 30 patients following hepatectomy, with liver transplantation occurring 6–41 hours later (the effect on ICP was not stated). It is impossible to draw conclusions from these anecdotal data. Temporizing hepatectomy has been criticized because of removing the option to perform an auxiliary transplant. Temporizing hepatectomy may have a role in severe liver trauma, with uncontrollable bleeding and primary graft non-function where there is no hope of recovery.

LIVER TRANSPLANTATION

Prognostic factors in fulminant hepatic failure and orthoptic liver transplantation

Hepatic transplantation in FHF has not been and never will be subjected to a controlled clinical trial. However, patients with FHF due to causes other than paracetamol poisoning who undergo transplantation have a 65% 2-month survival rate[11] compared to 20–25%

for patients managed with maximal medical therapy alone.[94] The survival without transplantation after paracetamol poisoning is higher than with FHF from other causes.

R
Grade B

The task for the doctors and surgeons looking after patients with FHF is to decide which of these patients will not survive without liver transplantation. The decision needs to be made as early as possible because there exists a "window period" during which a successful outcome can be expected.[95] Following paracetamol poisoning, time from ingestion to transplant was significantly longer in non-survivors following transplantation.[11]

In order to make an informed decision regarding the likelihood of spontaneous recovery from FHF an understanding of the natural history of the disease is necessary. Because FHF is a rare syndrome these data have only become available over the past 20 years, since the introduction of liver failure units around the world.

Poor prognostic markers developed from analysis of large databases from these liver units have been refined into clinically usable indications for transplantation. O'Grady *et al* developed criteria from a database of 588 patients presenting to King's College Hospital liver unit (see Box 28.2).[83] The time course of the illness is important. It has been known for many years that the time to encephalopathy from the onset of symptoms is important prognostically, the "hyperacute" patients having a better prognosis than the "sub-acute". Etiology and age are important in that different criteria were developed for FHF caused by paracetamol poisoning. The extremes of age are associated with a poor prognosis. A high serum creatinine and bilirubin were associated with a poor prognosis, as were prolongation of coagulation parameters.[83] Following paracetamol poisoning no particular prognostic cutoff level of INR has been found, but it has been noted that a rise of the INR from day 3 to day 4 is associated with a 7% survival as compared to a 79% survival in those whose INR fell from day 3 to 4.[85] Metabolic acidosis following fluid resuscitation was found to be highly specific for a poor outcome in paracetamol poisoning. A serum pH persistently less than 7.3 has become an independent transplant criterion regardless of grade of encephalopathy.[83]

A French group performed multivariate analysis of data from 115 patients with fulminant hepatitis B and found that a low factor V following the onset of grade III encephalopathy was the strongest predictor of a poor outcome (see Box 28.3).[96]

Box 28.2 King's College Hospital prognostic criteria

In *non-paracetamol induced* liver failure
Prothombin time >100 seconds (INR >6.5)
Or
pH <7.3
Or any three of the following:
Age <10 years
Age >40 years
Seronegative hepatitis (non A,B,C,E,F), halothane or other drug reaction
Duration of jaundice >7 days before encephalopathy
Prothrombin time >50 seconds (INR >3.5)
Bilirubin > 300 μmol/l
In *paracetamol induced* FHF
pH <7.3 (following fluid resuscitation)
Or the coexistence of:
Prothrombin time >100 (INR >6.5), creatinine >300 μmol/l and grade III or worse encephalopathy

Box 28.3 The Clichy criteria in viral FHF

Coma or confusion
and
Factor V <20% if under 30 years of age
or
Factor V <30% if over 30 years of age

Both sets of criteria are in common use around the world. Following the publication of the King's College Hospital data the criteria were evaluated retrospectively in a French liver unit. Eighty-one non-transplanted patients with non-paracetamol induced acute liver failure were studied. The mortality rate was 0.81. The predictive accuracies, respectively on admission and 48 hours before death, were 0.80 and 0.79 for the King's criteria and 0.60 and 0.73 for the Clichy criteria. The positive and negative predictive values, 48 hours before death, were 0.89 and 0.47 for the King's criteria and 0.89 and 0.36 for the Clichy criteria, respectively. The low negative predictive values (0.36 and 0.47) indicated that neither of these could identify a subgroup with a low risk of death.

While the above study compared prognostic criteria in non-paracetamol induced FHF, two recent studies compared general ICU scoring systems, the Acute Physiology and Chronic Health Evaluation (APACHE) scores, and the King's criteria for urgent liver transplantation.[11,97] Mitchell *et al* prospectively evaluated the APACHE II system in patients with FHF due to paracetamol poisoning. The study aimed to see whether the APACHE system is able to provide an accurate risk of hospital death in patients with paracetamol induced FHF or identify those patients needing transfer for possible hepatic transplantation and compared this to the King's College Hospital transplant criteria. A total of 102 patients were studied. An APACHE II score of >15 had the ability to predict death which was similar to that of the King's criteria (sensitivity 82% and 65%, respectively; specificity 98% and 99%, respectively) when evaluating those patients who were transplanted as "deaths". An APACHE II score of >15 was able to identify four more patients than the King's criteria on the first day of admission. The calculated risk of death according to the APACHE II score, using the original drug overdose coefficient, was poorly calibrated. This is probably due to the lower incidence of potentially life-threatening drug overdoses in the original calibration population. From these data the crude APACHE II score may be able to identify non-survivors at an earlier stage than the King's College Hospital criteria.[97]

Delays in listing patients for transplantation, and in organ procurement result in further patient deterioration. This altered status results in the withdrawal of patients from the urgent list. Withdrawal of patients is based on clinical experience. However, several authors have analysed the outcome from transplantation in FHF to help define contraindications to transplantation on the basis of poor outcome after transplantation. Devlin *et al*[11] used APACHE III data to look at 100 patients transplanted for FHF. They found that in the paracetamol group at the time of transplantation APACHE III score and serum bilirubin were significantly higher in the non-survivors. In the non-paracetamol group serum creatinine, organ system failure scores, and APACHE III scores were significantly higher in the non-survivors.[11] Bernal *et al*[98] studied the use of liver transplantation and the application of King's College Hospital transplant criteria in 548 patients presenting to the liver failure unit with severe paracetamol poisoning. Of 424 patients who did not fulfil criteria, 28 (7%) died. Of 124 who fulfilled the criteria, 68 (55%) were listed for transplant, and 44 underwent transplantation. Thirty-three of the transplanted patients left hospital. Of the 80 patients who satisfied criteria but were not transplanted, nine survived to leave hospital. The reasons why patients who satisfied criteria were not listed were multiple organ failure and cerebral edema.[98] These reasons also applied to the patients listed but withdrawn before a graft was available. In contrast to the report of Devlin *et al*,[11] the authors were unable to identify any preoperative factors predictive of death in the transplanted group. This suggests that patients unlikely to survive with a transplant are recognized and subsequently removed from the list. However, graft factors (identified by early markers of graft function, INR, and AST) were also significantly worse in the non-survivors.

Auxiliary OLT and regeneration

Auxiliary partial orthotopic liver transplantation holds potential advantages over conventional orthotopic liver transplantation in the setting of FHF. It has been known for many years that survivors from FHF often return to full health with normal or only slightly abnormal livers. The liver has great powers of regeneration and this has led to the introduction of partial liver transplantation in the hope of native liver regeneration and the eventual withdrawal of immunosuppression. A multicenter European study reported the results of 30 patients who underwent auxiliary transplantation for FHF.[99] After 3 months, 19 of the 30 patients survived; 13 had resumed normal native liver function with interruption of immunosuppression. The indications are not well defined, but the survivors off immunosuppression were aged less than 40 years and had FHF secondary to viral hepatitis and paracetamol poisoning.[99]

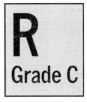

R
Grade C

REFERENCES

1 Trey C, Davidson LS. The management of fulminant hepatic failure. In: Popper H, Schaffner F (eds), *Progress in liver disease*. New York: Grune and Stratton, 1970, pp. 282–98.
2 Connors AF, Speroff T, Dawson NV *et al*. The effectiveness of right heart catheterization in the initial care of critically ill patients. *JAMA* 1996; **276**: 889–97.
3 Gimson AES, O'Grady J, Ede RJ *et al*. Late-onset hepatic failure: clinical, serological and histological features. *Hepatology* 1986; **6**: 288–94.
4 O'Grady J, Schalm SW, Williams R. Acute liver failure: redefining the syndromes. *Lancet* 1993; **342**: 273–5.
5 Trewby P, Williams R. Pathophysiology of hypotension in patients with fulminant hepatic failure. *Gut* 1977; **18**: 1021–6.
6 O'Grady J, Gimson AE, O'Brian CJ *et al*. Controlled trials of charcoal hemoperfusion and prognostic factors in fulminant hepatic failure. *Gastroenterology* 1988; **94**: 1186–92.
7 Rolando N, Harvey F, Brahm Jet *al*. Prospective study of bacterial infections in acute liver failure: an analysis of fifty patients. *Hepatology* 1990; **11**: 49–53.
8 Makin AJ, Wendon J, Williams R. A 7-year experience of severe acetominophen-induced hepatotoxicity (1987–1993). *Gastroenterology* 1995; **109**: 1907–16.
9 Lucke B, Mallory T. Fulminant form of epidemic hepititis. *Am J Pathol* 1946; **22**: 867–945.
10 McQuillan P, Pilkington S, Allan A *et al*. Confidential enquiry into quality of care before admission to intensive care. *Br Med J* 1998; **316**: 1853–8.
11 Devlin J, Wendon J, Heaton N *et al*. Pretransplantation clinical status and outcome of emergency transplantation for acute liver failure. *Hepatology* 1995; **21**: 1018–24.
12 O'Grady J. Acute liver failure. *J R Coll Phys Lond* 1997; **31**: 603–7.
13 Bihari DJ, Gimson AE, Williams R. Disturbances in cardiovascular and pulmonary function in fulminant hepatic failure. In: Williams R (ed), *Liver failure*. Edinburgh: Churchill Livingstone, 1986, pp. 47–71.
14 Schierhout G, Roberts I. Fluid resuscitation with colloid or crystalloid solution in critically ill patients: a systematic review if randomised trials. *Br Med J* 1998; **316**: 961–4.
15 Cochrane Injuries Group Albumin Reviewers. Human albumin administration in critically ill

patients: a systematic review of randomised controlled trials. *Br Med J* 1998; **317**: 235–40.
16 McClelland B. Albumin: don't confuse us with the facts. *Br Med J* 1998; **317**: 829–30.
17 Webb A. Journal Reviews. *Intensive Care Society Newsletter* 1998.
18 Shippy BR, Appel PL, Shoemaker WC. Reliability of clinical monitoring to assess blood volume in critically ill patients. *Crit Care Med* 1984; **12**: 107–12.
19 Hayes MA, Timmins AC, Yau EHS *et al*. Oxygen transport patterns in patients with sepsis syndrome or septic shock: influence of treatment and relationship to outcome. *Critl Care Med* 1997; **25**: 926–36.
20 Powers SR, Mannal R, Neckerio M *et al*. Physiologic consequences of positive end expiratory pressure (PEEP) ventilation. *Ann Surg* 1973; **178**: 265–72.
21 Bihari DJ, Gimson AE, Williams R. Cardiovascular, pulmonary and renal complications of fulminant hepatic failure. *Semin Liver Dis* 1986; **6**: 119–28.
22 Shoemaker WC, Appel PL, Kram HB *et al*. Prospective trial of supranormal circulatory values of survivors as therapeutic goals in high-risk surgical patients. *Chest* 1988; **94**: 1176–86.
23 Gasman JD, Ruoss SJ, Fishman RS *et al*. Hazards with both determining and utilizing oxygen consumption measurements in the management of critically ill patients. *Crit Care Med* 1996; **24**: 6–9.
24 Durham RM, Neunaber RN, Mazuski JE *et al*. The use of oxygen consumption and delivery as endpoints for resucitation in critically ill patients. *J Trauma* 1996; **41**: 32–40.
25 Third European Consensus Conference in Intensive Care Medicine. Tissue hypoxia: how to detect, how to correct, how to prevent? *Am J Respir Crit Care Med* 1996; **154**: 1573–8.
26 Gutierrez G, Palizas F, Doglio G *et al*. Gastric intramucosal pH as a therapeutic index of tissue oxygenation in critically ill patients. *Lancet* 1992; **339**: 195–9.
27 Silva E, DeBacker D, Créteur J. Effects of vasoactive drugs on gastric intramucosal pH. *Crit Care Med* 1998; **25**: 1749–58.
28 Olson D, Pohlman A, Hall J. Administration of low dose dopamine to nonoliguric patients with sepsis syndrome does not raise intramucosal pH nor improve creatinine clearance. *Crit Care Med* 1996; **154**: 1664–70.
29 Wendon J, Harrison P, Keays R *et al*. Effects of systemic hemodynamics on oxygen transport variables in patients with fulminant hepatic failure. *Hepatology* 1992; **15**: 1067–71.
30 Tighe D, Bradley C, Moss R *et al*. Alpha 1 adrenoceptor stimulation by dobutamine may amplify hepatic injury during sepsis. *Br J Intens Care* 1998; **8**: 150–6.
31 Tighe D, Moss R, Bennett D. Porcine hepatic response to sepsis and its amplification by adrenergic receptor alpha$_1$-agonist and beta$_2$-antagonist. *Clin Sci (Colch)* 1998; **95**: 467–78.
32 Larson FS, Ejlerson E, Hanson BA *et al*. Functional loss of cerebral blood flow autoregulation in patients with fulminant hepatic failure. *J Hepatol* 1995; **23**: 212–17.
33 Wendon JA, Harrison PM, Keays R *et al*. Cerebral blood flow and metabolism in fulminant liver failure. *Hepatology* 1994; **19**: 1407–13.
34 Baudouin SV, Howdle P, O'Grady JG *et al*. Acute lung injury in fulminant hepatic failure following paracetamol poisoning. *Thorax* 1995; **50**: 399–402.
35 Dreyfuss D, Saumon G. Ventilator-induced lung injury. *Am J Respir Crit Care Med* 1998; **157**: 294–323.
36 Amato MBP, Barbas CSV, Mederios DM *et al*. Effects of a protective-ventilation strategy on mortality in the acute respiratory distress syndrome. *N Engl J Med* 1998; **338**: 347–54.
37 Artigas A, Bernard GR, Dreyfuss D *et al*. The American-European Consensus Conference on ARDS Part 2: Ventilatory, pharmacologic, supportive therapy, study design strategies and issues related to recovery and remodeling. *Intens Care Med* 1998; **28**: 378–98.
38 Ramsay MAE, Savage TM, Simpson BRJ *et al*. Controlled sedation with alphaxalone-alphadone. *BrMed J* 1974; **2**: 656–9.
39 Hsiang JK, Chesnut RM, Crisp CB *et al*. Early, routine paralysis for intracranial pressure control in severe head injury: Is it necessary? *Crit Care Med* 1994; **22**: 1471–6.
40 Davis NA, Rodgers JE, Gonzalez ER *et al*.. Prolonged weakness after cisatracurium infusion: a case report. *Crit Care Med* 1998; **26**: 1290–2.
41 Road J. Reversible paralysis with status asthmaticus, steroids, and pancuronium: clinical electrophysiological correlates. *Muscle Nerve* 1997; **20**: 1587–90.
42 Chandra RK. Nutrition, infection and immunity: present knowledge and future directions. *Lancet* 1983; **i**: 688–91.
43 Shukla VK, Roy SK, Kumar J *et al*. Correlation of immune and nutritional status with wound complications in patients undergoing abdominal surgery. *Ann Surg* 1985; **51**: 442–5.
44 Baudouin S, Evans TW. Nutrition in the critically ill. In: Hall JB, Schmidt GA, Wood LDH (eds), *Principles of critical care*. New York: McGraw Hill, 1998, pp. 205–20.
45 Heyland D, Cook DJ, Winder B *et al*. Enteral nutrition in the critically ill patient: a prospective survey. *Crit Care Med* 1995; **23**: 1055–60.
46 Atkinson S, Sieffert E, Bihari D. A prospective, randomised, double-blind, controlled clinical trial of enteral immunonutrition in the critically ill. Guy's Hospital Intensive Care Group. *Crit Care Med* 1998; **26**: 1164–72.

47 Kudsk KA, Minard G, Croce MA *et al.* A randomised trial of isonitrogenous enteral diets after severe trauma. An immune-enhancing diet reduces septic complications. *Ann Surg* 1996; **224**: 531–40.
48 The Veterans Affairs Total Parenteral Nutrition Cooperative Study Group. Perioperative total parenteral nutrition in surgical patients. *N Engl J Med* 1991; **325**: 525–32.
49 Freeman J, Goldman DA, Smith NE *et al.* Association of intravenous lipid emulsion and coagulase-negative staphylococcal bacteremia in neonatal intensive care units. *N Engl J Med* 1990; **23**: 301–8.
50 Griffiths RD, Jones C, Palmer TE. Six month outcome of critically ill patients given glutamine-supplemented parenteral nutrition. *Nutrition* 1997; **13**: 295–302.
51 Houdijk AP, Rijnsberger ER, Janson J *et al.* Randomised trial of glutamine-enriched enteral nutrition on infectious morbidity in patients with multiple trauma. *Lancet* 1998; **352**: 772–6.
52 Macdougall BRD, Bailey RJ, Williams R. H2-receptor antagonists and antacids in the prevention of acute gastrointestinal haemorrhage in fulminant hepatic failure. *Lancet* 1977; **i**: 617–19.
53 Tryba M. Prophylaxis of stress ulcer bleeding. *J Clin Gastroenterol* 1991; **13**: S44–55.
54 Cook DJ, Reeve BK, Guyatt GH *et al.* Stress ulcer prophylaxis in critically ill patients. Resolving discordant meta-analysis. *JAMA* 1996; **275**: 308–14.
55 Cook D, Guyatt G, Marshall J, Leasa D, Fuller H, Hall R *et al.* A comparison of sucralfate and ranitidine for the prevention of upper gastrointestinal bleeding in patients requiring mechanical ventilation. Canadian Critical Care Trials Group. *N Engl J Med* 1998; **19**: 338(12): 791–7.
56 Rolando N, Philpott-Howard J, Williams R. Bacterial and fungal infection in acute liver failure. *Semin Liver Dis* 1996; **16**: 389–402.
57 Rolando N, Gimson AES, Wade JJ *et al.* Prospective controlled trial of selective parenteral and enteral antimicrobial regimen in fulminant hepatic failure. *Hepatology* 1993; **17**: 196–201.
58 Rolando N, Wade JJ, Stangou A *et al.* Prospective study comparing the efficacy of prophylactic parenteral antimicrobials, with or without enteral decontamination, in patients with acute liver failure. *Liver Transplant Surg* 1996; **2**: 8–13.
59 Liberati A, D'Amico R, Pifferi S *et al.* Antibiotic prophylaxis for respiratory tract infections in adult patients in intensive care units. In: *The Cochrane Library* (database on disk and CD-ROM). Issue 2, 1999. Oxford: Update Software.
60 Yang SS, Hughes RD, Williams R. Digoxin-like immunoreactive substance in severe acute liver disease due to viral hepatitis and paracetamol overdose. *Hepatology* 1988; **8**: 93–7.
61 Davenport A, Will EJ, Davison AM. Effect of posture on intracranial pressure and cerebral perfusion pressure in patients with fulminant hepatic and renal failure after acetaminophen self-poisoning. *Crit Care Med* 1990; **18**: 286–9.
62 Keays RT, Alexander GL, Williams R. The safety and value of extradural intracranial pressure monitors in fulminant hepatic failure. *J Hepatol* 1993; **18**: 205–9.
63 Blei AT, Olafsson S, Webster S *et al.* Complications of intracranial pressure monitoring in fulminant hepatic failure. *Lancet* 1993; **341**: 157–8.
64 Donovan JP, Shaw BW Jr, Langnas AN, Sorrell MF. Brain water and acute liver failure: the emerging role of intracranial pressure monitoring. *Hepatology* 1992; **16**(1): 267–8.
65 Davies MH, Mutimer D, Lowes J, Elias E, Neuberger J. Recovery despite impaired cerebral perfusion in fulminant hepatic failure. *Lancet* 1994; **28**: 343(8909): 1329–30.
66 Munoz SJ, Robinson M, Northrup B *et al.* Elevated intracranial pressure and computed tomography of the brain in fulminant hepatocellular failure. *Hepatology* 1991; **13**: 209–12.
67 Melot C, Berre J, Moraine JJ *et al.* Estimation of cerebral blood flow at the bedside by continuous jugular thermodilution. *J Cerebral Blood Flow Metabol* 1996; **16**: 1263–70.
68 Canalese J, Gimson AES, Davis C *et al.* Controlled trial of dexamethasone and mannitol for the cerebral oedema of fulminant hepatic failure. *Gut* 1982; **23**: 625–9.
69 Ede RJ, Williams RW. Hepatic encephalopathy and cerebral edema. *Semin Liver Dis* 1986; **6**(2): 107–18.
70 Prough DS, Zornow MH. Hypertonic maintenance fluids for patients with cerebral edema: does the evidence support a phase II trial? *Crit Care Med* 1998; **26**(3): 421–2.
71 Blei AT. Brain edema and intracranial hypertension in acute liver failure. In: Lee W and Williams R (ed), *Acute liver failure*. Cambridge: Cambridge University Press, 1997, pp 144–57.
72 Ede RJ, Gimson AE, Bihari D, Williams R. Controlled hyperventilation in the prevention of cerebral oedema in fulminant hepatic failure. *J Hepatol* 1986; **2**(1): 43–51.
73 Forbes A, Alexander GJ, O'Grady JG. Thiopental infusion in the treatment of intracranial hypertension complicating fulminant hepatic failure. *Hepatology* 1989; **10**: 549–55.
74 Louis PT, Goddard-Finegold J, Fishman MA *et al.* Barbiturates and hyperventilation during intracranial hypertension. *Crit Care Med* 1993; **21**: 1200–6.

75 Keays R, Harrison PM, Wendon JA *et al.* Intravenous acetylcysteine in paracetamol induced fulminant hepatic failure: a prospective controlled trial. *Br Med J* 1991; **303**: 1026–9.
76 Arroyo V, Ginès P, Gerbes AL *et al.* Definition and diagnostic criteria of refractory ascites and hepatorenal syndrome in cirrhosis. International Ascites Club. *J Hepatol* 1996; **23**(1): 164–76
77 Bersten AD, Holt AW. Vasoactive drugs and the importance of renal perfusion pressure. *New Horizons* 1995; **3**: 650–61.
78 Weisberg LS, Kurnik PB, Kurnik BRC. Risk of radiocontrast nephropathy in patients with and without diabetes mellitus. *Kidney International* 1994; **45**: 259–65.
79 Juste RN, Moran L, Hooper J *et al.* Dopamine clearance in critically ill patients. *Intens Care Med* 1998; **24**: 1217–20.
80 Van den Berghe G, de Zegher F. Anterior pituitary function during critical illness and dopamine treatment. *Crit Care Med* 1996; **24**: 1580–90.
81 Brenner RM, Chertow GM. The rise and fall of atrial natriuretic peptide for acute renal failure. *Curr Opin Nephrol Hypertens* 1997; **6**: 474–6.
82 Davenport A, Will EJ, Davison AM. Effect of renal replacement therapy on patients with combined acute renal and fulminant hepatic failure. *Kidney International (Suppl)* 1993; **41**: S245–S251.
83 O'Grady JG, Alexander GJM, Hayllar KM *et al.* Early indicators of prognosis in fulminant hepatic failure. *Gastroenterology* 1989; **97**: 439–45.
84 Smilkstein MJ, Knapp GL, Kulig KW *et al.* Efficacy of oral N-acetylcysteine in the treatment of acetaminophen overdose: analysis of the national multicenter study (1976–1985). *N Engl J Med* 1988; **319**: 1557–62.
85 Harrison P, O'Grady J, Alexander G *et al.* Serial prothrombin times: a prognostic indicator in acetaminophen-induced fulminant hepatic failure. *Br Med J* 1990; **301**: 964–6.
86 Harrison PM, Wendon JA, Gimson AE *et al.* Improvement by acetylcysteine of hemodynamics and oxygen transport in fulminant hepatic failure. *N Engl J Med* 1991; **324**: 1852–7.
87 Harrison P, Wendon J, Williams R. Evidence of increased guanylate cyclase activation by acetylcysteine in fulminant hepatic failure. *Hepatology* 1996; **23**(5): 1067–72.
88 Losgen H, Neumann E, Eisenbach G *et al.* Correction of increased plasma amino acid levels by dialysis with amino-acid-electrolyte-glucose solutions. In: Brunner G, Schmidt FW (eds), *Artificial liver support*. New York: Springer-Verlag, 1981, pp. 153–8.
89 Gimson AE, Braude S, Mellon PJ *et al.* Earlier charcoal haemoperfusion in fulminant hepatic failure. *Lancet* 1982; **ii**: 681–3.
90 Tygstrup N, Larson FS, Hansen BA. Treatment of acute liver failure by high volume plasmapheresis. In: Lee WM, Williams R (eds), *Acute liver failure*. Cambridge: Cambridge University Press, 1997, pp. 267–77.
91 Ellis AJ, Hughes RD, Wendon JA *et al.* Pilot-controlled trial of the extracorporeal liver assist device in acute liver failure. *Hepatology* 1996; **24**: 1446–51.
92 Watanabe FD, Mullon CJ, Hewitt WR *et al.* Clinical experience with a bioartificial liver in the treatment of severe liver failure. A phase I clinical trial. *Ann Surg* 1997; **225**(5): 484–91.
93 Ringe B, Lubbe N, Kuse E *et al.* Management of emergencies before and after liver transplantation by early total hepatectomy. *Transplant Proc* 1993; **235**: 1090.
94 Benhamou JP. Fulminant and sub-fulminant hepatic failure: definitions and causes. In: Williams R, Hughes RD (eds), *Acute liver failure: improved understanding and better therapy*. London: Mitre Press, 1991.
95 O'Grady JG, Wendon J, Tan KC *et al.* Liver transplantation after paracetamol overdose (see comments). *Br Med J* 1991; **303**: 221–3.
96 Bernuau J, Goudeau A, Poynard T *et al.* Multivariate analysis of prognostic factors in fulminant hepatitis B. *Hepatology* 1986; **6**: 648–51.
97 Mitchell I, Bihari D, Chang R *et al.* Earlier identification of patients at risk from acetaminophen-induced acute liver failure. *Crit Care Med* 1998; **26**: 279–84.
98 Bernal W, Wendon J, Rela M *et al.* Use and outcome of liver transplantation in acetaminophen-induced acute liver failure. *Hepatology* 1998; **27**: 1050–5.
99 Chenard-Neu MP, Boudjema K, Bernuau J *et al.* Auxiliary liver transplantation: regeneration of the native liver and outcome in 30 patients with fulminant hepatic failure – a multicenter European study. *Hepatology* 1996; **23**: 1119–27.

Liver transplantation: prevention and treatment of rejection

29

LUCY DAGHER, ANDREW K BURROUGHS

INTRODUCTION

Liver transplantation has been one of the most rapidly evolving clinical specialties in medicine over the past three decades. It may seem logical to consider liver transplant recipients as a homogeneous group of patients which should be managed using universally applicable protocols, but they are more likely to be a heterogeneous group of individuals, with different predisposing factors and cofactors for the development of rejection.[1] However, appropriate therapeutic approaches should be generated on the basis of evidence. In this review we attempt to elucidate the following:

- Do the severity, timing, and number of episodes of acute cellular rejection affect prognosis?
- Is it possible to predict which patients will develop clinically significant acute rejection?
- Can immunosuppression be tailored to the individual patient?
- What is the evidence from randomized controlled trials that supports the choice of an immunosuppressive agent?
- Is it possible to withdraw immunosuppression or to change to less toxic immunosuppression?

The success of hepatic transplantation has resulted in its widespread use for endstage and fulminant liver disease. One-year survival rates range from 70 to 90%, with 5- and 10-year survival rates of 80% and 62% respectively.[2] Improved short term survival is mainly a consequence of better prevention and treatment of both acute rejection and infection. Current immunosuppressive agents lack specificity and there is still a need to maintain a balance between over-immunosuppression, with its potential risk of life-threatening sepsis, and under-immunosuppression leading to graft loss from rejection. Despite the good short term and acceptable long term survival after hepatic transplantation, the morbidity and mortality associated with long term immunosuppression is significant. These include development of *de novo* malignancies or opportunistic infections as well as long term drug toxicity, mainly hypertension, renal dysfunction, and induction of diabetes and dyslipidemias.[3–8]. The most dramatic example is the development of nephrotoxicity due to cyclosporin. In a series reported from Birmingham 4% of patients surviving 1 year or more developed severe chronic renal failure, with a mortality of 44% in this group.[9] Moreover, the nephrotoxic effects, hypertension, and hyperlipidaemia of some immunosuppressive agents have been implicated in the pathogenesis of chronic allograft loss.[10] These problems have stimulated a re-evaluation of the ability of some patients to tolerate their liver graft without the need for long term immunosuppression, or with greatly reduced immunosuppression, with the benefits derived from the return of natural immunity and reduction in drug related toxicity.[11–13]

However, at present the vast majority of liver transplant recipients need to take life-long immunosuppressive therapy and this situation will not change until more reliable methods for predicting tolerance in individual patients are developed.

DEFINITIONS OF REJECTION

The gold standard for diagnosis of rejection is still a histological one. Clinical and laboratory findings in general lack both sensitivity and specificity, and liver histology is needed to confirm the diagnosis of acute rejection in the face of clinical and biochemical abnormalities.[14]

The histopathological features of acute rejection have been described in similar fashion by pathologists in all experienced liver transplantation centers.[15–20] A worldwide consensus on a common nomenclature[20] and grading for acute allograft rejection has been recently achieved.[17] It is based on a composite of the most frequent, reliable, and prognostically significant features available in currently existing schemes for liver allograft rejection.[17,18] According to this Banff schema for grading liver allograft rejection,[17] the characteristics are as follows.

Acute cellular rejection

DEFINITION

"Inflammation of the allograft elicited by genetic disparity between the donor and recipient, primarily affecting interlobular bile ducts and vascular endothelia, including portal veins and hepatic venules, and occasionally the hepatic artery and its branches."

CLINICAL AND LABORATORY FINDINGS

Usually acute cellular rejection first occurs between 5 and 30 days after liver transplantation, although earlier or later occurrence can be seen in pre-sensitized patients or in those who receive less than optimal baseline immunosuppression. Clinical findings are often absent in early or mild acute rejection, although in late or severe cases, fever, liver enlargement, and tenderness of the allograft may occur. Liver injury usually becomes recognized on the basis of non-selective serum elevations of some or all standard liver tests. Peripheral blood leukocytosis and eosinophilia are also frequently present.

THE HISTOPATHOLOGICAL FEATURES OF ACUTE REJECTION

The three main histopathological features are:

1 A predominantly mononuclear but mixed portal inflammation, containing blast-like or activated lymphocytes, neutrophils, and eosinophils (graded 1 to 3).
2 Subendothelial inflammation of portal or terminal hepatic veins (or both) (graded 1 to 3).
3 Bile duct inflammation and damage (graded 1 to 3).

Table 29.1 Banff schema for grading of acute liver allograft rejection[17]

Overall grade[a]	Criteria
Indeterminate	Portal inflammatory infiltrate that fails to meet the criteria for the diagnosis of acute rejection
Mild	Rejection infiltrate in a minority of the triads that is generally mild and confined within the portal spaces
Moderate	Rejection infiltrate that expands most or all of the triads
Severe	As for "moderate" but with spillover into periportal areas and moderate to severe perivenular inflammation that extends into the hepatic parenchyma and is associated with perivenular hepatocyte necrosis

[a]Verbal descriptions of mild, moderate, and severe acute rejection could also be labeled as grades 1, 2 and 3 respectively.

In general, at least two of the above histopathological findings and biochemical evidence of liver damage constitutes the minimal diagnostic criterion for hepatic rejection. The diagnosis is strengthened if >50% of the ducts are damaged or if unequivocal endothelitis of the portal vein branches or terminal hepatic venules can be identified.

GRADING AND STAGING

The Banff schema for grading acute liver allograft rejection represents a merger and simplification of many previously published studies (Table 29.1). The published quantitative scoring systems are recommended for evaluation of new immunosuppressive regimens.[15,17]

Chronic ductopenic rejection (CR)

DEFINITION

Chronic rejection usually does not occur within 60 days after transplantation, it is usually irreversible, and two main histopathological features define it: obliterative vasculopathy and loss of bile ducts. Although these two components usually coexist, they occasionally may occur independently. The process is elicited by genetic disparity between the donor and the recipient, but other cofactors may be involved.[20]

CLINICAL AND LABORATORY FINDINGS

Chronic rejection usually develops after an unresolved episode of acute rejection, or after multiple episodes of acute rejection, or indolently during a period of months to years with few or no clinically apparent acute episodes of cellular rejection. Unresolved or indolent rejection may become apparent only because of a persistent elevation of liver test values.[20]

Table 29.2 NIDDK definitions of grades for chronic rejection, and for rejection uncertain for chronicity (indefinite for bile duct loss)[20]

Rejection, uncertain for chronicity (indefinite bile duct loss)
No complicating lobular changes
Lobular changes, including one of the three findings: centrilobular cholestasis, perivenular sclerosis, or hepatocellular ballooning or necrosis or dropout
Chronic rejection[a]
Bile duct loss, without centrilobular cholestasis, perivenular sclerosis, or hepatocyte ballooning or necrosis and drop-out
Bile duct loss, with one of the following four findings: centrilobular cholestasis, perivenular sclerosis or hepatocellular ballooning or necrosis and drop-out
Bile duct loss, with at least two of the four following findings: centrilobular cholestasis; perivenular sclerosis or hepatocellular ballooning or centrilobular necrosis and drop-out

[a]Bile duct loss >50% of triads.

THE HISTOPATHOLOGICAL FEATURES OF CHRONIC REJECTION

Two main features characterize CR: damage or loss of small (less than 60 μm) bile ducts and obliterative arteriopathy. In biopsy specimens, the minimal diagnostic criteria suggested for CR are the presence of foam cell obliterative arteriopathy or convincing evidence of bile duct loss (more than 50% of the triads). Duct loss is determined by calculating the ratio between the number of hepatic artery branches and the number of bile ducts within a portal tract. Normally the ratio is greater than 0.7.[20] Obviously, the greater the number of portal tracts counted the more likely it is that the count is valid. The diagnosis is strengthened further if the patient had documented acute rejection that progressed to chronic disease and prolonged liver dysfunction, and had not responded to appropriate anti-rejection therapy.[20]

GRADING AND STAGING

There is a tentative scheme for grading chronic rejection proposed by the National Institute of Diabetes, Digestive, and Kidney disease (NIDDK)[16] (Table 29.2).

ACUTE CELLULAR REJECTION: PROGNOSTIC FACTORS

Do the severity, timing, and number of episodes of acute cellular rejection affect prognosis?

Number of episodes

In a recent abstract, Wiesner *et al*,[21] evaluating a liver transplant database with 870 patients followed for a median of 3 years, showed that the number of episodes of acute rejection and the histological severity were significantly associated with chronic rejection (P <0.001). Dousset *et al*,[22] in a prospective study with 170 liver transplant patients, showed that there was no difference in graft function between patients with a single episode of acute rejection (n = 56) and those without rejection (n = 84). Among patients treated for a single episode of acute rejection, late hepatic function was not influenced by the severity of acute rejection, and the response to corticosteroids. In contrast, patients with more than one acute rejection episode (n = 30) had significant impairment of liver function tests (aspartate aminotransferase $P<0.05$; alanine aminotransferase, $P<0.01$; alkaline phosphatase, $P<0.01$), lower dye clearances ($P<0.01$), and more severe histological damage ($P<0.001$). The authors concluded that a single episode of acute rejection does not impair long term hepatic function, whereas recurrent episodes can lead to damage to the liver allograft.

Severity

McVicar *et al*[23] describe a group of patients who had focal rejection in the hepatic allograft biopsy defined as lymphocytic infiltration involving less than 20% of portal tracts. In the follow-up of 41 patients showing focal or mild rejection, only six patients (15%) subsequently developed abnormal liver function tests and required treatment with additional immunosuppression for acute cellular rejection. The authors conclude that patients showing focal or mild rejection do not necessarily need additional immunosuppression and can be followed closely without immediate treatment.

In a follow-up in Birmingham of 151 patients to assess the effect of not treating mild acute rejection (protocol 7-day biopsies), 97 had histologically mild rejection: 50 had biochemical dysfunction and received prednisone for 3 days, while the remaining 47 cases with stable biochemistry had no additional treatment. Fifty-four patients with no rejection were included for comparison. The outcome at 3 months in all three groups was similar.[19]

Wiesner *et al*[24] using the Liver Transplantation Database in a cohort study of 762 consecutive adult liver transplantation recipients examined the association of histological severity of acute rejection and overall patient outcome. They showed, using univariate analysis, that acute rejection overall, including mostly the milder grades, was significantly associated with an increased patient survival (RR 0.71, $P = 0.05$) and a trend toward improved graft survival. Moreover, adjusting for other risk factors such as age and renal insufficiency, they found no significant decrease in survival among patients who had rejection. These findings were similar to those of Fisher *et al*,[25] who analyzed nine studies (comprising a total of 1473 patients), and found that there was no correlation between mortality and incidence of treated acute cellular rejection.

These findings in liver transplantation are in contrast to renal transplantation in which acute rejection is significantly associated with decreased patient and graft survival. Why acute cellular rejection in liver transplantation recipients is not associated with decreased patient and graft survival remains unexplained. It is possible that acute rejection in the setting of controlled alloreactivity exerts a tolerizing effect, making the graft less susceptible to further immunological attack. However, it should be noted that successful treatment for cellular rejection occurs in nearly all cases. Thus the correct interpretation of the finding reported above is that the occurrence and successful treatment of acute cellular rejection does not influence survival in liver transplant patients.

Timing

As regards timing of acute cellular rejection, there is no firm consensus to define what is early or late. In three different studies the timing and the outcome vary according to the definition of each centre.

In a multicenter retrospective analysis[21] of 623 liver transplants, the cumulative incidence of biopsy proven rejection was 59% for early episodes(<6 months) and 21% for late episodes (≥6 months). Patient and graft survival did not differ significantly between those who experienced an early acute rejection episode and those who did not ($P = 0.49$ and $P = 0.13$ respectively). Furthermore, they did not differ significantly between recipients who experienced a late acute rejection episode and those who did not (patient survival $P = 0.18$, and graft survival $P = 0.20$).

Wiesner *et al*[24] analyzed 762 consecutive adult liver transplantation recipients (Liver Transplantation Database) and found 367 (48%) who developed at least one acute cellular rejection episode within the first 6 weeks post transplantation (occurring at a median time of 8 days). Multivariate analysis indicated that acute cellular rejection had a trend to better survival (RR = 0.78, $P = 0.25$) and retransplantation free survival (RR = 0.86, $P = 0.44$). However, severe rejection doubled the risk of death or retransplantation compared to mild rejection. Using proportional hazards modeling, in the same study, seven factors were identified that were independently associated with an increased incidence of early acute hepatic allograft rejection: younger recipient age, lack of renal impairment, lack of edema, higher AST levels, fewer HLA DR matches, longer cold ischemic times, and older donors.

Mor *et al*[26] retrospectively reviewed 375 liver transplants, and defined late onset acute cellular rejection as that which occurred after 6 months. There were 315 episodes of early acute cellular rejection in 226 patients and 31 episodes of late acute cellular rejection in 26 patients. Low cyclosporin levels appeared to account for 58% of these late episodes. Most episodes of rejection responded to pulse corticosteroids, and chronic ductopenic rejection arose in only two patients. There was no difference in survival between patients experiencing early and late rejection.

Anand *et al*[27] reviewed late onset acute cellular rejection, defining it as rejection recognized after the first 30 days post transplantation. They evaluated 717 patients transplanted in Birmingham, between 1982 and 1994: 59 (8%) patients had 71 episodes of late rejection. They too found that the most common precipitating event was low levels of calcineurin antagonists, and that most acute episodes of rejection in this time frame were responsive to standard therapy. However, in contrast to Mor *et al*, Anand found that 16 of 59 (27%) patients developing late onset rejection progressed to chronic ductopenic rejection and graft loss. Delayed response to an earlier episode of acute rejection, and centrilobular necrosis or bile duct loss at the time of diagnosis of late rejection, were associated with high risk of progression to chronic rejection and graft loss.

These results regarding timing, severity, and number of episodes of early acute cellular rejection lead one to question whether an attempt to further reduce the incidence of early acute rejection in liver transplantation is either necessary or appropriate. This is especially questionable because increased immunosuppression theoretically could inhibit the development of donor-specific tolerance, increase the incidence of immunosuppressive elated complications, and result in poorer outcome. Indeed, it may be better not to treat certain mild acute rejection episodes. However, randomized controlled trials are needed to provide evidence supporting the latter approach.

PREDICTION OF ACUTE REJECTION

Is it possible to predict which patients will develop clinically significant acute rejection? Data from Birmingham[1,28] suggest that there is a lower incidence of acute rejection when there is no evidence of immune involvement in the pathogenesis of the original liver disease, eg fulminant hepatic failure from paracetamol. In contrast, in patients transplanted for primary biliary cirrhosis and sclerosing cholangitis, in which immune mediated damage of bile ducts is a feature of the original disease, acute rejection occurs more frequently and there is more frequent progression to ductopenic rejection. Wiesner *et al* in a study of 870 consecutive primary liver transplant recipients found that autoimmune liver disease was an independent risk factor for developing chronic rejection.[29] A similar conclusion was obtained in a second small series of 63 patients reported by Hayashi *et al.*[30] Patients with autoimmune hepatitis had a higher incidence of acute rejection than patients with alcoholic cirrhosis (81% vs 46.8%; $P<0.001$), regardless of the type of immunosuppression. In addition, steroid resistant rejection occurred more frequently in patients transplanted for autoimmmune liver disease (31.1% vs 12.8%; $P=0.003$). There was also a trend toward a higher incidence of chronic rejection. However, there was no difference in allograft or patient survivals at 1 and 3 years. Berlakovich *et al*[31] reported data from a group of 252 liver transplanted patients which showed that patients who had undergone transplantation for alcoholic cirrhosis ($n=60$), hepatoma ($n=91$) and post-hepatitic cirrhosis ($n=59$) had a lower risk for acute rejection and the need to receive rescue therapy than patients who had been transplanted for cholestatic disease ($n=42$). The cumulative rates of acute rejection episodes per patient per month at 6 months, when 94% of all acute rejection episodes occurred, were: 0.45 for alcoholic cirrhosis, 0.55 for post-hepatitic cirrhosis, 0.65 for hepatoma, and 1.0 for cholestatic disease.

The one group which has been consistently shown to have a lower incidence of acute and chronic rejection is chronic hepatitis B. It has been proposed that the reduced incidence of rejection in these patients might reflect the underlying defect in cell mediated immunity, which allowed the patients to become chronically infected with the virus in the first place.[32,33]

Farges *et al*,[33] in a retrospective analysis of the data obtained from 330 patients who were transplant recipients for chronic liver disease, found that the incidence of acute rejection (48 at 1 year) and chronic rejection (10% at 3 years) was comparable in patients who had undergone transplantation for primary biliary cirrhosis, sclerosing cholangitis, autoimmune cirrhosis, and hepatitis C cirrhosis. However, the incidence of acute (but not chronic) rejection was significantly lower in patients who had undergone transplantation for alcoholic cirrhosis (29% at 1 year). In patients who had undergone transplantation for HBV cirrhosis, the incidence of both acute (21% at 1 year) and chronic (0% at 3 years) rejection was significantly lower. They suggest that patients who undergo transplantation for alcoholic liver cirrhosis, because they are at high risk of sepsis and low risk of acute rejection, would probably benefit from a reduction in the level of immunosuppression. Because HBV replication is potentiated by immunosuppression, it could also prove beneficial to reduce the level of immunosuppression in these patients. However, Wiesner *et al*,[24] using multivariate analysis, showed that the 6-week incidence of acute rejection in a cohort of 762 consecutive adult liver transplant recipients was not dependent on the underlying disease.

Although it is difficult to draw firm recommendations from these studies, it should be possible to test the hypothesis that patients transplanted for HBV, HCV cirrhosis, alcoholic liver disease or hepatoma can be treated safely with early steroid withdrawal, or less intense immunosuppression, such as monotherapy, from the outset. Conversely, patients with autoimmune hepatitis, primary biliary cirrhosis, or primary sclerosing cholangitis may need steroid maintenance and heavier initial immunosuppression.

Table 29.3 Studies of steroid withdrawal in liver transplantation

Study	Immunosuppression	Interval at withdrawal	No. of patients	Follow-up (mth)	Steroid restarted	Acute rejection	Chronic rejection	Patient death	Graft loss
Late withdrawal									
Uncontrolled studies; prospective evaluation									
Punch, 1995[37]	CSA + AZA	>1 yr	51	13.8	6	2	0	0	0
Tchervenkov,1996[38]	CSA + AZA	1 yr	42 (33[a])	12	1	3 (9%)	0	0	1
Stegall, 1997[39]	CYA	>2 yr	28	12	5	2 (7.1%)	0	0	0
	CYA + S		24			1 (4.2%)	0		
Gomez,1998[41]	CYA	>1 yr	72	23±8		0	0	0	0
	CYA + A + S		14			0	0	0	0
Randomized trial									
McDiarmid, 1995[40]	CYA + A	>1 yr	33	19.7		2 (6%)	0	0	0
	CYA + A + S		31	17.6		2 (6.5%)	0	0	0
Early withdrawal									
Uncontrolled studies; retrospective evaluation									
Padbury, 1993[34]	CYA + AZA	≥3 mth	168	28	14	7 (4.5%)	6 (3.9%)	20	17
Fraser, 1996[36]	CYA + AZA	>3 mth	96	24.3±1	0	8 (8.3%)	3 (3%)	14 (14%)	4 (4%)
	CYA + AZA + S		18	8.4	0	7 (39%)	3 (17%)	8 (44%)	2 (22%)
Randomized trial									
Belli, 1998[35]	CYA + S	>3 mth	37	60	1	3 (8%)	1	9	
	CYA		1			2 (4%)	0	11	

[a]Only 33 of 42 patients were evaluated for steroid weaning.

WEANING IMMUNOSUPPRESSION

Steroid withdrawal

Steroid withdrawal has been studied in two different settings (Table 29.3): early withdrawal (3 months)[34–36] and late withdrawal (>1 year).[37–39,40,41]

In the early withdrawal group starting at 3 months after liver transplantation, there are two uncontrolled studies with retrospective evaluation, reported by Padbury *et al*[34] and Fraser *et al*.[36] The occurrence of rejection after steroid withdrawal was very similar in both studies (7.8% and 8.3% respectively). Grade C In the study by Fraser *et al* the incidence of acute cellular rejection was higher in the group remaining on steroids (38.9%), representing a group of patients in whom steroids could not be withdrawn because of a complicated clinical course. Thus there is a group of patients in whom steroids cannot be withdrawn. In both studies early withdrawal resulted in an improvement in the blood glucose control and fewer infections, but Fraser *et al* did not demonstrate an improvement in hypertension. Chronic rejection was not increased in the steroid withdrawal groups.

Belli *et al*[35] conducted a randomized trial in 104 patients to continue or stop steroids at 3 months after transplantation whilst continuing with cyclosporin. They found that the frequency of acute rejection after randomization was 8% (steroids) and 4% (no steroids). A single episode of chronic rejection was observed in a patient with long steroid therapy. Adverse effects of steroid therapy were less frequent in patients weaned off steroids, and when considering hypertension and diabetes, the difference between the two groups was statistically significant. After 5 years survival was similar in patients with or without steroids.

In the late steroid withdrawal group (after 1 year) there are four uncontrolled but prospectively evaluated studies[37–39,41] Grade B showing no increase in the incidence of acute rejection after steroid withdrawal, with no cases of chronic rejection and with an improvement in blood pressure, weight control, glycemic control, and lipid profile in the steroid withdrawal group. In one prospective controlled trial, McDiarmid *et al*[40] randomized 64 patients (42 adults, 22 children) at 1 year to steroid withdrawal (33 patients) or no withdrawal (31 patients). Grade A There was no difference in the incidence of biopsy proven acute rejection, but there was a difference in the frequency of steroid associated adverse effects.

Papatheodoridis *et al*[42] observed in an uncontrolled study that less immunosuppression is associated with less fibrosis in a small group of hepatitis C patients. Grade C Previous studies have shown that steroids increase replication of B and C viruses, accelerate recurrence of HCV hepatitis[42] in the liver graft, and worsen histology in patients with chronic hepatitis B.[43–45] Grade C

Total withdrawal and "subtherapeutic doses" of immunosuppression

Long term surviving liver transplant recipients are often systematically excessively immunosuppressed. Consequently, drug weaning is an important management strategy providing it is done gradually under careful physician surveillance. Devlin *et al*,[12] in 18 patients, showed that it was possible to either completely withdraw (five of 18 patients) or significantly reduce (nine of 18 patients) maintenance immunosuppression to levels previously considered subtherapeutic. Grade C Parameters associated with successful

Table 29.4 Randomized trials of tacrolimus vs cyclosporin (Sandimmune) with cumulative number or actuarial proportion of events at yearly follow-up intervals

Study	No. of patients	Initial dosage regimen (mg/kg/d)	Time of assessment (yr)	Results (% of patients) Graft survival (%)	Patient survival (%)	Acute rejection	Refractory rejection	Chronic rejection	Crossover for intractable rejection (*n*)
European FK506 Multicenter Liver Study Group[50]	264	Tacrolimus 0.075 mg/kg iv	1	77.5[a]	82.9[a]	107 (41%)	2 (1%)	4 (1.5%)	NA
		then 0.30 mg/kg oral	2	74.5[a]	80.6[a]	45.4 %[f]	3 (1%)	4(1.5%)	7
		+steroids (0.164 mg/kg)	3	70.6[a]	77.0[a]	45.4%[f]	1.2%[f]	2%[f]	NA
	265	Cyclosporin 1–6 mg/kg	1	72.6[a]	77.5[a]	132 (50%)	14 (5%)	14(5%)	14
		iv then 8–15 mg/kg	2	70[a]	74.8[a]	56%[f]	16 (6%)	14(5%)	27
		oral + AZA + steroids oral (0.168 mg/kg)+ ATG days 1–7[b]	3	65.2[a]	69.7[a]	55%[f]	5.9%[f]	7%[f]	NA
US Multicenter FK506 Liver Study Group[51]	263	Tacrolimus 0.075 mg/kg iv	1	82[a]	88[a]	154 (68%)	6 (3%)	5 (2%)	3
		reduced to 0.05 mg/kg	3	77	84[a]		NA	NA	NA
		then 0.15 mg/kg oral + steroids (90+65 mg/kg)	5	71.8	79[a]	17% 4.9%	0	0	6

	266	Cyclosporin 1–2 mg/kg iv, then 5 mg/kg oral + AZA + steroids (131+61 mg/kg)±ATG[c]	1	79[a]	88[a]	173 (76%)	32 (15%)	4 (1.5%)	22 (8%)
			3	72	79[a]	13%	NA	NA	NA
			5	66.4	73[a]	6%	0	0	22
Fung (Pittsburgh)[52]	79	Tacrolimus 0.1 mg/kg[d] iv + steroids 20 mg/day	4	78%[e]	84	50 (64%)	1 (1.2%)	NA	NA
	75	Cyclosporin 4 mg/kg IV then 8 mg/kg[d]+steroids 20 mg/day	4	70%[e]	84	62 (83%)	1 (1.3%)	13	47[g]

[a]Actuarial rates of survival.
[b]Antithymocite globulin (ATG) was administered at dose of 5 mg/kg per day for a week induction period post transplant in three centers.
[c]Regimen varied among centers.
[d]Ad hoc dose adjustments according to levels.
[e]Estimated from a graph.
[f]Kaplan–Meier estimates.
[g]47 patients crossed over to tacrolimus: seven before and 40 after rejection (one tacrolimus crossed into cyclosporin group).

drug withdrawal were transplantation for non-immune mediated liver disorders, fewer donor–recipient HLA A, B, and DR mismatches, and low incidence of early rejection. In a series of 95 patients from the University of Pittsburgh,[11–13] there were 18 (19%) patients who had been drug free from 10 months to 4.8 years, 37 (39%) patients were in an uninterrupted process of drug weaning, 28 (29%) patients had weaning interrupted because of rejection, and 12 (13%) were withdrawn from the protocol, eight of them because of non-compliance, two because of recurrent primary biliary cirrhosis, one for pregnancy, and one for renal failure necessitating kidney transplant. There were also five patients who had "self weaned" and three of the five remained well after a drug free interval of 14–17 years. A fourth patient died in a road traffic accident after 11 years off immunosuppression, and the fifth underwent re-transplantation because of hepatitis C infection after 9 drug free years. Although recurrence of autoimmune hepatitis has not yet been observed, two (15%) of 13 patients with PBC developed recurrence. In this study no patients were diagnosed with chronic rejection. However, according to these results in any given individual there are no criteria specific enough to indicate that total withdrawal of immunosuppression will be safe.

R
Grade C

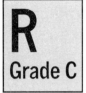

The optimal regimen of drug withdrawal is unknown. Criteria that can be used to select appropriate patients are required. Disorders with a well characterized immunological or viral basis appear to experience graft dysfuncion after withdrawal.[46,47]

Therefore the search continues for the ideal immunosuppressive agent – one that selectively inhibits alloantigen immune responses, prevents chronic allograft rejection, and is free of major adverse effects.[48]

CHOICE OF AN IMMUNOSUPPRESSIVE AGENT

What evidence is there from randomized controlled trials to support the choice of an immunosuppressive agent?

Calcineurin Inhibitors

Calcineurin inhibitors are currently the keystones of most immunosuppressive regimens used in clinical organ transplantation. Both cyclosporin and tacrolimus bind to cytoplasmic receptors (cyclophylin and FK-binding protein [FK BP-12], respectively) and resulting complexes inactivate calcineurin, a pivotal enzyme in T-cell receptor signaling. Calcineurin inhibition prevents IL-2 gene transcription, thereby inhibiting T-cell interleukin production.[48,49]

Three separate randomized trials have been conducted to compare the efficacy of tacrolimus and cyclosporin (Sandimmune) in primary liver transplant patients (Table 29.4).

1 European Multicentre Tacrolimus Trial (eight centers, 545 patients).[50]
2 US Multicenter Tacrolimus Liver Study Group (12 centers, 529 patients).[51]
3 University of Pittsburgh (single center, 154 patients).[52]

In all these trials tacrolimus was administered with corticosteroids, but no azathioprine. However, in the two large trials, the cyclosporin group received corticosteroids and azathioprine and, in some cases, antilymphocyte globulin. Moreover, the adjunctive immunosuppression was not the same in all centers that participated in the studies. These protocols of double therapy with tacrolimus versus triple or quadruple therapy with cyclosporin have been noted as being unbalanced and not representing therefore a comparison of tacrolimus versus cyclosporin.[53] However, the net non-specific immunosuppression in both arms seems to have been similar, since the frequency of cytomegalovirus infection in both arms did not differ.[54] Interpretation of the relative benefit of tacrolimus and cyclosporin is difficult in the framework of these studies.

PATIENT AND GRAFT SURVIVAL

In the multicenter studies the tacrolimus based regimen produced similar 1-year graft and patient survival rates to the cyclosporin based regimen. In the Pittsburgh trial, the 1-year patient and graft survival were not different when data were analyzed on an intention to treat basis, although as in the other two studies a trend was shown for a better survival in the tacrolimus group. Moreover, a recent long term follow-up of the US tacrolimus study group[55] has shown that cumulative 5-year patient and graft survival were comparable for the tacrolimus based regimen (79%, 71.8%) and cyclosporin based regimens (73.1%, 66.4%) but median patient survival was longer for tacrolimus treated patients (tacrolimus 25.1 ± 5.1 years, cyclosporin 15.2 ± 2.5 years). In the 3-year follow-up of the European multicenter trial[56,57] the analysis according to intention to treat at 3 years showed a significant difference in patient survival in favor of the tacrolimus based regimen[57] (tacrolimus 75.7%, cyclosporin 67.5%, $P = 0.036$).

R
Grade A

REJECTION

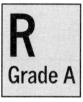

In the randomized trials a notable difference between tacrolimus and cyclosporin based regimens was the lower incidence of acute rejection with tacrolimus. In the European study acute rejection was less frequent in the tacrolimus based group (tacrolimus 56.6%, cyclosporin 46.4%, $P = 0.004$). Refractory rejection (tacrolimus 0.8%, cyclosporin 5.6%, $P = 0.005$) and chronic rejection (tacrolimus 1.5%, cyclosporin 5.3%, $P = 0.032$) were also less common with the tacrolimus regimen. These differences were observed despite higher concomitant use of corticosteroids or azathioprine in the cyclosporin group.

R
Grade A

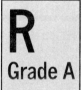

Data from the US multicenter study also showed less rejection with tacrolimus – acute rejection: tacrolimus 154 (68%), cyclosporin 173 (76%), $P < 0.002$; corticosteroid resistant rejection: tacrolimus 42 (16.3%) and cyclosporin 82 (30.8%), $P < 0.001$; refractory rejection: tacrolimus 6 (3%), cyclosporin 32 (15%), $P < 0.001$. The Pittsburgh group obtained similar results. In all three trials a large percentage of patients (see Table 29.4) were switched from cyclosporin to tacrolimus, mainly because of persistent rejection (European $n = 14$, US $n = 22$, Pittsburgh $n = 47$).

R
Grade A

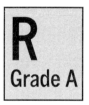

Ninety-one patients with chronic rejection that developed during cyclosporin based immunosuppression were converted to tacrolimus in an open label multicenter study[58] involving 17 liver transplant centers in the US. Sixty-four (70.3%) were alive with their initial hepatic allograft after a mean follow-up of 251 days. In this study patients with total bilirubin of ≤10 mg/dl at the time of conversion had a significantly better graft and patient survival than patients with total bilirubin >10 mg/dl. The time between liver transplantation and conversion also affected graft and patient survival. Patients converted to tacrolimus ≤90 days after transplantation had 1-year actuarial graft and patient survival of 51.9% and 65.9% respectively, compared with 73.2% ($P = 0.002$) and 87.7% ($P = 0.02$) for those converted >90 days after transplantation.

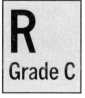

R
Grade C

Steroid sparing effect

R Grade A

In the US trial the cumulative dose of steroids for both prophylaxis and rejection was significantly less with tacrolimus than with the cyclosporin based regimen (90 vs 131 mg/kg, $P < 0.001$). Similarly, lower intravenous but not oral corticosteroid doses were required during maintenance therapy with tacrolimus versus cyclosporin in the European study at 1 year, and both oral and intravenous doses were lower with tacrolimus after 3 years ($P < 0.05$). At 3 years steroid therapy had been successfully withdrawn in 80% of tacrolimus and 68% of cyclosporin treated patients ($P = 0.025$).

Microemulsified cyclosporin

R Grade A

R Grade A

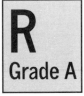

The recent development of a microemulsified formulation of cyclosporin (Neoral) addressed the major limitation of the previous oil based drug preparations, a highly variable partial and bile dependent gastrointestinal absorption process.[49,59–64] In two randomized controlled trials comparing Neoral with Sandimmune,[65,66] the Neoral group experienced less rejection, fewer episodes of steroid resistant rejection, and a lower incidence of moderate/severe histological rejection. Indeed the microemulsion formulation may remove or reduce the discrepancy in outcomes between cyclosporin and tacrolimus-based regimens seen in the randomized trials described above. In a randomized trial involving 71 patients, Stegall[67] observed a similar incidence of acute rejection episodes whether mycophenolate mofetil (MMF) was combined with Neoral or with tacrolimus. Fisher *et al*,[68] in a similar trial of MMF combined with Neoral or tacrolimus, also found similar rates of acute rejection (Neoral 46%, tacrolimus 42.3%), and there were no differences observed between treatment groups with respect to the incidence of diabetes mellitus, hypertension, or hyperglycemia.

Randomized trials comparing microemulsified cyclosporin with tacrolimus have been performed in Canada in approximately 180 patients and by the United Kingdom and Republic of Ireland Liver Transplant Study Group in over 600 patients. The results are awaited with interest.

Trials of mycophenolate mofetil

This drug is a selective inhibitor of the *de novo* pathway of purine biosynthesis, thereby providing a more specific and potent inhibition of T cell and B cell proliferation. Three large multicenter trials have compared mycophenolate mofetil with azathioprine or placebo in renal patients receiving cyclosporin and steroids. These studies showed that mycophenolate mofetil therapy is associated with a 50% reduction in acute rejection episodes in the first year after transplantation.[69,70] However, studies with longer term follow-up (>3 years) have not shown improved long term graft survival with mycophenolate mofetil. The principal adverse effects observed in these trials were bone marrow suppression and gastrointestinal toxicity. The experience in liver transplant is limited [71–74]

R Grade A

In liver transplantation Klupp *et al*[74] randomized 120 patients to receive Neoral/MMF, tacrolimus/MMF, or tacrolimus alone. All patients received concurrent low dose prednisone. After a mean follow-up of 18 months patient survival was similar in the three groups (82%, 95%, and 90% respectively) and graft survival was 72%, 95%, and

Table 29.5 Randomized trials of mycophenolate mofetil (MMF) for immunosuppression in liver transplantation

Study	No. of patients	Patient survival (%)	Graft survival (%)	Acute rejection	Steroid resistant rejection	Withdrawn MMF
Klupp, 1999[74]						
Neoral + MMF + steroids	40	82	72	33 (82.5%)	9 (22.5%)	23 (57.5%)
Tacrolimus + MMF + steroids	40	95	95	20 (50%)	5 (12.5%)	23 (57.5%)
Tacrolimus + steroids	40	90	85	20 (52.5%)	5 (12.5%)	—
Jain, 1998[73]						
Tacrolimus + MMF + steroids	101	83.1	79.2	32 (31.7%)	0	61 (61%)
Tacrolimus + steroids	99	85	80.2	41 (41.4%)	28[a]	—

[a]Received MMF to control ongoing acute rejection.

85% respectively ($P = 0.05$, for each comparison versus cyclosporin group). The incidence and severity of acute rejection were significantly different between the groups. Histologically confirmed rejection was observed in 33 patients (82.5%) in the Neoral/MMF group, 20 patients (50%) in the tacrolimus/MMF group, and 21 patients (52.5%) in the tacrolimus group ($P < 0.001$). OKT3 rescue therapy was necessary for nine (22.5%) patients in the Neoral/MMF group, for five (12.5%) in the tacrolimus/MMF group, and for five (12.5%) in the tacrolimus group. However, MMF was discontinued in both groups in a large proportion of patients (58%, 23 patients in each group) due to adverse events or refractory rejection. The authors concluded that the combination of MMF with tacrolimus and steroids offered no advantages compared with tacrolimus and steroid immunosuppression. However, graft survival was significantly worse in the Neoral group ($P = 0.05$), and in this group 48 patients were switched to tacrolimus due to rejection or toxicity (Table 29.5).

R Grade A

An interim report from a randomized trial comparing tacrolimus and prednisone versus tacrolimus, prednisone, and mycophenolate[75] in 200 patients described similar results (Table 29.6). During the study period 28 of 99 (28%) of patients randomized to tacrolimus plus prednisone received mycophenolate to control ongoing acute rejection, or reduce nephrotoxicity and/or neurotoxicity. However, 61 of 101 patients (61%) randomized to the tacrolimus/prednisone/mycophenolate regimen discontinued mycophenolate for infection, myelosuppression and gastrointestinal disturbances.

R Grade A

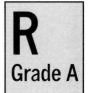

MMF may be a safe and potentially useful adjuvant immunosuppressive agent for initiation and maintenance therapy,[76] but to date there is no evidence that it is superior to tacrolimus and steroid immunosuppression. The use of MMF is limited by the adverse

Table 29.6 Randomized controlled trials of UDCA for prevention of liver transplant rejection

Study	Dose (duration)	Days after transplant	Acute rejection (%)
Pageaux, 1995[83]			
26 UDCA	600 mg/day	3–5	34
24 placebo	(2 mth)		37
Nordic Multicenter, 1997[81]		1	65
58 UDCA	15 mg/kg/d		68
48 placebo	(3 mth)		
Barnes, 1997[84]			
28 UDCA	10–15 mg/kg/d	3–5	61
24 placebo	(3 mth)		71
Fleckenstein, 1998[82]			
14 UDCA	15 mg/kg/d	1	79
16 placebo	(3–6 mth)		75

effects experienced in more than 50% of patients. More randomized controlled trials are needed to evaluate safety and efficacy.

Trials of ursodeoxycholic acid (UDCA)

Ursodeoxycholic acid is a hydrophilic bile acid that has been shown to protect the liver parenchyma in cholestatic states and possibly to slow the progression of primary biliary cirrhosis.[77,78] Additionally, UDCA has been shown to reduce the expression of major histocompatibility complex (MHC) class I antigens in patients with primary biliary cirrhosis and therefore may have immunomodulatory effects on T-cell dependent liver damage.[77–79]. During acute cellular rejection, there is an expression of MHC class I and II antigens on hepatocytes, although these are not primary target cells. Cholestasis itself may induce an increased expression of MHC class I antigens on hepatocytes, which can lead to lymphocyte $CD8^+$ dependent cytotoxicity.[80] Based on these theoretical considerations, UDCA could be used as adjuvant therapy to decrease acute cellular rejection episodes in liver transplant patients.

There are four randomized controlled trials evaluating UDCA (10–15 mg/kg) for prevention of acute allograft rejection in liver transplant patients.

1 The Nordic Multicenter double-blind randomized controlled trial of prophylactic UDCA in liver transplant patients[81] (54 UDCA, 48 placebo).
2 Fleckenstein *et al*[82] (14 UDCA, 16 placebo).
3 Pageaux G-P *et al*[83] (26 UDCA, 24 placebo).
4 Barnes *et al*[84] (28 UDCA, 24 placebo).

R
Grade A

Three randomized controlled trials[81–83] comprising a total of 182 patients showed that UDCA was not effective for prevention of acute rejection in liver transplanted patients. Although Barnes *et al*[84] found that there were significantly fewer patients in the UDCA treatment group who had multiple episodes of acute rejection (0 vs 6), the severity of rejection was not described. There is no good evidence to recommend UDCA as adjuvant therapy to prevent rejection (Table 29.6).

Table 29.7 Randomized controlled trials of tacrolimus and steroids with and without azathioprine for immunosuppression in liver transplantation

Study	Immunosuppression regimen	Patient survival (%)	Graft survival (%)	Acute rejection	Chronic rejection
Neuhaus, 1997[86]	Tacrolimus + steroids	79	76.5	24 (35.3%)	1
	Tacrolimus + steroids + azathioprine	88.7	80.6	27 (43.5%)	1
Samuel, 1998[85]	Tacrolimus + steroids	90.1	87.1	40 (39.6%)	0
	Tacrolimus + steroids + azathioprine	92.6	90.4	42(44.7%)	0

Trials comparing double (tacrolimus and prednisone) and triple (tacrolimus, prednisone, and azathioprine) therapy

Two randomized trials (Table 29.7), one reported by Samuel *et al*[85] (101 patients randomized to tacrolimus and steroids and 94 to tacrolimus, azathioprine, and steroids) and the second by Nehaus *et al*[86] (66 patients randomized to tacrolimus and prednisone, and 66 randomized to low dose of tacrolimus, azathioprine, and prednisone), revealed no statistically significant differences between these regimens with respect to graft or patient survival, the incidence of episodes of acute rejection, chronic rejection, or adverse events (Table 29.7), except for the higher incidence of hematologically related adverse events in the group of patients who received azathioprine.[85]

R
Grade A

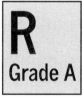

Trials comparing single agent immunosuppressive therapies

In a recent randomized controlled trial at the Royal Free Hospital,[87] 64 patients were randomized to receive single agent immunosuppressive therapy (with no maintenance steroids) with microemulsified cyclosporin (34 patients) or tacrolimus (30 patients). Survival at 1 and 3 years was similar in the two treatment groups. Biopsy evidence of acute cellular rejection (protocol biopsies were performed in all patients) was seen in 22 (70%) in the Neoral group and 20 (67%) in the tacrolimus group, but no graft was lost on account of acute or chronic rejection. All the episodes of acute cellular rejection responded to steroids.

This experience is extremely interesting because it is the first study comparing tacrolimus and Neoral "head to head", but also because it demonstrates for the first time that a single agent can be used with relative safety in terms of risk of graft loss. As one (and possibly two) episodes of acute rejection do not affect graft or patient survival, added immunosuppression could be given to those patients who have at least one or two acute rejection episodes, thus tailoring the maintenance regimen to the individual patient. However, initial monotherapy needs to be tested in larger studies. The advantage of not using maintenance steroids has been discussed above. Avoiding azathioprine will avoid cases of nodular regenerative hyperplasia[88] with portal hypertension, as well as cases of myelosuppression.

R
Grade A

RECOMMENDATION

The major evidence for determining the choice of primary immunosuppressive drug comes from randomized trials of cyclosporin (Sandimmune) versus tacrolimus. They have similar effects on graft survival in either short or long term, but the comparative evaluation is complicated by the conversion to tacrolimus of many cyclosporin patients because of persistent rejection. This analysis and the fact that that less steroids and azathioprine were used with tacrolimus regimens would favor tacrolimus. New trials of microemulsified cyclosporin versus tacrolimus, may lead to better evidence on which to base a choice of the main immunosuppressive agent. Currently the selection of the calcineurin inhibitor to be used first is generally based on either physician preference or patient intolerance to one of the drugs, eg due to cosmetic adverse effects, ill-defined pharmacodynamic resistance, and/or idiopathic nephrotoxic or neurotoxic sensitivity.[49] The advent of new immunosuppressive agents emphasizes the need for randomized controlled trials in this area.

Acknowledgements

Dr Lucy Dagher is supported by Fundagastro (Hospital General del Oeste) and Fundayacucho, and Fundacion Vollmer, Caracas-Venezuela.

REFERENCES

1 Neuberger J, Adams DH. What is the significance of acute allograft liver rejection? *J Hepatol* 1998; **29**: 143–50.
2 Abbasoglu O, Levy M, Brkic BB *et al.* Ten years of liver transplantation. *Transplantation* 1997; **64**: 1801–7.
3 Canzanello VJ, Schwartz L, Taler SJ *et al.* Evolution of cardiovascular risk after liver transplantation: a comparison of cyclopsorine A and tacrolimus (FK506). *Liver Transplant Surg* 1997; **3**: 1–9.
4 Canzanello VJ, Textor SC, Taler SJ *et al.* Late hypertension after liver transplantation: a comparison of cyclosporine and tacrolimus (FK506). *Liver Transplant Surg* 1998; **4**: 328–34.
5 Pham H, Lemoine A, Salvucci M *et al.* Occurrence of gammopathies and lymphoproliferative disorders in liver transplant recipients randomized to tacrolimus (FK506) or cyclosporine based immunosuppression. *Liver Transplant Surg* 1998; **4**: 146–51.
6 Jindal RM, Sidner RA, Milgrom ML. Post-transplant diabetes mellitus. The role of immunosuppression. *Drug Safety* 1997; **16**: 242–57.
7 Abouljoud MS, Levy MF, Klintmalm GB. Hyperlipidemia after liver transplantation: long-term results of the FK506/cyclosporine A US multicenter trial. *Transplant Proc* 1995; **27**: 1121–3.
8 Mor E, Facklam D, Hasse J *et al.* Weight gain and lipid profile changes in liver transplant recipients: long-term results of the American FK506 multicenter study. *Transplant Proc* 1995; **27**: 1126.
9 Fisher NC, Nightingale PG, Gunson B *et al.* Chronic renal failure following liver transplantation. *Transplantation* 1998; **66**: 59–66.
10 Pelletier RP, Orosz CG, Cosio FG *et al.* Risk factors in chronic rejection. *Curr Opin Organ Transplant* 1999; **4**: 28–34.
11 Mazariegos GV, Reyes J, Marino IR *et al.* Weaning of immunosuppression in liver transplant recipients. *Transplantation* 1997; **63**: 243–9.
12 Devlin J, Doherty D, Thomson L *et al.* Defining the outcome of immunosuppression withdrawal after liver transplantation. *Hepatology* 1998; **27**: 926–33.
13 Ramos HC, Reyes J, Abu-Elmagd K *et al.* Weaning of immunosuppression in long-term liver transplant recipients. *Transplantation* 1995; **59**: 212–17.
14 Wiesner R. Is hepatic histology the true gold standard in diagnosing acute hepatic allograft rejection? *Liver Transplant Surg* 1996; **2**: 165–7.
15 Gupta DS, Hudson M, Burroughs A *et al.* Grading of cellular rejection after orthotopic

liver transplantation. *Hepatology* 1995; **21**(1): 46–57.
16 Demetris AJ, Seaberg E, Batts KP *et al.* Reliability and predictive value of the national institute of diabetes and digestive and kidney diseases liver transplantation database nomenclature and grading system for cellular rection of liver allografts. *Hepatology* 1995; **21**: 408–16.
17 Demetris AJ, Batts KP, Dhillon AP *et al.* Banff schema for grading liver allograft rejection: an international consensus document. *Hepatology* 1997; **25**: 658–63.
18 Demetris AJ. Immune cholangitis: liver allograft rejection and graft versus host disease. *Mayo Clin Proc* 1998; **73**: 367–79.
19 Hubscher S. Diagnosis and grading of liver allograft rejection: a European perspective. *Transplant Proc* 1996; **28**: 504–7.
20 International Working Party. Terminology for hepatic allograft rejection. *Hepatology* 1995; **22**: 648–54.
21 Wiesner R, Goldstein R, Donovan J *et al.* The impact of cyclosporine dose and level on acute rejection and patient graft survival in liver transplant recipients. *Liver Transplant Surg* 1998; **4**: 34–41.
22 Dousset B, Conti F, Cherruau B *et al.* Is acute rejection deleterious to long-term liver allograft rejection? *J Hepatol* 1998; **29**: 660–8.
23 McVicar JP, Kowdley KV, Bacchi CE *et al.* The natural history of untreated focal allograft rejection in liver transplant recipients. *Liver Transplant Surg* 1996; **2**: 154–60.
24 Wiesner RH, Demetris AJ, Belle SH *et al.* Acute hepatic allograft rejection: incidence, risk factors, and impact on outcome. *Hepatology* 1998; **28**: 638–45.
25 Fisher LR, Henley KS, Lucey MR. Acute cellular rejection after liver transplantation: variability, morbidity and mortality. *Liver Transplant Surg* 1995; **1**: 10–15.
26 Mor E, Gonwa TA, Husberg BS *et al.* Late onset acute rejection in orthotopic liver transplantation-associated risk factors and outcome. *Transplantation* 1992; **54**: 821–4.
27 Anand AC, Hubscher S, Gunson B *et al.* Timing, significance and prognosis of late acute liver allograft rejection. *Transplantation* 1995; **60**: 1098–103.
28 Neuberger J. Incidence, timing and risk factors for acute and chronic rejection. Hepatic allograft rejection and evolving immunosuppressive strategies. *Proceedings, AASL and ILTS*, Chicago, 8 November 1998, pp. 31–9.
29 Wiesner R, Demetris A, Seabera EC. Chronic allograft rejection: defining clinical risk factors and assessing impact on graft outcome. *Hepatology* Abstract, AASL, 1998.
30 Hayashi M, Keeffe EB, Krams SM *et al.* Allograft rejection after liver transplantation for autoimmune liver diseases. *Liver Transplant Surg* 1998; **4**: 208–14.
31 Berlakovich GA, Rockenschaub S, Taucher S *et al.* Underlying disease as a predictor for rejection after liver transplantation. *Arch Surg* 1998; **133**: 167–72.
32 Adams DH, Hubscher SG, Neuberger J *et al.* Reduced incidence of rejection in patients undergoing liver transplantation for hepatitis B. *Transplant Proc* 1991; **23**: 1436–7.
33 Farges O, Saliba F, Farhamant H *et al.* Incidence of rejection and infection after liver transplantation as a function of the primary disease: possible influence of alcohol and polyclonal immunoglobulins. *Hepatology* 1999; **23**: 240–8.
34 Padbury R, Gunson B, Dousset B *et al.* Steroid withdrawal from long-term immunosuppression in liver allograft recipients. *Transplantation* 1993; **55**: 789–94.
35 Belli LS, De Carlis L, Rondinara G *et al.* Early cyclosporine monotherapy in liver transplantation: A 5-year follow-up of a prospective, randomized trial. *Hepatology* 1998; **27**: 1524–9.
36 Fraser GM, Grammoustinianos K, Reddy J. Long term immunosuppression without corticosteroids after orthotopic liver transplantation: a positive therapeutic aim. *Liver Transplant Surg* 1996; **2**: 411–17.
37 Punch JD, Shieck VL, Campbell Jr DA *et al.* Corticosteroid withdrawal after liver transplantation. *Surgery* 1995; **118**: 783–8.
38 Tchervenkov JI, Tector M, Cantarovich D *et al.* Maintenance immunosuppression using cyclosporine monotherapy in adult orthotopic liver transplant recipients. *Transplant Proc* 1996; **28**: 2247–9.
39 Stegall MD, Everson G, Schroter G *et al.* Prednisone withdrawal late after adult liver transplantation reduces diabetes, hypertension, and hypercholesterolemia without causing graft loss. *Hepatology* 1997; **25**: 173–7.
40 McDiarmid SV, Farmer DA, Goldstein LI *et al.* A randomized prospective trial of steroid withdrawal after liver transplantation. *Transplantation* 1995; **60**: 1443–50.
41 Gomez R, Moreno E, Colina F *et al.* Steroid withdrawal is safe and beneficial in stable cyclosporine-treated liver transplant patients. *J Hepatol* 1998; **28**: 150–6.
42 Papatheodoridis G, Patch D, Dusheiko GM *et al.* The outcome of hepatitis C infection after liver transplantation is influenced by the type of immunosuppression? *J Hepatol* 1999; **30**: 731–8.
43 Gane E, Naumov N, Qian S *et al.* A longitudinal analysis of hepatitis C virus replication following

liver transplantation. *Gastroenterology* 1996; **110**: 166–77.
44 McHutchinson JG, Wilkes LB, Pocros PJ *et al.* Pulse corticosteroids therapy increases viremia (HCV RNA) in patients with chronic HCV infection (Abstract). *Hepatology* 1993; **18**: 87.
45 Singh N, Gayowski T, Ndimbie O *et al.* Recurrent hepatitis C virus hepatitis in liver transplant recipients receiving tacrolimus: aasociation with rejection and increased immunosuppression after liver transplantation. *Surgery* 1996; **119**: 52–6.
46 Bird GLA, Smith HT, Portmann B *et al.* Acute liver decompensation on withdrawal of cytotoxic chemotherapy and immunosuppressive therapy in hepatitis B carriers. *Q J Med* 1989; **270**: 895–902.
47 Cakaloglu Y, Devlin J, O'Grady J *et al.* Importance of concomitant viral infections during acute liver allograft rejection. *Transplantation* 1995; **59**: 40–5.
48 Denton MD, Magee C, Sayegh MH. Immunosuppressive strategies in transplantation. *Lancet* 1999; **353**: 1083–91.
49 Hong JC, Kahan BD. Two paradigms for new immunosuppression strategies in organ transplantation. *Curr Opin Organ Transplant* 1998; **3**: 175–82.
50 Neuhaus P, Pichlmayr R, Williams R *et al.* Randomised trial comparing tacrolimus (FK506) and cyclosporin in prevention of liver allograft rejection. *Lancet* 1994; **344**: 423–8.
51 Busuttil RW, McDiarmid S, Klintmalm GB *et al.* A comparison of tacrolimus (FK 506) and cyclosporine for immunosuppression in liver transplantation. *N Engl J Med* 1994; **331**: 1110–15.
52 Fung JJ, Eliasziw M, Todo S *et al.* The Pittsburgh randomized trial of tacrolimus compared to cyclosporine for hepatic transplantation. *J Am Coll Surg* 1996; **183**: 117–25.
53 Starzl TE, Donner A, Eliasziw M *et al.* Randomised trialomania? The multicentre liver transplant trials of tacrolimus. *Lancet* 1995; **346**: 1346–50.
54 Morris ER, Brown, BW. Tacrolimus for prevention of liver allograft rejection: clinical trials and tribulations. *Lancet* 1995; **346**: 1310.
55 Wiesner RH. A long-term comparison of tacrolimus (FK506) versus cyclosporine in liver transplantation. A report of the United States FK506 study group. *Transplantation* 1998; **66**: 493–9.
56 Williams R, Neuhaus P, Bismuth H *et al.* Two-year data from the European multicentre tacrolimus (FK506) liver study. *Transplant Int* 1996; **9**: S144–S150.
57 Pichlmayer R, Winkler M, Neuhaus P *et al.* Three-year follow-up of the European Multicenter Tacrolimus (FK506) liver study. *Transplant Proc* 1997; **29**: 2499–502.
58 Sher LS, Consenza CA, Michel J *et al.* Efficacy of tacrolimus as rescue therapy for chronic rejection in orthotopic liver transplantation. A report of the US Multicenter study group. *Transplantation* 1999; **64**: 258–63.
59 Freise CE, Galbraith CA, Nikolai BJ *et al.* Risks associated with conversion of stable patients after liver transplantation to the microemulsion formulation of cyclosporine. *Transplantation* 1998; **65**: 995–7.
60 Hemming AW, Greig PD, Cattral MS *et al.* A microemulsion of cyclosporine without intravenous cyclosporine in liver transplantation. *Transplantation* 1996; **62**: 1798–802.
61 Holt DW, Johnston A. Cyclosporin microemulsion. A guide to usage and monitoring. *Biodrugs* 1997; **7**: 175–97.
62 Noble S, Markham A. Cyclosporin: a review of the pharmacokinetic properties, clinical efficacy and tolerability of a microemulsion-based formulation (Neoral™). *Drugs* 1995; **50**: 924–41.
63 Trull AK, Tan KKC, Tan L *et al.* Absorption of cyclosporin from conventional and new microemulsion oral formulations in liver transplant recipients with external biliary diversion. *Br J Clin Pharmacol* 1995; **39**: 627–31.
64 Perico N, Remuzzi G. Prevention of transplant rejection: current treatment guidelines and future developments. *Drugs* 1997; **54**: 533–70.
65 Graziadei IW, Wiesner RH, Marotta PJ *et al.* Neoral compared to Sandimmune is associated with a decrease in histologic severity of rejection in patients undergoing primary liver transplantation. *Transplantation* 1997; **64**: 726–31.
66 Otto MG, Mayer AD, Clavien PA *et al.* Randomized trial of cyclosporine microemulsion (Neoral) versus conventional cyclosporine in liver transplantation: MILTON study. *Transplantation* 1998; **66**: 1632–40.
67 Stegall MD, Wachs ME, Everson G *et al.* Prednisone withdrawal 14 days after liver transplantation with mycophenolate: a prospective trial of cyclosporine and tacrolimus. *Transplantation* 1997; **64**: 1755–60.
68 Fisher RA, Ham JM, Marcos A *et al.* A prospective randomized trial of mycophenolate mofetil with Neoral, or tacrolimus after orthotopic liver transplantation. *Transplantation* 1998; **66**: 1616–21.
69 The Tricontinental Mycophenolate Mofetil group. A blinded, randomized clinical trial of mycophenolate mofetil for the prevention of acute rejection in cadaveric renal transplantation. *Transplantation* 1996; **61**: 1029–37.
70 Mathew T. A blinded, long term, randomized, multicenter study of mycophenolate mofetil in cadaveric renal transplantation: results at three years: tricontinental mycophenolate mofetil renal

transplantation study group. *Transplantation* 1998; **65**: 1450–4.

71 Rudich SM, Riegler JL, Perez RV *et al.* Immunosuppression using tacrolimus, mycophenolate, and prednisone following orthotopic liver transplantation: a single-center experience. *Transplantation Proc* 1998; **30**: 1417–18.

72 Cai TH, Esterl RM Jr, Nichols L *et al.* Improved immunosuppression with combination tacrolimus (FK506) and mycophenolic acid in orthotopic liver transplantation. *Transplant Proc* 1998; **30**: 1413–14.

73 Jain AB, Hamad I, Rakela J *et al.* A prospective randomized trial of tacrolimus and prednisone versus tacrolimus, prednisone, and mycophenolate mofetil in primary adult liver transplant recipients: an interim report. *Transplantation* 1998; **66**: 1395–8.

74 Klupp J, Glanemann M, Bechstein KP *et al.* Mycophenolate mofetil in combination with tacrolimus versus Neoral after liver transplantation. *Transplant Proc* 1999; **31**: 1113–14.

75 Jain AB, Hamad I, Rakela J *et al.* A prospective randomized trial of tacrolimus and prednisone versus tacrolimus, prednisone, and mycophenolate mofetil in primary adult liver transplant recipients: an interim report. *Transplantation* 1998; **66**: 1395–8.

76 Klupp J, Bechstein WO, Platz KP *et al.* Mycophenolate mofetil added to immunosuppression after liver transplantation: first results. *Transplant Int* 1997; **10**: 223–8.

77 Angulo P, Batts KP, Therneau TM *et al.* Long term ursodeoxycholic acid delays histological progression in primary biliary cirrhosis. *Hepatology* 199; **29**: 644–7.

78 Lindor KD, Therneau TM, Jorgensen RA *et al.* Effects of ursodeoxycholic acid on survival on patients with primary biliary cirrhosis. *Gastroenterology* 1996; **119**: 1515–18.

79 Calmus Y, Gane P, Rouger P *et al.* Hepatic expression of class I and class II major histocompatibility complex molecules in primary biliary cirrhosis: effect of ursodeoxycholic acid. *Hepatology* 1990; **11**: 12–15.

80 Calmus Y, Arvieux C, Gane P *et al.* Cholestasis induces major histocompatibility complex class I expression in hepatocytes. *Gastroenterology* 1992; **102**: 1371–7.

81 Keiding S, Hockerstedt K, Bjoro K *et al.* The Nordic Multicenter double-blind randomized controlled trial of prophylactic ursodeoxycholic acid in liver transplant patients. *Transplantation* 1997; **63**(11): 1591–4.

82 Fleckenstein JF, Paredes M and Thuluvath PJ. A prospective, randomised, double blind trial evaluating the efficacy of ursodeoxycholic acid in prevention of liver transplant rejection. *Liver Transplant Surg* 1998; **4**(4): 276–9.

83 Pageaux GP, Blanc P, Perrigault PF *et al.* Failure of ursodeoxycholic acid to prevent acute cellular rejection after liver transplantation. *J Hepatol* 1995; **23**: 119–22.

84 Barnes D, Talenti D, Cammell G *et al.* A randomized clinical trial of ursodeoxycholic acid as adjuvant treatment to prevent liver transplant rejection. *Hepatology* 1997; **26**: 853–7.

85 Samuel D, Bismuth H, Boillot O *et al.* Tacrolimus (FK506)-based dual versus triple therapy following liver transplantation. *Transplant Proc* 1998; **30**: 1394–6.

86 Neuhaus P, Langrehr JM, Williams R *et al.* Tacrolimus-based immunosuppression after liver transplantation: a randomised study comparing dual versus triple low-dose oral regimens. *Transplant Int* 1997; **10**: 253–61.

87 Rolles K, Davidson BR, Burroughs A. A pilot study of immunosuppressive monotherapy in liver transplantation. *Transplantation* 1999, in press.

88 Gane E, Portmann B, Saxena R. Nodular regenerative hyperplasia of the liver graft after transplantation. *Hepatology* 1994; **20**: 88–94.

30 Liver transplantation: prevention and treatment of infection

NANCY ROLANDO, JIM J WADE

INTRODUCTION

The two major barriers to successful orthotopic liver transplantation (OLT) are rejection and infection. Infection dominates the early postoperative period, causing morbidity and mortality. Bacterial sepsis is the leading cause of death in several series[1–3] and is an independent risk factor for prediction of mortality.[4] There is a complex interplay between the immune system and infectious agents in the transplant recipient.

There is evidence that bacterial sepsis is a risk factor for fungal infection,[5–7] that cytomegalovirus (CMV) exerts an immunomodulatory effect and that CMV and hepatitis C virus are, respectively, risk factors for fungal [8] and bacterial infection.[9]

BACTERIAL INFECTION

The overall rate of bacterial infections following OLT is between 5% and 60%,[1,3,10–19] and related mortality is between 4.6% and 81%.[2,11] Comparing infection rates from different centers is difficult because of variable duration of follow-up,[20–24] inconsistent inclusion or exclusion of second or subsequent OLTs,[19,20,23] and the use of a variety of regimens for immunosuppression.[9,25–27] Some OLT series include data from both adult and pediatric patients[14,24,28,29] and from living related donors.[17,30] Lack of definitions of infection sometimes makes meaningful interpretation difficult.[1,12,23,31–34] These factors interfere with the interpretation of infection rates and of the efficacy of different regimens for prophylaxis.

Risk factors for bacterial infection

Identifying those patients most at risk for infection should allow more rational decisions concerning prophylaxis and treatment. Multivariate analysis has identified risk factors for bacterial infection (Table 30.1). Prior to OLT, elevated serum bilirubin is a risk factor for bacterial infection, although the reported cut-off values differ.[1,35] In the perioperative period the only surgical variable identified in more than one study as a risk factor is prolonged duration of surgery.[29,35] Following OLT, one or more episodes of cellular rejection,[19,22] and additional immunosuppression[22,36] are interrelated risk factors for bacterial infection demonstrated in more than one study.[22,36] Other risk factors include acute renal failure.[37]

Table 30.1 Risk factors for bacterial infection following orthotopic liver transplantation determined by multivariate analyses

Study	No. of patients	Risk factors
Cuervas-Mons *et al*, Pittsburgh, 1986[1]	93	Pre-creatinine ≥1.52 mg/%; pre-PMN ≥4847 cell/mm^3; pre-IgG ≥1546 mg/dl; pre-bilirubin ≥18.28 mg/dl; pre-WBC ≥7211 cell/mm^3
Murcia *et al*, Madrid, 1990[29]	30	Previous surgery; prolonged surgery; arterial thrombosis
George *et al*, Chicago, 1991[35]	79	Pre-OLT bilirubin ≥12.28 mg/dl; duration of surgery ≥8 h
Wade *et al*, London, 1994[19]	284	One or more episodes of acute cellular rejection; prolonged hospital admission
Saliba *et al*, Paris, 1994[37]	304	Pre-transplant thrombocytopenia; post-OLT acute renal failure; diabetes mellitus
Gotzinger *et al*, Vienna, 1996[22]	248	Increased immunosuppression; prolonged cold ischemia time, one or more rejection episodes; high blood replacement
Singh *et al*, Pittsburgh, 1997[9]	130	Early infections; portal vein thrombosis (100 days); late infections; hepatitis C
virus		recurrence
Whiting *et al*, Cincinnati, 1997[26]	102	Retransplantation
Gayowski *et al*, Pittsburgh, 1998[36]	130	Length of ICU stay; additional immunosuppression
Arnow *et al*, Chicago, 1996[28]	69	Pediatric; surgical complications

Perioperative antibacterial prophylaxis

Based on local experience and observational studies, there is a consensus that antibacterial prophylaxis should be used in the perioperative period. For a long surgical procedure requiring an extensive incision and both biliary and vascular anastomoses, this approach seems reasonable. However, there are no randomized controlled trials of perioperative prophylaxis. Most OLT centers use a regimen comprising a third generation cephalosporin with either ampicillin or tobramycin, with various combinations advocated for penicillin-allergic patients.[1,2,12,20,21,23,25,32,33,38] Cefotaxime has been described as "the antibiotic of choice", as its spectrum of activity encompasses most of the Gram-negative and Gram-positive bacteria implicated in early pneumonia, without affecting the anaerobic intestinal flora. Cefotaxime is also used by centers employing selective bowel decontamination (SBD). Some centers use the extremely broad spectrum carbapenem, imipenem.[39,40] Gaps in the spectrum of the carbapenems and third generation cephalosporins may result in superinfections with enterococci (including glycopeptide resistant *Enterococcus faecium*) or intrinsically resistant *Stenotrophomonas maltophilia*. Generally, the choice of regimen for perioperative antibacterial prophylaxis does not appear to determine the infection rates.

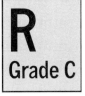

R
Grade C

Table 30.2 Infection rates in centers employing selective bowel decontamination in orthotopic liver transplantation

Study	No. patients	Antibiotic regimen	Timing of SBD	Total % infections
Wiesner, Mayo Clinic, 1987[48]	145	Polymyxin E, gentamicin, and nystatin	–3 → 21 days	24.1 early
Busuttil *et al*, UCLA, 1987[38]	100	Neomycin, erythromycin, and nystatin	Not stated	51
Paya *et al*, Mayo Clinic, 1989[12]	100	Polymyxin E, gentamicin, and nystatin	–3 → 21 days	25.5
Rosman *et al*, Groningen, The Netherlands, 1990[49]	39	Polymyxin E, tobramycin, amphotericin B	–6 h → ~ 36 days	45
Kuo *et al*, Baltimore, MD, 1997[50]	18	Ciprofloxacin, nystatin	High risk patients, admission to OLT ~ 23 days	55

Prophylaxis in the post-transplant period

For post-OLT prophylaxis of bacterial infection, the major difference between centers is in the use of SBD. The concept of SBD evolved from data suggesting that preservation of anaerobic gut flora limits colonization or overgrowth by aerobic Gram-negative bacilli,[41–43] which are major nosocomial pathogens. The topical, non-absorbable antibiotics of SBD regimens usually eradicate aerobic Gram-negative bacilli from the mouth in 2–3 days. However, eradication from the gut may take from 7 to 10 days,[44] and intravenous antibacterials may be used to cover this period. The rationale for SBD in OLT is the predominance of infections caused by Gram-negative bacilli,[3,32,35,45] and yeasts, both of which are targeted by SBD. Gram-negative bacillary infections may follow enterotomy,[31] or occur via translocation from the gut[46] or aspiration of pharyngeal secretions.[47]

R Grade C

The Mayo Clinic group were the first to adopt routine SBD for all OLT patients. The regimen is administered from 2 to 3 days pre-transplant and continued until discharge (21 days); a topical antibacterial paste is applied while the patient is ventilated.[7,12,48] Although the uncontrolled Mayo Clinic data consistently suggest that SBD reduces perioperative Gram-negative infections,[7,12,20,21] not all centers using this regimen (Table 30.2) have achieved similarly low infection rates.[38,49,50] The optimal timing,[7,12,21,23,24,48] duration, and composition of the SBD regimen remain to be determined. A regimen of gentamicin, nystatin, and polymyxin E is used at the Mayo Clinic,[7,12,20] while tobramycin replaces gentamicin at other centers. At the Mayo Clinic the SBD is initiated 3 days before transplantation. Initiating SBD in patients on a waiting list, when the time to transplantation is unknown, is difficult. Adverse effects on the gastrointestinal system, especially diarrhea, have been reported in up to a third of patients.[24,28,48] Poor compliance has been reported in up to 18% of patients.[28] The economic implications of SBD have been evaluated, and regimens containing amphotericin B are the most expensive.[28] The emergence of multiresistant bacteria during SBD is of increasing importance.

R Grade A

Data from three randomized controlled trials of SBD (Table 30.3) are inconclusive and controversial. An initial report from Birmingham[23] demonstrated a significant reduction in infection episodes during an observation period of 15 days, but the final report did not show a significant effect on the incidence of infection, the occurrence of endotoxemia, the development of organ system failure, or mortality.[51] A study from Chicago showed no statistically significant benefit of SBD on infection rates during a 28-day period of observation.[28] This study also highlighted the practical problems associated with the administration of SBD: adverse effects, poor compliance, and the difficulty of predicting the time of transplantation if initiating whilst the patient is on a waiting list. A study of 36 pediatric patients in Pittsburgh which used a short period of SBD did not show a statistically significant reduction in either the number of total episodes of infection or mortality,[24] although it did show a significant reduction in the number of patients experiencing Gram-negative infections. A meta-analysis of 22 randomized controlled trials involving 4142 patients in intensive care units showed that SBD reduces infection related morbidity (NNT to avoid one respiratory tract infection = 6; range 6–9).[52] However, no significant effect on mortality was demonstrated, except by subgroup analysis of those trials which employed combined topical and systemic antibiotics.

R Grade A

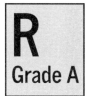

An alternative approach employed by some centers in the USA is the use of oral quinolones to eliminate the gut "pool" of aerobic Gram-negative bacilli.[50,53] The

Table 30.3 Randomized controlled trials of selective bowel decontamination in orthotopic liver transplantation

Study	No. of patients	Control	SBD antibiotic regimen	Infection rate controls	Infection rate SBD	*P*
[a]Badger *et al*, Birmingham, UK 1991[23]	30	Nystatin	Polymyxin E, tobramycin, amphotericin B 5 → 15 days	8/16	2/14	<0.05
[a]Bion *et al*, Birmingham, UK[51]	52	Nystatin	Polymyxin E, tobramycin, amphotericin B 5 → 15 days	12/31	3/21	ns
Arnow *et al*, Chicago, 1996[28]	69	Nystatin	Polymyxin E, gentamicin, nystatin, –3 → 21 days	14/33	14/36	ns
Smith *et al*, Pittsburgh, 1993 (pediatrics)[24]	36	Perioperative parenteral antibiotics only	Polymyxin E, tobramycin, amphotericin B 6 ± 4 days	19 episodes in 18 patients	32 episodes in 18 patients	ns

[a]Interim and final analyses of this series.

Cleveland group used quinolones in the interval between listing for transplantation and 28 days post transplant and reported a decrease in infection rates compared to historical controls.[53]

Since available data do not provide sufficient evidence to recommend SBD for all OLT patients, prophylactic regimens should target patients at high risk of infection (Table 30.1). Administration of SBD for 3 or more days *before* transplantation may be beneficial but there is only comparatively weak evidence to support this view.

Treatment of bacterial infections

Bacterial infections should be treated according to site of infection, confirmed or most likely pathogen, and local susceptibility patterns and antimicrobial policy.

FUNGAL INFECTION

The incidence of systemic fungal infection in liver transplant patients varies from 2.9% to 31%,[7,8,19,39,40,45,54–59] and fungal infection has a major impact on morbidity and mortality.[7,8,19,39,40,45,54,55,57–59] Difficulties in the clinical or laboratory confirmation of fungal infection make comparisons of infection rates problematical. Reports that only include cases confirmed by isolation of the organism, serological detection of antigens or antibodies, and/or histopathological evidence of invasion may underestimate the true incidence of fungal infection. In addition, as the diversity of interventions for prophylaxis increases, so does the difficulty in making meaningful comparisons between centers.

Fungal infections in OLT usually occur within the first month after transplantation, and are associated with mortality rates between 5.3% and 80%.[27,32,39,40,54,60,61] The proportion caused by *Candida* spp. was reported to be 87% in Boston,[8] 78% in Pittsburgh,[62] and approximately 50% in other centers.[7,19,59] *Aspergillus* spp. and the agents of mucormycosis are far less often implicated but these infections are associated with mortality rates ranging from 60% to 100%.[3,45,62–64]

Risk factors for fungal infections

Problems with diagnosing and attributing mortality to fungal infection have prompted attempts to identify those patients most at risk.[7,8,12,19,27,40,60,61] Multivariate analyses have identified risk factors related to the severity or complexity of the patient's pretransplant status (Table 30.4). Prolonged duration of surgery and an increase in transfusion requirements have been identified as risk factors by two or more centers.[8,12,27,45,61] It is impossible to ascertain whether these associations reflect severity of underlying illness or complexity of surgery. In the post-transplant period, retransplantation,[8,60] bacterial infection,[12,60] and return to the operating room[8,19] have been identified as risk factors (Table 30.4). Other risk factors associated with enhanced immunosuppression identified by multivariate analysis include corticosteroid use and CMV infection.[8,27,60,65,66] An association between CMV infection and fungal infection has also been reported[66,67] (see below).

Table 30.4 Risk factors for fungal infection following orthotopic liver transplantation – multivariate analyses

Study	No. patients	Pre-OLT variables	OLT variables	Post-OLT variables
Tollemar *et al*, Sweden, 1990[55]	29	Sex: male.	Prolonged surgery; ↑ transfusions	
Castaldo *et al*, Omaha, NB 1991[60]	303	Urgent status, RISK score	↑ Transfusions	Retransplantation; reintubation; bacterial infection; ↑ steroids; vascular complications; ↑ antibiotic use
Collins *et al*, NEDH, Boston, 1994[8]	158		↑ Operative time; renal failure	Retransplantation; reoperation; CMV infection
Briegel *et al*, Munich, Germany, 1995[40]	152			Hemofiltration or hemodialysis; ↑ FFP transfusion
Hadley *et al*, NEDH, Boston, 1995[27]	118	CMV infection	Choledochojejunostomy; ↑ transfusions	CMV infection ICU duration
Patel *et al*, Mayo Clinic, 1996[7]	405	Class II HLA partial or complete match	↑ Cryoprecipitates	Bacterial infection
Wade *et al*, King's College London, 1994[19]	284	↓ Hemoglobin ↑ Bilirubin		Return to surgery; prolonged therapy with ciprofloxacin

Table 30.5 Incidence of fungal infection following orthotopic liver transplantation in case series employing antifungal prophylaxis

Study	No. patients	Antifungal prophylaxis regimen	Fungal infection (%)
Mora *et al*, Bailor, Dallas, 1992[39]	150	In high risk patients: oral nystatin plus IV amphotericin B → 10–14 days	7.5
Collins *et al*, NEDH, Boston, 1994[8]	158	Nystatin oral → 3–6 months	21
Castaldo *et al*, Omaha, NB, 1991[45]	307	Nystatin oral → 3 months	23.8
Steffen *et al*, Virchow Klinik, Germany, 1994[54]	206	Nystatin, SBD	27.8
Briegel *et al*, Munich, Germany, 1995[40]	152	Amphotericin B SBD	16.5
Wade *et al*, King's College, London, 1995[19]	33	No prophylaxis	12
	198	Amphotericin B oral	7
	36	Nystatin	19
Patel *et al*, Mayo Clinic, 1996[7]	405	Nystatin, SBD	11

Interventions for prophylaxis against fungal infection

R Grade C

Due to the high mortality associated with fungal infection, all liver transplant centers use antifungal prophylaxis, most frequently with nystatin. A total of 1233 patients from six case series (Table 30.5) received nystatin. The average incidence of fungal infection with this intervention ranges from 11% to 34%, [7,8,19,54,55–58,68] and appears not to correlate with duration of antifungal prophylaxis.[7,8,19,68] When oral amphotericin B was used for prophylaxis in two case series, the observed incidence of fungal infection was 7%[19] and 16.5%.[40] The combination of low dose intravenous amphotericin B with nystatin did not prevent disseminated fungal infections in high risk patients.[9,69]

R Grade A

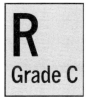

A randomized controlled trial compared the safety and efficacy of fluconazole (100 mg/d) and nystatin[58] (Table 30.6). Fluconazole was safe in OLT patients and there was no evidence of interaction with cyclosporin. Fluconazole resulted in fewer superficial fungal infections (fluconazole 13%, nystatin 34%, $P = 0.022$, ARR = 21%, NNT = 5). However, no statistically significant difference in systemic infection (fluconazole 2.6 %, nystatin 9.0%, $P = 0.12$) or mortality was demonstrated. The emergence of fluconazole resistant yeasts has been reported in patients undergoing bone marrow transplantation[70] and in AIDS patients.

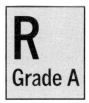

R Grade A

The randomized trial reported by Tollemar *et al*[71] in 86 OLT patients (Table 30.6) demonstrated that liposomal amphotericin B (1 mg/k/d for 5 days) significantly decreased early invasive fungal infections (amphotericin 0%, nystatin 16%, ARR = 16%, NNT = 6). Although liposomal amphotericin B is expensive, this approach to prophylaxis may still be cost-effective given the cost of treatment for fungal infection.

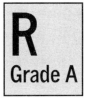

Recent data suggest that prophylaxis for CMV infection may also reduce the incidence of fungal infections[67] (see below).

The value of routine prophylaxis for *Pneumocystis carinii* has not been proven. In the absence of prophylactic therapy, the incidence of *P. carinii* pneumonia (PCP) has been reported to be between 3% and 11%.[3,12,39,72,73] Low dose cotrimoxazole appeared to be

Table 30.6 Randomized trials of interventions for prophylaxis against invasive fungal infection in OLT patients

Study	No. of patients	Experimental antifungal therapy	Control antifungal therapy	% invasive fungal infection		*P*
				Experimental	Nystatin	
Tollemar *et al*, Hussinge, Sweden, 1995[71]	86	Liposomal amphotericin B and nystatin until discharge	Nystatin	0/40	6/37	<0.01
Lumbreras *et al*, Madrid, Spain, 1996[58]	143	Fluconazole → 28 days	Nystatin	2/76	6/67	0.12

effective in reducing the incidence of PCP in a center with an incidence of 30% prior to its introduction, but the evidence for this benefit rests only on case series before and after introduction of the intervention.[74]

R
Grade C

Treatment of fungal infection

There are no controlled clinical trials of therapy for fungal infection in OLT patients. At most centers the standard therapy for invasive fungal infection is amphotericin B or liposomal amphotericin B, although 5-flucytosine is sometimes added.[61] A reduction in the level of immunosuppression has been recommended.[68] Alternatives to amphotericin B, such as fluconazole and itraconazole for yeast infections, need further evaluation. Novel agents should be evaluated in randomized controlled trials. Despite appropriate treatment the mortality remains high.

VIRAL INFECTION

Cytomegalovirus (CMV) is the most important and most studied opportunist infection following OLT. Infection may manifest as a syndrome of fever, leukopenia, and thrombocytopenia and result in disseminated infection with hepatitis, pneumonitis or gastrointestinal tract infection, usually within 3 months of transplantation. CMV infection is also implicated in acute and chronic rejection and, *via* its immunosuppressive effect, is a risk factor for bacterial and fungal infection. The serological status of donor and recipient are important factors: post-transplant CMV infection may be acquired from the graft or, less often, blood products, or result from reactivation of latent virus or superinfection with a new strain. Primary infections are more severe than reactivation infections or superinfection. Seronegative recipients of seropositive grafts (D+/R–) are at highest risk of CMV infection. Up to 80% of these graft recipients become infected and 60% develop CMV disease. Protective matching of the graft reduces the risk of CMV infection for seronegative recipients but the scarcity of donor organs makes this approach impractical. Retransplantation and the use of antilymphocyte globulin or OKT3 are also risk factors for CMV disease. Preventing CMV disease, especially in D+/R– patients, would be a major advance in liver transplantation.[75–77] The value of active immunization against CMV should be evaluated.

Interpretation of trials which compare different interventions for CMV prevention (Table 30.7) is complicated by variation with respect to patient population, immunosuppressive regimens, outcome measures, and even by variability among batches in human normal immunoglobulin (HN Ig) and CMV hyperimmune globulins (CMV Ig). Some studies evaluated interventions in all OLT recipients, while others studied 'pre-emptive therapy' for those with known risk factors for disease such as use of OKT3, D+/R– status or evidence of CMV shedding or viremia.

Passive immunization – immunoglobulin

R
Grade A

Human normal immunoglobulin (HN Ig) was not shown to be effective for prevention of CMV disease in a randomized double-blind trial which compared HN Ig with albumen in 50 patients.[78] By contrast, the small randomized trial of CMV hyperimmune globulin

Table 30.7 Randomized trials of interventions for prevention of CMV disease in OLT patients

Study	No. of patients	Patient selection	Experimental intervention	Control intervention	CMV disease		*P*
					Experimental	Control	
Cofer, Dallas, 1991[78]	50	No	HN Ig	Albumen	8/25	5/25	ns
Saliba, Villejuif, France, 1989[79]	22	D+/R–	CMV Ig	Nil	4/15	6/7	0.01
Snydman, Massachusetts, 1993[66]	141	No	CMV Ig	Albumen	21/169	41/72	ns
Saliba, Villejuif, France, 1993[80]	120	No	ACV × 3 mth	Nil	4/60	14/60	0.01
Green, Pittsburg, 1994[81]	29	No	GCV × 2 wk plus ACV × 1 yr	GCV × 2 wk	2/10	1/19	ns
Nakazato, San Francisco, 1993[82]	104	No	HN Ig plus GCV in hospital plus ACV after discharge	HN Ig plus ACV in hospital then ACV after discharge	2/52	8/52	0.046
Martin, Pittsburg, 1994[83]	139	No	GCV × 2 wk then ACV × 10 wk	ACV × 12 wk	6/68	20/71	0.0001
Cohen, London, 1993[84]	65	No	GCV in wk 3–4	GCV for therapy of established disease	9/33	11/32	ns
Winston, Los Angeles, 1995[85]	250	No	GCV × 100 days	ACV × 100 days	1/124	12/126	0.002
King, USA, Canada, 1997[86]	56	D+/R–	GCV × 30 d plus HN Ig	Saline plus HNIg	5/29	7/27	ns
Badley, USA, 1997[87]	167	No	GCV × 14 d then ACV × 106 d	ACV × 120 d	9/83	19/84	0.003
Stratta, Nebraska, 1992[88]	100	OKT3 treatment	HN Ig plus ACV × 3 mth	Nil	18/50	21/50	ns
Singh, Pittsburg, 1994[89]	47	CMV shedding	GCV with CMV shedding	ACV prophylaxis	1/23	7/24	0.048

(CMV Ig) conducted by Saliba *et al.*,[79] found that 4 of 15 (26.6%) D+/R– patients receiving CMV Ig post-OLT developed severe CMV disease, compared to 6 of 7 (85.7%) D+/R– control patients ($P = 0.01$). In a subsequent randomized, double-blind, placebo controlled trial Snydman *et al.* showed that CMV Ig decreased the incidence of severe CMV-associated disease (including invasive fungal disease with CMV infection) following OLT. Although subgroup analysis did not show a reduction in CMV disease or severe CMV-associated disease in D+/R– patients, there were only 19 such patients in each treatment arm and OKT3 was used more often in the CMV Ig arm.[66] In a further post hoc analysis of this trial, which also included patients from a further open label trial who received less OKT3, it appeared that the same CMV Ig regimen reduced severe CMV disease in the D+/R– subgroup.[90] A meta-analysis of 18 studies of HN Ig or CMV Ig prophylaxis in transplantation did not show benefit of CMV Ig over HN Ig. However, this analysis included patients with various solid organ transplants, as well as bone marrow transplants.[91] In summary there is evidence that CMV Ig but not HN Ig can prevent CMV disease in OLT patients other than in the high risk (D+/R–) group.

R
Grade A

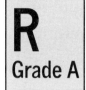

Antiviral prophylaxis:acyclovir and ganciclovir

Saliba *et al.*,[80] in a randomized controlled trial which included 120 CMV seropositive OLT recipients, showed that acyclovir (ACV) was well tolerated and was effective for prophylaxis against CMV reactivation, reinfection, and CMV disease. No differences in acute rejection, chronic rejection or mortality were demonstrated.[80] The randomized trial of Green *et al.*[81] in 29 children undergoing OLT did not show any reduction in CMV infection from one year of ACV therapy following an initial 2 weeks of GCV post-OLT.

R
Grade A

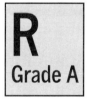

Nakazato *et al.*[82] randomized 104 patients to receive HN Ig plus either ACV or ganciclovir (GCV) while hospitalized. After discharge all patients received oral ACV. GCV reduced the incidence of CMV disease (GCV 3.8%, ACV 15%, $P < 0.05$) and rejection and the duration of hospitalization after OLT. Subgroup analysis of 16 D+/R– patients did not show any benefit of GCV.[82] In a randomized trial in which sequential GCV (14 days) and high dose ACV (10 weeks) was compared with high dose ACV alone for 12 weeks,[83] GCV delayed the onset and decreased the incidence of overall CMV infection, but neither regimen was shown to prevent primary CMV infection. Cohen *et al.*[84] randomized 65 patients to receive GCV prophylaxis given during weeks three and four post-transplant or GCV only as a therapeutic intervention. They did not find a difference in the incidence of CMV disease, although GCV prophylaxis was associated with a lower incidence of serologically diagnosed secondary infection.[84] Winston *et al.*[85] compared 100 days of therapy with GCV and ACV for prophylaxis and reported that GCV produced a highly significant reduction in CMV infection (GCV 5%, ACV 38%, $P < 0.0001$, ARR = 33%, NNT = 3) and disease (GCV 0.8%, ACV 10%, $P = 0.002$, ARR = 9.2%, NNT = 11). Subgroup analysis suggested that the benefit of GCV over ACV was observed in the R– patients (GCV 42%, ACV 11%, $P = 0.06$, ARR = 31 % NNT = 3) though not in the D+/R– patients.[85] In a subsequent uncontrolled study, the same group later followed 37 D+/R– OLT patients following administration of intravenous GCV for a mean of 15 months (range 5–38). None of these high risk patients developed CMV disease, while 4 of 10 D+/R– patients who received less than 7 weeks' GCV (mean duration 3 weeks) developed disease.[92] King *et al.*[86] randomized 56 D+/R– children to receive GCV plus HN Ig or placebo plus HN Ig and found a delay in the onset of CMV disease in the GCV group, but did not show a statistically significant decrease in incidence (GCV 17%, placebo 26%, $P = 0.429$).

R
Grade A

R
Grade A

R
Grade C

Badley *et al.*[87] randomized 167 OLT patients to receive either ACV for 120 days or GCV followed by oral ACV for 106 days. GCV was effective for reducing CMV infection (ACV 57%, GCV 37%, $P = 0.001$) and CMV disease (ACV 23%, GCV 11%, $P = 0.03$). Grade A The NNT, the number of patients needed to be treated with GCV rather than ACV to prevent one infection, is 5 and to prevent one occurrence of CMV disease is 8. The GCV regimen was effective even in D+/R– patients.[87]

Pre-emptive therapy for CMV disease

The purpose of 'pre-emptive therapy' is to prevent disease in those patients with known risk factors, viral shedding or viremia which place them at risk of subsequent CMV disease. This approach avoids administration of a prophylactic regimen to all OLT patients. It is recognized that some patients develop CMV disease without preceding detectable viremia or CMV shedding. More sensitive methods of detecting CMV, such as PCR, may improve the identification of patients at risk and the effectiveness of pre-emptive therapy.

Stratta *et al* randomized 100 patients receiving OKT3 to receive HN Ig plus oral ACV for 3 months after OKT3 therapy or no intervention and did not demonstrate any reduction in incidence or severity of CMV infections.[88] Grade A Lumbreras *et al* found that CMV disease occurred less frequently in a group of patients who received GCV prophylaxis than in a historical control group.[93] Grade C In a randomized controlled trial of 47 patients, Singh *et al.* showed that short course GCV therapy, administered only if CMV shedding occurred, was more effective than a prophylactic regimen of high dose ACV for the prevention of CMV disease.[89] Grade A This approach has been adopted in several transplant centers.

REFERENCES

1 Cuervas-Mons V, Millan J, Gavaler S *et al.* Prognostic value of preoperatively obtained clinical and laboratory data in predicting survival following orthotopic liver transplantation. *Hepatology* 1986; **6**: 922–7.

2 Cuervas-Mons V, Martinez AJ, Dekker A *et al.* Adult liver transplantation: an analysis of the early causes of death in 40 consecutive cases. *Hepatology* 1986; **6**: 495–501.

3 Kusne S, Dummer JS, Singh N *et al.* Infections after liver transplantation. An analysis of 101 consecutive cases. *Medicine* 1988; **67**: 132–43.

4 Martin M, Kusne M, Alessiani R *et al.* Infection after liver transplantation: risk factors and prevention. *Transplant Proc* 1991; **23**: 1929–30.

5 Castaldo P, Stratta RJ, Wood RP *et al.* Clinical spectrum of fungal infections after orthotopic liver transplantation. *Arch Surg* 1991; **126**: 149–56.

6 Patel R, Paya C. Infections in solid-organ transplant recipients. *Clin Microbiol Rev* 1997; **10**: 86–124.

7 Patel R, Portela D, Badley AD *et al.* Risk factors of invasive *candida* and non-*candida* fungal infections after liver transplantation. *Transplantation* 1996; **62**: 926–34.

8 Collins LA, Samore MH, Roberts MS *et al.* Risk factors for early invasive fungal infection complicating orthotopic liver transplantation. *J Infect Dis* 1994; **170**: 644–52.

9 Singh N, Gayowski T, Wagener M *et al.* Predictors and outcome of early versus late onset major bacterial infections in liver transplant recipients receiving tacrolimus (FK506) as primary immunosuppression. *Eur J Clin Microbiol Infect Dis* 1997; **16**: 821–6.

10 Kirby RM, McMaster P, Clements D *et al.* Orthotopic liver transplantation: postoperative complications and their management. *Br J Surg* 1987; **74**: 3–11.

11 Moulin D, Clement de Clety S, Reynaert M *et al.* Intensive care for children after orthotopic liver transplantation. *Intens Care Med* 1989; **15**: S71–2.

12 Paya CV, Hermans PE, Washington JA *et al.* Incidence distribution and outcome of episodes of infection in 100 orthotopic liver transplantations. *Mayo Clin Proc* 1989; **64**: 554–64.

13 Lumbreras C, Lizasoain M, Moreno E *et al.* Major bacterial infections following liver transplantation: a prospective study. *Hepatogastroenterology* 1992; **39**: 362–5.

14 Martinez-Ibañez V, Iglesias J, Llorret J *et al.* Experiencia de siete años en el transplante hepático pediátrico. *Cir Pediatr* 1993; **6**: 7–10.
15 Barkholt L, Ericzon BG, Tollemar J *et al.* Infections in human liver recipients: different patterns early and late. *Transplant Int* 1993; **6**: 77–84.
16 Kizilisik TA, Larsen IM, Bain VG *et al.* Liver transplantation at the University of Alberta Hospitals: a review of the first three years. *Transplant Proc* 1993; **25**: 2203–5.
17 Uemoto S, Tanaka K, Fujita S *et al.* Infection complication in living related liver transplantation. *J Pediatr Surg* 1994; **29**: 514–17.
18 Singh N, Gayowski T, Wagener M *et al.* Pulmonary infections in liver transplant recipients receiving tacrolimus. *Transplantation* 1996; **61**: 396–401.
19 Wade J, Rolando N, Hayllar K *et al.* Bacterial and fungal infection after liver transplantation: an analysis of 284 patients. *Hepatology* 1995; **21**: 1328–36.
20 Wiesner RH. The incidence of Gram-negative bacterial and fungal infections in liver transplant patients treated with selective decontamination. *Infection* 1990; **18**: S19–S21.
21 Wiesner RH. Selective bowel decontamination for infection prophylaxis in liver transplantation patients. *Transplant Proc* 1991; **23**: 1927–8.
22 Gotzinger P, Sautner T, Wamser P *et al.* Early post operative infections after liver transplantation, pathogen spectrum and risk factors. *Wien Klin Wochenschr* 1996; **108**: 795–801.
23 Badger IL, Crosby HA, Kong KL *et al.* Is selective decontamination of the digestive tract beneficial in liver transplant patients? Interim result of a prospective, randomised trial. *Transplant Proc* 1991; **23**: 1460–1.
24 Smith S, Jackson J, Hannakan CJ *et al.* Selective decontamination in paediatric liver transplants. *Transplantation* 1993; **55**: 1306–9.
25 Kusne S, Fung J, Alessiani M *et al.* Infections during a randomised trial comparing cyclosporine to FK506 immunosuppression in liver transplantation. *Transplant Proc* 1992; **24**: 429.
26 Whiting JF, Rossi SJ, Hanto DW. Infectious complications after OKT3 induction in liver transplantation. *Liver Transplant Surg* 1997; **3**: 563–70.
27 Hadley S, Samore MH, Lewis WD *et al.* Major infectious complications after orthotopic liver transplantation and comparison of outcomes in patients receiving cyclosporine or FK506 as primary immunosuppression. *Transplantation* 1995; **59**: 851–9.
28 Arnow PM, Carandang GC, Zabner R *et al.* Randomized controlled trial of selective bowel decontamination for prevention of infections following liver transplantation. *Clin Infect Dis* 1996; **22**: 997–1003.
29 Murcia J, Vasquez J, Hierro L *et al.* La infección como complicación del transplante hepático. *Cir Pediatr* 1990; **3**: 121–4.
30 Hasegawa S, Mori K, Inomata Y *et al.* Factors associated with post operative respiratory complications in paediatric liver transplantation from living-related donors. *Transplantation* 1996; **62**: 943–7.
31 Ascher NL, Stock PG, Bumgardner GL *et al.* Infection and rejection of primary hepatic transplant in 93 consecutive patients treated with triple immunosuppressive therapy. *Surg Gynecol Obstet* 1988; **167**: 474–8.
32 Colonna JO, Winston DJ, Brill JE *et al.* Infectious complications in liver transplantation. *Arch Surg* 1988; **123**: 360–4.
33 Jacobs F, van de Stadt J, Burgeois N *et al.* Severe infections early after liver transplantation. *Transplant Proc* 1989; **21**: 2271–3.
34 Raakow R, Steffen R, Lefebre B *et al.* Selective bowel decontamination effectively prevents Gram-negative bacterial infections after liver transplantation. *Transplant Proc* 1990; **22**: 1556–7.
35 George DL, Arnow PM, Fox AS *et al.* Bacterial infection as a complication of liver transplantation: epidemiology and risk factors. *Rev Infect Dis* 1991; **13**: 387–96.
36 Gayowski T, Marino IR, Singh N *et al.* Orthotopic liver transplantation in high risk patients; risk factors associated with mortality and infectious morbidity. *Transplantation* 1998; **27**: 499–504.
37 Saliba F, Ephraim R, Mathieu D *et al.* Risk factors for bacterial infection after liver transplantation. *Transplant Proc* 1994; **26**: 266.
38 Busuttil RW, Colonna JO, Hiatt JR *et al.* The first 100 liver transplants at UCLA. *Ann Surg.* 1987; **206**: 387–402.
39 Mora NP, Klintmalm GB, Solomon H *et al.* Selective amphotericin B prophylaxis in the reduction of fungal infections after liver transplant. *Transplant Proc* 1992; **24**: 154–5.
40 Briegel J, Forst H, Spill B *et al.* Risk factors for systemic fungal infections in liver transplant recipients. *Eur J Clin Microbiol Infect Dis* 1995; **14**: 375–82.
41 van der Waaij D, Berghuis-de Vries JM, Lekkerkerk-van der Wees JEC. Colonisation resistance of the digestive tract in conventional antibiotic-treated mice. *J Hyg* 1971; **69**: 405–11.
42 van der Waaij D, de Vries-Hospers HG, Welling GW. The influence of antibiotics on gut colonisation. *J Antimicrob Chemother* 1986; **18** (Suppl C): 155–8.
43 Vollard RJ, Clasener HAL, van Griethuysen AJA *et al.* Influence of cefaclor, phenethicillin, co-trimoxazole and doxycycline on colonisation resistance in healthy volunteers. *J Antimicrob Chemother* 1988; **22**: 747–58.

44 Stoutenbeek CP, van Saene HKF, Miranda DR *et al.* The prevention of superinfection in multiple trauma patients. *J Antimicrob Chemother* 1984; **14** (Suppl B): 203–11.
45 Castaldo P, Stratta RJ, Wood RP *et al.* Clinical spectrum of fungal infections after orthotopic liver transplantation. *Arch Surg* 1991; **126**: 149–56.
46 Wells CL, Maddaus MA, Simmons RL. Proposed mechanism for the translocation of intestinal bacteria. *Rev Infect Dis* 1988; **10**: 958–9.
47 Vallés J, Artigas A, Rello J *et al.* Continuous aspiration of subglotic secretions in preventing ventilator associated pneumonia. *Ann Intern Med* 1995; **122**: 179–86.
48 Wiesner RH, Hermans P, Rakela J *et al.* Selective bowel decontamination to prevent Gram-negative bacterial and fungal infection following orthotopic liver transplantation. *Transplant Proc* 1987; **19**: 2420–3.
49 Rosman C, Klompmaker IJ, Bonsel GJ *et al.* The efficacy of selective bowel decontamination as infection prevention after liver transplantation. *Transplant Proc* 1990; **22**: 2554–5.
50 Kuo PC, Bartlett ST, Lim JW *et al.* Selective bowel decontamination in hospitalised patients awaiting liver transplantation. *Am J Surg* 1997; **174**: 745–8.
51 Bion JF, Badger I, Crosby HA *et al.* Selective decontamination of the digestive tract reduces Gram-negative pulmonary colonization but not systemic endotoxemia in patients undergoing elective liver transplantation. *Crit Care Med* 1994; **22**: 40–9.
52 Selective Decontamination of the Digestive Tract Trialists' Collaborative Group. Meta analysis of randomised controlled trials of selective decontamination of the digestive tract. *Br Med J* 1993; **307**: 525–32.
53 Gorensek MJ, Carey WD, Washington JA *et al.* Selective bowel decontamination with quinolones and nystatin reduces Gram negative and fungal infections in orthotopic liver transplant recipients. *Cleve Clin J Med* 1993; **60**: 139–44.
54 Steffen R, Reinhartz O, Blumhardt G *et al.* Bacterial and fungal colonization and infections using oral selective bowel decontamination in orthotopic liver transplantation. *Transpl Int* 1994; **7**: 101–8.
55 Tollemar J, Ericzon BG, Holmberg K *et al.* The incidence and diagnosis of invasive fungal infection in liver transplant recipients. *Transplant Proc* 1990; **22**: 242–4.
56 Ruskin JD, Wood RP, Bailey MR *et al.* Comparative trial of oral clotrimazole and nystatin for oropharyngeal candidiasis prophylaxis in orthotopic liver transplant patients. *Oral Surg Oral Med Oral Pathol* 1992; **74**: 567–71.
57 Viviani MA, Tortorano AM, Malaspina C *et al.* Surveillance and treatment of liver transplant recipients for candidiasis and aspergillosis. *Eur J Epidemiol* 1992; **8**: 433–6.
58 Lumbreras C, Cuervas-Mons V, Jara P *et al.* Randomized trial of fluconazole versus nystatin for the prophylaxis of *Candida* infection following liver transplantation. *J Infect Dis* 1996; **174**: 583–8.
59 Grauhan O, Lohmann R, Lemmens P *et al.* Fungal infection in liver transplant recipients. *Langenbecks Arch Chir* 1994; **379**: 372–5.
60 Castaldo P, Stratta RJ, Wood RP *et al.* Fungal disease in liver transplant recipients: a multivariate analysis of risk factors. *Transplant Proc* 1991; **23**: 1517–19.
61 Tollemar J, Ericzon BG, Barkholt L *et al.* Risk factors for deep fungal infections in liver transplant recipients. *Transplant Proc* 1990; **22**: 1826–7.
62 Wajszczuk CP, Dummer JS, Ho M *et al.* Fungal infections in liver transplant recipients. *Transplantation* 1985; **40**: 347–53.
63 Plá MP, Berenguer J, Arzuaga FA *et al.* Surgical wound infection by *Aspergillus fumigatus* in liver transplant recipients. *Diagn Microbiol Infect Dis* 1992; **15**: 703–6.
64 Rossi G, Tortorano AM, Viviani MA *et al.* *Aspergillus fumigatus* infections in liver transplant patients. *Transplant Proc* 1989; **21**: 2268.
65 Kusne S, Torre-Cisneros J, Mañes R *et al.* Factors associated with invasive lung aspergillosis and the significance of positive Aspergillus culture after liver transplantation. *J Infect Dis* 1992; **16**: 1379–83.
66 Snydman DR, Werner BG, Dougherty NN *et al.* Cytomegalovirus immune globulin prophylaxis in liver transplantation: a randomized, double-blind, placebo-controlled trial. *Ann Intern Med* 1993; **119**: 984–91.
67 Snydman DR, Werner BG, Heinze-Lacey B *et al.* Use of cytomegalovirus immune globulin to prevent cytomegalovirus disease in renal transplant recipients. *N Engl J Med* 1987; **217**: 1049–54.
68 Castaldo P, Stratta RJ, Wood RP *et al.* Fungal infection in liver allograft recipients. *Transplant Proc* 1991; **23**: 1967.
69 Mora NP, Cofer JB, Solomon H *et al.* Analysis of severe infections (INF) after 180 consecutive liver transplants: the impact of amphotericin B prophylaxis for reducing the incidence and severity of fungal infections. *Transplant Proc* 1991; **23**: 1528–30.
70 Wingard JR, Merz WG, Rinaldi MG *et al.* Increase in *Candida krusei* infection among patients with bone marrow transplantation and neutropenia treated prophylactically with fluconazole. *N Engl J Med* 1991; **325**: 1274–7.
71 Tollemar J, Hickerstedt K, Ericzon BG *et al.* Liposomal amphotericin B prevents invasive fungal infections in liver transplant recipients. A randomised, placebo-controlled study. *Transplantation* 1995; **59**: 45–50
72 Hayes MJ, Torzillo PJ, Sheil AGR *et al.* *Pneumocystis carinii* pneumonia after liver transplantation in adults. *Clin Transplant* 1994; **8**: 499–503.

73 Colombo JL, Sammut PH, Langnas AN *et al.* The spectrum of *Pneumocystis carinii* infection after liver transplantation in children. *Transplantation* 1992; **316**: 621–4.

74 Torres-Cisneros J, de la Mata M, Lopez-Cillero P *et al.* Effectiveness of daily low-dose cotrimoxazole prophylaxis *for Pneumocystis carinii* pneumonia in liver transplantation. *Transplantation* 1996; **62**: 1519–21.

75 Patel R, Paya CV. Infections in solid-organ transplant recipients. *Clin Microbiol Rev* 1997; **10**: 86–124.

76 Patel R, Snydman DR, Rubin RH *et al.* Cytomegalovirus prophylaxis in solid organ transplant recipients. *Transplantation* 1996; **61**: 1279–89.

77 Kanj SS, Sharara AI, Clavien P-A *et al.* Cytomegalovirus infection following liver transplantation: review of the literature. *Clin Infect Dis* 1996; **22**: 537–49.

78 Cofer JB, Morris CA, Sutker WL *et al.* A randomized double-blind study of the effect of prophylactic immune globulin on the incidence and severity of CMV infection in the liver transplant recipient. *Transplant Proc* 1991; **23**: 1525–7.

79 Saliba F, Arulnaden JL, Gugenheim J *et al.* CMV hyperimmune globulin prophylaxis after liver transplantation: a prospective randomized controlled study. *Transplant Proc* 1989; **21**: 2260–2.

80 Saliba F, Eyraud D, Samuel D *et al.* Randomized controlled trial of acyclovir for the prevention of cytomegalovirus infection and disease in liver transplant recipients. *Transplant Proc* 1993; **25**: 1444–5.

81 Green M, Reyes J, Nour B *et al.* Randomized trial of ganciclovir followed by high-dose oral acyclovir vs ganciclovir alone in prevention of cytomegalovirus disease in paediatric liver transplant recipients: preliminary analysis. *Transplant Proc* 1994; **26**: 173–4.

82 Nakazato PZ, Burns W, Moore P *et al.* Viral prophylaxis in hepatic transplantation: preliminary report of a randomized trial of acyclovir and ganciclovir. *Transplant Proc* 1993; **2**: 1935–7.

83 Martin M, Manez R, Linden P *et al.* A prospective randomized trial comparing sequential ganciclovir–high dose acyclovir for prevention of cytomegalovirus disease in adult liver transplant recipients. *Transplantation* 1994; **58**: 779–85.

84 Cohen AT, O'Grady J, Sutherland S *et al.* Controlled trial of prophylactic versus therapeutic use of ganciclovir after liver transplantation in adults. *J Med Virol* 1993; **40**: 5–9.

85 Winston DW, Wirin D, Shaked A *et al.* Randomised comparison of ganciclovir and high-dose acyclovir for long-term cytomegalovirus prophylaxis in liver-transplant recipients. *Lancet* 1995; **346**: 69–74.

86 King SM, Superina R, Andrews W *et al.* Randomized comparison of ganciclovir plus intravenous immune globulin (IVIG) with IVIG alone for prevention of primary cytomegalovirus disease in children receiving liver transplants. *Clin Infect Dis* 1997; **25**: 1173–9.

87 Badley AD, Seaberg EC, Porayko MK *et al.* Prophylaxis of cytomegalovirus infection in liver transplantation. A randomized trial comparing a combination of ganciclovir and acyclovir to acyclovir. *Transplantation* 1997; **64**: 66–73.

88 Stratta RJ, Shaefer MS, Cushing KA *et al.* A randomized prospective trial of acyclovir and immune globulin prophylaxis in liver transplant recipients receiving OKT3 therapy. *Arch Surg* 1992; **127**: 55–63.

89 Singh N, Yu VL, Mieles L *et al.* High-dose aciclovir compared with short-course pre-emptive ganciclovir therapy to prevent cytomegalovirus disease in liver transplant recipients. *Ann Intern Med* 1994; **120**: 375–81.

90 Snydman DR, Werner BG, Dougherty NN *et al* and the Boston Center for liver transplantation CMVIG Study Group. A further analysis of the use of cytomegalovirus immune globulin in orthotopic liver transplant patients at risk for primary infection. *Transplant Proc* 1994; **26**: 23–7.

91 Glowacki LS, Smaill FM. Use of immune globulin to prevent symptomatic cytomegalovirus disease in transplant recipients – a meta-analysis. *Clin Transplantation* 1994; **8**: 10–18.

92 Seu P, Winston DJ, Holt CD *et al.* Long-term ganciclovir prophylaxis for successful prevention of primary cytomegalovirus (CMV) disease in CMV-seronegative liver transplant recipients with CMV-seropositive donors. *Transplantation* 1997; **64**: 1614–17.

93 Lumbreras C, Otero JR, Herrero JA *et al.* Ganciclovir prophylaxis decreases frequency and severity of cytomegalovirus disease in seropositive liver transplant recipients treated with OKT3 monoclonal antibodies. *Antimicrob Agents Chemother* 1993; **37**: 2490–2.

Index